Quick Reference to OB-GYN Procedures

Quick Reference to OB-GYN Procedures

Third Edition

Hugh R. K. Barber, M.D.

Director of Obstetrics and Gynecology
Lenox Hill Hospital
New York, New York

David H. Fields, M.D.

Associate Obstetrician/Gynecologist
Lenox Hill Hospital
New York, New York

Sherwin A. Kaufman, M.D.

Emeritus Attending Obstetrician/Gynecologist
Lenox Hill Hospital
New York, New York
Clinical Associate Professor, Ob/Gyn
New York Medical College
Valhalla, New York

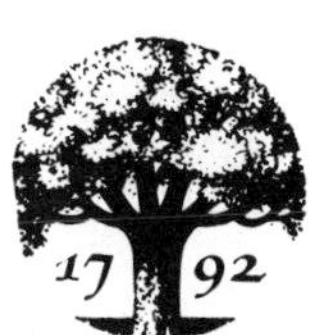

J. B. Lippincott Company • Philadelphia
Grand Rapids • New York • St. Louis • San Francisco
London • Sydney • Tokyo

To our wives, Mary Louise Barber, Claire Kaufman, and Ailene Fields, for their patience and help.

Third Edition

6 5 4 3 2 1

Library of Congress Cataloging in Publication Data

Barber, Hugh R.K., 1918–
Quick reference to ob-gyn procedure/Hugh R.K. Barber, David H. Fields, Sherwin A. Kaufman.— 3rd ed.
p. cm.
Includes index.
ISBN 0-397-50886-7
1. Gynecology—Handbooks, manuals, etc.
2. Obstetrics–Handbooks, manuals, etc.
I. Fields, David H. II. Kaufman, Sherwin A.
III. Title
[DNLM: 1. Gynecology—handbooks.
2. Obstetrics–handbooks.
3. Pregnancy Complications—handbooks.
WB 39 B234q]
RG110.B37 1990
618′.02′02—dc19
DNLM/DLC
for Library of Congress

The authors and publisher have exerted every effort to ensure that drug selection and dosage set forth in this text are in accord with current recommendations and practice at the time of publication. However, in view of ongoing research, changes in government regulations, and the constant flow of information relating to drug therapy and drug reactions, the reader is urged to check the package insert for each drug for any change in indications and dosage and for added warnings and precautions. This is particularly important when the recommended agent is a new or infrequently employed drug.

Preface

The warm reception given to the first edition of *Quick Reference to OB-GYN Procedures,* which presented material using a new outline format, attests to the success of our endeavors. It stimulated us to review our efforts for an even more successful second edition. We have kept the same format that was used in the first and second editions, while updating the material and including additional chapters. This has been the chief goal of this revision.

Since the publication of the first edition in 1969, the field of obstetrics and gynecology has made rapid and explosive advances. The fields of reproductive endocrinology and immunology, genetics, maternal-fetal medicine, oncology, the control of Rh sensitization, and the ability to create life in a test tube have literally created a new specialty. These staggering advances have challenged the imagination of students and have served to recruit them into the field of obstetrics and gynecology. The potential for contributions has made obstetrics and gynecology one of the most exciting specialties in the field of medicine today.

The volume of material, the changing concepts, and the almost daily additions to the literature make it difficult for the busy clinician to read the literature and organize and incorporate it into the everyday practice of medicine. The *Quick Reference* attempts to do this. We have tried to make each chapter concise without being superficial. The format should provide an overall review that can serve as a framework on which new knowledge may be placed and then used in clinical practice. The book is not designed for originality, but rather to present the basics, as well as updated material, in a readable format. It is truly the physician's assistant for giving patient care and is designed to save the doctor time without sacrificing the quality of care given to the patient. We have attempted to bring the art and science of medicine together for the benefit of the patient and to lighten the work of the busy physician. The book qualifies as an outline for each physician's continuing medical education.

We are grateful for the suggestions made by students, residents, practicing physicians, and our colleagues. The house staff at Lenox Hill Hospital has, as a group, made very helpful suggestions to us.

Other members of the Lenox Hill Hospital staff have also been most helpful. We would like particularly to thank the library staff, especially Chief Librarian Shirley Dansker, who has been extremely helpful in researching new material that we have incorporated into the book. Penelope Dell was indispensable to Dr. David Fields in the preparation of the second edition, without which there would be no third edition. Special thanks to Arlene Fields, whose patience and support eased the birth of the obstetrical chapters.

As always, we are most grateful to Elizabeth Armour and Ruzena Danek, who played a key role in typing and helping us to complete this book, and to Marcia Miller for her editorial assistance and dedication. Their superb efforts, above and beyond their routine work, have played a significant, if not major, role in bringing this third edition to fruition.

To J. B. Lippincott Company, a division of Harper & Row, we wish to express our appreciation for the opportunity to update *Quick Reference to OB-GYN Procedures.* We want to express our thanks to Mr. Stuart Freeman for his encouragement in undertaking the writing of the first and second editions of this book. Our thanks go also to Lisa McAllister, Editor, for the support and help she gave to us as we worked on the third edition of *Quick Reference To OB-GYN Procedures.*

We are most appreciative of the many doctors who have taken time from their busy practices to thank us for the help that the first and second editions of this book have provided them. It has made our work on this edition even more worthwhile.

To my co-workers, Bridie McGuire and Ann McGuire, who do such a wonderful job organizing my private practice and thereby allowing me time to devote to this text, I am most grateful.

To Dr. Irving Buterman and Dr. Alfred Fields I want to express my deep appreciation for the excellent coverage that they provided for my private practice while I was working on this book.

I am most grateful for the help given to me by my wife, Mary Louise. It has truly been a team effort.

Hugh R.K. Barber, M.D.

Contents

1 Embryology

Hugh R. K. Barber

THE EMBRYOLOGY OF THE GENITAL ORGANS

The genital organs develop in close association with those of the urinary tract. Both arise in the intermediate mesoderm on each side of the root of the mesentery beneath the epithelium of the coelom.

1. *The urinary system* develops from three successive systems.

a. The *pronephros* forms the cervical region and is vestigial. At the caudal end of the pronephros, however, an important duct develops which passes down the body to reach the cloaca. This is the *mesonephric (wolffian) duct.* It will connect some of the tubules of the mesonephros, which appear next.

b. The *mesonephros* forms in the thoracic and lumbar regions, is large, and is characterized by excretory units—nephrons—and its own collecting system, the mesonephric or wolffian duct. In the human it may function briefly, but most of the system disappears. It degenerates to different extents in the two sexes. Two important structures appear on the coelomic surface of the mesonephros: (1) the genital ridge in which the gonad will form, and (2) the paramesonephric (müllerian) duct.

c. The *metanephros,* or permanent kidney, develops from two sources. It forms its own excretory tubules or nephrons as do the other systems, but its collecting system originates from the ureteric bud, an outgrowth of the mesonephric duct. This bud gives rise to the ureter, the renal pelvis, the calices, and the entire collecting system. Connection between the collecting and excretory tubule systems is essential for normal development; failure to connect may cause congenital cystic disease and renal agenesis.

d. The *genital ridge* appears as a swelling on the medial aspect of the mesonephros; at first it covers the whole extent of the latter, but later it contracts to the central part only. The *paramesonephric duct* forms as a groove on the lateral aspect of the coelom, which then sinks below the surface and becomes a tube. This occurs in embryos of some 10 mm., crown-rump length (5 to 6 weeks).

2. *The genital system* consists of:

a. The *gonads,* or primitive sex glands

b. The *genital ducts*

c. The *external genitalia*

All three components go through an indifferent stage in which they may develop in a male or a female direction. Although the genetic sex of the embryo is established at fertilization, the influence of the chromosome complement of the primordial germ cells, which appear in the third week of development, pushes the indifferent gonad in a male or a female direction.

Development of the Ovary

The first sign of a primitive gonad may be seen at about five weeks.

1. The gonad has a triple origin from:

a. The coelomic epithelium of the genital ridge

b. The underlying mesoderm

c. The germ cells, which enter it from an extragonadal source

2. The sex of the embryo is determined genetically at the time of fertilization. However, the gonads do not acquire male or female morphological characteristics until the seventh week of development.

3. The gonads begin as a bulge on the medial aspect of the mesonephric ridge. This is a pair of longitudinal ridges, commonly called the genital or gonadal ridges. They are formed by the proliferation of the coelomic epithelium and condensation of the underlying mesenchymal tissue. Germ cells do not appear in the genital ridge until the sixth week of development.

4. In the human embryo, the *primordial germ cells* appear at an early stage of development among the endodermal cells in the wall of the yolk sac close to the allantois. They migrate by an ameboid movement along a Keinbahn and continue along the dorsal mesentery of the hindgut and invade the genital ridges in the sixth week of development. Failure of the primitive germ cells to reach the gonadal ridge results in the failure of the gonads to develop.

(It is interesting to note that the primitive germ cells migrate along the dorsal mesentery of the hindgut. It is known that there is an increased incidence of ovarian cancer when colon cancer is diagnosed, and vice versa.)

Indifferent Gonad

1. At about the time of the arrival of the primitive germ cells, the coelomic epithelium of the genital ridge proliferates and epithelial cells penetrate the underlying mesenchyma. Here they form the *primitive sex cords*. Since the sex cords are connected with the surface epithelium it is impossible to differentiate the male from the female gonad and, hence, it is called the *indifferent gonad.*

2. In the female embryo with an XX sex chromosome complement, the primitive sex cords are broken up into irregular cell clusters. They are mainly located in the medullary of the ovary and contain groups of primordial germ cells. Later they disappear and are replaced by a vascular stroma, which forms the *ovarian medulla.*

3. The surface epithelium of the female gonad, unlike that of the male, continues to proliferate. In the seventh week it gives rise to a second generation of cords, the *cortical cords,* which penetrate the underlying mesenchyma but remain close to the surface.

4. At about the fourth month these cords are split into isolated cell clusters, each surrounding one or more primordial germ cells. The germ cells subsequently develop into the *oogonia,* while the surrounding epithelial cells, descendants of the surface epithelium, form the *follicular cells.* It should be noted here that in the testis the surface epithelium disappears, while in the ovary it persists as mesothelial cells which give rise to the common epithelial ovarian cancers.

5. The XX sex chromosome configuration causes the medullary cords of the gonad to regress while a secondary generation of cortical cords develops. No tunica albuginea develops in the ovary.

Development of the Uterus and Fallopian Tubes

1. The paramesonephric ducts on each side extend caudally to reach the dorsal wall of the urogenital sinus by about 9 weeks. At this time the mesonephric and paramesonephric ducts are both present and capable of development (indifferent stage).

2. From this point on in the female the paramesonephric duct continues to develop, and the mesonephric to degenerate; in the male the opposite occurs.

3. As the paramesonephric ducts regress caudally, their lower portions come together in the midline and fuse; from this fused part the *uterus* and *cervix* develop, and from the separate upper part the *fallopian tubes* develop. It is to be noted that the müllerian ducts on either side grow in a caudal direction, extra-peritoneally. They bend medially and anteriorly and ultimately fuse in front of the hindgut. The mesonephric duct becomes involved in the walls of the paramesonephric ducts.

4. During the fourth month (12 to 16 weeks) proliferation of the mesoderm around the fused lower parts of the ducts forms the muscular walls of the uterus and cervix.

Descent of the Ovary

In the female, the *ovary* remains at the level of the pelvic brim until birth and gradually descends to its final position as the pelvis grows. The *vaginal process* is formed extending into the labium majus, but normally it atrophies completely. It may persist as the *canal of Nuck,* and remnants may remain as cysts in the inguinal canal. The gubernaculum of the ovary becomes the suspensory ligament of the ovary and the round ligament of the uterus.

The Vagina

1. Vaginal development is more complex. At the müllerian tubercle, where the paramesonephric ducts reach the urogenital sinus, a considerable growth of tissue occurs and the tubercle becomes obliterated.

2. This tissue growth forms the *vaginal plate,* which thus is composed of sinus epithelium and paramesonephric ducts.

3. The vaginal plate grows rapidly, pushing the remnant of the mesonephric duct, which has also reached the urogenital sinus cranially.

4. From this vaginal plate, the *vagina* forms. At first it is a solid organ, but after 16 to 18 weeks the central core begins to break down to form the vaginal lumen. Because of the great growth of the plate, it is not possible to be sure how much vagina is developed from the paramesonephric duct and how much from the urogenital sinus.

5. By the fifth month, the vaginal outgrowth is entirely canalized. The wing-like expansions of the vagina around the end of the uterus, the *vaginal fornices,* are of paramesonephric origin. Thus the vagina has a dual origin, with the upper one-third derived from the uterine canal and the lower two-thirds from the urogenital sinus.

6. The lumen of the vagina remains separated from that of the urogenital sinus by a thin tissue plate, known as the *hymen.* It consists of the epithelial lining of the sinus and a thin layer of vaginal cells. It usually develops a small opening during prenatal life.

7. After the paramesonephric ducts have fused in the midline, a broad transverse pelvic fold is established. This fold, which extends from the lateral sides of the fused paramesonephric duct toward the wall of the pelvis, is known as the *broad ligament of the uterus.* In its upper border is found the uterine tube, and on the posterior surface the ovary. The uterus and broad ligament divide the pelvic cavity into the *uterorectal* and *uterovesical pouches.*

The External Genitalia

1. The *urogenital sinus*—which forms the bladder, urethra, and vestibule—develops as a ventral diverticulum from the hindgut.

2. On the surface of the embryo, around the urogenital sinus, five swellings appear.

a. At the cephalic end a midline swelling grows—the *genital tubercle,* which will become the clitoris.

b. Posterior to the genital tubercle and on either side of the urogenital membrane, two folds are formed—urethral folds.

c. Lateral to each of these a further swelling appears—the *genital* or *labial* swelling. These swellings approach each other at their posterior ends, fuse, and form the *posterior commissure.* The remaining swellings become the *labia minora.*

3. Certain small but clinically important glands are formed in and around the urogenital sinus.

4. In the embryo, *epithelial buds* rise from the urethra and also from the epithelium of the urogenital sinus. In the male, these two sets of buds grow together and give rise to the glands of the prostate.

5. In the female, they remain separate; the urethral buds form the urethral glands and the urogenital buds give rise to the paraurethral *Skene's glands.* The ducts of the latter open into the vestibule on either side of the urethra.

6. Two other small glands arise by budding from the epithelium of the posterior part of the vestibule, one on either side of the vaginal opening. These are the *greater vestibular* or *Bartholin's* glands.

In summary, the urogenital sinus—which forms the bladder, urethra, and vestibule—develops as a ventral diverticulum from the hindgut.

7. At first the urogenital sinus and the hindgut open into a common cavity, the *cloaca,* which at this stage is separated from the exterior by the cloacal membrane.

8. Later the urogenital sinus is completely separated from the hindgut by a section of mesoderm which divides the cloacal membrane into a posterior part, which temporarily closes the future anus, and an anterior part, the *urogenital membrane.*

9. In front of this membrane arises a midline tubercle, the *phallic tubercle.*

10. On each side of the phallic tubercle two ridges develop, the inner called the *genital fold* and the outer the *genital swelling.*

11. Eventually the phallic tubercle forms the clitoris; the inner genital folds form the labia minora and the frenulum and prepuce of the clitoris; and the outer genital swellings give rise to the labia majora.

12. Finally the urogenital membrane disappears, so that the vestibule communicates with the exterior through the vulva.

2 Anatomy of the Reproductive Tract

Hugh R. K. Barber

ANATOMY OF THE FEMALE PELVIS

The Vulva

The *vulva* comprises the *mons pubis*, the *labia majora and minora*, and the *clitoris*, and it overlaps with the *vaginal vestibule*.

1. The Mons Pubis. The mons pubis is a pad of fatty tissue overlying the symphysis pubis and covered by skin and pubic hair. Inferiorly, it divides to become continuous with the labium majus of each side. The skin that covers it bears pubic hair, the upper limit of which is usually horizontal.

2. The Labia Majora

a. The labia majora form the lateral boundary of the vulva and extend from the mons pubis to the perineum; their medial aspects consist of stratified squamous epithelium with hair follicles, a thin layer of smooth muscle (tunica dartos), a layer of fascia, adipose tissue, and large numbers of sweat and sebaceous glands. The labia majora contain numerous nerve endings, some of which are free (pain sensitive), while others are in the form of corpuscles (that is, Meissner, Merkel, Pacini, and Ruffini corpuscles) (touch and pressure sensitive).

b. In the deepest part of each labium is a core of fatty tissue continuous with that of the inguinal canal. The fibers of the round ligament terminate here. During development, a diverticulum of the cavum peritonei, the processus vaginalis, accompanies the round ligament into the inguinal canal. It usually disappears but may persist as the canal of Nuck.

c. The nerves supplied to the vulva are mainly from T12 to S4.

d. The labia majora receive their nerve supply through the iliohypogastric, ilioinguinal, genitofemoral (supplying the dartos muscle), and posterior femoral cutaneous nerves carries sensation to the perineum. The pudendal nerve gives rise to the perineal nerve which gives sensory supply to the vulva.

e. The arterial supply comes from the internal and external pudendals and forms a circular rete. The venous drainage forms a plexus with extensive anastomosis to surrounding areas. The lymphatics of the upper two-thirds of the labia majora (superficial) go to the superficial inguinal nodes and to the deep, subinguinal nodes (Cloquet) to the external iliac chain. The lower one-third of the labia majora (superficial and deep) drain to the superficial inguinal nodes while posteriorly drainage is to the rectal lymphatic plexus of the inferior hemorrhoidal nodes.

3. The Labia Minora

a. The labia minora are two folds of skin which lie between the labia majora. Anteriorly, they divide into two parts, the upper of which unite over the clitoris to form the prepuce, and the lower of which unite to form the frenulum. The skin of the labia minora bears no hair follicles, although sebaceous glands and a few sweat glands are present. The labia minora are very sensitive and contain some erectile tissue. The labia minora have little or no subcutaneous fat. The epithelium is keratinized on the surface but changes to mucous membrane on the medial side.

b. The nerve endings are similar to those in the labia majora.

c. The arterial supply comes from the arterial freta of the labia majora and from the dorsal artery of the clitoris. The venous plexus drains to the labia majora and to the perineal vaginal inferior hemorrhoidal and clitoral vein. The lymphatic draining laterally is the same as that of the labia majora; superiorly as the lower one-third of the vagina; and in the middle, as the upper two-thirds of the labia majora.

4. The Clitoris

a. The clitoris consists of two small, erectile, cavernous bodies terminating in a glans consisting of erectile tissue covered by the prepuce. It is attached to the pubic arch by a suspensory ligament and is covered by stratified, squamous epithelium with numerous sweat and sebaceous glands (except on the glans itself). The nerve endings are similar to those of the labia minora; the nerve supply comes from the terminal branch of the pudendal S1 to S4.

b. The arterial supply is the dorsal artery of the clitoris (terminal branch of the internal pudendal), which divides into deep and dorsal branches as it enters the clitoris. A venous plexus beginning at the glans drains to the pudendal plexus and then to the pudendal vein. The lymphatic drainage of the clitoris is the same as that of the upper two-thirds of the labia majora, and there is some posterior drainage. The glans is covered with modified skin containing many nerve endings. The body and the crura are composed of erectile tissue. The ischiocavernosus muscles surround the crura and by their contraction produce erection of the clitoris.

The Vestibule

1. The vestibule is bounded anterolaterally by the labia minora and posteriorly by the fourchette. The urethra, the ducts of Bartholin's gland, and the vagina open into the vestibule.

2. The vestibular bulbs are two oblong masses of erectile tissue which lie on either side of the vaginal entrance from the vestibule. The bulb of the vestibule is a flask-shaped mass of erectile tissue covered by the bulbocavernosus muscle and homologous to the urethral bulb in the male. The skin of the vestibule is stratified squamous epithelium without hair follicles. The nerve supply is from the perineal branch of the pudendal S1 to S4.

3. The arterial supply is in the form of a plexus from the superficial transverse perineal artery, the interior hemorrhoidal artery, the dorsal artery of the clitoris, and the azygos artery of the vagina. The venous drainage is a plexus with extensive anastomosis of the surrounding area. The vestibule has a lymphatic drainage anteriorly, similar to the labia majora, and posteriorly goes to the rectal lymphatic plexus.

4. Bartholin's Glands (vestibular glands). These are two small racemose glands situated on either side of the vaginal orifice deep to the posterior ends of the labia minora. During sexual excitation, they secrete thin mucus, which serves as a lubricant. The duct on each side opens into the groove between the labia minus and the hymen. Each duct is about 0.5 cm. long, and, unless it is inflamed, the orifice usually cannot be seen. The gland cannot be palpated unless it is pathologically enlarged by inflammation or, as occurs very rarely, by new growth.

The Vagina

1. The vagina is 7 to 10 cm. long, the posterior wall being up to 2 cm. longer than the anterior. The long axis is at an angle of 90° to the cervix. The anterior vaginal wall is in direct relation to the bladder and the urethra throughout its length.

2. At the level of the junction between the urethra and the bladder are the pubourethral ligaments. The upper portion of the posterior vaginal wall is related to the peritoneal space (rectouterine pouch or pouch of Douglas) and the middle half of the rectum. The lower border is separated from the anal canal by the anal sphincters and the perineal body.

3. The cervix projects into the vaginal wall, which is described as having four fornices—anterior, posterior, and two lateral.

4. The vaginal walls are rugose with transverse walls. The vagina is normally kept moist by the secretion of the uterine and cervical glands, and by a watery transudate through its epithelial lining. It has no glands.

5. Laterally, the vagina is supported by the strong cardinal ligaments (transverse cervical ligaments) which form a sling extending from the side walls of the pelvis to the vaginal wall and supravaginal cervix. The vagina is also supported in the middle third by the medial edges of the levator ani muscle, from which fibers are given off to blend with the muscular coat of the vagina.

6. Posteriorly, the lower part of the vagina is supported by the perineal body, which is formed by decussating fibers of the levator ani muscle and of the superficial perineal muscles. In its middle third, the vagina is separated from the rectum only by a thin, rectovaginal septum of fascia. The rectovaginal pouch lies immediately behind the upper third of the vagina, where the peritoneum is reflected from the rectum over the posterior vaginal fornix to reach the supravaginal cervix in the body of the uterus.

7. The Hymen. The hymen is a membrane composed of connective tissue and covered by a stratified squamous epithelium on both aspects. It is perforated centrally, the opening varying in size from a pinhole to one that will admit two fingers. The hymen is partially ruptured at the first coitus and further disrupted during childbirth. Any tags remaining after rupture are known as *carunculae myrtiformes.*

Uterus

1. The uterus is 7.5 cm. long and consists of a main part (body or corpus), a constricted part which also includes the internal walls (isthmus), and a narrow terminal part (cervix): the portion lying above the opening of the fallopian tubes is known as the fundus.

2. The cervix penetrates the anterior wall but is divided into supra- and intravaginal portions. The uterus lies between the bladder and rectum; it weighs 50g. in the nullipara and 70g. in women who have had children.

3. Laterally, the uterus is related to the broad ligaments and the uterine arteries, which curve upward in the soft connective tissue of the broad ligaments.

4. The main blood supply is from the uterine artery, which may rise directly from the internal iliac or rise in common with another branch, especially the superior vesicle. The venous drainage of the uterus corresponds to the arterial supply.

5. The main lymphatic drainage of the uterus is into the external and internal iliac group of lymph nodes, although some lymphatics from the upper part of the uterus pass directly to the lateral aortic nodes, following the ovarian blood supply. A few small branches run up the round ligament into the superficial inguinal nodes.

Cervix Uteri

1. The cervix is cylindrical in shape and continuous above with the body of the uterus. It is described in two parts—supravaginal and vaginal. The vaginal part projects low into the vault of the vagina.

2. The cervical canal is spindle-shaped, being constricted above at the internal os and below at the external os, where it opens into the vagina.

3. The wall of the cervix consists of fibrous and elastic tissue. This is in contrast to the body of the uterus which is mostly smooth muscle.

The Fallopian Tubes

The fallopian tubes lie in the upper margin of the broad ligament and are 10 cm. long. The abdominal opening is at the base of the infundibulum, a trumpet-shaped expansion with fimbriated edge; one of the fimbriae is closely applied to the ovary. The tube consists of the following parts: the interstitial, which is about 1 cm. long and very narrow and is part of the uterus; the isthmus, which is 2 cm. long, straight and cord-like, 1 mm. in diameter; the ampulla, which is 5 cm. long, thin-walled and convoluted; and the infundibulum, which is 2 cm. long with a terminal expansion bearing fimbrial processes which help to attract the ovum.

Ovary

1. The ovary is about 3 cm. long and 1.5 cm. wide, roughly the size and shape of a date. It has its own mesentery, the mesovarium, which derives from the posterior leaf of the broad ligament. The ovary is attached to the corner of the uterus by the ovarian ligament, which is continuous with the round ligament, vestigial gubernaculum.

2. The ovary is developmentally an abdominal organ, and its blood supply is from the abdominal aorta. The ovarian vessels lie in the infundibulopelvic ligaments. The left ovarian vein empties into the left renal vein.

3. The free surface of the ovary has no peritoneal covering, only a surface epithelium. The part attached to the mesovarium, through which all vessels and nerves pass, is called the *hilum*.

4. The position of the ovary varies considerably, but it usually lies against the peritoneum of the lateral pelvic wall and the ovarian fossa, bounded above by the external iliac vein, and behind by the ureter, where it runs downward and forward in front of the internal iliac artery.

5. The most lateral part of the broad ligament is called the infundibulopelvic fold, and this supports the outer pole of the ovary.

BLOOD SUPPLY TO THE FEMALE PELVIS

The internal iliac (hypogastric) artery is a short vessel about 2 cm. in length which begins at the bifurcation of the common iliac artery in front of the sacroiliac joint. It soon divides into anterior and posterior divisions; branches which supply the pelvic viscera are all from the anterior divison.

The branches from the anterior trunk include the superior vesical, middle vesical, inferior vesical, middle hemorrhoidal, obturator, internal pudendal, inferior gluteal, and the uterine and vaginal arteries. The branches that arise from the posterior trunk include the iliolumbar, laterosacral, and the superior gluteal.

1. The Ovarian Artery. Because the ovary develops on the posterior abdominal wall and later migrates down into the pelvis, it derives its blood supply directly from the abdominal aorta. The ovarian artery arises from the aorta just below the renal artery and runs downward on the anterior surface of the psoas muscle to the pelvic rim, where it crosses in front of the ureter. It then passes into the infundibulopelvic fold of the broad ligament. The artery divides into branches which supply the ovary and tubes. The branches run on to reach the uterus, where they anastomose at the terminal branches of the uterine artery.

2. The Superior Hemorrhoidal Artery. This artery is the continuation of the inferior mesenteric artery and descends in the base of the pelvic mesocolon. It divides into two branches which run on either side of the rectum and supply numerous branches to it.

LYMPHATIC DRAINAGE OF THE FEMALE PELVIS

The lymphatic drainage of the pelvis begins as a plexus in the individual organs and generally follows the line of blood vessels. Major and fairly constant groups of nodes include the common iliac, the external iliac (collecting from the inguinal group), the internal iliac, the obturator, and the median and lateral sacral.

NERVES OF THE PELVIS

1. Nerve Supply of the Vulva and Perineum

a. The pudendal nerve arises from the second, third, and fourth sacral nerves. As it passes along the outer wall of the ischiorectal fossa, it gives off an inferior hemorrhoidal branch and divides into the perineal nerve and the dorsum nerve of the clitoris.

b. The perineal nerve supplies the sensory supply to the vulva; it also innervates the anterior part of the external anal sphincter and levator ani, and the superficial perineal muscle. The dorsal nerve of the clitoris is sensory.

c. Sensory fibers from the mons and labia also pass in the ilioinguinal and genitofemoral nerves to the first lumbar root. The posterior femoral cutaneous nerve carries sensations from the perineum to the small sciatic nerve, and thus to the first, second, and third sacral nerves. The main nerve supply of the levator ani muscles comes from the third and fourth sacral nerves.

2. Autonomic Nerve Supply to the Pelvis

a. Sympathetic fibers enter the pelvis via the lumbosacral chain and the mesenteric nerves. These fibers are called the presacral nerve at the bifurcation of the aorta. They pass forward in the uterosacral ligaments to reach the viscera and are known there as the hypogastric plexus or plexus of Frankenhauser.

b. Parasympathetic nerves (nervi erigentes) join the hypogastric plexus from sacral roots 2, 3, and 4. There is an additional sympathetic supply by the nerves accompanying the ovarian vessels.

c. The function of the autonomic nerves is not understood. In practice, it is possible to cauterize the cervix causing only a sensation of heat. The cervix or vagina may be grasped by forceps with only a momentary pricking sensation, and a sound in the uterine cavity causes a vague visceral discomfort.

d. Nevertheless, cervical dilatation must be done under anesthesia, and even then it has been known to cause a severe vasovagal collapse. Relief of pelvic pain by partial cordotomy has to be done well above the pelvis to be effective, and the level of choice is T2.

e. The myometrium of the uterus contains both alpha- and beta-adrenergic receptors as well as cholinergic receptors. In the non-pregnant uterus the balance of their action is uncertain, but during pregnancy strong stimulation of beta receptors with beta-mimetic drugs such as isoxsuprine will inhibit myometrial activity.

THE PERINEUM

1. *Perineum* refers to the anatomical region at the inferior end of the trunk, below the pelvic floor. With the thighs abducted, it is diamond-shaped. On the surface, it is bounded by the mons veneris in front, the buttocks behind, and the thighs laterally. More deeply, it is limited by the margins of the pelvic outlet, namely, the pubic symphysis and arcuate ligament, the ischial pubic rami, the ischial tuberosities, the sacrotuberal ligament, the sacrum, and coccyx. A transverse line joining the ischial tuberosities divides the perineum into an anterior urogenital and posterior angle triangle.

2. The perineal floor is composed of skin and two layers of superficial fascia, a superficial fatty layer, and a deeper membranous one. The former is continuous anteriorly with the superficial fatty layer of the abdomen (Camper's fascia) and posteriorly with the ischial rectal fat. The deeper, membranous layer of the superficial perineal fascia (Colles' fascia) is limited to the anterior half of the perineum. Laterally, it is attached to the ischial pubic rami, posteriorly it blends with the base of the urogenital diaphragm, and anteriorly it is continuous with a deep layer of superficial abdominal fascia (Scarpa's fascia).

3. The urogenital triangle contains the termination of the vagina and the urethra, the crura of the clitoris surrounded by the ischiocavernosus muscles, the bulb of the vestibule and the bulbocavernosus muscles, the greater vestibular glands and ducts, the urogenital diaphragm, the muscles which converge on the central point of the perineum and the superficial and deep perineal pouches, together with the blood vessels, nerves, and lymphatics in this region.

4. The urogenital diaphragm (triangular ligament) is a structure peculiar to man. It consists of a sheath of muscles enclosed between two triangular fascial membranes. The muscular sheath is formed by the transversus perinei profundus and the sphincter urethrae membranaceae muscles. The superior layer is the thin fascia bridging the gap between the anterior portions of the levator ani muscles. The inferior fascial layer is tough and fibrous.

5. The perineal body is the pyramidal mass of muscular tissue which lies between the anal canal and the lower third of the vagina. It is a fibromuscular mass into which the bulbocavernosus, transverse perinei, external anal sphincter, and levator ani muscles insert.

6. The perineal body is a fibromuscular mass between anus and vagina with attachments to eight muscles. These include a sphincter ani, a bulbocavernosus, two transverse perineal superficial muscles, two transverse perineal profundi muscles, and two levator ani.

7. The whole mass is what gynecologists mean when they talk about the perineum. If it is damaged during parturition and not properly repaired and healed, it will not function properly and the efficiency of the whole pelvic diaphragm may suffer.

8. The superficial perineal pouch is a potential space between the inferior fascia of the urogenital diaphragm (triangular ligament) and the fascia of Colles. It contains the Bartholins glands and the superficial perineal muscles. The roof of the superficial perineal pouch is formed by the inferior fascia of the urogenital diaphragm (triangular ligament) and its floor by the deep layer of superficial perineal fascia (Colles' fascia). Laterally, the superficial perineal pouch is bounded by the ischial pubic rami and posteriorly by the junction of the fascial layer around the superficial perinei muscles.

9. The deep perineal pouch is a potential space between the two fascial layers of the urogenital diaphragm and contains the membranous urethra surrounded by external sphincter and deep transverse perineal muscles. It is a strong, musculomembranous partition stretched across the anterior half of the pelvic outlet between the ischiopubic rami. It is composed of superior and inferior fascial layers between which are contained the deep perinei muscles, the sphincter of the membranous urethra, and the pudendal vessels and nerves. It is pierced by the urethra and vagina.

Muscles of the Perineum

1. The ischiocavernosus muscle arises from the medial aspect of the inferior ischial ramus and sheathes the crus clitoridis. This muscle compresses the root of the clitoris during sexual excitement, to produce erection by venous congestion.

2. The bulbocavernosus muscle originates in the perineal body, where it interdigitates with the external anal sphincter. This muscle conceals the vestibular bulb and the Bartholin's glands. Its function is to diminish the vaginal orifice during coitus.

3. The superficial transverse perineal muscle radiates from the perineal body to the ischial ramus. It is a feeble muscle which helps to fix the perineal body.

4. The deep transverse perineal muscle has the same origin and an insertion that lies deep to the inferior fascia of the urogenital diaphragm.

5. The sphincter ani externus normally is in a state of contraction to keep the anus closed. It also helps to fix the perineal body.

The Levator Ani Muscles (Pelvic Diaphragm)

1. The pelvic diaphragm forms a musculotendinous, funnel-shaped partition between the pelvic cavity and the perineum. It is composed of the levator ani and coccygeus muscles, sheathed in a superior and inferior layer of fascia. The muscles of the pelvic diaphragm extend from the lateral pelvic walls downward immediately to fuse with each other and are inserted into the terminal portions of the urethra, vagina, and anus. Anteriorly, they fail to meet in the midline and just behind the pubic symphysis, exposing a gap in the pelvic floor which is completed by the urogenital diaphragm. In this area, the inferior fascia of the pelvic diaphragm fuses with the superior fascia of the urogenital diaphragm.

2. The levator ani muscles may be subdivided into an anterior pubococcygeus and a posterior iliococcygeus portion. They originate on each side of the posterior aspect of the pubis, the tendinous arch, and the ischial spine. They are inserted into the coccyx, the anal coccygeal body, the lower end of the anal canal, the central point of the perineum, the lower vagina, and the posterolateral surface of the urethra. The levator ani muscles are primarily supporting structures, but also contribute a sphincteric action on the anal canal and the vagina. Contraction of the abdominal wall, as in straining or coughing, relaxes the levator muscles, and thus the angle between the rectum and the anus is diminished.

3. The coccygeus muscles are triangular in shape, rise from the ischial spine, and are inserted into the lateral borders of the lower sacrum and upper coccyx. They lie on the pelvic aspect of the sacrospinous ligaments.

4. Although they are not part of the pelvic diaphragm, two muscles cover the walls of the true pelvis—the obturator internus and the piriformis.

5. The nerve supply to the levator ani is from the third and fourth sacral nerves.

THE PELVIC FASCIAE

1. The pelvic fasciae of the pelvic diaphragm are continuous with the fascial layers of the perineal compartments, the endopelvic fascia, the obturator fascia, the iliac fascia, and the transversalis fascia of the abdomen.

2. The parietal layer comprises the aponeuroses and the fascial sheaths of the pelvic muscles. The visceral layer is the fascial sheath of the organs and the fatty tissue filling the space between them.

3. The relationships of the fascia are: the nerve trunks, which leave the pelvis, may be described as lying behind the fascia which gives them fascial sheaths. The vessels are in front of the fascia and lie between the fascia and peritoneum.

The Peritoneum and Ligaments of the Pelvis

1. The peritoneum is reflected from the lateral borders of the uterus to form on either side a double fold of peritoneum known as the *broad ligament.* It is not a ligament but a peritoneal fold, and it does not support the uterus. The fallopian tube runs in the upper free edge of the broad ligament as far as the point at which the tube opens into the peritoneal cavity; the part of the broad ligament which is lateral to the opening is called the infundibulopelvic fold, and in it the ovarian vessels and nerves pass from the sidewall of the pelvis and lie between the two layers of the broad ligament.

2. The peritoneum covers the uterus, with the exception of the anterior part of the supravaginal cervix and the intravaginal cervix. From the anterior surface of the uterus, the peritoneum is reflected onto the superior surface of the bladder, forming the uterovesical pouch. From the posterior surface of the uterus, the peritoneum continues onto the upper aspect of the vagina before it is reflected onto the anterior rectal surface, forming the rectouterine pouch (or pouch of Douglas). The lower extremity of this pouch is attached to the perineal body by connective tissue of the rectovaginal septum.

3. The portion of the broad ligament which lies above the ovary is known as the *mesosalpinx,* and between its layers are to be seen any wolffian remnants which are present.

4. Below the ovary, the base of the broad ligament widens out and contains a considerable amount of loose connective tissue called the *parametrium.* The ureter is attached to the posterior leaf of the broad ligament at this point.

5. The ovary is attached to the posterior layer of the broad ligament by a mesovarium, through which the ovarian vessels and nerves enter the hilum.

6. Vestigial remnants of the mesonephric bodies and ducts (wolffian ducts, duct of Gartner) are contained within the broad ligament. Remnants of the mesonephric body lie above and lateral to the ovary (epoophoron and hydatid of Morgagni) and between the ovary and uterus (paroophoron).

7. The ovarian ligament lies beneath the posterior layer of the broad ligament and passes from the medial part of the ovary to the uterus just below the point of entry of the fallopian tube.

8. The round ligament is the continuation of the same structure and thus runs forward under the anterior leaf of the peritoneum to enter the inguinal canal, ending in the subcutaneous tissue of the labia majora. Together, the ovarian and round ligaments are homologous with the gubernaculum testis of the male. The round ligament is seldom tense enough to prevent the uterus from becoming retroverted; it has no other supporting function.

9. The ligaments formed from pelvic fascia include the transverse cervical ligament (cardinal ligament), the pubocervical ligaments, and the uterosacral ligaments. All three ligaments insert into the upper vagina in the supravaginal cervix.

10. The essential support of the uterus and vaginal vault is provided by the cardinal ligaments (transverse cervical ligaments or ligaments of Mackenrodt). These are two strong, fan-shaped, fibromuscular expansions which pass from the cervix and vaginal vault to the sidewall of the pelvis on either side.

11. Uterosacral ligaments run from the cervix and vaginal vault to the sacrum. In the erect position, they are almost vertical in direction and support the cervix.

12. The bladder is supported laterally by condensations of the visceral pelvic fascia on each side, and there is also a sheet of pubocervical fascia which lies beneath it anteriorly.

THE FEMALE UROLOGIC SYSTEM

The Ureters

1. The ureters, commencing at the renal pelvis, are about 20 cm. long, the left one being a little longer than the right. Each crosses the posterior abdominal wall by running in an oblique medial direction behind the peritoneum and over the psoas muscle.

2. The ureter enters the pelvis retroperitoneally by crossing over or near the bifurcation of the common iliac artery.

3. It is itself crossed by the ovarian vessels and is near the fold of the peritoneum which forms the infundibulopelvic ligament.

4. The ureter passes down immediately behind the ovarian fossa and is in close relation to the internal iliac artery. In the healthy subject, its shape can be made out beneath the peritoneum and its movements observed.

5. The ureter then passes beneath the base of the broad ligament, through the transverse uterine ligament, and into the bladder. In this parametrial part of its course, it lies alongside the vaginal fornix and passes under the uterine artery.

6. Just before its termination in the bladder wall, the ureter is ensheathed by a part of the visceral layer of pelvic fascia known as the *fascia of Waldeyer.* In this fascia there are some plain muscle fibers derived from the longitudinal muscle coat of the ureter, which are capable of kinking the lower end of the ureter should the bladder become overdistended.

7. The blood supply comes from the abdominal aorta and the renal, ovarian, common and internal iliac, vesicle, and uterine arteries.

8. The nerve supplies are both sympathetic and parasympathetic and arise from the renal, aortic, and superior-inferior hypogastric plexuses (T10 to S4).

The Bladder

1. The bladder is derived in part from the urogenital sinus and in part from the ends of the mesonephric ducts. It is continuous with the allantoic duct, which persists as a partly canalized fibromuscular band, the urachus, joining the apex of the bladder to the umbilicus.

2. The bladder is a hollow, muscular organ lined by mucous membrane. The muscle wall is composed of a rich framework of plain muscle fibers. The submucosa is very loose, and this causes the mucous membrane and the greater part of the contracted organ to be thrown into a series of folds, giving it a trabeculated appearance.

3. The average capacity of the bladder is 400 ml.

4. The ureters open into the base of the bladder after running medially for about 1 cm. through the vesicle wall. The urethra leaves the bladder in front of the ureteric orifices; the triangular area lying between the ureteric orifices and the internal meatus is known as the *trigone.* With the internal meatus, the middle layer of the vesical muscle forms anterior and posterior loops around the neck of the bladder, some of the fibers of the loops being continuous with the circular muscle of the urethra.

5. The base of the bladder is related to the cervix with only a thin layer of connective tissue intervening. Below, it is separated from the anterior vaginal wall by the pubocervical fascia, which stretches from the pubis to the cervix.

The Urethra

1. The female urethra extends from the neck of the bladder to the external urethral orifice. It measures about 4 cm. in length and is embedded in the anterior wall of the vagina. The muscle layers are continuous with that of the bladder, and there is no internal sphincter at the junction of the bladder.

2. The urethra is lined with transitional epithelium near the bladder neck, grading to a non-keratinized, stratified, squamous epithelium near the external orifice.

3. As the urethra passes through the two layers of the urogenital diaphragm (triangular ligament), it is embraced by the striated fibers of the deep transverse perineal muscles (compressor urethrae), and some of the striated fibers form loops on the urethra. Between the muscular coat and the epithelium is a plexus of veins. There are a number of tubular mucous glands and, in the lower part, a number of crypts, which occasionally become infected.

4. In its upper two-thirds, the urethra is separated from the symphysis by loose connective tissue, but in its lower third it is attached to the pubic ramus on each side by strong bands of fibrous tissue called the pubourethral ligament. Posteriorly, it is related to the anterior vaginal wall, to which it is firmly attached in its lower two-thirds. The upper two-thirds of the urethra is mobile, but the lower third is relatively fixed.

5. The voluntary external sphincter (sphincter urethrae) is supplied by the perineal branch of the pudendal nerve (S2 to S4).

6. The arterial and venous blood supply to the upper third of the urethra is associated with that of the bladder, and the lower two-thirds with that of the anterior vaginal wall and clitoris.

7. Lymphatic drainage of the urethra is via the bladder to the external iliac chain.

8. The nerve supply comes from the hypergastric plexus.

The Rectum

1. The rectum is about 15 cm. long. It commences at the third sacral vertebra as a continuation of the pelvic colon. It is devoid of both tenia and appendices epiploicae. It descends in front of the sacrum and coccyx, and, just below the tip of the coccyx, it is kinked forward to form the anal-rectal flexure at the anal-rectal junction. The lower half of the rectum is ballooned to form the rectal ampulla.

2. In its upper third, its front and sides are covered by the peritoneum of the rectovaginal pouch; in the middle third, only the front is covered by the peritoneum.

3. In the lower third, there is no peritoneal covering, and the rectum is separated from the posterior wall of the vagina by the rectovaginal fascial septum. Lateral to the rectum are two uterosacral ligaments, beside which run some of the lymphatics draining the cervix and vagina.

The Anal Canal

1. The anal canal is about 2.5 cm. long. It commences below and in front of the coccyx and takes a sudden sweep backward to end at the anal orifice.

2. It is guarded by three sphincters; that is, the sphincter ani internus, which is a reduplication of circular muscle fibers of this part of the intestine, the levator ani (puborectalis), and the deep circular fibers of the sphincter ani externus. These three sphincters blend at the lower end of the anal canal.

3. Immediately in front of the anal canal is the perineal body, and immediately behind it is the anococcygeal body.

3 Infertility

Sherwin A. Kaufman

DEFINITIONS

1. *Infertility* is the inability to achieve pregnancy and carry through to live birth; thus a woman who has had only miscarriages may be considered infertile. *In primary infertility* no pregnancy has ever taken place, while in secondary infertility one or more previous conceptions have occurred.

2. *Sterility,* though technically synonymous with "infertility," implies that some absolute factor precludes conception; this may be temporary (previous tubal ligation) or permanent (previous hysterectomy). In general the term "infertility" is preferable to "sterility," because it has a less ominous connotation.

3. A couple is considered infertile if pregnancy has not occurred after one year of coitus without contraception. Normally, 75 per cent of women conceive during the first 6 months, and 85 per cent conceive in the first year. Therefore, if a couple has been trying to coneive for 1 year (or an older couple for 6 months), it is time to begin a workup.

BASIC PRINCIPLES

1. It is estimated that between 15 and 20 per cent of couples are either unable to initiate a preganancy or unable to carry to term.

2. This means that approximately 6 million couples in the U.S. are involuntarily childless, which makes infertility a common medical problem.

3. Management of infertility requires an organized plan of study, particularly because in the majority of couples more than one cause is found.

4. The various tests for infertility to be described are related to the basic prerequisites for fertility, which are as follows:

a. The male gonads must produce sperm of reasonable quantity and quality.

b. There must be no obstruction in the male genital tract.

c. The ejaculate must have access to the cervix.

d. The endocervical mucus must be favorable for sperm survival.

e. The tubes must be patent to allow for ascent of sperm and descent of the ovum.

f. The ovaries must produce and release normal ova.

g. There must be no obstruction between the ovaries and the fimbriated ends of the tubes.

h. The endometrium must be physiologically capable of permitting normal implantation of the fertilized ovum and continued embryonic growth.

Causes of Infertility

1. In the majority of cases, there are multiple causes for infertility.

2. About 40 per cent of infertility problems relate to the man (male factor) in whole or in part.

3. In the female, the most common causes of infertility, in order of frequency, relate to ovulation disturbances, tubal problems, and cervical factors; the last two are especially common in secondary infertility.

4. Less frequently, the cause is related to the uterine corpus, to metabolic factors, or to immunological problems.

5. In some cases no etiological factors are discernible despite complete investigation. (This is another way of saying that the causes remain elusive.)

6. Contrary to popular belief, psychological or emotional factors are actually an infrequent cause of infertility in those desiring children. Any psychosomatic aspects are generally results of frustration owing to barren marriage.

Doctor-Patient Relationship

1. Infertility is the only "illness" that involves two people. The physician must appreciate the sensitivities and frustrations of the couple.

2. It is wise to enlist the male's cooperation by having him present at the first interview and by explaining that infertility is considered a bilateral problem.

3. The terms "fault" and "blame" have no place in the management of infertility.

4. A well-organized and sytematic approach yields the best results. It saves time, and the rate of ultimate success is high.

5. The physician should outline the nature, scope, and purpose of the tests contemplated, the time involved (3 to 6 months), and the attendant costs.

6. If necessary, the gynecologist should utilize the services of a urologist, endocrinologist, and psychologist or psychiatrist.

7. The doctor's purpose is to determine first why the couple is infertile, then what treatment is indicated and the prognosis.

8. It is encouraging to note that from 50 to 70 per cent of infertility patients can be helped.

INFERTILITY INVESTIGATION OF THE MALE

Investigation of the male should be one of the first steps in the study. Detailed history and physical examination are of obvious importance when the semen quality is subnormal.

History

1. Past History

a. *Previous Marriage.* Fertility or infertility

b. *Previous Studies.* Previous infertility tests or treatments

c. *Medical.* Anomalies, varicocele, venereal disease, orchitis (e.g., mumps), chronic illness, obesity, endocrine disorders, allergies, drugs, recent febrile illness. (A recent flu, for example, can severely depress sperm quality for several weeks.)

d. *Surgical.* Varicocelectomy, herniorrhaphy, hydrocelectomy, genital injuries

e. *Occuptional.* Radiographs; chemicals (exposure to metals as in painting or printing); thermal factors (possible sources of excessive heat include febrile illness, prolonged or frequent hot baths, and tight scrotal supports). (Note: the deleterious effects of hyperthemia or viral illness—other than mumps orchitis—are completely dissipated after 3 months.) The ordinary pressures of life and work do not generally affect sperm quality; however, extreme stress can have a deleterious effect on male fertility and sexual functioning.

2. Present History

a. *Type of Problem.* Duration of infertility

b. *Habits.* Marijuana may depress the sperm count and can also cause chromosomal anomalies that can lead to genetic damage. Heavy tabacco smoking may cause some depression of sperm production, but no well-controlled studies have been reported. Excessive use of alchol may contribute to liver damage with resultant depression of sperm production. In addition, potency may be adversely affected by excessive use of alcohol or other drugs.

c. *Sexual History.* If the couple normally has intercouse two to three times a week it is unnecessary (and counterproductive) to belabor the question of timing. Only if intercourse is relatively infrequent is there merit in discussing the most fertile days in the woman's cycle (which can be quite variable). However, when the frequency of spontaneous coitus is very low, the reasons for the lack of desire (or response), or potency problems, should be explored. Here the unsatisfactory sexual relationship takes precedence over the infertility problem; solving the former may well solve the latter.

Physical Examination

1. The presence of varicocele may be significant. In addition, congenital disorders such as hypospadias, testicular atrophy, cryptorchidism, or absence of vas deferens must be ruled out.

2. In the general physical examination, special attention must be given to secondary sexual characteristics, poor nutrition, and evidence of any endocrinopathy.

Diagnostic Procedures

1. Semen Analysis

a. The period of abstinence should correspond to the couple's usual coital frequency (in order to obtain a representative sample).

b. The semen should be collected in a clean, dry glass or plastic wide-mouthed container by masturbation or coitus interruptus. A condom should not be used, but a commercially prepared plastic sheath with perforation is available for devout Catholics.

c. Examine within 3 hours of collection, preferably within 2 hours.

d. The normal standards against which to measure the semen are as follows:

(1) Liquefaction: usually complete in 5 to 20 minutes

(2) Volume: averages between 2 and 5 ml.

(3) Sperm count: a minimum of 20 to 40 million per ml.

(4) Motility at room temperature: Examination of several fields is done under high dry magnification. The numbers per high power field roughly correspond to millions per ml. At least 60 per cent of the sperm should have vigorous, progressive motion at initial examination. (Subsequent examinations in vitro are of no clinical significance.)

(5) Morphology: A simple stain test is to mix a drop of semen with a drop of 1-per-cent aqueous gentian violet. At least 60 per cent should be normal (oval) forms.

2. Urologic examination, especially for varicocele, if semen analysis is subnormal

3. Testicular biopsy when indicated. (Regarding azoospermia, the absence of fructose in the semen suggests congenital absence of vas deferens.)

4. Endocrine evaluation of pituitary, adrenal, and testicular function

5. Sex chromatin and chromosome analysis when indicated

INFERTILITY INVESTIGATION OF THE FEMALE

The importance of a detailed history cannot be overemphasized.

History

1. Past History

a. *Previous Marriage.* Fertility or infertility

b. *Medical.* Serious illnesses, endocrine disorders, psychiatric history

c. *Gynecological.* Menstrual irregularities, methods of contraception (e.g., IUD, Pill), pelvic inflammatory disease, possible endometriosis, venereal disease

d. *Surgical.* Pelvic operations, ruptured appendix

e. *Obstetrical.* Abortions (spontaneous or induced), deliveries, postpartum or postabortal complications

f. *Previous Studies.* Previous infertility tests and treatments

2. Present History

a. *Marital History.* Years married and duration of infertility

b. *Sexual History.* Coital frequency, and whether natural or "scheduled," use of lubricants, and postcoital habits such as arising immediately or douching

c. *Social Habits.* Excessive smoking or drinking, use of drugs or other medications

d. *Psychosomatic Evaluation*

Physical Examination

1. General physical examination
2. Gynecological examination

Diagnostic Procedures

1. Pap smears, urinalysis, blood count, serology, sedimentation rate, and cervical cultures for chlamydia, mycoplasma, and gonorrhea
2. Thyroid evaluation: TSH, T_3, and T_4
3. Basal body temperatures (BBT)
4. Tubal insufflation (Rubin test)
5. Hysterosalpingogram
6. Postcoital examinations (Sims-Huhner test), including evaluation of cervical mucus
7. Endometrial biopsy

Additional Studies That May Be Necessary

1. Serum progesterone, by radioimmunoassay (RIA), to establish occurrence of ovulation and to appraise adequacy of corpus luteum function
2. Ultrasound to detect degree of follicle maturation and determine whether ovum release has occurred or whether there is evidence of LUF (luteinized unruptured follicle) syndrome
3. Adrenal function studies: serum dehydroepiandrosterone sulfate (DHEA-S), cortisol, urinary 17-ketosteroids, 17-hydroxysteroids, pregnanetriol, dexamethasone suppression test. (See Chap. 27.)
4. Pituitary gonadotropins—i.e., serum follicle-stimulating hormone (FSH) and luteinizing hormone (LH)—by RIA to rule out hypopituitarism (decreased value) or premature menopause (elevated)
5. Metopirone test of pituitary reserve
6. Glucose tolerance test
7. Skull film, for visualization of sella turcica, and visual field examination to rule out pituitary tumor in amenorrheic or oligomenorrheic patients, combined with serum prolactin level (galactorrhea)
8. Progesterone withdrawal test (100 mg. progesterone in oil I.M.) in amenorrhea, to establish presence of endogenous estrogen and to demonstrate integrity of the endometrium
9. Sex chromatin test (Barr) to rule out chromosomal anomaly
10. In-vitro test of sperm–cervical mucus compatibility; determination of antisperm antibodies
11. Endoscopy, either culdoscopy or laparoscopy, to rule out endometriosis, tubal strictures or obstruction, peritubal or peri-ovarian adhesions, Stein-Leventhal syndrome (polycystic ovaries), ovarian dysgenesis

Determination of Ovulation

1. Evidence of Ovulation. Most indices of ovulation depend upon the elaboration of progesterone by the corpus luteum. Although they are not absolute evidence that ovulation has occurred, they are sufficient for practical, clinical purposes. The only direct signs that ovulation has taken place are: (1) visualization of the ovulation process at laparotomy or endoscopy, and (2) occurrence of pregnancy.

2. Methods for the Detection of Ovulation

a. *Basal Body Temperature (BBT).* A biphasic curve suggests ovulation. Progesterone is thermogenic, causing the typical elevation during the second half of the cycle.

b. *Cervical Mucus Changes.* Progesterone changes the mucus from profuse, clear, and watery to scant, cloudy, and viscous, and causes a gradual disappearance of microscopic ferning when the mucus is allowed to dry.

c. *Endometrial biopsy* for secretory changes, including "dating" of the endometrium according to the number of days past ovulation

d. *Serum progesterone* by radioimmunoassay, to establish the occurrence of ovulation and ascertain the adequacy of corpus luteum function

e. *Luteal surge,* as determined by currently available home kits for urine testing

f. *Serial sonography* to detect follicle maturation and release

g. *Endoscopy,* seeing a corpus luteum or corpus hemorrhagicum

Evaluation of Tubal Function

1. Purpose of Tubal-Function Tests. Tubal-function tests may be therapeutic as well as diagnostic, inasmuch as they may overcome minor degrees of phimosis, agglutination, or obstruction. Partial or complete tubal obstruction may be caused by pelvic inflammatory disease resulting from a wide variety of bacteria, including gonorrhea, postabortal or postpartum infections, or chlamydia. Obstruction may also be caused by adhesions resulting from endometriosis, appendicitis, or bleeding caused by a ruptured follicle or corpus luteum. Obstruction may, of course, be the expected result of tubal ligation or cauterization for sterilization.

2. Methods for Determining the State of the Tubes

a. *Tubal insufflation* (for tubal patency).

(1) The instrument should supply a constant source of carbon dioxide (never oxygen, which can cause air embolism). There should be a flowmeter, pressure gauge, and kymograph for recording pressure oscillations, which are thought to be related to tubal peristalsis.

(2) Under continuous observation, pressure may be permitted to reach a maximum of 200 to 250 mm. Hg if necessary. If gas is passing through, however, about 80 to 100 ml. of CO_2 is allowed to enter.

(3) The most frequent source of error is failure to secure a leakproof application of the cervical cannula; proper countertraction with a tenaculum on the cervix is helpful.

(4) Contraindications to Tubal Insufflation Test

(a) Local (vaginal) or pelvic infection. A white count and sedimentation rate are helpful to clarify, particularly if there is a history of previous infection.

(b) Uterine bleeding

(c) Abortion, spontaneous or induced, within the preceding 2 months

(d) Any possibility of a pregnancy having been initiated. (The test is normally done a few days after a normal menstrual period, not only to avoid this possibility but because there is least pelvic congestion at this time of cycle.)

(5) Evaluation of the Tubal Insufflation Test

(a) If normal patency is present there is usually an initial rise in pressure up to 80 to 120 mm. Hg, with a sudden drop to a lower level as gas passes into the peritoneal cavity.

(b) When either blockage or tubal (cornual) spasm is present, the kymograph shows a steady rise to 250 mm.; this maximum pressure should not be exceeded.

(c) Passage of CO_2 into the peritoneal cavity is confirmed by the presence of pain in one or both shoulders after the test, when the patient sits up. Without such pain, whether immediate or delayed, there is no proof that gas has gone through.

(d) If there is no passage (i.e., maximum pressure required throughout and no shoulder pain following), owing to spasm or obstruction, the test should be repeated at another time, after administration of a sedative or tranquilizer.

(e) In essence, a positive test shows only that there is a free communication between the uterine cannula and the peritoneal cavity. It does not show that both tubes are patent, because the same result can be obtained with one patent tube as with two. Most important, it does not show if the tubes (though patent) are physiologically *normal.* Tubes may be partially occluded, or be bound down by adhesions and unable to pick up or transport an expelled ovum, and yet show a "normal" Rubin test.

(f) Conversely, if the test is consistently negative, it does not mean that the tubes are necessarily occluded. A hysterosalpinogram should be done.

b. *Hysterosalpingogram*

(1) A radiograph of the uterine cavity and tubes is not competitive with a Rubin test. Each has its own value and is capable of revealing things that the other may not. A Rubin test remains a good screening procedure and can prove immediately that at least one tube is open, which is of great reassurance to the anxious patient.

(2) A hysterosalpingogram is helpful in clarifying a questionable or abnormal tubal insufflation test. *Many physicians prefer to use the radiograph alone, omitting the Rubin test.*

(3) However, a hysterosalpingogram has its own limitations. It can indicate that dye has passed through both tubes, but one cannot be certain from this information that the tubes are anatomically normal, because dye can pass through partially strictured or adherent tubes as well.

(4) Nevertheless, the radiograph can provide further information:

(a) Determination of the site of tubal obstruction if it exists

(b) Delineation of suspected adhesions in the event of pooling of dye near the fimbriated ends

(c) Detection of uterine malformations (anomalies), submucous leiomyomata, endometrial polyps, synechiae

(d) Delineation of cervical canal, as in incompetent cervix, cervical stenosis, isthmic synechiae

(e) Capability of overcoming minor obstructions by the force of hydrostatic pressure employed

(5) Contraindications: The same as for tubal insufflation

(6) Technique

(a) Like a Rubin test, radiography is performed 3 to 5 days after cessation of menses.

(b) An oil medium or a water-soluble medium may be used. Most clinicians prefer the simplicity of the latter, even though tubal outline may be overshadowed by too-rapid spillover into the pelvis if the injection of the dye is not methodically slow.

(c) A sterile technique is used, and the same instruments are used as for the tubal insufflation test. A scout film is taken first. The cannula must be emptied of air by a filling of dye before insertion. The guard at the tip of the cannula is tightened so that the tip enters the external cervical os for a distance of 1 cm., in order to get a picture of the cervical canal. Fractional amounts (0.5 to 2 ml.) are injected and the film is taken and developed after each instillation. Attachment of a television screen during the procedure is helpful. In instances of uterine flexion, it is important to apply traction in order to straighten out the uterus.

(d) If cornual or fimbrial blockage is seen, it is helpful to shift the patient's position from side to side, permitting a more adequate dispersion of dye.

(e) As stated, the Rubin test and hysterosalpingography are not competitive tests; each can give information the other cannot. Moreover, it has been amply demonstrated that both these procedures can reveal "normal" tubes that are later shown to be pathological at endoscopic examination. Therefore, no firm conclusions should be drawn from either procedure. It should also be kept in mind that both of these procedures, although primarily diagnostic, may be therapeutic in clearing out minor degrees of phimosis and agglutination.

c. *Endoscopy* (culdoscopy or laparoscopy). *Culdoscopy* is the direct visualization of the pelvic organs through the vagina. *Laparoscopy* is the direct visualization of the pelvic organs through the abdomen.

(1) Indications For Endoscopy

(a) Endoscopy is the definitive method for ruling out suspected or unsuspected tubal pathology, peri-adnexal adhesions, endometriosis, polycystic or other ovarian disease, or abnormalities in uterine contour in the infertile patient.

(b) Endoscopy is an essential prerequisite to any tubal plastic or ovarian (wedge) procedure for infertility.

(c) An integral part of the procedure is tubal perfusion of indigocarmine dye (chromotubation) under direct vision through the endoscope. Unlike the Rubin test or salpingography, this clarifies whether dye is passing through freely or whether there are phimosis, agglutination, occlusion, or adhesions. Moreover, in an operating-room setting, much more pressure can be exerted, which may be therapeutic in overcoming lesser degrees of phimosis and agglutination.

(2) Contraindications to Culdoscopy

(a) Fixed retroverted uterus or other mass in the cul-de-sac

(b) Acute pelvic infection

(c) Orthopedic or other disorder that precludes placing the patient in the knee-chest position

(3) Technique of Culdoscopy

(a) Best performed in a hospital operating room

(b) Preoperative Preparation: Low enema the night prior to surgery and perineal prep only. Benadryl, 50 mg. I.M., 1 hour before surgery.

(c) Proper placement in the knee-chest position is of paramount importance for satisfactory examination. Padded shoulder braces should be used to prevent movement.

(d) Sterile technique is used throughout.

(e) The following combination has been found most satisfactory in the prevention of discomfort: (a) local infiltration of the uterosacral ligaments with 2 ml. of 1-per-cent lidocaine without epinephrine on each side; (b) Demerol, 50 mg. to 100 mg., and diazepam (Valium), 2.5 to 5 mg., given intravenously, very slowly. The dosages should be individualized according to the degree of patient anxiety.

(f) The actual technique of cul-de-sac puncture and visualization cannot be learned by description; it should be taught in the operating room. A cervical cannula is also positioned in order to instill dilute indigo-carmine dye under direct vision. This is an integral part of the procedure.

(g) A fractional D & C is easily performed at the end of the procedure without requiring any change in the patient's position. This will rule out cervical or uterine pathology.

(h) After culdoscopy it is important, for later comfort, to expel the air that has entered the abdomen by the sucking in of negative pressure. As much air as possible is expelled by abdominal pressure as the patient assumes the prone position, while the cannula is still in place. The puncture site in the cul-de-sac requires no stitches, as a rule. The patient may feel sleepy the rest of the day but is usually quite comfortable except, perhaps, in the upright position. Some shoulder pain may remain. She may have diet as tolerated, be ambulated ad lib, and go home in a few hours.

(4) Indications for Laparoscopy

(a) For infertility patients, the indications are the same as those described for endoscopy.

(5) CONTRAINDICATIONS TO LAPAROSCOPY

(a) Previous abdominal or pelvic surgery where intestinal adhesions are suspected near the parietal peritoneum

(b) Contraindication of general anesthesia, so that local anesthesia cannot be supplemented if necessary

(c) Extreme obesity (relative)

(6) TECHNIQUE OF LAPAROSCOPY

(a) Patient is in a modified dorsal-lithotomy position

(b) After examination under anesthesia, a fractional D & C is performed, followed by insertion of a special cannula into the cervix, which can be attached to a tenaculum already on the anterior cervical lip.

(c) Dilute, sterile indigo-carmine dye in a 20-ml. syringe is attached to the cannula for instillation during the subsequent laparoscopy. The cannula is also useful in moving the uterus into different positions.

(d) With the patient now in the supine position, the laparoscopy may proceed. As with culdoscopy, the technique cannot be learned from description but must be carefully taught in the operating room. In this procedure, about 3 L. of suitable gas are first instilled into the abdominal cavity to distend it; then the laparoscope is thrust through the enlarged opening at the lower margin of the umbilicus.

(e) Numerous complications of laparoscopy have been documented; they tend to be proportional to the experience of the operator. These include minor problems such as hematoma of the abdominal wall and subcutaneous emphysema (especially in obese patients), or—more serious—the perforation of a viscus or vessel. Anesthetic complications may also occur; hence the need for an experienced anesthetist.

d. *Comparison of Culdoscopy and Laparoscopy*

(1) Choice is usually the operator's preference, according to his or her own experience.

(2) Visibility is generally *much better at laparoscopy,* especially the view of the cul-de-sac.

(3) The position for laparoscopy is more convenient if laparotomy is to be performed immediately after the procedure.

(4) Culdoscopy has the significant advantage of no risk from general anesthesia, because none is employed.

(5) The puncture site for culdoscopy (cul-de-sac) is far less risky than the abdominal puncture site for laparoscopy.

(6) In over 20,000 culdoscopic examinations reported over the past 20 years in the world literature, there have been no deaths. Complications are rare.

e. *Hysteroscopy.* Endoscopic visualization of the uterine cavity has attracted greatly renewed interest in recent years.

(1) Although hysteroscopy can often be done in an office setting under local anesthesia, it is more frequently *combined with laparoscopy.*

(2) Indications include detection (or confirmation) of uterine polyps, submucous myomas, synechiae, or septal defects.

(3) Hysteroscopes have a diameter of 6 to 8 mm. with optional channels for operative work. For uterine distension, various fluids have been employed (5-per-cent glucose in water, normal saline, or dextran), or CO_2 gas at no more than 100 ml. per minute at a maximum pressure of 200 mm. Hg. By operating during the proliferative phase of the cycle one avoids the obscuring of the tubal ostia by endometrial growth.

(4) Several kinds of uterine pathology have been successfully managed under hysteroscopic control. These include polyps, synechiae, certain cases of uterine septum in secondary infertility, and even cases of small submucous fibroids.

(5) The procedure is not without complications, especially for the inexperienced operator. These include cervical lacerations, uterine perforation, exacerbation of unsuspected pelvic inflammatory disease, and the potential risk of pulmonary embolism from the medium.

Endometrial Biopsy

1. Purposes

a. Provision of evidence of the occurrence of ovulation

b. Evaluation of the adequacy of endometrial maturation ("dating") in preparation for ovum implantation

c. Ruling-out of unsuspected endometrial pathology, such as chronic endometritis or tuberculosis

2. Contraindications

a. Acute pelvic inflammatory disease

b. Possible pregnancy

3. Procedure

a. The ideal time for an endometrial biopsy is about 7 to 10 days after presumptive ovulation (days 21 to 24). Large surveys have shown that the risk of interrupting a pregnancy is extremely small. If either the doctor or the patient is concerned about this, the patient can abstain from coitus or use contraception during the cycle leading up to the biopsy. Another way to reduce anxiety is to obtain a serum quantitative beta subunit 24 to 36 hours prior to the procedure. Some doctors defer the procedure until there is a premenstrual basal temperature drop or even until the first day of the period, but the tissue obtained that late will be less informative.

b. When there is a suspected inadequate luteal phase (poorly sustained rise or short, 8- to 10-day rise), it is best to take the biopsy 7 to 8 days after ovulation for more precise "dating." If the histological dating differs from the chronological by more than 2 days (as determined by the onset of the *oncoming* period), a luteal phase defect is suggested. A serum progesterone measurement taken at the same time is also helpful.

c. An endometrial biopsy can be an extremely uncomfortable procedure, particularly in the nulligravida. The use of an extra-thin, malleable curette, which some instrument companies make, is appreciated by the patient.

Evaluation of Cervical Mucus

Certain physical and chemical characteristics of the cervical mucus change according to the phase of the menstrual cycle, reflecting the effects of estrogen and progesterone. The endocervical glands are stimulated by estrogen and inhibited by progesterone. During ovulation, the condition of the cervical mucus becomes most favorable for sperm penetration. Under estrogenic influence the mucus changes from scant, viscous, and acidic to profuse, watery, and alkaline.

1. Parameters for the Evaluation of Cervical Mucus

a. *Spinnbarkeit, or Stretchability.* At ovulation the maximum length may be 10 to 15 cm.

b. *Fern Phenomenon.* Under estrogenic influence, cervical mucus forms a fern-like pattern when allowed to dry on a slide. After ovulation, under the influence of progesterone, the fern pattern gradually disappears.

c. *Leukocytes.* There are very few (0 to 4 per high power field) at ovulation time. Greater numbers at midcycle suggest endocervicitis, though they may be present in greater quantity normally at other times of the cycle.

d. *pH.* Alkalinity is at a maximum at the time of ovulation.

2. Postcoital Test (Sims-Huhner test)

a. *Purpose.* The test provides information regarding the quality and quantity of cervical mucus, the degree and quality of sperm penetration into the cervical canal, and (indirectly) coital technique.

b. *Timing of the Test*

(1) The test should be done at ovulation time, but because this is not precisely known, especially in advance, it is best performed on alternate days during a typical ovulatory phase (e.g., days 10, 12, 14). Once the basal temperature has risen for 2 days or more, ovulation is presumed to have occurred, and there is no point in repeating the test. (The last drop before the sustained rise marks the ideal time.)

(2) The question of the optimal time interval between coitus and examination is unsettled, probably because surveys using widely varying intervals have reported comparable results. It would seem reasonable to suggest that the test be done within 12 hours after coitus, preferably within 6 hours. The longer interval would accommodate couples who are not "morning" people as far as intercourse is concerned, so that they may have coitus the night before.

(3) When there is a moot question as to whether the semen is being properly deposited in the vagina, the husband's semen may be artificially placed against the cervix, and the patient asked to return in several hours for the same test.

c. *Instructions to the Patient*

(1) Intercourse under normal conditions within 12 hours preceding the office visit

(2) No precoital lubricants

(3) No postcoital douching

d. *Procedure*

(1) The speculum must be dry.

(2) Samples aspirated from the posterior vaginal fornix, the external cervical os, mid cervical canal, and the area of the internal os should be separated. The external cervix is wiped before the last two samples are taken.

(3) The observer should note the volume of mucus as well as its color, *spinnbarkeit*, and viscosity. A portion is allowed to dry for evaluation of ferning. The remaining samples are separately examined under high dry magnification for spermatozoa and cellular content.

d. *Evaluation*

(1) It must be stressed that results are interpreted in light of (1) quality of cervical mucus, (2) sperm quality, and (3) relation to time of ovulation. If it turns out that the same test done 2 to 4 days later is closer to ovulation, then the initial findings are discarded in favor of those closest to midcycle. Thus interpretation may be retrospective.

(2) There is no unanimity of opinion regarding the minimum qualifications of a good postcoital test. However, it would be reasonable to say that if there are 5 to 20 actively motile sperm per high power field in the low- and midcanal samples (there may be fewer at the internal os level), then the result is favorable.

(3) It should be emphasized that a single observation, even at midcycle, is not necessarily conclusive; several cycles should be similarly studied to see if this is a consistent pattern (when the results are poor). On the other hand, if the initial results are excellent, there is no point in repeating the test at a more favorable time of the cycle, because that result would only be expected to be even better.

(4) The vaginal-pool sample should show only dead sperm, because vaginal secretions are hostile to sperm motility. The only cause to view this sample would be a complete absence of sperm in the endocervical sample. This would suggest extreme oligospermia (or azoospermia) or faulty coital technique.

(5) A consistently fair-to-poor result in cervical samples may be caused by (*1*) poor sperm quality (a semen analysis would clarify this), (*2*) poor quality of cervical mucus ("hostile mucus"), (*3*) poor timing of the test in relation to ovulation, (*4*) immunological factors, or (5) a combination of these. Poor quality of cervical mucus may be caused by (*1*) endocervicitis, or (*2*) poor estrogen production.

MANAGEMENT OF THE MALE

General Measures

1. Adequate sleep, rest, diet, and exercise

2. Moderation in use of alcohol and tobacco

3. Relief of emotional tension

4. Avoidance of regimented coitus, as long as spontaneous exposures average two to three times a week

5. Weight reduction in obesity

6. Treatment of any chronic illness or metabolic disorder

7. Avoidance of excessive or prolonged heat to scrotum

8. A patient with azoospermia, significant oligospermia, or poor motility should have a urologic consultation. The following tests are indicated: urinary gonadotropins assay, 17-ketosteroids, thyroid function, and testicular biopsy in certain cases. Testicular failure is suggested by high urinary gonadotropins and low 17-ketosteroids.

9. Varicocele should be excluded. If varicocele is found in a patient whose specimens are subnormal, varicocelectomy may be helpful in improving motility and reducing immature and tapering sperm forms. Some studies report a 75-per-cent improvement rate and a pregnancy rate of 45 per cent. Careful selection of patients is stressed in these reports.

10. A patient with abnormal external genitals or poorly developed secondary sex characteristics warrants chromosomal study to rule out Klinefelter's syndrome (seminiferous tubule dysgenesis). Eunuchoidism, gynecomastia, and elevated urinary gonadotropins are variable findings with this syndrome. The cardinal finding is the characteristic histology, showing hyalinization of the seminiferous tubules and Leydig-cell clumping.

Treatment of Azoospermia

1. A patient with azoospermia but with normal-appearing testes and normal spermatogenesis on testicular biopsy may have an obstruction of the distal epididymis or proximal vas deferens. Vasoepididymostomy may be considered.

2. Artificial insemination with donor semen (therapeutic donor insemination) may warrant consideration.

Treatment of Oligospermia

1. With *demonstrable* thyroid deficiency, the use of triiodothyronine (Cytomel) is justified. Too often thyroid therapy is given on a purely empirical basis, without evident benefit.

2. The use of clomiphene citrate (Clomid) for oligospermia has been generally disappointing, with some patients showing an early increase in sperm count followed by a decline during continuation of the treatment. Actually, the use of clomiphene citrate in the oligospermic male must at present be considered experimental, as it has not yet been approved by the FDA. There are ongoing studies to determine if clomiphene citrate may be of some value in men with diminished FSH, 17-ketosteroid, or testosterone secretions.

3. Similarly disappointing results have been found after the experimental use of human menopausal gonadotropin (Pergonal).

4. Injections of human chorionic gonadotropin (HCG) have been reported, in some cases, to increase sperm motility. The usual dosage is 2,500 to 3,000 I.U. given I.M. every 5 days. Some doctors have employed HCG empirically in patients with idiopathic oligospermia and after varicocelectomy in patients who had preoperative counts below 10 million per ml. Some improvement in semen quality was noted about 3 months after completion of a series of injections of 4,000 I.U., twice weekly for 10 weeks. A more constant result was an increase of libido.

5. The so-called testosterone-rebound phenomenon has had a long and generally disappointing history; it fell into disuse because some oligospermic men became permanently azoospermic as a result of therapy. In addition, methyltestosterone was shown to be hepatotoxic. However, another oral androgen, fluoxymesterone (Halotestin) has more recently been tried in doses of 10 mg., twice daily for 6 weeks, with reported improvement in sperm motility for at least a limited time after cessation of therapy. The sperm count should nevertheless be watched carefully, because some patients may develop spermatogenic depression even at this dosage level.

6. Cortisone therapy has proved generally unsuccessful for poor sperm quality and should probably be reserved for suppression of the adrenal cortex in those patients with oligospermia secondary to the adrenogenital syndrome. (The use of high-dosage cortisone for certain immunological problems is mentioned on p. 32.)

7. Arginine, an amino acid, has received some attention but has been a generally ineffective approach for the treatment of poor semen quality.

8. The *split-ejaculate technique for homologous artificial insemination (A.I.H.)* is based on the fact that, in 90 per cent of males, the first portion of the ejaculate contains at least 75 per cent of all the sperm and also those of best quality. (In 5 per cent of males there is no difference between the first portion and the remainder of the ejaculation, and in another 5 per cent the findings are reversed.) Insemination of the superior portion of the husband's ejaculate into the cervix of the wife during her most fertile day or days may be of value in cases of oligospermia or hypomotility, or in couples with repeatedly poor postcoital tests who do not respond to the usual measures. This method is the quickest way of obtaining instant improvement in sperm quality and utilizing it to advantage.

9. In recent years the use of processed ("washed") sperm, from which seminal irritants have been removed, has permitted insemination directly into the uterine cavity. Although this approach is more refined than intracervical insemination, the success rate has not been notably high where oligospermia has been the main problem.

10. The technique of freezing and storing subnormal sperm, then combining several samples for insemination, has proved to be unrewarding.

11. Another option if sperm are subnormal is in-vitro fertilization, wherein only a relatively small number of sperm are needed for fertilization outside the body prior to embryo transfer.

MANAGEMENT OF THE FEMALE

Ovarian Factor

Major factors to be considered include ovulation defects, endometriosis, periovarian adhesions, and an inadequate luteal phase.

1. Ovulation Defects

a. General defects include: nutritional deficiencies, metabolic disorders (hypopituitarism, hypothyroidism, hyperthyroidism, diabetes mellitus, adrenogenital syndrome, Cushing's disease), chronic illness, neurogenic disorders, psychogenic disorders, and specific ovarian disorders (polycystic ovarian disease, ovarian dysgenesis, ovarian tumors).

b. Because failure of ovulation (anovulation), faulty ovulation, or infrequent ovulation (oligo-ovulation) can be the result of deficiencies in other endocrine organs, the pituitary, thyroid, and adrenal glands must be investigated. Psychosomatic factors should also be considered, particularly in women who have had a normal menstrual history prior to deciding to conceive.

c. Pituitary, thyroid, and adrenal dysfunctions are treated as indicated (see Chap. 27).

d. Polycystic or sclerocystic ovaries (Stein-Leventhal syndrome) should be treated with clomiphene citrate (Clomid), the nonhormonal drug of choice, starting with 5 mg. daily for 5 days, from the fifth day of the cycle. It may be necessary to increase the dosage gradually to 200 mg. daily, but in all instances there should be careful monitoring by pelvic examination to make sure that overstimulation (cystic enlargement) of the ovaries does not occur. Ovulation is presumed to have occurred if the basal temperature graph becomes normally biphasic, if the endometrial biopsy shows secretory endometrium, or if there is significant plasma progesterone. (It is definitely confirmed if the patient becomes pregnant). If clomiphene fails in such cases after several months of trial, and if there is a specific preference not to initiate human menopausal gonadotropin (HMG) therapy, then wedge resection of the ovaries—preceded by endoscopy to confirm the diagnosis of sclerocystic ovaries—may be considered.

e. Patients with demonstrable pituitary-gonadotropic (FSH) failure, normal ovaries, and no other causes for infertility may be candidates for Pergonal (HMG) in combination with HCG. With dosages and frequent monitoring carefully worked out on an individualized basis, a high percentage of patients will ovulate with such therapy. However, the medication is expensive, the incidence of multiple births can be high, and potential side effects include cystic enlargement of the ovaries including rupture, ascites, and hydrothorax. Such side effects can be minimized by careful patient selection, preliminary evaluation of ovarian (hormonal) function, utilization of minimal effective doses, and frequent examination of the patient with ultrasound and measurement of serum estradiol levels.

2. Endometriosis

a. The ovary is the most common site of external endometriosis.

b. Endometriosis is associated with infertility in 30 to 40 per cent of patients even when lesions are minimal with no gross anatomic changes, for reasons that remain obscure.

c. The more obvious cases of infertility associated with endometriosis are caused by interference with tubo-ovarian motility and disturbance in ovum pickup, related to demonstrable adhesions around the tubes and ovaries.

d. Endometriosis should be considered in all patients who have been unable to conceive despite a "normal" infertility investigation. The diagnosis is confirmed by direct visual endoscopic examination.

e. The diagnosis of endometriosis is suggested in patients with menstrual irregularities, progressive dysmenorrhea, dyspareunia, fixed retroverted uterus, and nodularity of the uterosacral ligaments. However, a patient may also have a normal menstrual history and pelvic findings, yet have fairly extensive endometriosis. As stated above, endoscopy is the only way to establish the diagnosis with certainty.

f. The treatment of endometriosis associated with infertility is varied and depends upon the patient's age, the extent of the disease process, and the presence and degree of other symptoms. The use of progestational steroids (e.g., an oral contraceptive in sufficient daily dosage to prevent menstruation and breakthrough bleeding) to induce pseudopregnancy provides good symptomatic relief and has a salutary effect upon the disease process. More commonly, instead of steroids, one may employ a mildly androgenic preparation, danazol (Danocrine), daily in the same manner to induce pseudomenopause. Since this drug, unlike the steroids, is neither estrogenic nor progestational, it has not been implicated in thromboembolic complications. Minor side effects are common, however, and the drug is expensive. Whichever drug is used, it requires many months to obtain a beneficial effect, during which time the patient, of course, remains infertile. More often, endoscopy will demonstrate tubal or peritubal problems associated with the disorder; if all other factors are normal, laparotomy is useful not only to correct the tubal abnormalities but to excise any major implants. Some doctors employ progestational steriods or danazol prior to such contemplated surgery, others afterward, and still others rely on surgery alone if the endometriosis is not too extensive (though its effects on the tubes may be considerable.) Each patient, therefore, must be considered individually.

g. Recent work suggests that Gn-RH (a gonadotropin-releasing hormone agonist) may provide an alternative treatment for endometriosis by its inhibiting effect on the pituitary-ovarian axis, which suppresses endogenous stimuli to endometriotic tissue.

3. Peri-ovarian Adhesions

a. These may result from pelvic inflammatory disease, appendicitis, endometriosis, previous surgery, or the process of monthly rupture of the ovarian follicle.

b. Peri-ovarian adhesions diminish fertility either by blocking the extrusion of the ovum or by interfering with the pickup of the ovum by the tube.

c. Such adhesions often involve the tube, uterus, lateral pelvic wall, or intestine.

d. The diagnosis is confirmed by endoscopy.

e. Treatment consists of:

(1) Lysis of adhesions

(2) Suspension of the uterus, if it is retroverted, brings the tubes and ovaries forward and may be of value in preventing new adhesions.

(3) Corticosteroids such as dexamethasone are sometimes used during the operation and postoperatively, in the hope that future adhesions will be minimized.

4. Inadequate Luteal Phase

a. The condition usually results from inadequate progesterone production by the corpus luteum and has been associated with both infertility and early miscarriage.

b. In turn, it is believed to give insufficient hormonal support to the endometrium, which then cannot properly support nidation.

c. The diagnosis is suspected from studies of the basal temperature graph (short, 8- to 10-day luteal phase), endometrial biopsy (off phase, by dating), blood progesterone level (relatively low), and cervical mucus changes, plus vaginal smears, to determine whether estrogen stimulation is inadequate.

d. *Treatment* of inadequate luteal phase is often difficult but essentially depends upon the specific hormone deficiency involved.

(1) General constitutional measures (e.g., for nutritional deficiencies, emotional tension, or metabolic disease) should not be overlooked.

(2) Clomiphene citrate is helpful in creating a better ovulatory cycle, and hence a better luteal response. Dosage usually starts at 50 mg. daily for 5 days from the fifth day of the cycle, and may be increased depending upon the response.

(3) Low-dosage estrogen (e.g., estrone sulfate 0.3 mg. or ethinyl estradiol 0.02 mg.) given from day 5 until midcycle is ordinarily not enough to interfere with ovulation, but is aimed at maintaining a normal follicular-phase endometrium in preparation for the oncoming progestational stimulation by the corpus luteum.

(4) For progesterone deficiency, the safest treatment is to make up pure progesterone as 25-mg. vaginal suppositories (in glycol or other suitable base), to be inserted twice daily during the second half of the cycle and continued if the menstrual period is missed.

(5) HCG has also been used to stimulate endogenous progestrone secretion. A dosage of 3,000 to 5,000 I.U. every third day from the twelfth (i.e., pre-ovulatory) day to the twenty-fourth day, a total of five injections, has been employed.

Tubal Factor

1. Functions of the Fallopian Tubes

a. Permit ascent of spermatozoa to the site of fertilization

b. Pick up the ovum and transport it to the site of fertilization

c. Nurture the zygote as it is transformed into a blastocyst, during transport to the uterine cavity

2. Etiology of Abnormal Function of the Tubes

a. Alteration in ovum pickup (e.g., hydrosalpinx, fimbrial occlusion or phimosis, peritubal adhesions)

b. Damaged cilia secondary to endosalpingitis, interfering with normal ovum transport

c. Midportion or cornual occlusion of tubes secondary to inflammation or a sterilization procedure

d. Restriction of normal tubal motility (e.g., peritubal adhesions secondary to pelvic inflammatory disease, endometriosis, appendicitis, or previous pelvic surgery)

3. Classification of Tubal Pathology

a. *Peritubal Adhesions.* Related perisalpingitis or peritonitis

b. *Fimbrial End Obstruction.* The result of endosalpingitis or perisalpingitis

c. *Middle-Third Obstruction.* Generally the result of tubal sterilization

d. *Cornual Obstruction.* This may result from salpingitis isthmica nodosa, endosalpingitis, adenomyosis, or pressure from myomata.

4. Classification of Operative Techniques

a. *Fimbriolysis.* Separation of agglutinated fimbria that are otherwise grossly fairly normal

b. *Salpingolysis.* Lysis of peritubal adhesions

c. *Salpingostomy.* The creation of a new ostium or opening

d. *Resection and anastomosis* of midtubal obstruction

e. *Tubal implantation* for cornual obstruction

5. Tubal Plastic Sugery

a. Assuming that the rest of the diagnostic infertility workup is normal, the prognosis for conception and live birth after tubal sugery will depend on the type and the extent of pathology, the type of surgery performed, the skill of the surgeon, and postoperative care.

b. The couple should be thoroughly informed about the statistical possibilities of conception following tuboplasties. The only criterion for success is term live birth. Because tuboplasty is a major procedure for damaged tubes, the true success rate is not notably high—30 to 40 per cent term live births is considered acceptable, and, with some tubal desease, pregnancy rates are considerably lower. When only periadnexal adhesions are present, the rate may be as high as 60 per cent within 3 years of sugery. In general, the results with distal tubal disease are not as good because there is usually more tubal destruction; in proximal disease, the rest of the tube is often basically normal. When both proximal and distal occlusions are present in both tubes, the prognosis is so poor that tubal surgery should probably not be considered. Also, tubal surgery is generally not considered in women beyond the age of 40, because of the lessened fertility owing to age alone. The possibility of an ectopic pregnancy should also be mentioned.

c. In genaral, pregnancy rates are roughly one-half the patency rates in long-term follow-up.

d. Statistically, the peak success rate occurs relatively late—between 12 and 24 months after surgery. The reason for this long lapse is not precisely known, but it is believed to represent the long healing time and recanalization that apparently are needed.

6. Surgical Technique

a. For simple dilatation and phimosis, a pediatric (no. 8) Foley catheter, or the thinner Fogarty catheter, may often be used to advantage by delicately swelling and deflating the inner "bolus" in order to exert uniform atraumatic pressure in all directions.

b. In those instances where the agglutinated fimbriated folds require it, a better ostium may be created by the eversion of the tips of several folds to the serosal surface of the tube with very thin (e.g., 6–8 vicryl) sutures.

c. The merits of different types of prosthesis have been debated for years. Unfortunately, comparison of results has been difficult or impossible because of the variability in etiology and extent of tubal damage, and because of the different techniques used. Many surgeons use no prostheses at all for distal disease, while others use polyethylene, Silastic, or Teflon in various shapes.

d. Microsurgery (surgery with the use of magnification) has been recognized as beneficial for more precise dissection and reduction of trauma. Most operators prefer loupes of 4 to 8 power. Some use a microscope, which increases operative time but may be of aid in special instances such as end-to-end anastomosis of tubes that have been previously ligated. (Tubes that have been sterilized by coagulation are often too damaged for salvage.) The use of a microscope requires elaborate, expensive apparatus and considerable experience.

e. The use of a laser may be helpful to those who are comfortable with this procedure. Whether it enhances accuracy and reduces postoperative adhesions (compared to magnification techniques) in terms of "success" rates is difficult to say, since such statistics are always influenced by patient selection, other fertility factors, and the skill of the operator.

7. Postoperative Care

a. Because even a slight infection would probably negate the benefits of surgery, it seems advisable to use prophylactic broad-spectrum antibiotics just before surgery and for 1 to 3 days postoperatively.

b. There is no unanimity of opinion regarding the parenteral use of dexamethasone (Decadron), ostensibly to minimize postoperative adhesions. Some doctors use it intraperitoneally at the conclusion of surgery, while others give it (or oral prednisone) for several days postoperatively.

c. Some doctors use hydrotubation during the proliferative phase of the cycle—e.g., using a combination of hydrocortisone and a suitable antibiotic. Others prefer to leave the tubes alone postoperatively. As stated, it is difficult to assess (not to mention compare) the results obtained by different investigators, because of the general lack of meaningful classification of procedures relative to the precise pathology present.

d. Whether or not postoperative hydrotubations are done, it is common to perform a hysterosalpingogram about 3 to 6 months after surgery if pregnancy has not intervened.

8. In-Vitro Fertilization. Since the pioneering work of Steptoe and Edwards in 1978, the process of in-vitro fertilization and embryo transfer has been gradually refined; it is currently available in most major medical centers. Indications have broadened to include not only damaged tubes but also oligospermia, hostile cervical mucus, unsuccessfully treated endometriosis, immunological problems, and a broad category of "unexplained" infertility.

(a) The complex procedure involves induction of multiple ova, with ovulatory stimulants such as HMG and clomiphene citrate, and monitoring by ultrasonography and serum estradiol levels.

(b) When appropriate follicular size and estradiol levels are reached, HCG is given to trigger ovulation.

(c) Oocyte retrieval is performed about 36 hours after HCG administration, just before anticipated ovulation. The retrieval used to be by laparoscopy, but more recently there is a definite preference to avoid the abdominal procedure and general anesthesia, instead retrieving oocytes transvaginally under ultrasonographic guidance.

(d) Retrieved oocytes are immediately exposed to sperm in an adjoining laboratory. If fertilization and cleavage occur, the embryos are transferred transcervically into the patient's uterus, usually about 48 to 72 hours after insemination.

(e) Although the "pregnancy" rate may be as high as 30 to 40 per cent per cycle, the actual success rate (live births) is disappointingly lower, perhaps 10 to 15 per cent in most experienced centers, the rates being higher with successive attempts. It is hoped that this rate will rise further as more experience is gained.

9. Gamete Intrafallopian Transfer. This relatively new procedure requires at least one normal tube. Ova are aspirated from stimulated follicles and, together with sperm previously collected from the male, are deposited in the ampullary segment of the tube. In this "GIFT" procedure, as many as four ova can be replaced in each patient, provided that both tubes are patent (i.e., two ova in each tube).

Uterine Factor (Corpus)

1. Leiomyomata Uteri

a. Most uterine fibroids do not prevent conception.

b. Although the spontaneous miscarriage rate is higher in women with myomata, it is difficult to prove a cause-and-effect relationship.

c. Submucous fibroids, diagnosed by hysterography or hysteroscopy, may interfere with implantation or may cause cornual occlusion.

d. If a thorough investigation reveals no other cause for the infertility, and if the myomata are of sufficient size and appropriately located (submucous or cornual), myomectomy may be considered.

e. Postoperatively, contraception is advisable for at least 3 months to allow for complete healing.

f. If the endometrial cavity has been entered during the operative procedure, subsequent pregnancy is likely to be delivered by elective cesarean section.

2. Retroversion

a. A movable retroversion is common, and does not have a causative role per se in infertility.

b. A fixed retroversion is often associated with infertility, not from the position of the uterus but from the underlying cause of the fixation (e.g., pelvic inflammatory disease or endometriosis).

c. A fixed retroversion noted at laparotomy for pathology of the corpus, tubes, or ovaries in an infertile patient may be treated by uterine suspension. This minimizes further peri-adnexal adhesions and permits the uterus to rise out of the pelvis should pregnancy occur.

3. Anomalies

a. Uterine anomalies are related to varying degrees of failure of fusion of the müllerian ducts.

b. The three most common anomalies are uterus didelphys, bicornuate uterus, and septate uterus (not to be confused with a slight arcuate tendency, which is common).

c. It is the septate type that is most often associated with secondary infertility. Primary infertility is rarely associated with uterine anomalies.

d. Even if there is a history of repeated miscarriages or premature births with a uterine anomaly present, it is still important to rule out metabolic, endocrine, and genetic causes before attempting surgical reconstruction.

e. One generally makes the diagnosis on hysterography, using both lateral and oblique views while pulling down on the cervix.

f. As stated, it is the septate uterus that is usually associated with secondary infertility. With this anomaly, bimanual examination reveals one uterus, while the radiograph shows two cavities.

g. The three procedures used for septate uterus are wedge excision of the septum, a vertical incision without removal of the septum, and the classic Strassmann operation, which fuses the two halves.

h. A high percentage of patients who undergo a unification operation carry subsequent pregnancies to term.

4. Traumatic Intrauterine Synechiae (Asherman Syndrome)

a. A significant number of these cases are probably undiagnosed.

b. Synechiae may occur in the corpus alone, in the cervix, or in both.

c. They are usually related to postpartum or postabortal curettage.

d. *Symptoms.* Amenorrhea or hypomenorrhea, dysmenorrhea, infertility, or habitual abortion

e. *Diagnosis.* By hysterography, probing the cervix or corpus, or by hysteroscopy (direct visualization).

f. *Treatment*

(1) *Cervical or isthmic synechiae* sometimes respond to gentle, gradual dilatation of the cervix.

(2) *Uterine (corpus) synechiae* can be gently lysed with thin sounds, preferably under hysteroscopic visualization during the proliferative phase.

(3) *Postoperative Treatment.* Antibiotics and an intrauterine device such as a tipless, inflated Foley catheter, which projects slightly into the vagina, are advisable for 1 or 2 weeks. Postoperative administration of estrogen for 2 or 3 cycles will help to proliferate the endometrium. The use of progesterone cyclically will help shed the endometrium at appropriate intervals.

(4) *Prognosis.* Most reported series give a generally unfavorable prognosis regarding term pregnancy. Repeated surgery often is required. The prognosis is particularly poor when intrauterine synechiae are associated with amenorrhea from destruction of the endometrium.

5. Endometrial Polyps, Hyperplasia. The diagnosis of endometrial polyps can be made on hysterography or hysteroscopy. Treatment is by uterine curettage, particularly with the use of polyp forceps, or by direct removal during hysteroscopy. Hyperplasia is generally the result of unopposed estrogen stimulation, as with anovulation, and treatment is directed to correction of the cause.

Cervical Factor

The problems to be considered are (1) failure in sperm deposition or ascent, (2) poor or hostile cervical mucus, and (3) local cervical pathology.

1. Improvement in Coital Techniques. In history taking, inquiry should be made regarding coital techniques. Surprisingly many women, despite their wish to conceive, get back on their feet immediately after intercourse and even douche. While this may not totally prevent conception, it is at least a deterrent that the couple may be unaware of. Some couples use large amounts of lubricating jelly, which can act as a sperm barrier.

2. Poor or hostile cervical mucus may be caused by:

a. Endocervicitis from inflammation, with destruction of endocervical glands and resultant alteration in mucus quality.

b. Inadequate estrogenic stimulation of the cervical glands. This may also be combined with endocervicitis.

c. Immunological problems, such as reaction of sperm antigen with antibody in the cervical mucus or in the serum

3. Treatment of These Conditions

a. Endocervicitis may be treated with antibiotics, electrocautery (very gentle), or cryosurgery. When the condition is chronic and does not respond well to therapeutic measures, the area may be "bypassed" by artificial insemination, with the male's semen, to the level of the internal os (A.I.H.), or by intrauterine insemination with processed ("washed") sperm.

b. Hypoestrinism (inadequate estrogenic stimulation) can often be remedied by the administration of small doses of estrogen (e.g., estrone sulfate 0.3 mg., or ethinyl estradiol 0.02 mg.) daily from about day 5 until midcycle. This dose generally does not interfere with ovulation. Another method which may help cervical mucus is the administration of a cough expectorant (guaifenesin) in palatable capsule form (200 mg t.i.d.) from day 5 of the cycle until ovulation is over. This may be given instead of, or in addition to, estrogen. If endocervicitis is also present, appropriate antibiotic therapy is given as well. There is often a marked improvement in the postcoital test after a few cycles of such measures.

c. Although many studies and reports have appeared over more than two decades, the basic question of how circulating antibodies in the female inhibit or prevent conception remains unanswered. Because of inconclusive results and different interpretations, the role of immunology in infertility remains controversial. The common test employed is the sperm agglutination test, which relates the husband's sperm against the wife's serum. If such a test is strongly positive (in the absence of other causes for infertility), the recommended treatment is the use of condoms for about 6 months, to prevent sperm contact. This also requires avoidance of semen exposure through oral-genital or anal contact. When repeat agglutinating antibody reaction disappears or becomes minimal, the couple is permitted unprotected intercourse around the time of ovulation, to minimize overall exposure. Because pregnancies have been reported following such a regime, it is worth trying.

d. Sperm-immobilizing antibodies are another vexing problem. High dosages of cortisone have been recommended by some doctors as a counter to this tendency.

e. In recent years, newer therapeutic measures have been advocated for infertility thought to be due to immunological factors. These include intrauterine insemination with processed sperm and in-vitro fertilization. It is apparent that there are still many unanswered questions about the role of immunology; ongoing research in the field may help to clarify this issue.

4. Local Cervical Pathology

a. *Endocervical polyps* should be twisted off or excised, and their bases lightly cauterized to minimize regrowth. Sometimes a prolapsed endometrial polyp (or even a submucous myoma) is mistaken for an endocervical polyp. Thus, when the polyp is large, with a broad base whose extent cannot be easily determined at office examination, excision is best performed in the hospital. However, the common variety of small endocervical polyp is easily removed in the office and is almost invariably benign.

b. *Cervical stenosis,* whether congenital (rare) or after overly vigorous cauterizations or frequent cervical infections, is suspected when it is not possible to pass a small probe through the cervix (e.g., in attempting to do an endometrial biopsy). Treatment is by gentle, careful sounding, beginning with very thin (2-mm.) graduated sounds. Paracervical infiltration with 1-per-cent lidocaine is often helpful to facilitate dilatation as well as reduce discomfort. One should be mindful that with an acute flexion of the uterus, the internal os may normally be difficult to bypass unless there is strong traction on the tenaculum to straighten the uterus. In rare instances, when the stenosis does not respond to any of the above procedures or maneuvers, dilatation may need to be done under anesthesia in the operating room.

c. *Cervical erosions* (often eversions) are not generally associated with infertility; in any event, the postcoital test will clarify this (a normal postcoital test means that erosions play no role in the infertility). If there is interference, it is more likely the result of the associated endocervicitis. As mentioned above, the treatment of endocervicitis must be most gentle in order not to destroy or scar the canal. Electrocautery, for example, should be done only in stages at intervals of 4 to 8 weeks, with use of a nasal-tip cautery in one or two areas only. This permits normal endocervical tissue to grow in gradually, and does not compromise the whole canal.

d. *Synechiae* and *hypoestrinism* have been discussed on pages previously

e. *Incompetent Cervix.* The typical history is that of repeated, painless abortions during the second trimester, usually preceded by bulging amniotic membranes. Diagnosis in the nonpregnant state is suggested by the ability to pass a #9 Hegar dilator easily through the internal os. Hysterography, which should be performed during the secretory phase (when the cervical canal width is smallest), may also be suggestive if the isthmic width is 8 mm. or more. Whenever incompetent cervix is suspected, weekly bimanual examinations are performed to note if there is any gradual dilatation of the internal cervical os. In some carefully selected cases, once the diagnosis has been made and there have been signs of cervical widening during pregnancy, operative cerclage of the internal os by one of several methods has been successfully employed. In selected cases, many operators prefer to do a cerclage procedure at about 14 weeks rather than await dilatation, which can take place with very little warning.

4 Maternal Adaptations To Pregnancy

David H. Fields

BASIC PRINCIPLES

1. Pregnancy results in great changes in the functions of most of the body's organ systems.

2. These changes are manifested as alterations in normal values of both physical examination and laboratory testing and result in maternal symptoms which would be considered pathologic outside of pregnancy. See Table 4-1.

The normal ranges for many laboratory values are altered by pregnancy. Below is a list of the most commonly used tests, how they are altered by pregnancy, and why, if the reason is known.

3. These changes are caused by

a. Alterations in maternal endocrine function

b. Superimpostion of fetal and placental endocrine function

c. Fetal metabolic and physical demands

So that the physician can properly evaluate maternal complaints and physical and laboratory data during pregnancy, these changes will be reviewed system by system.

GENITAL SYSTEM

The female reproductive tract is the system most intimately involved with pregnancy, and the changes it undergoes are most familiar to physican and patient alike. Therefore, patient complaints referable to these organs are usually ascribed to pregnancy rather than disease, and rightly so.

Uterus

1. The uterus enlarges almost 1,000 times in volume and 30 times in weight, to become a 1-Kg. organ with a capacity of approximately 5 L. It enlarges steadily throughout pregnancy to occupy most of the abdominal cavity. The pressure it exerts is responsible for changes in the gastrointestinal, respiratory, cardiovascular, and urinary systems (see specific areas).

2. The blood flow to the uterus increases 60 times, to approximately 600 ml. per minute (about 10 per cent of cardiac output) at term, and is accommodated by huge increases in the size of the uterine and ovarian vessels.

Vagina and Cervix

1. The vagina and cervix respond to the same increases in blood flow by becoming engorged. This may be seen as a bluish coloration of both organs (Chadwick's sign) and a softening of the cervix (Hegar's sign).

2. Occasionally one sees what appears to be a cervical polyp. This is frequently decidual tissue. Usually this spontaneously resolves by the beginning of the second trimester.

3. Many pregnant women experience a great increase in vaginal discharge, usually secondary to increased cervical secretion caused by high estrogen levels. Unless a

Table 4-1. Laboratory Interpretation

Test	*Alteration in Limits of Normal*	*Mechanism*
Hematology		
Hemoglobin	Decreased to 10 g./100 ml.	Hemodilution secondary to increased blood volume
Hematocrit	Decreased to 30%	
WBC count	Increased up to 15,000/cu. mm.	? Increased corticosteroids
Platelets count	Unchanged	—
Fibrinogen	Increased 50%, up to 300–600 mg./100 ml.	Increased estrogen
PT, APTT	Shortened slightly	?
Fibrin split products	Increased slightly	Hyperdynamic coagulation system
Erythrocyte sedimentation rate	Increased up to 40 mm./hr.	Increased fibrinogen; hemodilution
Blood Chemistry		
Potassium	Decreased to 3 mEq./L.	Respiratory alkalosis
Sodium, Chloride	No change	—
BUN	Decreased to 5–10 mg./100 ml.	Increased GFR; hemodilution
Creatinine	Decreased to 0.3–0.8 mg./100 ml.	Increased GFR; hemodilution
Creatinine clearance	Increased to 150 ml./min.	Increased GFR; hemodilution
Albumin	Decreased to 2.5–3.0 g./100 ml.	?
Fasting blood sugar	Upper limit decreased to 90 mg./100 ml.	Increased insulin
2-hr. postprandial sugar	Upper limit increased to 145 mg./100 ml.	HPL, estrogen
Alkaline phosphatase	Increased up to twice normal	Placental production
T_4	Increased up to 16 g./100 ml.	Estrogen effect causing increased thyroid-binding globulin
T_3 resin uptake	Decreased up to 30%	
Thyroid-binding globulin	Increased up to 30%	
Free thyroxide	No change	—
Free thyroxide index	No change	—

specific pathogen (*Trichomonas vaginalis, Candida albicans, Hemophilus vaginalis*) can be identified, treatment is usually unrewarding and unnecessary.

Ovaries

The corpus luteum usually begins to regress by the eighth week of pregnancy, and the ovaries become largely inactive because placental estrogen and progesterone production inhibits pituitary gonadotropins. Any ovarian cyst which persists into the second trimester should be treated surgically (see Chap. 38, "Benign Tumors of the Ovary").

Any ovarian cyst discovered at cesarean section should be resected and treated appropriately. Frequently the ovaries at term will be covered with a pink frothy material which is decidual reaction secondary to high progesterone levels. This is not pathologic and may cover the tubes as well.

Breasts

1. Both acinar and ductal breast growth are greatly accelerated by steadily increasing production of estrogen, progesterone, and prolactin throughout pregnancy. Because of the rapid growth in size, the overlying skin may develop striae. In addition, the areola (like all pigmented skin in pregnancy) becomes darker, and the nipple itself increases in erectile capacity.

2. In spite of the very high prolactin levels near term, lactation does not occur until after delivery, most likely because placental progesterone prevents prolactin from stimulating the production of lactalbumin.

ENDOCRINE SYSTEM

The hormonal changes associated with pregnancy are attributable to the production of huge amounts of placental estrogen and progesterone, as well as other placental hormones. In addition, the fetus contributes several hormones to the maternal circulation. Finally, the maternal endocrine system responds to the placental and fetal systems by altering its hormonal output.

Placental Hormones

All are thought to be made by the syntrophoblast.

1. Estrogen. Placental estrogen production increases steadily throughout pregnancy, so that at term, maternal estrogen levels are 100 times nonpregnant values. Most of this is estriol converted by placental sulfatase from fetal precursors. Dehydroepiandrosterone sulfate (DHEAS) produced by the fetal adrenal directly from cholesterol is hydroxylated in the fetal liver to 16-hydroxyDHEAS, (16-OH-DHEAS), which is the substrate for placental sulfatase. Smaller amounts of estriol are also produced from maternal 16-OH-DHEAS. Estradiol is similarly, although in much smaller amounts, converted from fetal and maternal DHEAS. There is no interconversion of estriol and estradiol. These high estrogen levels have far-reaching effects (see below).

2. Progesterone. The placenta produces even more progesterone than estrogen, so that near term, it is producing approximately 250 mg. daily. Progesterone's major functions appear to be inhibition of uterine contractions and decreasing sensitivity of the vascular tree, allowing expansion of both these organs. It also has effects on many maternal organ systems (see below).

3. Human Chorionic Gonadotropin (HCG). HCG is detectable in maternal serum several days after conception. Its measurement is the basis of all pregnancy tests. Peaking at about 60 days of gestation, its major function seems to be maintenance of the corpus luteum, although it may also play a role in placental immunology. In healthy pregnancies, HCG levels double every 48 to 72 hours during the first few weeks. This knowledge is useful for distinguishing normally implanted pregnancies from ectopics.

4. Human Placental Lactogen (Placental Growth Hormone, Human Chorionic Somatomammotropin, HPL). HPL also steadily increases throughout pregnancy, so that daily production near term may be as much as 2 g. HPL's major effects are metabolic. It has actions antagonistic to insulin; in effect, it creates a diabetogenic state in the mother, presumably to make more glucose available for fetal use.

Maternal Hormones

1. Pituitary. The gland itself enlarges significantly during pregnancy (rarely enough to cause symptoms), mostly because increased estrogen levels stimulate increased production of prolactin by acidophilic cells.

a. *Gonadotropins.* Follicle-stimulating hormone and luteinizing hormone are maintained at very low levels throughout pregnancy by negative feedback of placental estrogen and progesterone.

b. *Prolactin (see above).* Produced in increasingly large amounts throughout pregnancy, secondary to high estrogen levels, it causes increased breast growth. Lactation is blocked by progesterone until after placental expulsion.

c. *Somatotropic Hormone (Growth Hormone).* Present at very low levels throughout pregnancy, it probably is suppressed by very high levels of its placental counterpart, HPL.

d. *Thyroid-stimulating hormone, adrenocorticotropic hormone and melanocyte-stimulating hormone* are largely unaffected by pregnancy.

2. Thyroid Hormone. The gland hypertrophies significantly during pregnancy. Although production of thyroxine T_4 and tri-iodothyronine T_3 are both increased, unbound levels remain essentially unchanged, the extra hormone being bound by increases in thyroid-binding globulin caused by high levels of estrogen (see Table 4-1). The only thyroid hormone which undergoes significant, real increase is calcitonin, whose function is maintenance of bone calcium.

3. Adrenal Hormones

a. There is a large increase in bound cortisol secondary to an increase in estrogen-mediated levels of transcortin, the cortisol-binding hormone. Free cortisol may be slightly increased.

b. Aldosterone, renin, and angiotensin tend to increase intravascular volume. These are all increased in normal pregnancy, although angiotensin sensitivity (vasospasm) is decreased. Increase is probably secondary to the natriuretic effect of the large amounts of progesterone produced, and to the relative lack of vascular reactivity to angiotensin.

4. Insulin. The beta cells of the islets of Langerhans undergo significant hypertrophy, and insulin levels, both fasting and non-fasting, are increased in pregnancy. There is, however, a cellular resistance to insulin action which results in higher postprandial glucose levels. Many of the hormones of pregnancy, including estrogen, progesterone, and HPL, tend to increase insulin needs.

5. Parathormone. Although there may be some increase in the size of the parathyroid glands, their function seems to be largely unchanged during pregnancy.

CARDIOVASCULAR SYSTEM

Many physiological effects of pregnancy duplicate otherwise pathologic conditions. Basic to the cardiovascular changes are an increase in circulating blood volume by up to 50 per cent and in cardiac output by 30 to 40 percent. In addition, blood pressure typically drops during mid-pregnancy by up to 30 mm. Hg systolic and 15 mm. Hg diastolic. These changes appear to be mediated largely by progesterone. Furthermore, in the second half of pregnancy, the large uterus serves as a functional obstruction to venous return. The following complaints and abnormal physical findings simulating heart disease may occur:

Complaints

1. Dyspnea, either at rest or on exertion, is probably secondary to the hyperventilatory drive of progesterone, or is perhaps secondary to the large uterus raising the diaphragm.

2. Palpitations, etiology unknown

3. Orthopnea, secondary to large intra-abdominal mass

4. Orthostatic hypotension, secondary to vascular pooling

Abnormal Physical Findings

1. Heart rate increase of 10 beats per minute

2. PMI of heart pushed laterally by the growing uterus

3. Apparent increase in cardiothoracic ratio on radiograph to more than one-half

4. Systolic murmurs secondary to increased cardiac output are found in almost all pregnant women.

5. Diastolic and continuous murmurs, while much less common and more often indicative of pathology, may also be physiological.

6. Third-heart sound, etiology unknown

7. Lower extremity edema, secondary to partial venous obstruction by a large uterus

8. Lower extremity and trunk varicosities, secondary to increased venous pressure

9. Supine hypotension, caused by aortocaval compression from the large uterus in the second half of pregnancy

HEMATOLOGIC SYSTEM

1. Intravascular volume increases by 40 to 50 per cent but RBC mass increases by only 30 per cent, so that there is a relative hemodilution. Hemoglobin levels as low as 10 g./100 ml. and hematocrits as low as 30 per cent are physiological.

2. Normal leukocyte counts increase to 12,000 to 15,000/mm^3.

3. Many coagulation factors, including fibrinogen and Factors II, VII, VIII, IX, and X, increase by up to 50 per cent, probably mediated by high levels of estrogen.

4. Conversely, thrombolytic activity also increases.

RESPIRATORY SYSTEM

The major respiratory changes are an increased tidal volume and minute ventilation (secondary to progesterone drive and metabolic demand) in the face of decreased diaphragmatic excursion (secondary to the enlarging uterus). Dyspnea is a very common complaint and may be due to the slight respiratory alkalosis induced by high levels of progesterone.

URINARY SYSTEM

Renal

1. The glomerular filtration rate (GFR) and renal plasma flow (RPF) are increased up to 50 per cent, secondary to increased cardiac output.

2. Mild hydronephrosis and hydroureter occur (right more than left), most likely secondary to decreased muscle tone and to pressure from the enlarging uterus.

Bladder

1. Urinary frequency is primarily due to traction exerted on the bladder by the enlarging uterus but is compounded by increases in urine production secondary to increased GFR.

2. Stress incontinence in the second half of pregnancy is secondary to changes in the urethrovesical angle when the bladder is pulled up to become an intra-abdominal organ.

GASTROINTESTINAL SYSTEM

Most of the gastrointestinal changes are secondary to the effect of an enlarging intra-abdominal mass (uterus) and to high levels of progesterone.

1. Heartburn and Belching. Secondary to changes in position of the stomach and reflux of stomach acid into the lower esophagus, compounded by decreased esophageal sphincter tone secondary to high levels of progesterone. Stomach acid production in fact decreases, and ulcers are less common.

2. Nausea and Vomiting of the First Trimester. Probably secondary to HCG.

3. Ptyalism. The cause of excess salivation is controversial and may be a failure to swallow rather than excess production.

4. Pica. Although abnormal cravings in diet may be signs of nutritional failure, some feel they are more likely cultural aspects of pregnancy.

5. Constipation. Frequent and due to increased progesterone levels resulting in decreased gastrointestinal motility.

6. Hemorrhoids. Varicosities of the anal sphincter are secondary to increased venous pressure in the lower body and are exacerbated by constipation.

SKELETAL SYSTEM

1. The enlarging uterus increases the normal lordosis and probably contributes to frequent backaches.

2. Demineralization of the bones (but not the teeth) may occur in severely calcium-deficient women.

3. The joints, especially of the pelvis, may become more mobile, and slight pubic separation may occur.

SKIN

1. There is an increase in skin pigmentation secondary to high levels of melanocyte-stimulating hormone. This is most notable in the areola and linea nigra but may be seen in the more generalized form known as chloasma.

2. High levels of adrenal steroids combined with rapid stretching of skin over the abdomen, buttocks, and breasts may give rise to striae.

3. Rapid increase in abdominal girth causes diastasis recti, midline separation of the rectus muscles, especially in multiparas.

5 Ectopic Pregnancy

Hugh R. K. Barber

DEFINITION

1. Ectopic pregnancy is pregnancy in which the products of conception are developing outside the uterus. By far the most common site is the fallopian tube.

2. Combined heterotopic pregnancy is characterized by the existence of simultaneous intrauterine and extrauterine pregnancies.

3. Cornual pregnancy is gestation that has developed in a rudimentary horn of the uterus (rudimentary horn pregnancy).

BASIC PRINCIPLES

1. Ectopic pregnancy is the leading cause of maternal death. Chlamydial infections have become epidemic in the United States, and the incidence of ectopic pregnancy has paralleled the rise in chlamydial infections. In view of the role of ectopic pregnancy as a cause of maternal death, there is no substitute for awareness of the possibility of ectopic pregnancy and its protean manifestations.

a. Fatalities and complications relating to ectopic pregnancy result almost uniformly from delay or outright failure in making the diagnosis.

b. Physicians miss 50 per cent of all ectopic pregnancies on first examination, and allow some 25 per cent of patients to progress to frank shock before determining that ectopic pregnancy is present.

c. The average time between the patient's first request for medical intervention and the establishment of a correct diagnosis is often as much as ten days, making a ruptured ectopic pregnancy a more common finding than an unruptured one.

d. As unsettling as these statistics are, their cause is clear: ectopic pregnancy is one of the most difficult diagnoses for physicians to establish.

(1) An ectopic pregnancy clinically may mimic numerous other abdominal or pelvic conditions.

(2) Objective tests do not often provide clear-cut clues, especially in cases where the pregnancy is early or where physicians interpret results incorrectly.

2. Any woman of childbearing age with an acute abdominal pain or with anemia out of proportion to external blood loss should be considered to have an ectopic until it is ruled out.

3. It is better to operate and be proved wrong in the diagnosis of ectopic pregnancy than to lose a patient by not operating.

4. Laparoscopic examination is very helpful in making the diagnosis.

5. A *primary ectopic* is one in which the process continues at the site of original nidation.

6. A *secondary ectopic* is one in which the initial nidation is changed either by rup-

Relative Incidence of Tubal Ectopic Pregnancies	
Ampullar	42 per cent
Isthmic	28 per cent
Interstitial	13 per cent
Fimbrial	7 per cent
Ovarian	less than 1 per cent
Cervical, Peritoneal	Very rare

ture or by continued development at a secondary site in the abdomen.

7. Ectopic pregnancies are manifested in two forms:

a. Acute: intraperitoneal hemorrhage, acute pain, and shock.

b. Chronic: obscure symptomatology, less pain, and absence of shock.

8. Ectopic implantation must be regarded as fortuitous; but there are some recognized predisposing factors:

a. Preceding tumor or pelvic inflammation with residual chronic infection and distortion by adhesions.

b. Migration of an ovum across the pelvic cavity to the fallopian tube on the side opposite to the follicle from which ovulation occurred.

c. Congenital abnormality of the tube, such as hypoplasia, elongation, or diverticula. Diverticula are occasionally seen and, in theory, present a cul-de-sac in which the ovum may lodge.

9. The rising ratio of extrauterine to intrauterine pregnancies is traceable to the changing mores of sexually active young people, the rising incidence of venereal disease, and the effectiveness of modern antibiotic therapy in preventing total tubal occlusion after salpingitis.

10. The widespread use of the IUD has had a remarkable influence on the occurrence of extrauterine pregnancies. There are reports showing that a high percentage of extrauterine pregnancies occurring in IUD users are ovarian ectopics. It seems clear that the IUD affords good protection from intrauterine implanation but has little power to prevent extrauterine pregnancies. Consequently, the ratio of extrauterine to intrauterine pregnancy is destined to increase with renewed use of the IUD. Although the IUD has been largely withdrawn from the market in the United States, there are two American companies still marketing versions of the device. In addition, women are still going out of the country for insertion of IUDs. Therefore one must ask whether an IUD is in place when taking the history.

11. Among patients taking progesterone-only oral contraceptives, studies in this country and abroad show a disproportionately high incidence of ectopic pregnancies (4.1 per cent).

12. Induced abortion appears to be associated with an increased risk of ectopic pregnancy. The mechanism of this complication seems clear: subclinical endometritis associated with induced abortion produces secondary perisalpingitis and peritubal adhesions leading to partial oviduct obstruction. Because there is no decidual membrane in tubal mucosa, and no submucosa, the ovum rapidly burrows through the mucosa and embeds in the muscular wall of the tube, opening maternal blood vessels and causing necrosis and the proliferation of connective tissue.

13. The uterus may enlarge in the first 3 months of an ectopic pregnancy. The uterine decidua grows abundantly; when the ovum or embryo dies, bleeding occurs as the decidua degenerates. Rarely it is expelled entirely as a decidua cast, and it is replaced within a few weeks (perhaps before clinical diagnosis) by normal endometrium.

14. Arias-Stella reaction is an atypical glandular proliferation of the endometrium associated with ectopic pregnancy. A decidual cast containing no villi may be expelled.

15. Signs and symptoms include amenorrhea, pain, and vaginal bleeding, which may present as spotting. The urge to have a bowel movement, followed by fainting while straining at stool ("bathroom sign"), is almost diagnostic of ectopic pregnancy. Unfortunately these signs and symptoms are often obscure. A high degree of suspicion is required in their evaluation.

16. The differential diagnosis must include salpingitis, abortion, appendicitis, torsion of pedicle of ovarian cyst, rupture of corpus luteum or follicular cyst, and lateral displacement of a gravid uterus.

17. The diagnostic measures include a careful history taking and physical examination. Thorough abdominal, pelvic, and rectal examinations must be carried out. Also recommended are immunological and biological pregnancy tests, culdocentesis, colpotomy, culdoscopy, laparoscopy, and ultrasonography.

18. There is no substitute for the carefully elicited history and the physical examination followed by surgical abdominal exploration if suspicion is high. Always take a thorough history and always think of ectopic pregnancy!

19. Bolt's sign—severe tenderness when the examiner lifts the uterine cervix—is associated with ruptured tubal pregnancy.

ETIOLOGY OF ECTOPIC PREGNANCY

Possible Causes

1. Pelvic infection. (Chlamydia, which is now epidemic, causes submucosal scarring of the fallopian tubes. This interferes with peristalsis. Since the infection is often associated with a very mild clinical presentation of infection, it may be overlooked. Furthermore, only recently has an easy and inexpensive way of diagnosing chlamydia been introduced.)

2. Narrowing of the fallopian tubes

3. Transmigration of the fertilized ovum

4. Use of an IUD

PATHOGENESIS

1. Ectopic pregnancies implant by the same mechanism as intrauterine pregnancies—that is, by erosion of tissues. The differences between the features of the ovum's embedding in the uterus and those of its embedding in the fallopian tube are related to the differences between the respective structures of the two organs.

2. In the uterus is a thick decidua in which the fertilized ovum can embed. The bleeding points on blood vessels in the decidua are opened by the trophoblasts; this bleeding is small in amount and is seldom a source of danger to the embryo. In a normal intrauterine pregnancy there is always a layer of decidua between the trophoblasts and the uterine muscle.

3. In the tube there is only a very thin layer of connective tissue separating the epithelium from the muscle, so it is easy for the trophoblast to erode into the muscle of the tube.

4. The fertilized ovum comes to lie in a cavity in the tube wall. This cavity is bounded on the outer side by peritoneum and a thin layer of muscle, and on the inner side by the tubal mucous membrane and an incomplete sheet of muscle.

5. As the trophoblast burrows into the muscle it meets some large vessels. When these are opened, hemorrhage occurs around the embryo and into the surrounding tubal muscle. The blood may burst through the sac surrounding the embryo—either into the lumen of the tube (intratubal rupture) or through the wall of the tube and into the peritoneal cavity (extratubal rupture). Ocassionally, extratubal rupture occurs between the layers of the broad ligament.

6. In cases of tubal pregnancy, the uterus is enlarged; in advanced cases it becomes nearly as large as the normal pregnancy of eight weeks. The endometrium undergoes decidua changes indistinguishable from those that occur in normal pregnancy. An Arias-Stella reaction—an atypical glandu-

RANGE OF HCG CONCENTRATIONS DURING PREGNANCY

Gestational Age	*I.mU. per ml.*
First week	5–50
2 weeks	40–1,000
3 weeks	100–5,000
4 weeks	600–10,000
5–6 Weeks	1,500–100,000
7–8 Weeks	16,000–200,000
2–3 Months	12,000–300,000
Second Trimester	24,000–55,000
Third Trimester	6,000–48,000

LOWER LIMITS OF POSITIVE REFERENCE SENSITIVITY OF VARIOUS PREGNANCY TESTS

Test Type	*Lower Limits of Positive Reference Sensitivity (I.mU. per ml. of HCG)*
Urine slide test	1,500
Urine tube test	750
Serum radioreceptors (RRA)	200
Urine enzymatic immunoassay	50
Serum immunoradiometric assay (IRMA)	25
Serum radioimmunoassay (RIA)	25

lar proliferation of endometrium associated with the ectopic pregnancy—is often found. A decidua cast containing no villi may be expelled. After the death of the embryo the decidua may be thrown off as a cast in the uterus, or may come away in fragments.

INVESTIGATION OF SUSPECTED TUBAL PREGNANCY

When the diagnosis of tubal pregnancy on clinical grounds is in doubt, the following investigations may be performed:

Pregnancy Test

1. The standard immunological pregnancy tests that demonstrate the presence of chorionic gonadotropin (HCG) in the urine are not helpful; the tubal pregnancy may not produce enough HCG to give a positive result.

2. Estimation of the concentration of the beta subunit of HCG in the serum is of greater value, especially when used in conjunction with ultrasonic scanning.

3. If the level of beta HCG is above 6,000 I.mU. per ml., the patient is likely to have a normal intrauterine pregnancy, especially if the level rises rapidly. Absence of beta HCG virtually eliminates pregnancy, but levels below 6,000 I.mU. per ml. are suggestive of tubal pregnancy or a missed abortion.

4. If the beta HCG is above 6,500 I.mU. per ml. and the ultrasound demonstrates a gestational sac or a fetal heartbeat (usually a later finding), the patient can be assumed to have an intrauterine pregnancy. Further ultrasound study is warranted only if symptoms persist. This assumption can be made because ectopic pregnancy coexists with intrauterine pregnancy in only one in 30,000 cases.

5. Conversely, if ultrasound fails to demonstrate a gestational sac, the patient is very likely to have an ectopic pregnancy; immediate laparoscopy is recommended.

Pelvic Ultrasound

1. At 4 to 5 weeks of gestation the decidua reaction of the endometrium in an ectopic pregnancy may be hard to distinguish from an intrauterine sac.

2. In a normal pregnancy there is a double sac sign; this is due to echo-separation of the decidua vera and the decidua capsularis.

3. Ultrasonic demonstration of fetal cardiac activity within the uterus is undeniable evidence of an intrauterine pregnancy, but one can rarely be certain until the eighth week, 1 to 2 weeks after recognition of the gestational sac.

4. If a transonic area surrounded by an echogenic rim is present in the uterus and the beta HCG level is above 6,000 I.mU. per ml., it is very probable that the pregnancy is intrauterine.

5. Lower levels of beta HCG are likely to be associated with tubal pregnancy or missed abortion; in this case the sac in the uterus is formed by the decidua. From the seventh week onward it may be possible to show a gestational sac and fetal cardiac echoes besides the normal uterus, thus giving direct confirmation of ectopic pregnancy.

Laparoscopy

1. If there is any doubt about the diagnosis, laparoscopy should be performed. It allows direct visualization of the tubes and ovaries. The risk of doing a laparoscopy that may only show a normal pelvis is far less than the risk of a missed ectopic pregnancy.

2. With laparoscopy an almost certain diagnosis of tubal pregnancy can be made, but it involves giving the patient an anesthetic, which is undesirable if the pregnancy is intrauterine. Estimation of beta HCG levels and the use of ultrasound, as described above, may help to reveal an intrauterine pregnancy and thus obviate an unnecessary laparoscopy.

3. When the clinical evidence is clear-cut, laparoscopy should not be advised—it will only delay laparotomy. But if the diagnosis is in doubt laparoscopy may be valuable in preventing laparotomy from being performed on patients with certain conditions, such as salpingitis, that should be treated medically.

Culdocentesis

1. This test is useful, in patients presenting acutely with pelvic pain, abnormal bleeding, syncope, or shock, to determine whether there is free blood in the peritoneal cavity.

2. Aspiration of the cul-de-sac should produce some fluid material. The normal contents are slightly yellowish and clear, with a volume of 3 to 5 ml.

3. The presence of non-clotting blood in the syringe is diagnostic of free blood in the peritoneal cavity and supports the diagnosis of ectopic pregnancy.

4. Some physicians believe that culdocentesis has very little to offer in the diagnosis of a patient with suspected ectopic pregnancy.

Endometrial Histology

1. In patients undergoing dilatation and curettage for abnormal uterine bleeding, as in suspected spontaneous abortion, the finding of decidua in the endometrial sample without chorionic villi indicates ectopic pregnancy until proved otherwise.

2. An additional finding in such an endometrium may be the Arias-Stella reaction, an endometrial response to the hormonal stimulation of pregnancy which produces a patchy, hyperactive, often hypersecretory pattern. It may be seen in patients treated with progesterone-like drugs.

48-Hour Observation

If ultrasound fails to demonstrate either a gestational sac or an adnexal mass in the patient with a beta HCG titer below 6,000 I.mU. per ml., the differential diagnosis does not change; it is still between normal intrauterine pregnancy, on the one hand, and abnormal pregnancy—either impending spontaneous abortion or ectopic pregnancy—on the other. For these patients a 48-hour observation is recommended, during which serial beta HCG determinations are used to distinguish normal from abnormal pregnancies. The waiting period has not led to any increased morbidity, and has allowed physicians to further confine the use of laparoscopy to those cases in which the procedure is absolutely necessary to establish the diagnosis.

ECTOPIC TUBAL PREGNANCY

Basic Principles

Ectopic tubal pregnancy is a difficult diagnosis to make. Few patients present with the classic signs and symptoms. It should always be considered as a possibility in a patient with salpingitis, threatened abortion, appendicitis, torsion of ovarian cyst or rupture of corpus luteum or follicular cyst, infertility of 3 or more years, or a history of previous ectopic pregnancy. The tubes should be carefully examined when any cyst is excised from the ovary. The three most common signs and symptoms are: abdominal pain, vaginal bleeding or spotting, and amenorrhea.

Ampullar Pregnancy

1. Ampullar pregnancy is an ectopic pregnancy in the ampullar portion of the fallopian tube. This is the most common site of implantation.

2. It generally ends in tubal abortion if it is within 1 cm. of the fimbriated end of the tube. There is a trickle of bleeding into the peritoneal cavity, and this may collect as a clot in the pouch of Douglas. It is then called a *hematocele.*

3. These ectopics may be situated 1 to 4 cm. from the fimbriated end of the tube, and rupture in 8 to 12 weeks. This may occur spontaneously or from pressure (such as from straining at stool, from coitus, or from pelvic examination) and occurs at about 8 to 12 weeks. Hemorrhage may be severe.

4. Sometimes rupture is retroperitoneal between the leaves of the broad ligament—this is *broad ligament hematoma.* Hemorrhage in this site is more likely to be controlled.

Isthmic Pregnancy

1. Isthmic pregnancy is an ectopic gestation in the narrow portion of the tube. After the ampullary ectopics it is the next most common ectopic. It occurs in the middle third of the tube.

2. Rupture usually occurs at 8 weeks. The hemorrhage is severe and often is accompanied by shock. Diagnosis prior to rupture is rare.

Interstitial Pregnancy

1. Interstitial pregnancy is pregnancy in the interstitial portion of the fallopian tube (angular pregnancy, tubo-uterine pregnancy). (This portion of the tube lies within the uterus and is 1 to 3 cm. long).

2. It is rare but very dangerous, because it ends in rupture of the uterine muscle with severe hemorrhage. It may rupture into the peritoneal cavity or into the upper part of the uterus.

Management

There are several ways to manage an ectopic tubal pregnancy. (These have included salpingo-oophorectomy: the rationale for this management was that all subsequent ovulations would occur from an ovary with an adjacent tube, thus increasing the patient's potential intrauterine pregnancy rate per cycle. However, this is no longer considered justifiable.)

1. Salpingectomy: This is the most common treatment of ectopic pregnancy. It consists of cross-clamping the broad ligament and removing the whole tube. This form of surgical management is most appropriate in the event of ruptured ectopic pregnancy, which involves considerable bleeding. One must take care to close off the tube at the level of the uterus, to guard against a future ectopic pregnancy in the stump of a tube.

Management of the unruptured ectopic pregnancy allows a greater number of options. These include:

2. Milking: An unruptured tubal pregnancy may be milked from the fimbriated end of the tube. If there is no undue bleeding after the products of conception have been milked from the end of the tube, nothing further need be done.

3. Salpingostomy: If the pregnancy is at the midpoint of the tube, a linear salpingostomy—an opening-up of the tube, followed by removal of the ectopic pregnancy and closure of the tube—may be performed.

4. Segmental Resection of the Tube: The segment of the tube involved may be removed and an anastomosis of the tubal ends performed. Alternatively the cut ends of the tube may be ligated, and anastomosis done at a later date.

5. Interstitial (cornual) pregnancy may present a more difficult problem in management. Rupture usually takes place later than in cases of ampullary pregnancy, but bleeding may be unusually profuse as the uterine wall is extremely vascular. The treatment is to excise the cornu by a wedge-shaped incision, or sometimes, if the uterus is extensively damaged, to perform hysterectomy.

6. Pregnancy in the rudimentary uterine horn is not really extrauterine, but is mentioned here for convenience. The comparatively thick muscular wall of an undeveloped uterine horn may accommodate the gestation for a time, but it usually ruptures at about the sixteenth week, with severe intraperitoneal hemorrhage.

a. If the connection between the rudimentary cornu and the developed half of the uterus is not too intimate, it is possible to remove only the former.

b. In the case of pregnancy in the rudimentary horn, the round ligament will be attached on the outer side of the gestational sac. On tubal pregnancies it is inserted on the inner side of the gestational sac, between it and the uterus. Hysterectomy may be necessary for these patients.

Preoperative Orders

1. Nothing per os, no catharsis, no enemas

2. CBC, hematocrit every 4 hours, erythrocyte sedimentation rate, urinalysis, blood volume

3. Type and crossmatch 1,500 ml. of whole blood.

4. Complete bed rest

5. Radioreceptor assay

6. Infusion of 1,000 ml. Ringer's lactate. Use a large No. 16 or No. 18 needle at two sites.

7. If the vein is not available, do an immediate cutdown.

8. If shock is present treat it, but do not delay surgery.

9. Check vital signs every 15 minutes.

10. Notify the O.R. staff and anesthetist as soon as the diagnosis is suspected.

11. Culdocentesis

12. Abdominal and perineal preparation

13. Preoperative medication: Demerol, 50 mg. and atropine, 0.4 mg. This is given one-half hour before surgery.

Postoperative Orders

1. Nothing per os until bowel sounds indicate normal peristalsis beyond 24 hours after the operation

2. Fluid balance sheet (measure of fluid intake and output, and record)

3. Replacement of blood loss

4. Hematocrit 12, 24, and 48 hours after surgery

5. Replacement of fluids and electrolytes as indicated

6. Vital signs every 30 minutes for 6 hours

7. Monitoring of primary urinary output on an hourly basis. An output of 40 ml. per hour indicates adequate tissue perfusion.

8. Demerol, 75 mg., every 3 hours p.r.n. for pain

9. Seconal, 100 mg., I.M. and repeated if needed (option) p.r.n. for sleep

10. Compazine, 10 mg., I.M. every 6 hours p.r.n. for nausea

ECTOPIC OVARIAN PREGNANCY

Basic Principles

1. Primary ovarian pregnancy is a rare form of ectopic pregnancy in which impregnation of the ovum by the spermatozoon occurs before the former is extruded from the ovary.

2. The association of use of the IUD and ovarian pregnancy has been reported several times.

3. Ovarian pregnancy probably is not an uncommon entity, as previously reported. It may be overlooked clinically in unexplained cases of hematoperitoneum or because it is of too little interest to warrant publication.

4. These pregnancies frequently rupture before the end of the third month, and almost never reach viability.

5. Their preoperative diagnosis is impossible because the clinical signs and symptoms are the same as those of tubal pregnancy.

6. At operation ovarian pregnancy resembles a ruptured ovarian cyst. Diagnosis is made on histological examination if placental and fetal elements cannot be identified.

7. For a valid diagnosis of this rare form of ectopic pregnancy the postulates of Spiegelberg are mandatory:

a. The tube, including the fimbria, must be intact and clearly separate from the ovary.

b. The gestation sac must occupy the normal position of the ovary.

c. The sac must be connected to the uterus by the ovarian ligament.

d. Ovarian tissue should be demonstrable in the walls of the sac.

8. Ovarian pregnancy may become abdominal pregancy if the fetus survives and reimplants after rupture.

9. Secondary ovarian pregnancy is a rare form of ectopic pregnancy in which the blastocyst implants on the surface of the ovary.

Management

The choice of appropriate management depends on how much ovary is destroyed, the number of children the patient has, and her age.

ECTOPIC CERVICAL PREGNANCY

Cervical pregnancy is gestation that develops when the fertilized ovum becomes implanted in the cervical canal of the uterus.

Basic Principles

1. This form of pregnancy is so rare that even responsible physicans usually do not consider the diagonsis.

2. The bleeding is profuse, and the patient usually goes into shock.

3. Usually the physician makes a diagnosis of incomplete abortion. When an attempt is made to remove the products of conception that present at the os, the bleeding becomes profuse.

Criteria for Diagnosis

1. There must be cervical glands opposite the placental attachment.

2. The attachment of the placenta to the cervix must be intimate.

3. Fetal elements are not recovered from the corpus of the uterus.

4. The whole placenta is implanted below the internal os of the cervix.

5. Cervical pregnancy should be suspected in any patient with first trimester painless vaginal bleeding who has a large ballooning cystic-like cervix that feels flush

with the vault and that has a firm uterus sitting on top.

6. Early abortion fortunately is the rule, but some cervical pregnancies continue for more than 16 weeks.

7. These patients have profuse hemorrhage and shock. Hemostasis is a problem.

Management

1. Finger curettage and tight cervical packing make up the preferred mode of treatment.

2. If the therapy proves inadequate, ligation of the descending cervical branches of the uterine artery may be indicated.

3. If bleeding cannot be controlled, a total hysterectomy may be necessary.

4. Delayed hemorrhage may occur as late as 6 weeks after evacuation of the cervical pregnancy.

5. Preoperative and postoperative orders are the same as for tubal pregnancy.

Prognosis

1. Patients with ectopic pregnancy must be told that the prognosis for future fertility is decreased and that approximately 40 per cent of patients never conceive again.

2. Of the 60 percent who do achieve another pregnancy, 12 per cent will have another ectopic pregnancy, and another 15 to 20 per cent will abort spontaneously.

3. Because of the high risk in women with previous ectopic pregnancies, every patient should be instructed to notify her physician as soon as she misses her menses so that the location of the new pregnancy can be detected by serial testing of the serum HCG beta subunit and by ultrasound.

4. If another tubal pregnancy is diagnosed early, surgical management to preserve the remaining tube is still a possibility.

5. Patients with ectopic pregnancy do run the risk of Rh symptomatization; therefore Rh typing of their blood is important. If a patient is Rh-negative, she should receive 50 μg. of RhD immune globulin.

ABDOMINAL PREGNANCY

Abdominal pregnancy is gestation occurring within the peritoneal cavity (intraperitoneal pregnancy).

Primary Abdominal Pregnancy

This is growth of the fetus and placenta within the peritoneal cavity. Fertilization and embryonic growth occur before entrance into the fallopian tube. This is a rare condition.

Secondary Abdominal Pregnancy

This is pregnancy that develops in the abdominal cavity following tubal abortion or rupture. The fetus may continue to grow until term or may become macerated, skeletonized, or mummified.

Basic Principles

1. Unlike other ectopic pregnancies, these frequently approach term.

2. Abdominal pregnancy is very rare.

3. Most abdominal pregnancies begin initially as ectopic tubal pregnancies that are expelled from the tube and implant elsewhere in the pelvis; or implantation occurs primarily in the peritoneum.

4. The ovum may be expelled intra- or retroperitoneally. The trophoblast develops its connection with the nearest blood supply (usually on the broad ligament and back of the uterus); in the retroperitoneal situation, the proximity of great vessels will increase the risk of hemorrhage.

5. For the first 6 weeks the history is similar to that of tubal ectopic pregnancy, but after a few months gastrointestinal and genitourinary symptoms develop.

Clinical Features

1. There is a history of threatened abortion with irregular bleeding.

2. Continued abdominal discomfort is felt, and fetal movements are painful.

3. Fetal abnormality is common and the rate of fetal mortality is high. Fetal death may be followed by suppuration with abscess pointing into bowel or bladder, and then by calcification and lithopedion formation.

4. The suggestive symptoms and signs are:

a. Painful fetal movements

b. Palpable fetal parts in the cul-de-sac

c. Absence of Braxton Hicks contractions

d. Abnormal presentation and abdominally palpable fetal parts

e. A pelvic mass (uterus) may be felt separately from the fetal mass

5. Diagnosis is difficult; palpation is unreliable even when fetal limbs are easily felt.

a. X-ray findings should include a fetus in an abnormal position in the abdominal cavity, absence of the uterine and placental shadows from their normal position, unusual clarity of the fetus and fetal parts, unchanged position of the fetus on serial studies, presence of pelvic or lower abdominal mass, close proximity of the fetus to the anterior abdominal wall, and fetal parts that overlie the maternal vertebral column.

b. Hysterography and aortography have been employed in the past to help confirm the diagnosis, but recent advances in technology have made these studies unnecessary in most cases.

c. Serial sonographic studies may be helpful and may spare the patient x-ray exposure.

d. The fetus is "small for dates."

e. Estriol excretion levels are below normal.

Management

1. Many physicians advocate early treatment once the diagnosis is made.

2. The chief risk in continuing pregnancy is hemorrhage. Very few babies survive beyond 36 weeks, because of placental insufficiency.

3. The fetus is removed, the cord tied, and the abdomen closed.

4. No attempt is made to detach the placenta. (The absence of a contractile uterus leaves no means of controlling hemorrhage.)

Preoperative Orders

1. CBC and hematocrit. Urinalysis, ESR. Blood sugar, urea, and creatinine levels.

2. Standing and reclining, A.P. and lateral x-rays of the abdomen

3. Chest x-ray and EKG

4. Ultrasound and/or MRI

5. Uterogram, in cases in which it is indicated

6. Fetal EKG

7. Type and crossmatch 4,000 ml. of whole blood.

8. Cantor tube through the pylorus

9. Foley catheter

10. Nil per os 12 hours preoperative

11. Intestinal preparation with Neomycin

12. Abdominal and perineal preparation

13. Infusion of 1,000 ml. Ringer's lactate with a No. 18 or a No. 16 needle at two sites

Surgery

1. Great care must be taken in opening the abdomen.

2. The incision should not be made near the placenta if there is any choice.

3. Remove the fetus gingerly and steady the insertion of the placenta.

4. Do not separate the placenta unless it is attached to an organ to which the blood supply can be controlled.

5. Do not pull on the cord.

6. Do not remove the placenta from bowel or mesentery.

7. Ligate the cord at its insertion and leave the placenta in situ.

8. Close the abdomen without drainage.

Postoperative Orders

The postoperative orders are the same as for tubal pregnancy.

MANAGEMENT BY METHOTREXATE

Management of ectopic pregnancy by the use of methotrexate has been suggested. This should be condemned except in very highly selected cases resting in the hands of physicians with expertise in the field and access to well-structured back-up teams.

It has been suggested that in abdominal pregnancy the placenta be managed by the use of postoperative methotrexate. There are too few reported cases to support any positive statement at present.

6. Antepartum Care

David H. Fields

DEFINITION

The aim of antepartum care is to safeguard the health of the mother and fetus and to smooth the transition to parenthood. Since many of the factors which adversely affect the fetus do so in the very early weeks, often before the mother is aware she is pregnant, optimal antepartum care must begin before conception.

BASIC PRINCIPLES

1. Pregnancy is not a disease. It is, however, a physiologic process which places increasingly severe metabolic and nutritional demands on the mother as gestation advances. These demands must be met to ensure a healthy outcome for both mother and infant. Because they become progressively more severe, they are best satisfied in advance, rather than by playing catch-up throughout the pregnancy.

2. A safe and satisfying pregnancy requires not only maternal physical adjustments, but also mental and psychic preparation on the part of both parents.

3. The cornerstones of good pre-conception and antepartum care are:

a. Good nutrition

b. Early detection and treatment of illness.

c. Adjustment to physical limitations of pregnancy, if any

d. Education of the prospective parents about the normal and abnormal events of pregnancy

e. Avoidance of substances harmful to the fetus

All of these can be best achieved by the maintenance of open communication between the woman and her obstetrician.

PRE-CONCEPTION CARE

For the most part, pre-conception care should be directed toward detecting conditions which are likely to have teratogenic or other negative effects on pregnancy. Much of the information sought and the advice given is the same as used to be sought and given in early pregnancy, simply sooner.

Essentials of History

Specific inquiry should be made about:

1. Drug use, especially alcohol, tobacco, and illicit drugs

2. Genetic history, especially Tay-Sachs (European Jews), β-thalassemia (Mediterranean origin), sickle cell and related hemoglobinopathies (blacks), and retardation or abnormal children in either family

3. Medical diseases which adversely affect early pregnancy, especially diabetes and heart disease

Essentials of Physical Examination

Generally, there are no findings which adversely affect early pregnancy which will not be found during a routine gynecological exam.

Laboratory Screening

The following laboratory tests are performed by many or all obstetricians before conception:

1. At the very least, rubella immune status should be determined and vaccination performed if appropriate.

2. Screening for overt diabetes, preferably as part of a blood profile, or as part of a urinalysis for glucose. Very strict control of diabetes in the first few weeks after conception is probably the only method of decreasing the congenital anomalies associated with it.

3. Determination of hematocrit

4. Screening for Tay-Sachs, β-thalassemia, etc., if indicated, as above.

5. More and more, screening is being done for HIV antibody status, especially for women in high-risk categories. The best time to do this is before conception, when the decision to avoid pregnancy is possible.

6. Many physicians now do all the routine prenatal tests before conception, if possible (see below).

THE INITIAL VISIT

The initial visit should be made as early in pregnancy as possible and should include a complete history, physical examination, and laboratory screen, to establish as many baseline parameters as possible.

Essentials of History

1. Information regarding the current pregnancy, including date and character of last menstrual period and normal frequency of menstruation

2. Previous obstetric history, including weight, condition, timing, and type of previous deliveries

3. Medical history, especially regarding diabetes, hypertension, and cardiovascular disease

4. Surgical history, especially with reference to abdominal or uterine surgery

5. Medications used during this pregnancy (including alcohol, tobacco, and marijuana)

6. Any problems encountered during this or previous pregnancy

Essentials of Physical Examination

1. General examination with special emphasis on:

a. Weight, height, blood pressure

b. Heart murmurs, breasts

c. Lower extremity edema or varices

d. Pelvic examination. (While many physicians gauge pelvic architecture on the first visit, it may be preferable to defer this to the third trimester, when both the patient and her perineum are more relaxed.)

Laboratory Screening

1. CBC

2. Blood type and Rh identification with antibody screening

3. VDRL

4. Rubella titer

5. Serum glucose

6. Clean-catch urinalysis, for sugar, acetone, and albumin, and a microscopic exam

7. Papanicolaou smear

8. Cervical culture or antibody smear (Gonozyme) for gonorrhea

9. Cervical smear for *Chlamydia trachomatis* (either antibody detection by Microtrak or Chlamydiazyme or by culture)

10. Tine test or PPD for tuberculosis; if positive, follow-up chest x-ray with abdominal shielding may be done to rule out active tuberculosis.

11. Many obstetricians now do antibody screening for a variety of infections which may adversely affect pregnancy, including *Toxoplasma gondii,* cytomegalovirus, herpes simplex virus (1 & 2), hepatitis B, and human immunodeficiency virus (HIV).

Advice to the Prenatal Patient at the First Visit

1. Diet. A normal diet consisting of meats, eggs, milk, and vegetables should be encouraged for the woman of normal pre-pregnancy weight. The following requirements should be met:

a. Kilocalories. Approximately 2,400, as three good meals per day

b. Protein. 75 to 125 g./day; supplied by meat or fish daily, eggs several times per week, and 1 quart of milk daily

c. Minerals

(1) All basic mineral needs except that for iron may be met by adequate vegetable, fruit, and milk intake.

(2) Iron must be supplied as ferrous sulfate (or gluconate or fumarate) tablets at least once daily.

(3) Many physicians recommend prenatal vitamins, all of which have supplementary minerals, including calcium.

(4) If the patient cannot drink adequate amounts of milk, her needs may be met by calcium supplement of 1 to 2 g. daily.

d. Vitamins

(1) All vitamin needs are met by adequate vegetable and fruit intake but are usually supplemented by any of the prenatal vitamins.

(2) In addition, many physicians prescribe supplementary folic acid (0.5 to 1.0 mg. daily), although the need for this has not been proven.

2. Weight Gain

a. Normal pregnancy is associated with a minimum weight gain of 20 pounds. This breaks down more or less as follows:

(1) 11 pounds: intrauterine contents

(2) 7 pounds: uterus, breasts, intravascular volume

(3) 2 pounds: extravascular fluid retention

b. Weight gains from 25 to 30 pounds are associated with optimal fetal growth and minimal maternal complications.

c. Weight gain greater than 30 to 35 pounds is associated with an increase in maternal morbidity, especially with abnormal glucose tolerance, and with difficulty losing the extra fat after delivery.

d. Obese women should still gain the minimum 20 pounds, with all attempts at dieting strictly watched for the development of ketosis.

3. Activity

a. Unless there is a risk of premature labor (e.g., twins), the normal pregnant woman may carry out virtually any activity with which she is comfortable. She should not undertake dangerous sports (e.g., skiing, sky diving) and should avoid extreme overexertion, as this may cause hyperthermia. Similarly, prolonged sauna and steam bath exposure should be avoided.

b. She may continue to work at her job until she cannot easily physically perform it, as long as it does not involve specifically dangerous conditions (e.g., exposure to radiation or chemicals). Many women remain at work until they go into labor.

c. There are no restrictions on travel, with the understanding that the woman should not sit in positions that compromise lower extremity circulation for long periods of time. She should move about every 1 or 2 hours. Avoiding locales where dangerous diseases are common is an exercise of common sense. Many vaccinations are safe during pregnancy, but each must be verified separately.

4. Sexual Intercourse

a. Coitus may be unrestricted in normal pregnancy as long as the cervix is not significantly dilated. It should be forbidden in pregnancies complicated by vaginal bleeding, ruptured membranes, or premature labor.

b. Under no circumstances should air be blown into the vagina if cunnilingus is performed. This has resulted in fatal air embolus.

c. Although its significance is unknown, fetal bradycardia has been reported after orgasm, presumably secondary to uterine contraction. Perhaps orgasm should be advised against in pregnancies at high risk for fetal distress.

5. Drug Use

a. All recreational drug use should be discussed. Alcohol, in even moderate amounts, is known to cause fetal alcohol syndrome, a constellation of neurological, craniofacial, and skeletal defects. Tobacco use is associated with higher perinatal mortality and lower birth weight. Narcotics and cocaine have effects on the fetus at least as deleterious as those on the mother. While there are no hard data on fetal injury from marijuana use, in an age when pregnant women are leery of taking acetaminophen, the physician should discourage use of essentially all recreational drugs.

b. Any prescription item should be researched and its benefits weighed against its potential hazards. A good reference for this is the Physicians' Desk Reference, which is very wary of drug use in pregnancy.

c. Most physicians allow limited use of acetaminophen for headache and encourage its use for fever.

6. Genetic Screening

a. Amniocentesis, usually performed at 16 to 18 weeks for detection of chromosomal anomalies, should be discussed with every pregnant woman. In most parts of the country, it is a standard part of care for every gravida 35 or older. This makes sense since, at 35, the risk of a chromosomally abnormal fetus is approximately 1/180 (of which half are Down syndrome), which is greater than the risk of a miscarriage from the amniocentesis (commonly quoted at no higher than 1/200). Many younger women also elect to have the procedure. The fluid is also tested for alpha-fetoprotein (AFP) to screen for neural tube defects (NTDs).

b. Chorionic villus sampling (CVS) enables one to detect chromosomal anomalies in the first trimester, making termination of pregnancy much less traumatic. However, because the pregnancy loss rate is currently higher than with amniocentesis (1 to 4 per cent), it is usually recommended for women who are at very high risk for anomalies. As CVS becomes safer with experience and technological advance, it may replace amniocentesis.

c. Serum AFP screening for NTDs should be performed on all gravidas who do not plan to have amniocentesis. It is usually begun after the fifteenth week.

7. Clothing

a. Common sense should dictate comfortable clothes. The only real caveats are:

(1) Constriction of venous return below the waist, most commonly caused by tight girdles or socks (stockings) with elastic tops, and

(2) High-heeled shoes

b. Adequate support of the breasts with a brassiere usually adds to maternal comfort.

8. Hygiene

a. Normal hygiene is encouraged.

b. Tub baths and showers are acceptable as long as the mother is not at risk of falling.

c. Douching should be avoided unless specifically indicated for medication delivery. If necessary, it must be performed gently and carefully.

d. Dental care should be sought early in pregnancy. All necessary work may be done with local anesthesia.

9. Prepared Childbirth Classes.

a. These are now readily available throughout the country and should be attended by every patient whether or not she intends to have "prepared childbirth."

b. The preparation given and the knowledge gained about labor and delivery will serve to decrease anxiety, cutting down on intrapartum medication in almost all cases.

c. The exercises and toning in preparation for labor will make labor easier for most women.

d. The involvement of the husband in the pregnancy and delivery will usually serve to make both a more enjoyable "family experience" and may result in a smoother transition to the postpartum period.

10. Warning Signs
Certain symptoms or signs may be of grave importance. The pregnant woman should be encouraged to report any of the following:

a. Vaginal bleeding
b. Leakage of fluid from the vagina
c. Blurring of vision
d. Persistent headache or dizziness
e. Fever or chills
f. Abdominal pain
g. Recurrent vomiting
h. Swelling of hands or face

Follow-up Visits

1. The normal obstetric patient should be seen at least at 4-week intervals from the first visit until approximately 30 to 32 weeks gestation. Many physicians see their patients monthly until 26 weeks, then at 3-week intervals until 32 weeks. From 32 to 36 weeks, visits should be bi-weekly, and after 36 weeks, weekly.

2. The following information should be obtained at every visit: weight, blood pressure, urine sugar and protein, uterine size, and fetal lie and heart rate, if possible, after 12 weeks gestation.

3. Unless there is a specific contraindication, vaginal examination for cervical dilatation and presenting part should be performed weekly from the thirty-sixth week. While custom has decreed that pelvic exams not be routinely performed between the first visit and the thirty-sixth week, there seems to be no good reason for such a policy. Certainly the exam is harmless (we do not interdict sex). Furthermore, information on the state of the cervix may be useful in cases of premature rupture of the membranes or even to detect early effacement and dilatation.

4. Pelvic architecture, if not evaluated previously, should be thoroughly examined at the thirty-sixth week.

5. The following laboratory work should be routinely obtained after the first visit in normal pregnancy.

a. Hemoglobin/hematocrit, at least once each in the second and third trimester

b. Repeat blood type, Rh, and antibody screen—at 26 to 28 weeks and at 36 weeks gestation

c. Serologic test for syphilis (VDRL, STS), in the third trimester

d. Mini glucose tolerance test (MGTT) consisting of a fasting and a 1-hour glucose determination with a 50-g. glucose load between. This is an attempt to detect the approximately 8 per cent of gravidas who are chemical diabetics. Most obstetricians are screening at least once at 28 to 32 weeks, while some advocate testing twice (at 22 to 24 and at 30 to 34 weeks).

e. In high-risk populations, late-third-trimester screening for cervical gonorrhea and chlamydia is probably worthwhile.

Special Diagnostic Studies

Any special diagnostic studies may be performed as long as they do not require the administration of medication or exposure to radiation. If either of these is necessary, the benefits must be weighed against the risks.

1. Radiographic Studies. With the exception of x-ray pelvimetry and the single flat plate of the abdomen to determine fetal lie, x-ray studies for obstetric indications have been largely supplanted by ultrasonography, which may be used to document fetal death, fetal maturity, fetal abnormality, and placental location.

2. Chest Radiography. Delivers minimal radiation, especially when performed with an abdominal shield. It should be obtained in cases of suspected pulmonary tuberculosis (in all positive Tine tests), as well as on suspicion of pneumonia.

3. Radiographic Contrast Studies. Intravenous pyelograms, barium enemas, and upper GI series can usually be postponed until the postpartum period. If the need to know is great enough, all can be performed with less than 10 rads of exposure by keeping the number of films and fluoroscopy to a minimum.

4. Radioactive scanning of the lung, liver, and thyroid should be avoided unless the situation is life threatening.

5. Ultrasonography has been in use for over 25 years and is so far considered safe. The indications for its use expand almost daily and currently include placental localization, determination of fetal size, age, lie, growth patterns, and well-being (biophysical profile and detection of fetal abnormalities).

Commonly Encountered Problems in Antepartum Care

1. Nausea and Vomiting. Possibly a reaction to high levels of HCG, this is essentially a problem of the first trimester. So-called morning sickness is probably the most commonly encountered side effect of pregnancy and is covered in great detail in Chap. 7.

2. Fatigue. Another common complaint, extreme tiredness is also a first and early second trimester problem. If anemia or chronic disease is not present, the physician should explain the need for extra rest during pregnancy.

3. Ptyalism

a. When excessive salivation occurs, the most reasonable approach is to reassure the patient that it is harmless. Attempts at treatment with anticholinergic agents such as propantheline are usually unsuccessful.

b. Some investigators have suggested that ptyalism is actually failure to swallow, rather than increased salivary gland production.

4. Pica

a. Although the ingestion of bizarre substances (most commonly clay or starch) is probably more a social custom than anything else, investigation of the diet for a specific deficiency should be made.

b. It is rarely a problem unless huge quantities of the particular substance are eaten.

5. Heartburn

a. This is due to reflux of gastric acid into the esophagus secondary to upward pressure on the stomach by the growing uterus. It is probably made worse by the decreased gastric motility of pregnancy.

b. Tremendous relief is obtained with antacids, which should be of the magnesium or aluminum salt types. Amphojel and Gelusil are constipating, while milk of magnesia, Maalox, and Mylanta have the opposite effect.

c. Sodium bicarbonate antacids should be avoided because of the large sodium load which may be involved.

6. Constipation

a. This frequent complaint is best treated by diets high in fiber, fluid intake, and cathartic substances (prunes, raisins), combined with retraining of bowel habits.

b. If necessary, commercial cathartics and stool softeners may be used.

c. It is not a problem unless the stool is especially hard and bowel movements become painful.

7. Hemorrhoids

a. These inevitable results of pregnancy are made worse by constipation and are eased by soft, regular bowel movements without straining.

b. Surgical treatment during pregnancy is only indicated for acutely thrombosed hemorrhoids and then should usually be limited to clot evacuation under local anesthesia.

c. Hemorrhoidectomy is not indicated since hemorrhoids regress spontaneously postpartum and recur with the next pregnancy.

8. Lower Extremity Varicosities

a. Like hemorrhoids, these are due to increased venous pressure from the growing uterus.

b. Treatment is almost always conservative, consisting of support elastic stockings (perferably the pantyhose type) and elevation of the legs while sitting or lying.

9. Excessive Vaginal Discharge

a. The key to treatment of leukorrhea during pregnancy is identical to that outside of pregnancy: identification of the causative organism.

b. This is best done by a wet mount preparation in saline to check for trichomonads and "clue cells" (*Hemophilus vaginalis*) followed by a 10% KOH or NaOH preparation to detect candidiasis.

c. If the above are not revealing or if therapy is unsuccessful, cultures for *Candida albicans* (on Nickerson's medium), *H. vaginalis* (standard "culturette"), and gonorrhea (Thayer-Martin medium, Transgro), or smear for chlamydia (Microtrak, Chlamydiazyme) may be performed. Trichomonads are best identified on Pap smear.

d. Therapy should be directed toward a specific etiology:

(1) *Candida:* Nystatin (Mycostatin) suppositories b.i.d., 10 to 14 days; miconazole (Monistat) cream or suppositories hs, 3 to 7 days; clotrimazole (Gyne-Lotrimin, Mycelex G) cream or suppositories h.s., 3 to 7 days.

(2) *H. vaginalis:* sulfa cream (Sultrin, AVC) b.i.d. × 1 week; ampicillin (P.O.) 500 mg. every 6 hrs. × 1 week. Although metronidazole (Flagyl, Protostat) is currently the drug of choice for *H. vaginalis,* its use is contraindicated during the first trimester, and most avoid it throughout pregnancy, since this infection is of questionable importance. Treating the male partner is essential.

(3) *Trichomonas:* Although metronidazole (Flagyl) is the drug of choice for this, it is contraindicated in first-trimester pregnancy. It should probably be reserved during later gestation for cases which MUST be treated and do not respond to local povidone-iodine (Betadine) application or other creams. If metronidazole is used, the dosage is 250 mg. t.i.d. × 7 days.

(4) Gonorrhea: Best treated in pregnancy with probenecid 1 g. P.O. followed by either 4.8 million units of procaine penicillin I.M. or 3.5 g. of ampicillin or 3 g. of amoxicillin P.O. The P.O. regimens do not cure pharyngitis. In the penicillin allergic, spectinomycin (Trobicin) 2 g. I.M. is used. Treatment of the male partner is essential to prevent reinfection.

(5) Chlamydia: Best treated in pregnancy with erythromycin 500 mg. q.i.d. 10 to 21 days. Treatment of the male partner is essential to prevent reinfection.

10. Abdominal Cramping

a. This is common in the third and fourth months of pregnancy as the uterus rises out of the pelvis, and is commonly ascribed to the "round ligament syndrome."

b. It can be distinguished from urinary and gastrointestinal problems by careful history, examination, and urinalysis.

c. Benign in nature, it usually responds well to mild bed rest and local application of heat.

11. Backache

a. Usually caused by the exaggerated lordosis of pregnancy, low back pain responds well to relief of the strain.

b. If conservative measures do not afford relief, orthopaedic consultation should be sought.

12. Headaches

a. Very common in early pregnancy, these should respond well to simple analgesia.

b. If they persist beyond the first few weeks of gestation, are not relieved by aspirin, or are accompanied by neurologic symptoms, they should be thoroughly investigated.

13. Edema

a. Swelling of the feet or legs during the course of the day is normal for pregnancy. The swelling responds well to elevation.

b. Swelling of the face or hands is less likely to be normal, and preeclampsia should be suspected.

c. Diuretics and salt restriction are not indicated for simple edema of pregnancy since it is a hydrostatic phenomenon.

7 Nausea and Vomiting of Pregnancy

Hugh R. K. Barber

BASIC PRINCIPLES

1. Nausea and vomiting is probably the most common disorder seen in the first 12 weeks of pregnancy. It is estimated that about one-half of all pregnant women have some nausea or vomiting; but of this group, only about one-half need any treatment.

a. As a rule, nausea and vomiting in pregnancy begins at the sixth week and stops spontaneously before the fourteenth week. Although it is generally limited to the early morning, it may occur at other times of the day.

b. Usually the symptoms are slight; excessive or prolonged vomiting is certainly pathological, and its cause uncertain.

c. From about the sixth to the twelfth week of pregnancy, nausea or vomiting in the early morning is so common that it is accepted as a symptom of normal pregnancy. It usually occurs soon after waking, and consists of retching rather than vomiting.

d. It nearly always stops before the 14th week and does not disturb the patient's health or her pregnancy.

e. Since morning sickness sometimes occurs when a woman does not yet know that she is pregnant, it seems to be caused by something other than a psychological reaction to pregnancy; the increased symptoms of vomiting in cases of twins and hydatidiform mole have led to the theory that it is the result of higher levels of chorionic gonadotropin (HCG) or of higher sensitivity to it.

f. The vomiting occurs at the time of peak output of HCG in normal pregnancy, but studies comparing hormone levels and sensitivities in cases of excessive vomiting with those of normal control subjects have not consistently supported this theory.

g. If the vomiting is persistent and disturbs the patient's health, it is called *hyperemesis gravidarum*. In these severe cases the only biochemical abnormalities that have been found are those secondary to vomiting, starvation, and dehydration; namely, ketosis, electrolyte imbalance, and vitamin deficiency.

h. In the past 20 years the incidence of hyperemesis gravidarum has greatly diminished.

i. In some persistent cases there may be psychological factors. Mere removal to the hospital, without any other treatment, often leads to dramatic and immediate improvement. Hyperemesis is almost unknown in so-called underdeveloped countries.

j. It is important to detect other diseases—for example, gastroenteritis, cholecystitis, hepatitis, peptic ulcer, and pyelonephritis.

2. Treatment can usually be given on an ambulatory basis. However, about one gravida in 300 requires hospitalization.

3. The criteria for hospitalizing a patient with vomiting of pregnancy are:

a. Acetone or diacetic acid in urine

b. Weight loss of 5 per cent or more

c. Heart rate of 120 b.p.m. or more

d. Elevated temperature with signs of dehydration

e. Elevated specific gravity of the urine with low urinary output

4. It is important to be certain of the diagnosis. Marked vomiting in early pregnancy may be associated with twins or a hydatidiform mole. More serious problems such as hepatitis, diabetic acidosis, or acute porphyria may be mistaken for vomiting of pregnancy.

5. The average case of vomiting in pregnancy presents a picture of electrolyte and water imbalance not unlike that seen in the nonpregnant patient. Although the hydrochloric-acid content of the vomitus is reduced below nonpregnant values, there is still enough loss of chlorides in the early phases of vomiting to lead to hypochloremic alkalosis. Vomiting leads to starvation with the initiation of ketosis. It is not unusual to find hypochloremic alkalosis and ketosis coexisting in the early stage of vomiting.

6. If therapy is not instituted, dehydration becomes marked; there is a reduction in the extracellular fluid, with a drop in glomerular filtration. The urine output drops, the specific gravity of the urine is increased, and sulfates and phosphates accumulate in the extracellular space. The resultant acidosis represents a very serious problem, which demands prompt and intelligent therapy.

MANAGEMENT

1. In any case of severe or persistent vomiting it is essential to make an accurate and positive diagnosis.

2. Ordinary morning sickness can be simply treated by reassurance, and sometimes by giving one of the antiemetics that have been proved nonteratogenic, such as Meclozine 25 mg., Cyclizine 50 mg., or Promezathine 25 mg., all three times daily. However, in the present litigious climate in the United States most physicians hesitate to give any medication in the first trimester. Bendectrin has been withdrawn from the market in the United States.

3. If the vomiting is severe the patient is admitted to the hospital. If it continues, dehydration, ketosis, and electrolyte imbalance require treatment by intravenous infusion. The basic fluid and electrolyte requirements are:

a. 1,000 ml. of 5% glucose and water

b. 500 ml. of 5% glucose and saline

c. 1,000 ml. of 5% glucose and water

4. To this should be added the replacement of fluid and electrolytes lost in vomitus. Inasmuch as the vomiting is almost entirely gastric, it can be replaced in the ratio of two-thirds 5-per-cent glucose and saline and one-third 5-per-cent glucose and water. This replacement is satisfactory, even though the gastric juice in a pregnant patient usually contains less hydrochloric acid than is seen in the normal nonpregnant patient.

5. As soon as the urinary output is improved to about 1,000 ml. per day, it is important to replace the daily requirement of KCl (30 to 40 mEq.) plus another 20 mEq. of KCl for each 1,000 ml. of vomitus that is replaced.

6. The use of amino acids has very little place in the therapy of the patient with acute vomiting of pregnancy and may, of itself, cause vomiting. Because the enzyme systems concerned with the utilization of the amino acids are functioning poorly, the amino acids are often excreted in the same concentrations in which they are infused. The liver in the pregnant patient with acute vomiting may have central necrosis and lesions that resemble the hepatic lesions of starvation. Liver insufficiency is not conducive to the utilization of infused amino acids.

7. Severe cases present a real challenge to the institution of intelligent therapy. The problem of acidosis occurring as a late phase of vomiting of pregnancy may be accompanied by some degree of liver insufficiency, and attempts to correct acidosis with sodium lactate are to be discouraged. The poorly functioning liver is unable to adequately metabolize the lactate, and it accumulates in the extracellular space. In situations of this kind the use of sodium bicarbonate is preferred. When sodium bicarbonate is given, the bicarbonate ion (HCO_3^-) dissociates, and the CO_2 is blown off by the lungs, while the sodium ion remains in the extracellular space and carries out its functions as a cation.

8. The problem of ammonium toxicity has not been investigated in cases of vomiting of pregnancy. Whether present research in the field of ammonium toxicity will find any application in evaluating these problems remains to be determined. However, certain of these cases have some liver insufficiency, and it has been shown that ammonium toxicity is frequently associated with liver insufficiency. Sodium glutamate may be substituted for sodium bicarbonate in these cases. The rationale behind this plan is that the glutamate reacts with ammonium to form the easily metabolized glutamine, while the sodium combines with the metabolically available CO_2 to form sodium bicarbonate. Sodium glutamate is given in 30- to 40-g. doses and is added to the glucose-and-water solution.

9 In summary, the fluid regimen to be used in severe cases of vomiting of pregnancy is as follows:

a. 1,500 to 2,000 ml. of 5-per-cent glucose and water. Five-per-cent glucose and water may be used as all or part of the infusion in order to increase the caloric intake.

b. 500 ml. of 5-per-cent glucose and saline

c. Replacement of the vomitus (replace as two-thirds 5-per-cent glucose and saline, and one-third 5-per-cent glucose and water)

d. 30 to 40 mEq. of potassium chloride (only after the urinary output reaches 1,000 ml. per day)

e. 20 mEq. of potassium chloride for each 1,000 ml. of vomitus replaced

f. 44 to 88 mEq. of sodium bicarbonate in cases of marked acidosis (run frequent EKG determinations so that any dangerous fall in potassium can be detected)

g. 30 to 40 g. of sodium glutamate in glucose and water (if liver insufficiency or ammonium toxicity is present)

10. The total infusion should be divided into morning and late afternoon infusions. This cuts down the period of starvation between the end of one infusion and the start of the next. Because the body can only utilize 0.5 g. of glucose per Kg. of body weight, it is wise to run the infusion slowly. This means that the body can only utilize about 30 to 50 g. of glucose per hour. If the infusion is run at a more rapid rate, dehydration secondary to the osmotic diuresis may result.

11. The above regimen is concerned only with the replacement of fluids and electrolytes. In treatment of these cases, the standard regimen—which includes sedation, vitamins, psychotherapy, and antiemetics—should be employed.

12. Only rarely is it necessary to interrupt the pregnancy.

8 Antepartum Fetal Evaluation

David H. Fields

DEFINITION

1. Tests performed on the fetus before the onset of labor may be to evaluate morphology, well-being, growth, and/or maturity.
2. They may be invasive or noninvasive, and chemical or biophysical.

TESTS TO EVALUATE FETAL MORPHOLOGY OR GENETIC STRUCTURE

Basic Principles

1. It has become increasingly possible to detect abnormalities of fetal development during the first few months of pregnancy. With this ability has come the demand for such information.
2. The two most commonly sought pieces of information concern fetal chromosomal abnormalities and open neural tube defects (NTDs), although many other diseases are detectable (see below).
3. Several procedures are available to determine if fetal structural development is normal. Some of these may be used to obtain more than one type of information.
4. Sometimes abnormalities are found whose significance is not certain. In these cases, the parents are faced with difficult decisions regarding their course of action.

KARYOTYPING

Basic Principles

1. Chromosomal abnormalities are not rare. They account for more than 50 per cent of all spontaneous abortions and almost 1 per cent of all unscreened live births.
2. Although some anomalies are repeatedly inheritable (e.g., balanced translocations), most occur in cases where the mother has no such history.
3. Chromosomal abnormalities occur with greater frequency as maternal age increases. To a much lesser extent, they are also related to paternal age. The overall risk of a chromosomally abnormal baby parallels maternal age roughly as follows:

Maternal age	Risk
under 30	<1/500
30	1/450
31	1/400
32	1/350
33	1/300
34	1/225
35	1/185
36	1/150
37	1/110
38	1/90
39	1/70
40	1/50

4. Approximately half of all chromosomally anomalous babies have Down's syndrome (trisomy 21).
5. These abnormal fetuses are detectable by karyotyping fetal cells obtained antenatally.

6. The methods for obtaining these cells (amniocentesis and chorionic villus sampling [CVS]) are not without risk.

Indications

1. Standard of care dictates that karyotyping be recommended to all of the following women:
   a. Age 35 or over
   b. Parental chromosomal anomaly
   c. Previous child with chromosomal anomaly
   d. Risk of a sex-linked disorder, requiring fetal sex determination
2. Many women not in these categories opt for kayotyping even if their risk for bearing a chromosomally abnormal fetus is lower than their risk for a miscarriage from amniocentesis.

Timing

1. Sampling should be done as early as possible to allow for early termination of pregnancy, if necessary.
   a. By CVS, usually between the seventh and tenth weeks
   b. By amniocentesis, usually between the sixteenth and eighteenth weeks

Methods and Interpretation

1. Cells for culture may be obtained by
   a. Amniocentesis
   b. CVS
2. Using banding techniques, abnormal and missing chromosomes may be identified and fetal sex determined.

Pitfalls

1. Karyotyping is > 99 per cent accurate. If a 46, XX complement results, there is a small possibility that maternal cells have been mistakenly harvested.
2. Occasionally fetal cells fail to grow in culture and another sample needs to be obtained. This is rare today.
3. The risk of the test is that of the method used to obtain the cells (CVS or amniocentesis).

FETAL SEX DETERMINATION

Basic Principles

The fetal sex may be determined either by karyotyping or by ultrasonic visualization of the genitalia.

Indications

When there is a considerable risk of a sex-linked hereditary disorder such as Duchenne's muscular dystrophy or hemophilia.

Timing

As early as possible, depending on the method used.

Methods

1. CVS or amniocentesis for karyotyping
2. Ultrasound for visualization of fetal genitalia

ALPHA-FETOPROTEIN (AFP) DETERMINATION

Basic Principles

1. AFP is made by the fetal yolk sac and liver and secreted into the fetal serum. It then passes into the amniotic fluid (AF) and, finally, into the maternal serum.
2. Certain fetal abnormalities lead to increased levels of AFP in both the AF and the maternal serum. These include:
   a. Open NTDs
   b. Ventral abdominal wall defects, esophageal and duodenal atresias
   c. Pilonidal sinus and sacrococcygeal teratoma
   d. Fetal urinary tract disease, such as congenital nephrosis, renal agenesis, and bladder neck obstruction
   e. XO karyotype
   f. Fetal death

3. While elevations of maternal serum AFP do not reliably identify these abnormalities, normal maternal serum AFPs reduce the likelihood of these abnormalities to almost zero.

Indications

1. Maternal serum AFP screening is indicated in all pregnancies.

2. Women who have had a previous pregnancy complicated by an NTD have up to a five-per-cent risk of another.

Timing

1. Standardized curves for normal AFP levels are available for between 15 and 22 weeks.

2. Since the technique (see below) may require two samples and follow-up amniocentesis, obtain the first sample as soon as possible after the fifteenth week.

Method and Interpretation

1. Obtain the first sample of maternal blood as soon as possible between 15 and 22 weeks. If this is in the normal range the fetus is almost certainly without an open NTD or other predisposing abnormality (see above). Of 1,000 samples, 950 will be normal.

2. If the first sample is elevated (50 out of 1,000 will be), repeat the sample. If the repeat sample is in the normal range, this is statistically the same as if the first sample were normal. Of the 50 repeated samples, 30 will be normal.

3. If both samples have been elevated (20 of the original 1,000), perform ultrasound. If an explanation for the elevation is discovered (larger, older fetus than suspected, twins, visible defect), either recompute or act appropriately. Ultrasonography will be explanatory in 5 of these 20 cases.

4. If the ultrasound examination is not explanatory (15 of the 20), perform an amniocentesis and analyze the fluid for AFP and acetylcholinesterase.

5. If the amniotic fluid AFP and AChE are normal, the fetus may be assumed to be free of open NTD or associated anomaly (13 or 14 out of the 15 remaining cases). If either is abnormal, there is a presumptive NTD, ventral wall defect, or other abnormality (1 or 2 of the 15). The presence of acetylcholinesterase in the amniotic fluid may be considered diagnostic for an NTD.

Pitfalls

1. Most maternal serum AFPs are not associated with disease. AFP may be elevated spuriously by

- **a.** A mistake in gestational dating
- **b.** Macrosomia
- **c.** Multiple gestation
- **d.** Unknown: of 1,000 initial samples, 50 will be elevated. There will be no explanation for approximately 90 per cent of these.

2. AF AFP may be falsely elevated by a bloody tap.

OTHER PRENATALLY DETECTABLE DISEASES

Basic Principles

A host of inheritable diseases may be detected by analysis of either fetal cells, fetal blood, or amniotic fluid.

Indications for Testing

1. If both parents are heterozygous for a recessive gene which is dangerous if present homozygously.

2. If one parent carries a dominant or sex-linked gene which is dangerous.

3. A partial listing of hundreds of disorders follows:

- **a.** Inborn errors of metabolism
- **b.** Hemoglobinopathies
- **c.** Hemophilias

Timing

Usually between the sixteenth and nineteenth weeks, at the time of amniocentesis or fetoscopy.

Indications

A high index of suspicion, based on either parental history or previously affected pregnancy.

TESTS OF FETAL WELL-BEING

General Principles

These tests indirectly assess placental function, since antepartum fetal jeopardy is usually secondary to placental insufficiency. There are four basic categories of tests:

1. Biochemical measurement of substances produced by healthy placentas (estriol, human placental lactogen)

2. Functional evaluation of fetal oxygen reserve (stress and nonstress testing, fetal activity determination, biophysical profile)

3. Evaluation of serial fetal growth (serial ultrasonography)

4. Direct observation of fetus and amniotic fluid to detect signs of distress such as meconium (amnioscopy, fetoscopy)

BIOCHEMICAL TESTS OF FETAL WELL-BEING

Biochemical assessment of the feto-placental unit has largely been replaced by functional tests of fetal well-being because of inaccuracies and delays inherent in these techniques. The two major assays, for estriol and for human placental lactogen, are discussed briefly below but are rarely employed in clinical practice.

Estriol Measurement

1. Basic Principles

a. Estriol, estetrol, and quinestrol are three estrogen products of the feto-placental unit which reflect fetal health. Most work has been done with estriol.

b. Made in the placenta from precursors supplied by the fetus, estriol is secreted into the maternal circulation, then conjugated by the maternal liver and excreted into the maternal urine.

c. It may be measured in either the maternal plasma or the maternal urine.

d. Serial measurement of estriol levels would seemingly be a useful tool for evaluating the fetus. In practice, however, it is subject to limitations which make it less than ideal.

e. Its use has been largely replaced by functional testing.

2. Pitfalls

a. Deteriorating placental condition cannot be diagnosed in fewer than several days, because of the need to establish baseline measurements.

b. Estriol measurements may be artefactually lowered by maternal liver or kidney disease, incomplete urine collection, many drugs (e.g., ampicillin), or decreases in the supply of fetal precursors.

Human Placental Lactogen (HPL)

HPL is a substance produced solely by the placenta and secreted into maternal serum where its levels continue to increase until approximately the thirty-sixth week of gestation.

1. Pitfalls

a. Attempts to correlate HPL levels with fetal well-being have not been as promising as was originally hoped, largely because the presence of HPL reflects placental mass more than fetal condition. Consequently, large placentas may be associated with high levels of HPL, even when the fetus is in jeopardy, and small placentas with falsely low values.

b. Like estriol measurement, HPL assay is subject to wide fluctuation and delay in diagnosis of deteriorating fetal condition.

c. Like estriol measurement, it has been largely replaced by functional testing.

FUNCTIONAL TESTS OF FETAL WELL-BEING

Nonstress Test (NST)

1. Basic Principles

a. The healthy fetus moves with regularity.

b. In response to these movements, there is acceleration of the fetal heart rate (FHR).

c. The healthy fetus exhibits a certain amount of variability (5 to 15 b.p.m.) in its baseline FHR.

d. Changes in these parameters may be detected before fetal damage from hypoxia occurs.

2. Indications

a. Suspicion of uteroplacental insufficiency

(1) Decreased fetal movement

(2) Post-dates pregnancy

b. Monitoring high-risk pregnancies complicated by

(1) Preeclampsia, hypertension

(2) Diabetes

(3) Active Rh disease

(4) Other medical conditions (e.g., hyperthyroidism, collagen vascular diseases, cardiovascular disease)

(5) Previous stillbirth

3. Timing

a. NSTs are begun as soon as a problem is suspected and delivery is an alternative.

b. For monitoring a high-risk pregnancy, they are usually begun between the twenty-eighth and thirty-second weeks.

c. If reassuring, they are repeated every 2 to 7 days, depending on the condition being monitored.

4. Procedure

a. Begin with electronic FHR monitoring and uterine contraction monitoring.

b. Instruct the mother to depress the tocodynamometer each time the fetus moves.

c. Continue the test for 20 minutes if the criteria for a reactive test (see below) are met and for at least 40 minutes if they are not.

5. Interpretation

a. *Reactive NST.* Indicates a healthy fetus.

(1) Good baseline variability and rate.

(2) Two fetal movements within 10 minutes, each accompanied by acceleration of the FHR by at least 15 b.p.m. for at least 45 seconds.

b. *Nonreactive NST.* Fetal status is uncertain, perform contraction stress test (CST).

(1) Baseline is abnormal or variability is lacking.

(2) Fetus will not move sufficiently.

(3) FHR does not change with fetal movement.

6. Pitfalls

a. A sleeping fetus exhibits less activity and less FHR reactivity. A nonreactive NST must be continued for at least 40 minutes to be sure of traversing one whole fetal sleep-wake cycle.

b. If the mother is hypoglycemic, a nonreactive NST may result. Try repeating the test after a sugar load (orange juice?).

c. A nonreactive NST is suggestive of a compromised fetus but is not sufficient evidence by itself to mandate delivery. The situation must be further evaluated by CST or by biophysical profile (BPP).

7. Contraindications

None.

Contraction Stress Test (CST)

1. Basic Principles

a. This test is based on the fact that a fetus suffering the effects of even borderline placental insufficiency will show evidence of hypoxia via FHR monitoring during minimal stress.

b. This stress is applied in the form of contractions, during which blood flow to the placenta, and hence oxygen to the fetus, are cut off.

c. We can thus unmask those fetuses in such poor condition that they cannot tolerate 30 seconds of "breath-holding."

2. Indications

a. *Nonreactive NST.* Since most fetal jeopardy is investigated initially using the NST, the CST is used primarily to investigate those fetuses who cannot be certified as healthy by the simpler test.

b. *Oligohydramnios and Post-Dates Pregnancy.* In these two conditions cord compromise is as important a consideration as placental insufficiency. The contractions of the CST will reveal these more effectively than will an NST.

3. Timing

a. Like the NST, the CST may be used at any time in the third trimester when delivery is an option for the distressed fetus.

b. Also like the NST, it is repeated every 2 to 7 days, depending on the condition being monitored.

4. Methods

a. Contractions may be spontaneous or induced, either by nipple stimulation or by intravenous oxytocin in minute amounts.

b. Perform pelvic exam for cervical assessment.

c. Establish a baseline of 15 to 20 minutes by monitoring the fetus using an external FHR transducer and tocodynamometer (this is an NST). Pay particular attention to maternal position (reclining at about 45 degrees with perhaps a slight tilt to the side) since the production of aortocaval compression and maternal supine hypotension may artefactually decrease placental perfusion and result in a false-positive test.

d. If there are no contractions or fewer than 3 contractions per 10 minutes which are not associated with abnormal FHR patterns, begin either nipple stimulation or IV oxytocin drip by infusion pump. If using oxytocin, begin at 1 mU./minute and double every 20 minutes until 3 contractions of 40 to 60-second duration occur in 10 minutes or until repetitive late decelerations (usually 3 in a row) occur.

5. Interpretation

a. *Negative Test.* There are no late (Type II) decelerations in the FHR while the mother is having 3 contractions per 10 minutes. A negative test is very good evidence of a fetus not in distress at that moment who will tolerate continued intrauterine existence for one week. IT DOES NOT PREDICT THE OUTCOME OF LABOR, which involves much greater stress.

b. *Positive Test.* The FHR exhibits repetitive late decelerations while being stressed by NO MORE THAN 3 contractions per 10 minutes. Presumably, the fetus that shows this response with less stress is in greater jeopardy. A positive CST has been associated with a significant incidence of intrauterine death within 1 week and even within 72 hours. There is also, however, a 25-per-cent likelihood of a false-positive test.

c. *Suspicious Test.* If the FHR shows late decelerations after some but not all contractions, at a contraction rate of not more than 3 per 10 minutes, the meaning of the test is not clear; it should be repeated in 24 hours.

d. *Hyperstimulation.* If uterine contractions occur too frequently (more than 4 per 10 minutes) or last too long (greater than 90 seconds), one cannot interpret the significance of late deceleration. Under these circumstances the test should be repeated within 24 hours. If on repeat there are no late decelerations, the test is negative.

e. *Unsatisfactory.* The test cannot be interpreted if:

(1) There is a poor quality FHR recording, so that late deceleration cannot be determined.

(2) There are fewer than three contractions per 10 minutes (unless the test is positive), so that the fetus has not been stressed enough to call the test negative. Repeat in 24 hours.

f. *Additional Interpretive Refinements*

(1) FHR variability greater than five beats per minute reflects a healthy fetus and rarely is associated with a positive test.

(2) Other Decelerations. Early (Type I) and/or variable (Type III) decelerations should not be interpreted as a positive test or as indicative of fetal jeopardy. Repeated variable decelerations, however, may reflect oligohydramnios or cord compression.

(3) Acceleration. Speeding of the FHR with contractions is generally considered to be a favorable sign.

6. Contraindications

Because the CST requires the production of uterine contractions, any condition under which this might be dangerous should preclude the use of this test. Common contraindications include:

a. Placenta Previa. Risk of hemorrhage

b. Previous Classic Cesarean Section. Risk of uterine rupture

c. Multiple Gestation. Risk of premature labor

d. Premature Rupture of Membranes. Risk of premature labor

e. Hydramnios. Risk of premature labor

f. Previous Premature Labor. Risk of premature labor

Biophysical Profile (BPP)

1. Basic Principles

a. Real-time ultrasound enables the obstetrician to obtain a sort of antenatal Apgar score on the fetus.

b. By assessing fetal tone, reactivity, breathing, and amniotic fluid, an indication of fetal well-being may be obtained.

2. Indications

a. Nonreactive NST and inconclusive CST.

b. Some are using the BPP to assess the well-being of all post-dates fetuses.

3. Timing

Same as for NST and CST.

4. Methods and Interpretation

a. Using real-time ultrasound, the fetus is observed for 30 minutes.

b. Two points are allotted for:

(1) An episode of extension and flexion

(2) Three body or limb movements

(3) 30 seconds of breathing movements

(4) One 1-cm. pocket of amniotic fluid

c. The sum of these scores is combined with either 2 points for a reactive NST or none for a nonreactive NST. A total of 8 or more points is indicative of a healthy fetus. A score below 6 indicates fetal jeopardy, and 6 is equivocal.

5. Contraindications

None.

EVALUATION OF FETAL SIZE AND GROWTH BY ULTRASONOGRAPHY (USG)

Basic Principles

1. The healthy fetus grows at a predictable rate when one corrects for different-sized fetuses.

2. The healthy fetus grows proportionally—i.e., head, body, and femur grow according to established norms.

3. By establishing a growth curve for the average fetus and also for the individual (see "Interpretation," below), placental supply may be indirectly evaluated by ultrasound.

4. The growth-retarded fetus may have symmetric intrauterine growth retardation (IUGR) (head, body, and limb growth all equally decreased) or asymmetric IUGR (growth of the head appears normal while body growth is stunted). Symmetric IUGR tends to be due to constitutional factors or congenital infection, while asymmetric IUGR usually reflects placental supply problems.

Indications

1. Uterus smaller or larger than dates by abdominal exam

2. All conditions under which abnormal fetal growth is suspected.

a. Common conditions predisposing to retarded growth (IUGR)

(1) Preeclampsia or chronic hypertension with vascular involvement

(2) Diabetes with vascular involvement

(3) Multiple gestation

(4) Conditions resulting in hypoxia, including severe maternal anemia and sickling disease, cyanotic heart disease, pregnancy at very high altitude, and maternal smoking

(5) Conditions resulting in poor fetal nutrition, including poor maternal weight gain and drug addiction (heroin, cocaine, alcohol)

(6) Intrauterine infections such as congenital rubella and cytomegalovirus

b. Common conditions predisposing to accelerated growth (macrosomatia)

(1) Diabetes without vascular disease

(2) Excess maternal weight gain

Timing

1. Obtain USG whenever

a. There is a discrepancy between gestational age by dates and size by exam.

b. One of the above maternal conditions is present

2. Repeat USG at 3- to 4-week intervals to assess continued growth.

Interpretation

1. Fetal size correlates with gestational age progressively less as the pegnancy advances, due to genetic and environmental factors affecting "normal" growth.

a. *First trimester.* Measurement of gestational sac and crown-rump length may date the pregnancy accurately to within 2 or 3 days.

b. *Second trimester.* BPD, trunk and femur length may date the fetus to within 7 to 10 days.

c. *Third trimester.* BPD, trunk and femur length measurements may be accurate to within 2 weeks.

2. The fetus is the right size for its age (within the limits above). Placental supply is probably acceptable.

3. The fetus is too small symmetrically. This may be due to any of the following:

a. Gestational age is less than expected. Reconsider.

b. Fetus is constitutionally small. One or both parents are small or there is history of small, otherwise normal babies.

c. Fetus is growth retarded. Suspect poor maternal nutrition, smoking, drug use, congenital infection, or chromosomal anomaly.

4. The fetus is too small asymmetrically. This suggests IUGR based on placental insufficiency until proven otherwise.

IUGR may diagnosed by any of three criteria:

a. The fetus is found by USG to be below the tenth percentile in size for its age, which has been previously and accurately established.

b. It has failed to grow in accordance with its own previously established growth curve.

c. Asymmetric IUGR is demonstrated on sonography.

5. The fetus is larger than expected. This may indicate

a. An older fetus than expected

b. A constitutionally large fetus

c. Macrosomia. Suspect gestational diabetes.

TESTS OF FETAL MATURITY

These are designed to predict the fetus's ability to survive in the outside world. They fall into two groups: tests on amniotic fluid, designed to assess functional maturity, and USG, which attempts to date the pregnancy accurately and enable the physician statistically to predict maturity based on age.

TESTS ON AMNIOTIC FLUID—LECITHIN/SPHINGOMYELIN RATIO (L/S RATIO)

The most commonly accepted test of fetal maturity is determination of the L/S ratio of amniotic fluid. Since the major cause of morbidity and mortality in premature infants is respiratory distress syndrome (RDS), the most reasonable measure of fetal "survivabililty" is lung function.

Basic Principles

1. As the fetal lungs begin to mature, Type II pneumocytes within the alveoli produce increasing amounts of surfactant, actually a combination of surface tension-reducing phospholipids, called lecithins, which prevent atelectasis after birth. Initially, two lecithins, phosphatidylcholine (PC) and phosphatidylinositol (PI), are produced. Four to five weeks before term, however, PI production is replaced by phosphatidylglycerol (PG) production.

2. PC, PI, and PG are secreted by the pneumocytes and carried by the fetal breathing movements into the amniotic fluid. The likelihood of RDS may be estimated by measuring the concentrations of these lecithins in the amniotic fluid.

3. These concentrations are expressed in relation to the amount of another phospholipid, sphingomyelin, as the lecithin/sphingomyelin ratio, or L/S ratio. Additionally, a separate measurement of the amount of PG is made.

4. If the L/S ratio and the total amount of PG are high enough, the likelihood of RDS is extremely small.

Indications

Either planned or likely early delivery for any reason. Most commonly for:

1. Maternal diabetes
2. Preeclampsia
3. Premature rupture of membranes
4. Repeat cesarean section
5. Rh-sensitized pregnancy

Contraindications

The only contraindication to amniocentesis is a relative one, the anterior placenta. Its importance varies conversely with the need to know about fetal maturity.

Interpretation

1. An L/S ratio greater than 2 indicates a fetus with mature lungs. The incidence of RDS is very small (less than 2 per cent) and of fatal RDS virtually nil (0.1 per cent), and is largely limited to fetuses that suffer intrapartum hypoxic distress or whose mothers are diabetic. Now that PG can be measured directly, its presence is known to be associated with an extremely small risk of RDS, even in diabetic pregnancies.

2. If the L/S ratio is between 1.5 and 2, RDS may occur in 25 to 40 per cent of births but will rarely be fatal.

3. If the L/S ratio is below 1.5, up to 75 per cent of fetuses will develop RDS, often severe. Because of advances in neonatal management, fatal RDS is much less common, so that most fetuses with L/S ratios greater than 1 will survive.

Pitfalls

1. Infants of diabetic mothers seem to develop RDS more often than other infants in the face of an L/S ratio of 2 or even higher. This risk may be obviated by measurement of PG, the presence of which seems to accurately predict lung maturity even in diabetic pregnancies.

2. Meconium staining lowers the L/S ratio at any level. The detection of PG, however, is NOT affected by contamination of the AF with either blood or meconium.

3. Contamination with maternal blood (serum) lowers the L/S ratio, if it is above 1.3.

4. Contamination of amniotic fluid with maternal urine (bladder tap) lowers both the L/S ratio and PG level at any level.

FOAM TEST

This is a test to functionally assess surfactant activity, which the physician may easily do himself.

Basic Principles

If the amniotic fluid contains enough surfactant, it will form a stable ring of bubbles upon shaking in a test tube. By diluting its concentration and repeating the test several times, one can measure surfactant activity.

Method

1. To five test tubes, add 1.0, 0.75, 0.50, 0.25, and 0.20 ml. of amniotic fluid, respectively. Then dilute the volume of the last four tubes to 1 ml. using normal saline.

2. Add 1 ml. of freshly prepared 95-per-cent ethanol to each tube.

3. Shake well, then rest in a stand. Do not move before reading.

4. Observe each tube for a stable ring of bubbles around the periphery.

Interpretation

1. Negative. No complete ring of bubbles in any tube; this usually correlates with L/S ratio of less than 1.5.

2. Intermediate. A complete ring of bubbles in one or two tubes; this usually correlates with an L/S ratio of 1.5 to 2.

3. Positive. A complete ring of bubbles in three tubes; this usually correlates with an L/S ratio greater than 2.0. *N.B.* A positive test is a very good predictor of a fetus that will not develop RDS. A negative or intermediate test is less reliable and should be checked by L/S ratio measurement.

Pitfalls

1. False-negative results may occur from any of the following:

- **a.** Dirty glassware
- **b.** Old alcohol
- **c.** Failure to shake sufficiently
- **d.** Wrong diameter test tubes (8 to 14 mm. is acceptable)

2. False-positive tests may occur in the presence of meconium, vaginal secretions, or enough blood to result in a 3-per-cent hematocrit.

AMNIOTIC FLUID—CREATININE

Basic Principles

1. As the fetus grows and its kidneys mature, creatinine levels in the AF increase. High-enough levels usually indicate a fetus large enough to be mature.

2. Because of the relatively inconstant relationship between fetal size and lung maturity, this test has been largely replaced by the L/S ratio and PG determination.

Interpretation

Levels greater than 2 mg. per 100 ml. have been associated with a mature fetus.

Pitfalls

Amniotic fluid creatinine level concentration varies directly with maturity of fetal kidney, muscle mass of fetus, and maternal serum creatinine levels. Falsely high levels may occur with high maternal creatinine or with a macrosomic fetus.

AMNIOTIC FLUID BILIRUBIN DETERMINATION

Basic Principles

1. In the second half of pregnancy, amniotic fluid bilirubin tends to decrease, reaching zero at term. The absence of bilirubin in AF has therefore been used to infer fetal maturity.

2. Like AF creatinine, however, it correlates much less well with lung maturity than do the L/S ratio and PG concentration, measurements of which have largely replaced it.

Method

1. Obtain amnoitic fluid.

2. Protect from light since bilirubin may be broken down from exposure to light.

3. Laboratory determination of bilirubin levels by spectrometry.

Interpretation

Levels of zero usually indicate a mature fetus; otherwise, prediction is very unreliable.

Pitfalls

1. Varies with maternal bilirubin
2. Increased in fetal hemolytic disease

ULTRASONOGRAPHY (USG)

Basic Principles

1. Except in pregnancies complicated by diabetes, lung function can almost always be presumed to be mature at 37 completed weeks.
2. Fetal age may be gauged either by early dating or by measurement of fetal size later.

Early Dating

1. Early accurate dating of the pregnancy is the best method for determining fetal age.
2. In most cases, physical examination in the first 8 to 10 weeks which correlates with a known last menstrual period (LMP) and regular menses (or often, these days, a known date of conception) is sufficient.
3. In the absence of any of these, USG measurement of the amniotic sac or of the fetal crown-rump length in the first trimester may effectively date the gestation to within 2 or 3 days.

Later Size Determination

1. After this early period, environmental and hereditary factors affecting growth progressively loosen the correlation between fetal size and age.
2. During most of the second trimester, BPD, trunk and femur length may date the fetus to within 7 to 10 days.
3. By the middle to late third trimester, these measurements (BPD, trunk and femur length) may be accurate only to ±2 weeks, rendering this method less useful unless the values obtained are far beyond 37 weeks.

SPECIFIC PROCEDURES

Amniocentesis

1. Definition

Puncture of the amnion and aspiration of amniotic fluid (AF)

2. Indications
   a. For Morphological Screening
      (1) Fetal karyotype from cultured cells
      (2) Presence or absence of NTD by measurement of AF alpha-fetoprotein (AFP) and acetylcholinesterase
      (3) Presence or absence of many inborn errors of metabolism by biochemical testing (e.g., for Tay-Sachs disease, Lesch-Nyhan syndrome, the aminoacidurias)
      (4) Presence or absence of hemoglobinopathies by enzyme restriction analysis
   b. For Fetal Well-being
      (1) Detection of fetal infection by culture of AF (e.g., for cytomegalovirus, rubella)
      (2) Determination of AF delta OD_{450} in erythroblastosis fetalis
   c. For Fetal Maturity
      (1) Determination of AF L/S ratio and phosphatidylglycerol
      (2) Determination of AF creatinine and bilirubin
3. Timing
   a. For genetic screening: 16 to 18 weeks is ideal, as there is a sufficient number of shed fetal skin cells and adequate AF. Such timing also allows the 3 to 4 weeks necessary to culture the cells and still have time to terminate the pregnancy, if necessary.
   b. For AFP determination: after the two serum AFPs have been performed and have failed to rule out an NTD. Since they are usually begun at 15 weeks, this is usually in the same time frame as for genetic studies (17 to 19 weeks).

c. For other studies: when the need arises, usually during the third trimester.

4. Technique

a. Determine position of fetus, placenta, cord, and suitable pocket of fluid with ultrasound. For third trimester amniocentesis, puncture site may be either fundal or suprapubic. If the suprapubic site is chosen, the mother must urinate before the procedure to avoid obtaining urine instead of AF.

b. Prep skin with an antiseptic such as povidone-iodine.

c. Inject skin and abdominal wall with 1 to 2 ml. of local anesthetic (some physicians skip this step).

d. Perform amniocentesis with long (6 in.) 20 or 22 gauge needle with stylet in predetermined area to predetermined depth.

e. Upon removal of stylet, free flow of AF should occur. Aspirate desired amount (usually 10 to 20 ml.) of AF.

f. Apply pressure to puncture site for several minutes after withdrawal of the needle.

g. If a third trimester tap, monitor FHR for 30 minutes afterward (longer if there is any evidence of the tap being traumatic).

h. Administer Rh immune globulin, 300 μg., if the mother is Rh (−).

5. Risks

a. Spontaneous abortion occurs in approximately 0.5 per cent, usually secondary to intrauterine infection or hemorrhage.

b. Inadvertent puncture of the fetus or cord is an extremely rare complication, especially since the introduction of real-time sonography.

c. Feto-maternal bleeding may occur with sensitization in Rh (−) women.

Chorionic Villus Sampling (CVS)

1. Definition

Aspiration of chorionic tissue from the first trimester pregnancy, usually transcervically

2. Indications

a. To obtain fetal cells for culture and analysis

b. For karyotyping and genetic studies which are performed on cells rather than on AF

c. May not be used to evaluate the risk of an NTD or any other disease which requires AF analysis

d. Because of the higher loss rate, CVS is currently recommended for women who are at high risk for an abnormality (and for whom early detection may be especially important) and who are willing to accept the higher risk of a miscarriage. For example, a woman who has a balanced translocation at chromosome 21 and who therefore runs a 50-per-cent risk of having a Down's syndrome fetus is an ideal candidate, while a woman who has been an infertility patient and has succeeded in conceiving after 2 years of trying is not.

3. Timing

Between the seventh and tenth weeks after the LMP, once fetal heart activity is certain and before filling of the uterine cavity

4. Technique

a. Establish fetal heart motion by ultrasound.

b. Prep the cervix with an antiseptic.

c. Insert a small (16–20 gauge) plastic catheter transcervically to the edge of the chorion under sonographic guidance.

d. Aspirate a small quantity of chorion with a syringe.

e. Verify the presence of chorionic villi with low-power magnification.

f. Remove the catheter.

g. Administer Rh immune globulin if the mother is Rh (−).

5. Risks

a. Spontaneous abortion is the essential risk. The likelihood of this is being lowered rapidly in many centers. Only a year or two ago it was as high as 5 to 8 per cent; many centers are now claiming loss rates as low as 1 to 2 per cent.

b. Feto-maternal transfusion with Rh sensitization is a smaller risk.

Fetoscopy

1. Definition

Visualization of the fetus by insertion of a scope into the amniotic sac

2. Indications

a. Primarily when fetal blood (or occasionally tissue) is required for genetic testing

b. May also be used to visualize the fetus when abnormalities are suspected but not definitely confirmable on ultrasound

3. Timing

Same as for amniocentesis, usually after the seventeenth week

4. Technique

a. As for amniocentesis, except that, instead of a long needle, a fiberoptic scope is used

b. Fetal blood may be obtained either from a vein on the fetal surface of the placenta or from an umbilical vein.

5. Risks

Essentially those of amniocentesis, except at a higher level. The spontaneous abortion rate following fetoscopy with blood sampling may be as high as 5 to 10 per cent, and the risks of infection and Rh sensitization are greater.

9 Conduct of Normal Labor

David H. Fields

DEFINITION

Normal labor is defined as periodic uterine contractions with progressive effacement and dilatation of the cervix.

BASIC PRINCIPLES

Labor is an acute event terminating the chronic process of pregnancy. Its object is the delivery of a healthy baby to a healthy mother (and father). Today, labor has become a social event as well, to be shared by the family unit. The aim of the obstetrician is to integrate all of the above factors to the benefit of all participants.

PREPARATION FOR LABOR

1. The patient and her husband should be advised to take part in a childbirth preparation course. She may not desire "prepared childbirth," but the physical exercises and psychological preparation from the course will ease her way, regardless of her needs during labor.

2. She should be advised to notify her physician early in the course of labor, so that careful observation of labor and preparation for delivery may be initiated with time to spare. *It is preferable to have a patient arrive in false labor rather than to have her arrive in the delivery room "fully dilated and pushing."*

3. She should be instructed in differentiating labor from Braxton Hicks contractions via the time-honored criteria:

a. Regular contractions at

b. Progressively shorter intervals which are

c. Painful in the fundus and

d. Not alleviated by walking around

e. A useful guide is six contractions in 1 hour, of 45 seconds' duration each.

ARRIVAL IN THE DELIVERY ROOM

1. A rapid but appropriate history should include the following information:

a. Expected date of confinement—last menstrual period

b. Time of onset of labor

c. Frequency of contractions

d. Presence or absence of amniotic fluid leakage

e. Presence or absence of abnormal bleeding

f. Past obstetrical history, especially size, presentation, and mode of delivery of previous children

g. Past medical history that may affect labor and delivery, especially diabetes, heart disease, epilepsy, respiratory disease, allergic history

2. A rapid but appropriate physical examination should include the following:

a. Vital signs

b. Abdominal examination to determine fetal lie and fetal heart rate (FHR).

Brief electronic fetal monitoring (EFM) to ascertain fetal well-being before proceeding with other measures is appropriate.

c. Sterile vaginal exam (not performed if there is a suspicion, by history or observation, of placenta previa) to assess:

(1) Cervical dilatation and effacement

(2) State of membranes—if necessary, via use of nitrazine paper or microscopic exam for ferning

(3) Fetal presenting part

(4) Pelvic architecture

(5) The sterile vaginal exam, almost an oxymoron, is most nearly achieved if one uses two hands—one to hold open the labia so that an antiseptic can be applied INSIDE them, and the other to do the exam with.

d. Routine examination of the heart, lungs, extremities, and neurologic condition

3. Routine orders for conduct of normal vertex labor are increasingly being questioned as inappropriate to the status of childbirth as a natural event, rather than a medical one. Each of those presented below is recommended for what we consider good reasons.

a. Modified nil per os. Because of decreased gastric motility, the likelihood of vomiting, and the ever-present risk of cesarean section, intake should be limited to small amounts of clear fluids and sucking candies.

b. Bed rest. If this is necessary, it should be in the left lateral recumbent position, especially for the patient who has received analgesia. For the unmedicated patient, sitting or semi-reclining is both more comfortable and preferable to lying supine since it prevents the hypotension associated with uterine compression of the vena cava. Intermittent ambulation is acceptable for short periods of time if the fetal condition has been demonstrated to be good.

c. The partial perineal preparation should be used merely to remove the hair from the likely area of episiotomy, if this is anticipated.

d. A mild cleansing or Fleet's enema may be used to empty the rectum to prevent fecal soilage of the delivery area as the fetus descends in the second stage of labor. While some consider it "adding insult to injury," the enema gives the additional benefits of a cleaner field of delivery and obviation of the need for a bowel movement for a couple of days postpartum. These advantages seem to outweigh the minor and brief discomfort imposed early in labor.

e. Contraindications to enema are:

(1) Ruptured membranes with unengaged fetal head and dilated cervix

(2) Imminent delivery

f. Bladder function: Spontaneous voiding should be encouraged; catheterization should be employed if necessary, but should not be routine.

g. Hematocrit should be determined, if not already known, on every patient on admission. If the hematocrit is less than 30, two units of crossmatched packed red blood cells should be available.

h. Urinalysis for sugar, acetone, and protein, on admission, to check for diabetes, starvation ketosis, and preeclampsia

i. Maternal vital signs should be recorded every hour.

j. The FHR and uterine contractions should be monitored continuously and electronically, if possible. If this is not possible, the FHR should be checked and recorded immediately at the end of a contraction, at least every 15 minutes in the first stage of labor, and every 5 minutes during the second stage. (For details of fetal monitoring, see Chap.11.)

k. I.V. fluids may be administered during a long labor to prevent dehydration. Since glucose may make the fetal brain more susceptible to hypoxic damage, glucose solutions should be used with caution. The fluids of choice are 0.9N NaCl (NS) or lactated Ringer's solution (RL) at 80 to 125 ml. per hour, with piggyback supplementation with D_5W as needed to prevent ketosis and hypoglycemia.

l. Analgesia/anesthesia should be administered as necessary. (See Chap. 12.)

m. Subsequent vaginal examinations:

(1) To assess progress of labor, usually at 1- to 2-hour intervals

(2) Immediately upon rupture of membranes, to rule out cord prolapse and assess cervical dilatation

(3) Upon notation of any FHR abnormality, to rule out cord prolapse and assess cervial dilatation

CRITERIA FOR FOLLOWING LABOR WITHOUT INTERVENTION

1. Progressive cervical dilatation of at least 1 to 2 cm. per hour after effacement.

2. Progressive descent of the fetal head and delivery within 1 to 2 hours after full cervical dilatation.

3. No ominous FHR changes, either by auscultation or by electronic monitoring.

4. No excessive vaginal bleeding.

5. If any of the above criteria are not met, the obstetrician will need to either stimulate or interrupt labor, or provide additional support for the fetus (see Chap. 11.)

10 Augmentation and Induction of Labor

David H. Fields

DEFINITIONS

1. *Augmentation:* Increasing the frequency or strength of contractions during labor already in progress.

2. *Induction:* Artificially producing contractions to terminate pregnancy when labor does not yet exist. There are two basic types of induction:

a. Third-trimester induction, the purpose of which is usually delivery of a live infant; and

b. Second-trimester induction, which is usually for purposes of abortion.

AUGMENTATION OF LABOR

Basic Principles

1. Should be performed when inadequate contractions seem to be the cause of poor progress in labor.

2. Is best accomplished using a quick-acting agent with a very short half-life, the dosage of which may be minutely adjusted.

3. Requires constant fetal (EFM) and maternal surveillance to avoid trauma to either.

Indications

1. Hypotonic labor. Contractions of less than optimal intensity or frequency in the face of an apparently adequate pelvis suggest the need for stimulation of labor, IF CERVICAL DILATION IS NOT PROCEEDING AT 1 to 2 CM./HOUR. If the labor pattern seems inadequate, but the cervix is dilating, the smart physican will keep hands off.

Contraindications

1. Cephalopelvic disproportion (CPD). If CPD is seriously suspected, augmentation of labor is contraindicated. In most cases, the situation is not so clear, and a cautious trial of augmentation may be preferable to the radiation exposure of x-ray pelvimetry or to immediate cesarean section (C/S). This presupposes good fetal condition and no other relative contraindications (see below).

2. Abnormal fetal presentation. If one has chosen to attempt vaginal delivery of a breech, one of the prerequisites is an easy labor. If labor does not progress well, this is an indication for C/S, not augmentation.

3. Conditions which predispose to uterine rupture. Common sense tells one that if labor is permissible for women who have had previous C/S and for grand multiparas, then augmentation, if one is careful, should be equally so. *Medically,* this is probably mostly true. *Medicolegally,* if uterine rupture were to occur under these circumstances, the physician would most likely be defenseless.

4. **Fetal distress.** This is an absolute contraindication to augmentation of labor.

Agents for Augmentation of Labor

1. At present, there is only one chemical agent for augmentation of labor: oxytocin

(Pitocin, Syntocinon). It is well suited for this purpose because it:

a. Is rapidly effective (within 10 to 20 minutes)

b. Has a short half-life (90 seconds)

c. May be dissolved in crystalloid solution for I.V. administration (so the dosage is finely tunable.)

This means that if labor becomes too strong because of overstimulation, the drug may be withdrawn and its effect will abate within 5 minutes.

2. While oxytocin may be administered nasally, transbuccally, and intramuscularly as well as I.V., these routes have all fallen by the wayside because I.V. administration affords much more control. For even greater safety, it should be administered by infusion pump, which guarantees precisely the desired rate of flow.

Technique for Augmentation of Labor

1. Prepare infusion by adding 10 units oxytocin to 1,000 ml. normal saline (NS) or Ringer's Lactate (RL). Each ml. will then contain 10 milliunits of oxytocin.

2. Begin the infusion, using a pump, at 0.5 to 1 mU./min. (3 to 6 ml./hr.)

3. Increase the infusion rate by 1 mU./ml. every 20 minutes until adequate labor is obtained or fetal distress occurs.

4. If adequate labor cannot be obtained with less than 20 mU./min., re-evaluate, since it is likely that the labor is adequate and cervical dilatation is not occurring for other reasons. If 20 mU./min. is not sufficient, more usually is not better.

Risks

1. Hyperstimulation. Too much oxytocin will produce contractions which are too frequent, too long, and too strong. Contractions should not:

a. Last longer than 45 to 60 seconds

b. Occur more often than every 2 to 3 minutes

c. Be less than 1 minute apart

d. Be stronger than 60 mm. Hg (if intrauterine tocodynamometry is used)

2. Fetal distress. This is the major danger of hyperstimulation. The best way to avoid it is to avoid hyperstimulation. However, it may occur in the face of seemingly normal labor. If adequate fetal surveillance with EFM is performed, it should be detected early.

Appropriate action is, first of all, to stop the oxytocin. Then, immediately begin other measures described in Chap. 9

3. Uterine rupture. Almost never occuring in the absence of previous uterine trauma or superimposition of too much stimulation on unrecognized CPD for too long, this is a disaster best avoided by careful monitoring of contractions and maternal condition.

4. Hyponatremia. Oxytocin hinders free water clearance so that administration of large amounts (more than 40 mU./min.) in D_5W (no salt) may result in an inability to excrete the water. The resultant hyponatremia may cause coma and convulsions and is avoidable by administering the oxytocin in a salt solution (NS or RL).

5. Postpartum hemorrhage. There seems to be an increased likelihood of uterine atony after long, hard, oxytocin-driven labors. This may best be avoided by continuing the oxytocin for 1 hour after delivery.

THIRD-TRIMESTER INDUCTION

Basic Principles

1. Should be performed when the physician wants to terminate pregnancy and there is no contraindication to labor

2. Is best controlled using a quick-acting agent with a very short half-life, whose effects can be turned on and off quickly, i.e., intravenous oxytocin via continuous infusion

3. Must be continuously monitored by a physician in attendance

Indications

1. Maternal Jeopardy. Severe preeclampsia/eclampsia, severe cardiovascular disease, placental abruption, premature rupture of membranes, intrauterine fetal death with coagulation abnormalities, or maternal malignancy, to name a few.

2. Fetal Jeopardy. Hemolytic Rh disease, placental abruption, fetal distress as determined by tests of fetal well-being, regardless of etiology.

Although fetal jeopardy makes successful induction less likely, it does not make it impossible. Before beginning the induction, all possible measures to improve fetal condition should be implemented, including maternal hydration and oxygenation and intensive EFM. Additionally, C/S should be prepared for in advance so that if fetal distress does occur, there need be no delay in delivery. Approximately 25 per cent of fetuses that have a positive CST may successfully withstand labor induced under such conditions.

3. High-Risk Pregnancy, Easily and Safely Delivered. If continued pregnancy poses a significant but not immediate risk to either mother or fetus (diabetes, premature rupture of membranes, mild preeclampsia, post-dates pregnancy) and if the fetus is mature (L/S ratio >2, PG present, positive foam test, biparietal diameter >37 weeks) and if the cervix is easily inducible (soft, midposition to anterior, somewhat effaced), induction of labor should probably be undertaken.

4. Elective induction of labor for the convenience of either the patient or the obstetrician has become a very controversial area. If the fetus is unquestionably mature and the cervix ripe (see above) and if the labor is carefully conducted and monitored, elective induction should be as safe as spontaneous labor. However, the risks should be discussed with the patient in advance.

Contraindications

Since a carefully conducted induced labor should mimic an ideal labor, the contraindications to induction should be identical to the contraindications to labor and vaginal delivery:

1. Known or suspected cephalopelvic disproportion

2. Placenta previa

3. Abnormal fetal presentation or lie

4. Previous cesarean section

5. Previous vaginal reconstructive surgery

6. Grand multiparity—medically, this condition demands a very careful and gentle induction. Medicolegally, if uterine rupture were to occur, the physician would probably be defenseless.

Agents for Induction of Labor

1. Chemical

a. At present, as for augmentation of labor, there is only one chemical agent available for induction of labor: oxytocin (Pitocin, Syntocinon).

b. For details of its use, see "Agents for Augmentation of Labor," above.

c. Prostaglandins of the E and $F_{2\alpha}$ classes are currently under investigation for third-trimester induction of labor. They may be administered orally, nasally, intravenously, vaginally, or intramuscularly. Due to the high incidence of disturbing side effects (nausea, vomiting, diarrhea, fever, flushing, and sweating), they may offer no advantage over oxytocin.

d. Prostaglandin E gel applied vaginally has great promise as an agent to ripen the cervix. Pretreatment will certainly convert many failed inductions into successful ones as soon as it is approved for general use.

2. Physical: Amniotomy

a. Initially used as a method of induction by itself, artificial rupture of the membranes has become an adjunct to oxytocin-induced labor. Traditionally performed at the beginning of an induction, this practice often results in long labors with ruptured membranes, which are then complicated by amnionitis.

b. It makes more sense to postpone amniotomy until after good contractions have been established and some cervical change produced.

Techiques for Induction of Labor

1. Before Induction

a. All preparations as for natural spontaneous labor (see "Conduct of Normal Labor," Chap.9)

b. External fetal heart rate and uterine-contraction monitoring should precede induction to document fetal condition and absence of labor.

2. Intravenous Oxytocin

a. Prepare infusion by adding 10 units oxytocin to 1,000 ml. NS or RL. Each ml. will then contain 10 milliunits of oxytocin.

b. Begin the infusion, using a pump, at 0.5 to 1 mU./min. (3 to 6 ml./hr.).

c. Increase the infusion rate by 1 mU./ml. every 20 minutes until adequate labor is obtained or fetal distress occurs.

d. Many will double the infusion rate every 20 to 30 minutes until a nearly satisfactory labor pattern is obtained, then revert to 1 mU./ml. every 20 minutes for fine tuning.

e. If adequate labor cannot be obtained with 20 to 30 mU./min., more is not likely to suffice either, and the induction will fail. If this happens, one has the option of C/S (usually) or serial induction, which amounts to trying again tomorrow.

3. Amniotomy

a. Standard prep for sterile vaginal examination

b. Check fetal heart rate, preferably with continuous monitoring.

c. Feel amnion through dilated cervix and locate fetal head.

d. Rupture membranes as anteriorly as possible with Amnihook or similar device.

e. Allow fluid to escape while maintaining or guiding fetal head against the cervix using fundal pressure and intravaginal hand.

f. DO NOT REMOVE INTRAVAGINAL HAND UNTIL FETAL HEAD IS FIRMLY APPLIED TO CERVIX AND OVERT CORD PROLAPSE HAS BEEN RULED OUT.

g. Recheck fetal heart rate.

How to Judge the Quality of Induced Labor

1. If the monitor shows no evidence of fetal distress (late decelerations, fetal tachycardia or bradycardia) the labor is not too strong. Obviously, if there is evidence of fetal distress, the labor, no matter how poor, is too vigorous.

2. If the cervix is showing the effects of labor (progressive effacement and dilatation), the labor is not too weak.

3. If the cervix is not dilating and contractions seem to be of good quality and frequency, two steps should be taken:

a. Re-evaluate for CPD.

b. Institute internal uterine contraction monitoring to measure the actual strength of contractions.

Risks of Induction

1. Fetal Prematurity. Traditionally, the most common complication of induced labor. If induction is for medical reasons, the risk of prematurity should be weighed against that of continued pregnancy. Before elective induction, fetal maturity should be documented by ultrasonography or L/S ratio.

2. Uterine Hypertonus. Early in induction, oxytocin may result in elevated resting uterine tone, rather than rhythmic contractions. This may be seen on the monitor as so-called pit contractions lasting upwards of several minutes. Unless there is an associated fetal bradycardia, the physician may observe, and it will pass as contractions become regular.

3. Hyperstimulation. See "Augmentation of Labor," above.

4. Fetal Distress. See "Augmentation of Labor."

5. Uterine Rupture. See "Augmentation of Labor."

6. Hyponatremia. See "Augmentation of Labor."

7. Postpartum Hemorrhage. See "Augmentation of Labor."

SECOND-TRIMESTER INDUCTION

Basic Principles

1. Usually done between 16 and 24 weeks gestation. There is rarely expectation of delivering a live child.

2. All considerations are for avoiding maternal morbidity and mortality.

3. The cervix is tremendously resistant to dilatation in the second trimester.

Indications

1. Elective abortion (16 to 20 weeks gestation)

2. Maternal jeopardy (16 to 24 weeks), usually severe cardiovascular or renal disease or malignancy

3. Abnormal fetus documented by amniocentesis (16 to 24 weeks)

Contraindications

1. *To all methods.* Previous uterine surgery predisposing to uterine rupture.

2. *To saline infusion.* Severe cardiac or renal disease, coagulopathy.

Agents

1. Hypertonic saline, intra-amniotic instillation

2. Hyperosmolar urea, intra-amniotic instillation

3. Prostaglandins ($F_{2\alpha}$, E), intra-amniotic instillation, extra-amniotic instillation, vaginal suppositories, intravenous infusion, oral ingestion

4. Intravenous oxytocin, usually used in combination with one of above agents

Intra-amniotic Hypertonic Saline: 20-per-cent NaCl

1. Methods

a. Prepare patient as for labor (N.P.O., S.S.E., bladder evacuation).

b. Begin sedation prior to instillation, usually a narcotic/tranquilizer combination (meperidine/promazine; morphine/diazepam).

c. Prepare and drape abdomen.

d. Infiltrate site of injection (usually 1 in. from midline and midway between symphysis pubis and top of fundus) with local anesthetic.

e. Perform amniocentesis using 14 or 16 gauge needle, and insert polyethylene tubing through needle into amnion. Remove needle.

f. Remove 100 to 300 ml. of amniotic fluid (as much as possible up to 300 ml.) and replace with an equal volume +50 ml. of 20-per-cent saline.

g. Begin infusion of high-dose oxytocin (50 to 100 milliunits/min.) intravenously within several hours.

h. Continue oxytocin infusion until at least 1 hour after delivery.

i. Delivery usually occurs within 48 hours. Instillation of intra-amniotic saline may be repeated once after 2 days if there has been little effect.

j. If after two instillations delivery cannot be effected, hysterotomy should be performed.

2. Risks

a. Hyperosmolar crisis (precipitated by hypertonic saline infusion)

b. Congestive heart failure (saline loading)

c. Disseminated intravascular coagulation (saline loading and placental necrosis)

d. Water intoxication (high-dose oxytocin without electrolyte solution)

e. Postpartum hemorrhage

f. Septic shock (prolonged labor)

g. Incomplete abortion (Approximately 20 to 50 per cent of patients will require curettage for complete removal of the placenta).

Intra-amniotic Hypertonic Urea: 30- to 40-per-cent Urea in 5-per-cent Glucose

1. Method

a. Prepare patient as for labor (N.P.O., S.S.E., bladder evacuation).

b. Begin sedation prior to instillation, usually a narcotic/tranquilizer combination (meperidine/promazine; morphine/diazepam).

c. Prepare and drape abdomen.

d. Infiltrate site of injection (usually 1 in. from midline and midway between symphysis pubis and top of fundus) with local anesthetic.

e. Perform amniocentesis using 14 or 16 gauge needle, and insert polyethylene tubing through needle into amnion. Remove needle.

f. Remove 100 to 300 ml. of amniotic fluid.

g. Replace with an equal volume of 30- to 40-per-cent urea in D_5W.

h. Begin infusion of high-dose oxytocin (300 to 400 mU./min.) intravenously.

i. Continue oxytocin until 1 hour after delivery.

2. Risks

a. Water intoxication (high-dose oxytocin)

b. Postpartum hemorrhage

c. Septic shock (prolonged labor)

d. Incomplete abortion

Unlike hypertonic saline, hypertonic urea crosses membranes easily. Therefore the risk of hyperosmolar crisis and congestive heart failure is much less. Disseminated intravascular coagulation is also much less likely than with saline.

Prostaglandins

1. Intra-amniotic Instillation

a. Prepare patient as for labor (N.P.O., S.S.E., bladder evacuation).

b. Begin sedation prior to instillation, usually a narcotic/tranquilizer combination (meperidine/promazine; morphine/diazepam).

c. Prepare and drape abdomen.

d. Infiltrate site of injection (usually 1 in. from midline and midway between symphysis pubis and top of fundus) with local anesthetic.

e. Perform amniocentesis using 14 or 16 gauge needle, insert polyethylene tubing through needle, and insert polyethylene tubing through needle into amnion. Remove needle.

f. Inject a test dose of 5 mg. (1 ml.) of prostaglandin $F_{2\alpha}$ (Prostin F2 alpha) slowly. Observe for reactions such as chest pain, vomiting, or bronchospasm.

g. After 5 minutes, inject an additional 35 mg. (7 ml.). Tape the catheter in place. Await labor.

h. If abortion is not imminent within 24 hours, a second dose of $PGF_{2\alpha}$ may be injected in the same fashion after verifying the catheter placement.

i. If labor and delivery are not imminent 24 hours after the second injection, or if the membranes rupture, oxytocin infusion is added until 1 hour after delivery.

2. Risks

a. Water intoxication (if oxytocin must be added)

b. Incomplete abortion (slightly higher than for hyperosmolar saline)

c. Nausea, vomiting, diarrhea, flushing, tachycardia, chest pain, and bronchospasm (all side effects of prostaglandins)

d. Sepsis (prolonged labor)

e. Postpartum hemorrhage

3. Other Routes for Prostaglandin Administration

Currently, these other methods of prostaglandin administration are experimental. In the near future they may be available.

a. *Extraovular.* Prostaglandin $F_{2\alpha}$ may be injected via pump through a balloon catheter inside the cervix, or placed there in a gel. This may be useful when amniotic fluid is scant, as from 13 to 15 weeks gestation.

b. *Vaginal Suppository.* PGE_2 is currently under investigation as a vaginal suppository. Its side effects are basically those of prostaglandins.

c. *Intravenous and Oral Prostaglandins.* At present, these seem to be characterized by a higher rate of side effects than the intra-amniotic or extraovular routes of administration.

11 Intrapartum Fetal Monitoring

David H. Fields

BASIC PRINCIPLES

1. The most stressful and dangerous part of pregnancy for the fetus is labor and delivery.

2. Fetal damage during labor is due to interruption of the fetal oxygen supply. This is usually (but not always) a progressive series of hypoxic events.

3. The fetal heart is more sensitive to oxygen deprivation than the fetal brain, so the fetal heart rate (FHR) changes secondary to hypoxia and asphyxia precede brain damage and death and can be used as an early warning system.

4. Continuous electronic FHR monitoring is a sensitive *screening* method for detecting these changes. Determination of fetal *p*H is an accurate method for evaluating the extent of oxygen deprivation and overall fetal condition.

5. These two methods, in combination, allow the doctor to detect fetal distress and correct it or terminate labor before permanent fetal damage occurs.

6. The gadgetry of fetal monitoring IS NOT a substitute for clinical judgment. It is a tool to provide the information one must have in order to exercise clinical judgment.

GLOSSARY OF FETAL MONITORING

Fetal Distress

Danger to the welfare of a fetus, usually on the basis of hypoxia, acidosis, or asphyxia

Biochemical Terms

Hypoxia—pO_2 below normal (for fetus, less than 20 torr)

Acidosis—*p*H below normal (for fetus, less than 7.20 to 7.25)

Asphyxia—Combined hypoxia and acidosis

Electronic Fetal Heart Rate Monitoring

Instantaneous fetal heart rate—The number of beats that the heart would make in 1 minute, calculated from the interval between any two consecutive beats (e.g., two beats are 1 second apart → IFHR of 60 b.p.m.; two beats are 1/2 second apart → IFHR of 120 b.p.m.)

Baseline fetal heart rate—The heart rate of an unstressed fetus between uterine contractions

Acceleration—Transient increase of fetal heart rate; usually associated with either fetal movement or mild stress, as seen in partial cord occlusion (see below); considered a sign of a fetus not in distress

Deceleration—Transient slowing of fetal heart rate

(Early) Type I deceleration (dip)—Repetitive, gradual decrease and recovery of fetal heart rate which inversely patterns associated uterine contraction (UC). Usually caused by increased vagal tone secondary to pressure exerted on the fetal head by the contraction, it reaches its nadir AT the peak of the contraction and recovers as the contraction wanes.

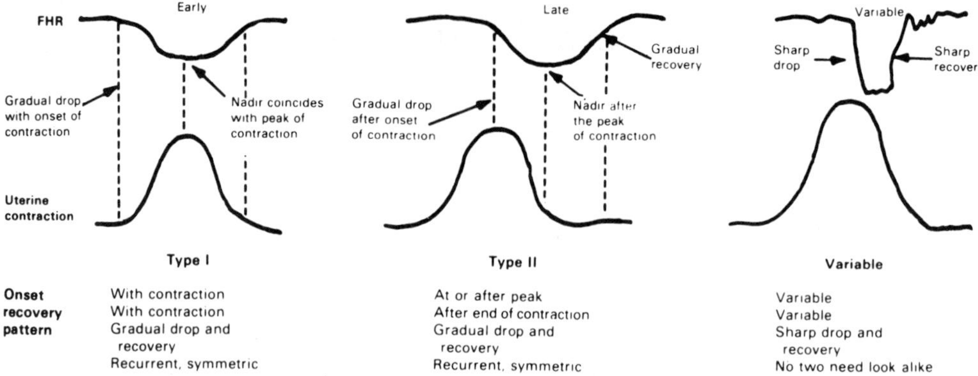

Fig. 11-1. Pattern of Contractions.

Type II deceleration—Repetitive, gradual drop and recovery of fetal heart rate which begins after beginning of UC, peaks near end of UC, and recovers after UC. The timing of this deceleration reflects the fact that placental flow is cut off early in the UC, resulting in hypoxia and deceleration by the middle or latter part. Since blood flow is not restored until late in the UC, recovery from the hypoxia cannot begin until near its end, so return to baseline begins AFTER its end.

Type III deceleration—Variable, sharp drop and recovery of fetal heart rate which may occur in any temporal relation to fetal heart rate and may or may not recur. Reflects complete occlusion of the umbilical cord, which results in a rapid rise in fetal blood pressure because umbilical arteries are occluded. A baroceptor response to the elevated blood pressure causes a very rapid decline in FHR, seen as a precipitous drop on the strip, with a ragged bottom. When the occlusion is relieved as the pressure of the UC wanes, the recovery is also extremely rapid.

Incomplete cord occlusion results in umbilical artery patency but in obstruction of the umbilical vein, so that venous return to the fetus is cut off. This causes fetal hypotension and tachycardia, and probably explains the minor accelerations that frequently precede and follow variable decelerations.

Combined—A late extension (functional Type II) may be superimposed over Types I or III if they are complicated by hypoxia.

Bradycardia—Persistent slowing of fetal heart rate to less than 100, OR baseline of less than 100

Tachycardia—Persistent increase of fetal heart rate to more than 180, OR baseline of more than 180

Variability

Short-term—Beat-to-beat variability (BBV) of instantaneous fetal heart rate reflects an interplay between the sympathetic and parasympathetic systems. Good variability (5 to 15 b.p.m.) is usually an indication of a healthy fetus, but typically increases and decreases in 20- to 30-minute cycles with the fetal sleep-wake cycle in utero.

Long-term—Undulations of baseline over several minutes

CONDUCT OF FETAL MONITORING DURING LABOR

External Electronic Monitoring (EEM)

1. All Labors

a. Begin monitoring of all labors with external fetal heart and uterine contraction sensors.

b. If adequate facilities are not available to monitor all labors, special consideration should be given to the following conditions, with initiation of electronic monitoring:

(1) Preeclampsia/eclampsia/chronic hypertension

(2) Diabetes mellitus

(3) Postdates labor

(4) Prematurity

(5) Suspected intrauterine growth retardation

(6) Oxytocin-induced or stimulated labor

(7) Prolonged labor

(8) Prolonged rupture of membranes

(9) Maternal cardiac or pulmonary disease likely to predispose to hypoxemia

(10) Labors requiring epidural anesthesia

2. Clear Recording/Reassuring Patterns

a. Continue EEM as long as the recording is clear and only reassuring patterns (see Table 11-1) are noted. This is acceptable because a normal FHR recording is very good evidence of a fetus not in distress. IT IS ALSO NONINVASIVE.

3. Unclear Recordings

a. Unclear FHR recording

(1) The Doppler or phonosensor may not be in good apposition to the mother's skin. REAPPLY THE SONOLUCENT JELLY.

(2) The fetus may have descended in the birth canal during the course of labor.

(a) RESEARCH MATERNAL ABDOMEN FOR AREA OF BEST RECORDING.

(b) ADJUST THE DEPTH FOCUS OF YOUR SENSOR IF YOUR EQUIPMENT HAS THIS FEATURE. Optimal depth is usually 8 to 12 cm.

(3) If it is impossible to obtain a clear recording of the FHR externally, SWITCH TO INTERNAL FHR MONITORING.

b. Unclear uterine contraction (UC) recording

Table 11-1. **Reassuring FHR Patterns**

a) Baseline FHR between 120 and 160 beats per minute (b.p.m.). 100 and 120 and 160 and 180 b.p.m., although not usual, are acceptable ranges if no other abnormal conditions are present.
b) Good short-term baseline variability (5 to 15 b.p.m.)
c) No change in FHR baseline with contractions
d) Accelerations of FHR with contractions or with fetal movement
e) Mild to moderate Type I decelerations

(1) The tocodynamometer may be too tightly or too loosely applied to the mother's abdomen. CHECK BY MANUAL PRESSURE ON THE TOCODYNAMOMETER TO MIMIC A UC.

(2) Shifts in maternal position tend to change the pressure against the tocodynamometer. TRY SHIFTING MATERNAL POSITION.

(3) If an adequate recording cannot be obtained, and there are periodic FHR changes which must be correlated with contractions, SWITCH TO INTERNAL UC MONITORING.

4. Ominous Patterns (See Table 11-2). Any ominous pattern present on EEM must be investigated further. The first step is to rule out an artefact by switching to internal electronic monitoring (IEM). In addition to being more reliable, IEM also gives more precise information regarding beat-to-beat variability.

Internal Electronic Monitoring (IEM)

1. When to Initiate. IEM should be used whenever an unclear recording or an ominous FHR pattern is obtained using EEM. Some physicians routinely use internal FHR monitoring when the fetal membranes are ruptured.

Table 11-2. **Nonreassuring FHR Patterns**

a) Tachycardia (more than 180 beats per minute [b.p.m.])
b) Bradycardia (less than 100 b.p.m.)
c) Decreased beat-to-beat variability (less than 5 b.p.m., unless this is the only abnormality or the mother received sedation or analgesia)
d) Severe early (Type I) deceleration (FHR drops to less than 60 b.p.m.)
e) Late (Type II) deceleration of any magnitude
f) Variable (Type III) deceleration of moderate to severe magnitude (FHR drops to less than 90 b.p.m. for more than 30 seconds.)

2. Clear Recording/Reassuring Patterns. If IEM is instituted and a clear recording and reassuring patterns are noted, continue until delivery. Like EEM, a normal FHR recording is very good evidence of a fetus not in distress.

3. Unclear Recording

a. Unclear FHR Recording

(1) Most monitors are keyed to respond to the R spike of the fetal EKG. If the electrode wires are reversed on the ground plate of the mother's legs, this may be read as a Q by the machine and not recorded properly. TRY REVERSING THE ATTACHMENT OF THE ELECTRODE WIRES TO THE GROUND PLATE. This is the simplest adjustment to make and should be tried first.

(2) Another common cause of an unclear FHR record using IEM is poor application of the electrode. CHECK THE APPLICATION OF THE ELECTRODE BY VAGINAL EXAM AND REAPPLY IF NECESSARY.

(3) If the recording is intermittently unclear and cannot be improved by the above measures, it may represent transient fetal arrhythmia. CHECK WITH A FETAL EKG STRIP.

b. Unclear UC Recording

(1) The problem easiest to remedy is a plug in the catheter. FLUSH THE SYSTEM WITH NORMAL SALINE AND RECALIBRATE.

(2) If the above does not work, the catheter may be out of position. ATTEMPT TO REPOSITION THE CATHETER.

4. Ominous Patterns. If IEM confirms the presence of an ominous pattern, a fetal scalp *p*H should be obtained and appropriate steps (see specific patterns below) taken immediately to correct the cause of the abnormal pattern (while awaiting *p*H results).

a. *Tachycardia*

(1) *Causes*

(a) Fetal Hypoxia/acidosis

(b) Maternal or fetal fever (amnionitis)

(c) Fetal arrhythmia—especially paroxysmal atrial tachycardia (PAT)

(c) Maternal medication such as scopolamine and atropine

(e) Prematurity

(2) *Diagnostic Steps*

(a) Perform pelvic examination to rule out cord prolapse and evaluate cervical dilatation.

(b) Obtain fetal *p*H.

(c) Take maternal temperature.

(d) Obtain fetal EKG to rule out PAT.

(e) Consider medications given.

b. *Bradycardia*

(1) *Causes*

(a) Hypoxia

(b) Arrhythmia (congenital heart block)

(c) Mistaken measurement of maternal heart rate

(2) *Diagnostic Steps*

(a) Perform pelvic examination to rule out cord prolapse and evaluate cervical dilatation.

(b) Obtain fetal *p*H.

(c) Obtain fetal EKG.

c. *Decreased Beat-to-Beat Variability (BBV)*

(1) *Causes*

(a) Asphyxia/acidosis

(b) Sedation and anticholinergic agents

(c) Tachycardia

(d) Sleeping baby

(2) *Diagnostic Steps*

(a) If decreased BBV occurs in the absence of any other ominous signs (HR normal, no decelerations), observe for 20 minutes to rule out sleeping baby.

(b) Review medications.

(c) If the mother has received no narcotics or anticholinergics, perform scalp *p*H.

d. *Late Deceleration*

(1) *Causes:* Hypoxia. Late decelerations, no matter how slight, are evidence of a fetus already in distress.

(2) *Diagnostic Steps*

(a) Perform pelvic examination to rule out cord involvement and assess cervical dilatation.

(b) Obtain fetal *p*H, pO_2.

(c) Obtain maternal blood pressure.

e. *Variable Deceleration, moderate to severe*

(1) *Causes.* Cord occlusion

(2) *Diagnostic Steps*

(a) Perform pelvic examination to rule out cord prolapse.

(b) Shift maternal position to see if pressure is relieved.

(c) Test fetal *p*H to determine severity of fetal compromise.

Scalp *p*H

1. Indications

a. Any of the conditions listed under "Ominous Patterns," above

2. Contraindications

a. Fetal coagulopathy (usually also a contraindication to labor)

3. Technique

a. Perform a sterile vaginal exam. If cervical dilatation is at least 3 to 4 cm., scalp sampling may be attempted.

b. Using a standard cone with light source, place the cone against the fetal scalp to prevent accumulation of amniotic fluid.

c. Swab the fetal scalp clean.

d. Apply silicone gel to facilitate beading of blood.

e. Perform puncture using depth-limited blade. Often a single puncture will not create an adequate drop of blood. In this case, two punctures in a cruciate pattern are usually adequate.

f. Collect the blood in a heparinized microliter capillary tube.

g. Observe the puncture site for bleeding. Apply pressure if necessary.

h. Insert the tube into the previously prepared *p*H meter.

3. Risks

a. Fetal hemorrhage from scalp puncture. Observe and apply pressure, if necessary.

b. Scalp infection. Use sterile technique. Clean puncture sites with antiseptic after delivery.

Continuous *p*H

Continuous *p*H electrodes are just now becoming commercially available. Their primary use will likely be in labors where repeated *p*H measurements are necessary; they should obviate the need for repeated fetal scalp punctures.

THERAPY FOR ABNORMAL PATTERNS

While Awaiting *p*H Results

Once fetal compromise is suspected or diagnosed, begin conservative therapeutic measures pending return of *p*H results. These therapeutic measures are based on strengthening the following links in the maternal-to-fetal oxygen chain.

1. To increase maternal pO_2:

a. Nasal O_2 at 10 L. per min.

2. To increase maternal cardiac output:

a. Place mother in left lateral position, relieving great vessel compression.

b. If regional anesthesia has been used, elevate legs and fluid load with Ringer's lactate solution.

c. Rule out shock.

3. To increase uterine blood flow:

a. Decrease intensity and frequency of uterine contractions by stopping oxytocin stimulation, if any.

b. In the near future, β-adrenergic uterolytic agents may be generally available to stop or slow spontaneous labors.

4. To increase placental function—NO MEASURES AVAILABLE.

5. To relieve obstruction of umbilical cord:

a. Change maternal position, usually to left lateral, then right lateral or Trendelenburg.

6. To increase fetal cardiac output—NO MEASURES AVAILABLE.

After Obtaining *p*H Results

1. If *p*H is more than 7.25, continue conservative therapeutic measures and repeat *p*H only if ominous patterns persist.

2. If *p*H is between 7.20 and 7.25, continue conservative measures and repeat *p*H in 20 to 30 minutes.

3. If *p*H is less than 7.20, repeat immediately and if confirmed, perform immediate delivery unless abnormal FHR patterns have reverted to normal. In this case, repeat *p*H in 15 minutes.

If *p*H Monitoring Is Not Available

If *p*H monitoring is not available, the abnormal FHR may be watched unless there are late decelerations, severe variable decelerations, or severe bradycardia or tachycardia. If any of these are present, the conservative therapeutic measures outlined above ("While Awaiting *p*H Results") should be applied for 15 to 30 minutes. If the FHR patterns have not reverted to normal by this time, immediate delivery should be performed—by forceps if safe, or by cesarean section.

12 Anesthesia and Analgesia

David H. Fields

DEFINITIONS

1. Analgesia. Pain relief without loss of sensation

2. Anesthesia. Loss of all sensation

3. General Anesthesia. Anesthesia by induction of loss of consciousness, usually via a combination of injectable and inhalation agents

4. Conduction Anesthesia. Anesthesia created over an area of the body by anesthetizing a major nerve trunk, also known as *regional anesthesia*

5. Local Anesthesia. Anesthesia in a given area by injection in that area

BASIC PRINCIPLES

1. Obstetrical anesthesia and analgesia are complicated by the attempt to provide the mother relief without affecting the fetus, treating "two patients at one time." This attempt is never wholly successful.

2. While anesthesia usually is needed for a given period of time, for a specific operative procedure, analgesic requirements during labor frequently seem open-ended.

3. The choice of analgesic agent or anesthetic method should be made taking into consideration such factors as:

a. Duration of action

b. Likelihood of causing fetal depression

c. Effect on mother's cardiorespiratory status (especially in women whose labors are complicated by hypertension, hemorrhage, or fetal distress)

d. Effect on labor

4. The need for analgesia during labor may be significantly decreased or eliminated by antepartum prepared-childbirth classes.

ANALGESIA

The basic purpose of analgesia during labor is to prevent undue maternal suffering. This is usually accomplished by using a narcotic analgesic, with or without a tranquilizing agent, or by epidural block (see "Anesthesia," below).

NARCOTIC ANALGESICS

Basic Principles

1. All agents in this class have essentially the same effects: pain relief and central nervous system depression (especially on consciousness and respiration).

2. Their effects are roughly proportional to dosage.

3. They all cross the placenta to cause fetal neurologic depression and sedation.

Advantages

1. They have a rapid onset of action and their effects are short-lived. When given in reasonable doses (meperidine 50 to 100 mg., morphine 5 to 10 mg.) their effects peak within 5 to 10 minutes (I.V.) or 30 to 60 minutes (I.M.), and are gone in 2 to 4 hours.

2. They have no effect on established labor.

3. They are easily and completely reversible. Virtually instantaneous and complete reversal of narcotic depression is obtained with naloxone (Narcan), a pure narcotic antagonist.

4. They may be administered by any physician.

Risks

1. Fetal respiratory depression at birth may be severe. Narcotic analgesics are a major cause of low Apgar scores.

2. Fetal heart-rate patterns as seen on electronic monitoring lose variability.

3. Complete pain relief is not obtained without loss of consciousness.

4. They create reflex nausea and vomiting of short duration.

Administration

1. Given either intravenously (quicker onset, shorter duration) or intramuscularly, doses of 50 to 100 mg. of meperidine (5 to 10 mg. of morphine) may be used either alone or with a tranquilizer (e.g., promethazine) as needed.

2. One should attempt to use as little as possible, but enough to do the job. A good end-point is no discomfort between contractions, combined with easily tolerable contractions.

3. Avoid giving a dose within 1 to 2 hours of delivery, if possible, to avoid neonatal depression. Since the fetal liver is not fully functional at birth, narcotic effects tend to persist in the neonate once he or she is separated from the mother's metabolic system.

4. Avoid administration too early in labor. Heavy doses of analgesia before 3 or 4 cm. cervical dilatation may slow or even stop early labor.

NARCOTIC ANTAGONISTS

1. Until recently, all narcotic antagonists (e.g., nalorphine, levallorphan) also had an agonist effect, severely limiting their usage and effectiveness.

2. Today, naloxone (Narcan), a pure antagonist with no depressive effect of its own, offers a safe effective method for reversing narcotic depression, both in the mother and in the neonate.

3. NALOXONE DOES NOT REVERSE DEPRESSION CAUSED BY ANY OTHER MEDICATIONS OR SITUATIONS. IT IS ONLY EFFECTIVE FOR COUNTERACTING NARCOTICS.

4. Dosage for naloxone is as follows:

a. Adult: one ampule containing 0.4 mg.

b. Neonatal: one ampule containing 0.02 mg.

5. These drugs should be administered in the following manner:

a. Intravenously: onset of action in less than 1 minute

b. Intramuscularly: onset within 2 to 3 minutes

c. In cases of severe neonatal depression suspected of being secondary to narcotics, naloxone should be administered via the umbilical vein, if it is readily available; otherwise it should be given intramuscularly.

d. If severe neonatal respiratory depression is anticipated because of heavy maternal narcosis, the physician may give the mother an intravenous dose (0.4 mg.) several minutes before delivery.

TRANQUILIZERS

1. The most commonly used agents are phenothiazine derivatives (such as promethazine in dosages of approximately 25 mg.).

2. They are usually used in combination with a narcotic.

3. They offer the advantages of nausea relief and reduction of maternal anxiety.

4. They have the disadvantage of not being reversible.

5. Agents of the benzodiazepine group (e.g., Valium, Librium) generally have long-lasting (several days) depressive effects on the fetus and should not be used in labor.

ANESTHESIA

AGENTS FOR REGIONAL OR LOCAL ANESTHESIA

1. For most regional and local anesthesia in obstetrics, the injectable agents are largely interchangeable.

2. All agents listed below are indicated for all types of regional and local anesthesia except spinal, with the exception of procaine and tetracaine, which may be used for spinal anesthesia as well.

3. All should be used without epinephrine for two reasons:

a. Epinephrine may slow labor.

b. If oxytocin becomes necessary, it may cause severe hypertension when used in the presence of a vasopressor.

4. The side effects and risks of all the agents are essentially the same, with the exception of prilocaine, which in addition to its other effects, may precipitate an acute attack of methemoglobinemia or exacerbate a preexistent case.

5. The agents, with their average durations in hours, are listed below:

Table 12-1. **Duration of Action of Anesthetics**

chloroprocaine	(Nesacaine)	1/2–1 hr.
procaine	(Novocaine)	1/2–2 hrs.
piperocaine	(Metycaine)	1–1 1/2 hrs.
lidocaine	(Xylocaine)	1 1/2–2 1/2 hrs.
mepivacaine	(Carbocaine)	1 1/2–2 1/2 hrs.
prilocaine	(Citanest)	1 1/2–3 hrs.
tetracaine	(Pontocaine)	1 1/2–6 hrs.

6. Allergy to any one "-caine" contraindicates use of any local anesthetic.

ANESTHESIA FOR LABOR

Paracervical Block

1. Indication. Relief from the pain of uterine contraction and cervical dilatation. Additional anesthesia is necessary for delivery. Because of its frequent undesirable consequences and because it provides no anesthesia for delivery, paracervical block is less commonly used than it was, especially if epidural block is available.

2. Risks

a. Maternal toxicity with rapid absorption of repeated doses of large amounts of anesthetic agent is a real risk.

b. Fetal bradycardia has been described shortly after injection in up to 25 per cent of paracervical blocks. This is most likely secondary to high fetal levels of anesthetic.

c. If a large paracervical vein is lacerated, a considerable hematoma may result.

d. Inadvertent injection of the drug directly into the fetus is a real and very dangerous risk.

e. Allergic reaction may occur to any of the "-caine" drugs.

3. Contraindications. The following conditions should prevent one from performing a paracervical block.

a. Fetal distress

b. Full cervical dilatation

c. Allergies to the "-caine" drugs

4. Method

a. Prep the vagina with povidone-iodine (Betadine).

b. Determine cervical dilatation.

c. Use a needle director (e.g., the Iowa trumpet, which allows no more than 0.5 to 1 cm. of the needle to project beyond it).

d. Place the guide in the lateral vaginal fornix somewhere between the 3 and 4 o'clock positions (or 8 to 9 o'clock). If injections are made at the 3 and 9 o'clock positions, this is called a paracervical block. If they are at 4 and 8 o'clock, it is termed a uterosacral block. They are functionally the same.

e. Aspirate to be sure there is no blood.

f. Inject 10 ml. of anesthetic solution.

g. Repeat on the other side.

h. Observe the fetus with continuous fetal heart rate (FHR) monitoring.

i. Since this anesthesia typically lasts 1 to 2 hours, it may have to be repeated.

Continuous Lumbar Epidural Anesthesia

1. Indications

a. Complete relief of the pain of both labor and delivery, whether vaginal or transabdominal, may be obtained using epidural anesthesia.

b. It is most useful during labor when extended pain relief is required, since an indwelling catheter in the epidural space enables one to reinforce the block as often as necessary. If used only for delivery, a catheter does not have to be placed.

c. Because of the risks and complexity of the method it is usually not used for short labors.

2. Advantages

a. Epidural anesthesia offers complete pain relief for both labor and delivery in up to 90 per cent of patients, without altering sensorium. It is ideally suited to today's climate of patient participation in childbirth as a social event.

b. Through the indwelling catheter, its effect may be extended throughout labor.

c. Because relatively small amounts of anesthetic are used, the risk of direct toxicity for mother and child is small.

d. Distribution of the anesthesia can be controlled by dosage and maternal positioning to provide relief from contractions during labor, perineal anesthesia for vaginal delivery, or abdominal anesthesia for C/S.

3. Risks

a. *Hypotension.* Maternal hypotension occurs much less frequently than with spinal anesthesia, but it is not rare. Because vascular pooling in the lower half of the body secondary to sympathetic blockade results in decreased venous return, cardiac output falls, resulting in hypotension. It is both more common and more dangerous in women who are hypovolemic, usually from hemorrhage or preeclampsia.

The best treatment is to avoid the problem by preloading with saline. If hypotension occurs, it is usually corrected by rapid infusion of 500 to 1,000 ml. of Ringer's lactate or normal saline, combined with elevation of the mother's legs or shifting her to the left lateral position. Vasopressors are rarely necessary but should always be available. Ephedrine 5 to 10 mg. by I.V. push is usually effective within 2 to 3 minutes after administration.

b. *Fetal Distress.* Fetal heart rate changes suggestive of distress occur commonly for a short while after institution of epidural anesthesia. They may be due to maternal hypotension resulting in decreased uteroplacental blood flow. They are best avoided by preloading the mother with normal saline or Ringer's lactate to avoid hypotension. Additionally, some physicians routinely hyperoxygenate (mask 10 L. min.) all mothers for 20 to 30 minutes after placement of the epidural.

If such changes do occur, combined treatment as for hypotension and for fetal distress usually reverses them within a few minutes.

c. *Interference with Labor.* If administered before active labor and cervical dilatation of 3 to 4 cm. have occurred, epidural anesthesia may considerably slow labor, perhaps by interference with Ferguson's reflex. It may also interfere with "pushing" in the second stage by eliminating sensations of rectal pressure and uterine contractions.

Early dysfunction can be overcome with oxytocin infusion. Interference with pushing in the second stage may be avoided by timing the reinforcement so that it wears off at about the time the second stage is entered. Should that timing be off, an attendant telling the patient when a contraction is beginning and enthusiastically urging her to "push" is usually sufficient to compensate for the lack of rectal pressure. If it is not, forceps rotation may be required.

Curiously, sometimes epidural anesthesia, if it does not inhibit contractions, seems to speed the course of active labor. Perhaps it interferes with some neurological communication with the cervix which ordinarily maintains cervical tone or resistance.

d. *Postpartum bladder distension* frequently results if there is no catheter, because the patient is not aware of the urge to urinate. This is compounded by the large amounts of fluid infused to avoid hypotension.

e. *Inadvertent Spinal Puncture.* Inadvertent placement of the needle in the spinal canal may cause two complications:

(1) *Spinal Blockade.* If the puncture is not recognized, injection of the relatively large amounts of anesthesia needed for epidural anesthesia into the small space of spinal canal may cause total spinal blockade, resulting in cardiorespiratory arrest. This may be avoided by injecting a test dose.

(2) *Postspinal Headache.* Because epidurals are done with a large needle, inadvertent puncture of the arachnoid may result in continued leakage of CSF from the spinal canal for several days afterward, causing headaches upon standing. The incidence of postspinal headache is about one per cent. If it occurs, it may be managed either by hydration, analgesia, and bed rest or, more effectively, by a "blood patch." Some anesthesiologists will perform a "blood patch" immediately upon recognition of the puncture.

f. *Inadvertent I.V. Injection of Anesthetic.* In some women, the epidural veins are extremely dilated during pregnancy, and it is possible to place either the needle or the catheter within one. If anesthetic is injected directly into a vein, convulsions and cardiorespiratory arrest may occur. This is best avoided by always aspirating before injecting.

4. Contraindications

a. Absolute Contraindications

(1) Maternal hypotension

(2) Maternal hemorrhage, either present or anticipated

(3) Maternal coagulation disorder

(4) Fetal distress

(5) "-caine" allergy

(6) Local infection

b. Relative Contraindications

(1) Neurologic disease

(2) Maternal hypertensive disease, especially preeclampsia, although with increasing refinement of technique and adequate fluid loading, many anesthesiologists feel they can safely use epidural blockade in these patients.

(3) Need for immediate anesthesia

5. Method. Epidural anesthesia is usually performed by an anesthesiologist, especially in major centers.

a. Fluid-load the patient with at least 1,000 ml. of Ringer's lactate before performing the puncture. Keep a running I.V. throughout.

b. Institute continuous EFM, if not already in use, preferably with internal electrode, since the mother frequently requires positional shifting which interferes with external FHR recording.

c. Measure the patient's blood pressure before performing the puncture. If it is not normal, stop.

d. Prep and drape the woman either sitting or lying on her left side with her legs flexed and back straight. Her shoulders should be aligned perpendicularly to the table, to prevent spinal rotation.

e. Anesthetize the skin and underlying tissues of any one of the lumbar interspaces.

f. Introduce a Tuohy needle (16 gauge) with stylet into the center of the anesthetized space until the ligamentum flavum is punctured. This will be accompanied by a sudden loss of resistance.

g. Attach a syringe and first aspirate. If neither blood nor spinal fluid is obtained, inject 2 to 3 ml. of air. It should enter without resistance.

h. Insert a plastic catheter (18 to 20 gauge) through the needle and advance it either up or down the canal. As stated in the section "Caudal Anesthesia," below, never withdraw the catheter through the needle inside the canal.

i. After again aspirating and checking position of the catheter, remove the needle and tape the catheter in place.

j. Inject a test dose of 2 to 5 ml. of anesthetic and wait 2 to 3 minutes.

k. If no evidence of spinal anesthesia occurs (rapid anesthesia, lower extremity paralysis), inject an additional 10 to 25 ml. of anesthetic solution.

l. Turn the patient to her back and begin to check her blood pressure every 1 to 2 minutes for at least 20 minutes.

m. Administer additional anesthetic agent as required.

ANESTHESIA FOR DELIVERY

Local Infiltration

1. Indications

a. Episiotomy

b. Cesarean section is rarely done using local anesthesia.

2. Advantages

a. There is essentially no risk of anesthetic mortality.

b. Performed in the delivery room, there is essentially no effect on the fetus if recommended dosages are used.

c. It is easily and quickly administered by any physician.

3. Risks. The complications of local anesthesia are rare and usually minor:

a. Allergic reaction to "-caine" drugs

b. Local hematoma

c. Systemic toxicity, if too much is used, rarely

4. Contraindications. The only contraindications to local anesthesia are:

a. Allergy to the "-caine" drugs

b. Local infection

5. Method

a. After sterilely prepping and draping the perineum, infiltrate each side of the area requiring anesthesia with 10 to 20 ml. of local anesthetic.

b. Avoid injection directly into a blood vessel by attempting to aspirate through the needle before every injection. If blood is obtained, reposition the needle and try again.

Pudendal Block

1. Indications. Relief of perineal pain during birth or episiotomy

2. Advantages

a. By blocking the pudendal nerve with its branches of the second through fourth sacral nerves, the perineum can be effectively anesthetized for delivery.

b. If recommended anesthetic dosages are not exceeded, and intravascular injection does not occur, maternal and fetal drug effects are essentially none.

c. It may be easily administered by any physician.

3. Risks

a. See "Risks" under "Local Infiltration," above.

b. If the pudendal artery or vein is lacerated, a sizable hematoma may occur. This is usually prevented by the pressure applied by the descending fetal head. However, if the block is performed after delivery, for repair of the perineum, this safety precaution is absent.

4. Method

a. Holding a needle guard (e.g., Iowa trumpet) between two fingers of one hand, it is guided intravaginally to the lower edge of the ischial spine on one side.

b. A long 20- to 22-gauge needle which protrudes from the end of the guard by no more than 0.5 cm. is then passed through the vaginal mucosa and to the sacrospinous ligament.

c. Three to four ml. of anesthetic is injected after first attempting to aspirate blood (see "Local Anesthesia," above).

d. The needle is then advanced past the ligament and another 3 to 4 ml. injected after aspiration is attempted.

e. The needle is then withdrawn, a second puncture made slightly higher up the ischial spine, and another 3 to 4 ml. injected.

f. The procedure is then repeated on the other side.

Caudal Anesthesia

1. Indications

a. Relief of perineal pain during delivery or episiotomy, when lumbar epidural anesthesia cannot be performed. This is essentially low epidural anesthesia.

b. If a greater volume of more dilute anesthetic solution is given, the level of anesthesia rises and relief from the pain of labor may be obtained.

2. Advantages. Inadvertent spinal puncture during placement of caudal anesthesia is extremely unlikely.

3. Risks. Being a form of epidural anesthesia, caudal block carries all the risks of same, including hypotension, drug toxicity from large volumes of anesthetic, and impaired labor. See "Continuous Lumbar Epidural Anesthesia," above, for a discussion of these.

4. Contraindications. These are the same as for lumbar epidural anesthesia.

5. Method

a. Prep and drape the sacrum and coccygeal area with the patient in the left lateral Sims' position.

b. After making a skin wheal over the sacral hiatus, the needle (17 to 18 gauge) is passed through the skin at a 90° angle until it has entered the sacral hiatus. The sacrococcygeal membrane will be felt as it is pierced.

c. A syringe is now used to aspirate and to inject a small amount of air. No blood or spinal fluid should be obtained on aspiration. No resistance should be encountered on injecting the air. If there is resistance, the needle may be either in maternal soft tissue, or in the fetus. Remove it.

d. Once entry to the caudal space has been verified, depress the needle almost parallel to the skin and advance it approximately 1 in. into the canal.

e. Now thread approximately 2 to 3 in. of a plastic catheter (19 to 20 gauge) through the needle into the caudal space. If resistance is met, try angulating the needle somewhat. *Never pull back on or attempt to withdraw the catheter through the needle*—the bevel of the needle may cut the catheter, leaving a piece inside the canal.

f. Once the catheter is placed, withdraw the needle, tape the catheter down, and inject a test dose of approximately 5 ml. of anesthetic agent.

g. If no evidence of spinal anesthesia, such as lower extremity paralysis, occurs in 5 min., an additional 20 to 25 ml. of anesthetic is injected.

h. The catheter is left attached to a syringe and may be left in place for additional anesthesia as required.

i. Maternal blood pressure and fetal heart rate are closely monitored.

Spinal Anesthesia

1. Indications

a. Introduction of an anesthetic directly into the spinal canal may be performed for either vaginal or abdominal delivery.

b. Because it is a single injection technique, it is not indicated for labor itself.

c. Epidural anesthesia is preferable if it can be achieved, since the incidence of side effects is lower.

2. Risks

a. *Postspinal Headache.* Continued leakage of fluid from the puncture site may occur for several days and result in headaches which are very resistant to treatment. It is best to avoid this as much as possible by using a very small needle (25 or 26 gauge) for the puncture. Many physicians also keep the woman flat for 12 hours after spinal anesthesia.

Once headaches have begun to occur, treatment by abdominal binders or placement of "spinal patches" yields variable degrees of success.

b. *Hypotension.* This tends to be more common, more severe, and more sudden than with epidural anesthesia.

c. *Fetal Distress.* See "Risks" under "Continous Lumbar Epidural Anesthesia," above.

d. *Interference with Labor.* See "Risks" under "Continous Lumbar Epidural Anesthesia," above.

e. *Bladder Dysfunction.* See "Risks" under "Continous Lumbar Epidural Anesthesia," above.

f. *Arachnoiditis/Meningitis.* With the advent of sterile technique, disposable equipment, and single-dose containers of anesthetic, these have become rare complications.

3. Contraindications. The reasons to avoid spinal anesthesia are the same as those for not performing epidural blocks.

4. Method

a. Fluid-load the patient with Ringer's lactate or normal saline. Keep a running I.V. in place.

b. Measure the patient's blood pressure. If it is not normal, stop.

c. With the patient sitting over the edge of a bed or table, her whole spine flexed (and held by an assistant), prep the area around the L3–L4 interspace.

d. Anesthetize the skin and underlying tissues.

e. Perform a "spinal tap" with a small-gauge spinal needle and stylet.

f. Obtain a free flow of spinal fluid from the needle.

g. Inject a small amount of an appropriate anesthetic agent. For vaginal delivery 1.0 to 1.5 ml. will suffice, while 2.0 to 2.5 ml. may be needed to obtain a level high enough for cesarean section.

h. Remove the needle, apply pressure to the puncture site for a moment and turn the mother to the supine position with her head elevated slightly.

i. Measure maternal blood pressure every minute for 10 to 15 minutes after placement of the anesthetic.

j. Adjust the level of anesthesia as it develops, by tilting the patient up or down.

General Anesthesia

1. Indications

a. *Vaginal Delivery.* While general anesthesia used to be commonly used for vaginal delivery, it is now much less resorted to. The wide availability of prepared-childbirth classes supplemented by local and regional anesthesia for operative vaginal deliveries has reduced the need for general anesthesia tremendously. It is now routinely used if:

(1) Anesthesia is needed on a moment's notice, e.g., repair of a cervical laceration or operative delivery for fetal distress.

(2) Intrauterine manipulation is attempted, e.g., delivery of a second twin, or difficult manual removal of a placenta.

(3) Postpartum curettage is necessary.

(4) Delivery of a malformed or stillborn child is anticipated.

b. *Cesarean Section.* General anesthesia is acceptable anesthesia for any cesarean section, unless the mother has eaten very recently. It is the anesthesia of choice for abdominal delivery under the following circumstances:

(1) Any emergency delivery where anesthesia is needed quickly, e.g., cord prolapse, fetal distress.

(2) Any condition which contraindicates regional anesthesia, e.g., fetal distress, maternal hypotension or hemorrhage.

2. Risks

a. Aspiration of gastric contents is the most common cause of obstetric anesthetic death. Since gastric emptying is so delayed in pregnancy, and especially during labor, there is a grave risk of aspirating acidic stomach contents during the reflex vomiting which may occur during anesthesia induction and reversal.

(1) *The following steps may be taken to reduce the risk:*

(a) Enforce at last an 8-hour, and preferably longer, fast before general anesthesia, if possible.

(b) Administer 30 ml. of an antacid before anesthesia. Even if she has fasted, never assume the patient has an empty stomach. Sodium citrate is preferable to something like Maalox or Mylanta, since particulate matter may be as dangerous as acidic fluid, if aspirated.

(c) Perform endotracheal intubation as soon as possible after induction of anesthesia.

(d) Extubate her when the patient is awake enough to cough and keep her head down and to the side.

(2) *If aspiration of gastric contents does occur, the following maneuvers should be taken:*

(a) Immediate removal of all particulate matter in the pharynx followed by examination of the vocal cords for other material. Bronchial lavage is no longer practiced.

(b) Immediate administration of large doses of corticosteroids, e.g., 1 g. of hydrocortisone I.V. followed by 250 mg. I.V. q. 6h. Although the efficacy of this regime is not proven, there is a general feeling that it may help. If it is to be of any use, it must be given early in the course.

(c) Antibiotic coverage with a broad spectrum agent, e.g., ampicillin 1 g. I.V. every 6 hrs. or an appropriate dose of cephalosporin.

(d) Immediate chest radiograph, for baseline evaluation.

(e) Immediate blood gas measurement.

(f) Oxygen by mask, cannula, or reintubation, if necessary, in concentrations sufficient to maintain pO_2 above 60 torr.

(g) Close observation of the patient for 24 hours, even if her condition does not seem to require it.

3. General Anesthetic Agents

a. *Inhalation Anesthetics*

(1) NITROUS OXIDE

(a) By itself, nitrous oxide cannot provide anesthesia. Used in a 40- to 50-per-cent mixture with oxygen for analgesia, it does not provide surgical anesthesia or relaxation until concentrations reach 80 to 85 per cent. At this level, maternal-fetal hypoxia is inevitable.

(b) However, in 60- to 70-per-cent mixtures with oxygen it may be used very effectively for "balanced anesthesia" (see below) in combination with other agents.

(2) HALOTHANE (FLUOTHANE), METHOXYFLURANE (PENTHRANE), AND ENFLURANE (ETHRANE)

(a) These are all halogenated agents used for general anesthesia.

(b) All are potent myometrial relaxants and may be used for intrauterine manipulation, although halothane and enflurane seem more effective. They also cause increased intrapartum and postpartum blood loss.

(c) All cause severe respiratory depression in both mother and fetus and are usually not used for delivery.

(d) Halothane may be hepatotoxic.

(e) Methoxyflurane may be nephrotoxic.

b. *Intravenous Agents.* The ultrashort-acting barbiturates, such as thiopental when given intravenously, induce virtually instantaneous loss of consciousness without unpleasant sensations. Unfortunately, they do not provide adequate muscle relaxation or anesthesia for surgery, and would rapidly cross the placenta to cause severe fetal depression if used to maintain unconsciousness.

c. *Balanced Anesthesia*

(1) For cesarean section, the use of a short-acting barbiturate, a muscle relaxant, and a combination of nitrous oxide/oxygen with narcotic analgesia has evolved.

(2) It is used as follows:

(a) When everyone is ready to begin surgery, the patient is "put to sleep" with a dose of short-acting barbiturate, e.g., thiopental, after a small dose of *d*-tubocurarine to prevent fasciculation.

(b) She is then paralyzed with succinylcholine and intubated.

(c) Anesthesia is maintained with a nitrous oxide/oxygen mixture until the baby is born.

(d) After birth of the baby, anesthesia is continued with nitrous oxide/oxygen supplemented with intravenous narcotic analgesics, while muscle relaxation for surgery is maintained using a paralytic agent.

(3) It offers the advantages of:

(a) Rapid, pleasant induction

(b) Minimal fetal depression

(c) Easy, safe reversal

13 Immediate Care of the Newborn

David H. Fields

BASIC PRINCIPLES

1. The most immediately important aspect of making the transition from intrauterine to extrauterine life is the ability to breathe. If a newborn is breathing well, most likely he or she is not seriously ill. A newborn who is not breathing adequately will need resuscitation.

2. Next most important is the rapidity with which the newborn infant loses heat to the environment. He or she must be kept warm.

3. Apgar scoring at 1 minute gives a good indication of the need for resuscitation. At 5 minutes, it is used to prognosticate subsequent perinatal course.

4. Since neonatal resuscitation and intensive care has become a specialty, if one suspects the likelihood of a problem at birth it is prudent to have on hand a pediatrician skilled in such measures. In our hospital, pediatricians attend the following deliveries:

a. Those following fetal distress in labor

b. Breech deliveries

c. Cesarean sections

d. Deliveries involving multiple infants

e. Midforceps deliveries

f. Preterm deliveries

MANAGEMENT

1. Upon delivery of the infant's head, the obstetrician may choose to suction the nose and pharynx. If the delivery is complicated by the presence of thick meconium in the amniotic fluid, this should be done before the infant breathes. If there is no meconium, it may be postponed until the delivery of the infant is completed.

2. After completion of the delivery the infant is held, head down, and suctioned if this has not already been done. If the amniotic fluid has been meconium-stained, the infant's vocal cord should be visualized to rule out aspiration.

3. Next the cord is clamped and cut. There has been considerable controversy in the past regarding delayed or immediate clamping of the cord. In most cases of otherwise normal babies it makes no particular difference. If there is reason to suspect fetal anemia, delaying the clamping and holding the infant below the level of the perineum will infuse him or her with extra volume and extra red cell mass. On the other hand, if the infant is premature, extra volume may overload him or her. One should not intentionally "transfuse" the premature infant.

4. If the infant does not require resuscitation, he or she may be wrapped in a warm blanket and given to the parents or placed in slight Trendelenburg position in a warmer, to prevent heat loss to the environment. Radiant heating devices have been found to be best for this.

5. At this time the 1-minute Apgar scoring is done. See Table 13-1.

Table 13-1 Apgar Scoring.

Sign	0	1	2
Heart rate	absent	below 100	over 100
Respiratory effort	absent	slow; weak cry	good
Muscle tone	flaccid	some flexion of extremities	well flexed active motion
Reflex irritability	none	grimace	viorous cry
Color	blue	body pink; extremities blue	completely pink

6. Immediate further care is based on the Apgar score.

a. If the score is 7 or above, no resuscitation is needed. Routine care is instituted.

b. If the score is 4 to 6, the infant is considered moderately depressed and probably needs some stimulation, but not active resuscitation.

c. If the score is below 4, the infant is seriously depressed. Active immediate resuscitation should be started.

CARE OF THE NEWBORN

Care of the Moderately Depressed Infant

1. Mild mechanical stimulation may "wake up" the infant. Tapping the soles, rubbing the back, or "puffing" him or her with air from a suction bulb is acceptable. Sphincter dilatation, thoracic compression, and vigorous slapping of the back may do more harm than good.

2. Simultaneously bathing the infant's face in a flow of oxygen, without applying the mask to his or her face, may be of help.

3. If neither of the above has sufficient effect and there is any question of narcotic suppression because of maternal medications, one ampule (0.02 mg.) of naloxone neonatal should be given I.M.

4. The above will almost always serve to "resuscitate" the moderately depressed infant; if so, routine care may resume.

Care of the Severely Depressed Infant

1. As noted above, this is best done by someone skilled in neonatal resuscitation.

2. The severely depressed infant has a slow heart rate and poor respiration and is neurologically depressed. Usually these conditions are due to hypoxia, so immediate resuscitation after clearing the pharynx and nose should consist of administration of oxygen via face mask. This should be administered as short "puffs" in rapid sequence at a pressure of about 15 to 20 cm. of water.

3. If after 1 minute of this therapy the infant's condition has not improved, endotracheal intubation with a search for a site of obstruction should be performed. Oxygen should then be administered, as described above, via the endotracheal tube.

4. While this is in progress a second attendant should be placing an intravenous line, preferably in the umbilical vein. This line may then be used for administration of the following medications:

a. Naloxone 0.02 mg, I.V., if narcotic suppression is suspected

b. Sodium bicarbonate 3 to 4 mEq. initially; if resuscitation is not rapidly successful, further doses are guided by blood gas and *p*H measurements drawn from the umbilical artery line, which should also be placed at this time.

4. Resuscitation may continue in this fashion as long as the infant is ventilated and has a cardiac output, as estimated by heart rate.

5. In the event of cardiac arrest, artificial ventilation is continued at the rate of 30 to 40 "breaths" per minute. This is best done by light pressure with two fingers on the lower sternum. If there is a palpable femoral pulse in response to massage, effective circulation is being maintained. Intracardiac epinephrine may also be given in treating cardiac arrest.

6. If resuscitation is successful, the infant is transferred to a neonatal intensive care unit.

Resumption of Routine Care

If the infant needs no resuscitation, or only mild stimulation, routine care may be finished in the delivery room. This consists of:

1. Drying the infant

2. Applying a clamp and shortening the remaining umbilical cord

3. Applying an antibacterial ointment to the infant's eyes to prevent ophthalmitis. Years ago penicillin and silver nitrate were the agents of choice, because *Neisseria gonorrhoeae* was the most common etiology. Now, because of the increasing incidence of *Chlamydia trachomatis,* tetracycline and erythromycin are increasingly used.

4. Permanently identifying both fetus (footprint) and mother (fingerprint), on a single piece of paper, before either leaves the delivery room

5. Conducting a rapid physical examination for congenital anomalies

14 Routine Postpartum Care

David H. Fields

IMMEDIATE POSTPARTUM CARE

Definitions

1. Care rendered after the third stage of labor, but before the completion of the puerperium, is termed *immediate postpartum care.*

2. The puerperal period begins directly after the delivery of the placenta and ends with the return of the reproductive tract to a normal nonpregnant condition, usually by 6 weeks postpartum.

3. Postpartum care may be divided into immediate postpartum care, subsequent in-hospital care, and late postpartum care, generally rendered at home.

Basic Principles

1. The most common early postpartum problem is hemorrhage, which most frequently becomes manifest during the first hour after delivery.

2. To focus awareness on the need for constant attendance with the mother during this period, it is sometimes called the "fourth stage of labor." It is usually managed in a "recovery room."

3. Like problems at other times during pregnancy, immediate postpartum problems are best dealt with before they occur.

Routine Immediate Postpartum Management

1. Account for all sponges and gauze pads before the patient leaves the delivery room. Always perform a final vaginal examination to ensure the removal of any sponges.

2. Be certain the uterus is well contracted and the amount of blood draining from the vagina is normal before removal of the patient from the delivery table.

3. Check lochia, pulse, and blood pressure every 15 minutes for the first hour. If any begins to rise, further investigation is warranted.

4. Check firmness and height of the uterine fundus every 15 minutes for the first hour. If it begins to rise or soften, massage to enhance uterine contraction.

5. Many physicians routinely continue an infusion of oxytocin through the first hour, thereby avoiding the most common cause of postpartum hemorrhage, uterine atony. This may consist of 10 to 20 units of oxytocin per 1,000 ml. of salt solution. It may be infused at the rate of 100 to 200 ml. per hour. Others prefer 10 units I.M.

6. Ergot alkaloids (Ergotrate, Methergine) 0.2 mg. may be given I.M. immediately postpartum in place of the oxytocin, or in addition to it, if necessary. Usually, if this is begun immediately postpartum, it is continued for 24 hours, 0.2 mg. q. 4h., either I.M. or P.O. Ergot alkaloids are contraindicated in hypertensive women.

7. Many women desire to nurse immediately after delivery. If the mother and child are in good condition, this should be encouraged. It will be satisfying to the new mother and will facilitate uterine contraction.

8. Even if all seems well, allow no food during the first hour. Sips of water may be taken.

9. If blood loss during labor was considered excessive, but vital signs are stable, measure hematocrit in the first hour.

10. Be alert for difficulty in urinating. The patient can usually void using a bedpan or if allowed to the bathroom with assistance. If she cannot, however, a full bladder may predispose to uterine atony.

If necessary, perform catheterization.

ROUTINE IN-HOSPITAL CARE AFTER THE FIRST HOUR POSTPARTUM

Basic Principles

1. As hospital stays have become shorter, more postpartum management must be conducted at home. Whereas women were previously routinely watched for several days to a week, most are now home within 2–3 days.

2. The major problems in the first days after delivery are:

a. Postpartum bleeding and/or shock

b. Infection, especially of the uterus, episiotomy site, and bladder

c. Urinary difficulty

d. Poor return of bowel function

e. Breast problems, especially engorgement

f. Postpartum hypertension

g. Thrombophlebitis

3. Care at this time is directed toward avoiding these problems or detecting them early if they do occur.

Routine Postpartum Orders

1. Bed rest for several hours after delivery, then ambulation as soon as tolerated by the patient. Early ambulation is of singular importance in avoiding phlebitis.

2. Regular diet. The sooner a normal diet is resumed, the sooner normal bowel function begins.

3. Vital signs four times daily

4. Fundal palpation several times daily, with attention to quantity and quality of lochia

5. Void or catheterize every 6 to 8 hours, p.r.n. The use of catheterization can frequently be avoided if the patient is encouraged to use the bathroom rather than the bedpan. Sometimes, attempting to urinate while standing in a warm shower may be of help. If necessary, periodic catheterization or even an indwelling Foley catheter for a day or so is preferable to prolonged bladder distension.

6. Perineal care, consisting of cleansing and drying several times daily

a. Frequent use of an ice pack in the first 24 hours helps avoid swelling.

b. After the first 24 hours, witch hazel pads or a heat lamp may provide additional comfort.

7. Breast and abdominal binders, as needed for the patient's comfort

8. Hemoglobin and hematocrit determination on the second postpartum day

9. Analgesia sufficient to maintain maternal comfort will almost never affect the nursing infant. A range of options should be supplied, beginning with acetaminophen 650 to 1,000 mg. or aspirin 650 mg. P.O. q. 4h. p.r.n., and extending up to a narcotic such as codeine 30 to 60 mg. or meperidine 50 to 100 mg. P.O. q. 4h. p.r.n. Many practitioners prefer a combination agent such as Percocet or Percodan on a similar schedule.

10. Sleeping medication (e.g., Seconal 100 mg., Dalmane 15 to 30 mg., or Halcion 0.25 mg. P.O. h.s. p.r.n.)

11. Cathartic (milk of magnesia 30 ml. P.O. h.s.) on the second night and, if necessary, an evacuatory suppository (e.g., Dulcolax) or enema on the third day

12. Rh_o D Immune Globulin (Rho GAM), 300 μg. should be administered to all unsensitized Rh_o (D) negative or D^u negative mothers who deliver Rh positive infants, within 72 hours.

13. Agents to Suppress Lactation. Several days after delivery and the removal of progesterone blockade, the mother's milk will "come in." This creates breast engorgement to a degree sufficient to cause fever in a few and moderate-to-severe discomfort in most. If she is not nursing, the mother may benefit from lactation suppression. Although there are several available agents for this, one has come to the forefront.

a. *Bromocryptine (Parlodel).* A specific inhibitor of prolactin production, this seems to be the most sensible method for suppressing lactation. Begun within 24 hours of delivery (2.5 mg. P.O. b.i.d.), it will almost always block milk production sufficiently to avoid engorgement. To avoid significant rebound after therapy, it must be continued for 10 to 14 days. The most common side effect of general use is nausea, but this is much less frequent during the postpartum period. Although bromocryptine seems to be safe for most women, recent reports have indicated a slightly increased risk of cardiovascular accident in hypertensive postpartum women who use it.

b. *Deladumone OB 2 ml. I.M.* This combination of 180 mg. of testosterone enanthate and 8 mg. estradiol valerate, if given shortly before or directly after delivery, suppresses lactation in more than half of postpartum women and decreases it in almost all. There is a risk of masculinization from the testosterone and possibly of an increased incidence of postpartum phlebitis and thromboembolism secondary to the estrogen. Since the introduction of bromocryptine, Deladumone has been used much less often than in the past.

c. *Ice Packs, Support, and Compression.* While not as comfortable as hormonal suppressives, these simple mechanical measures will, when combined with mild analgesia, provide a safe method for dealing with engorgement. The patient usually tolerates them well if their safety is explained.

DAILY POSTPARTUM ROUNDS

Abnormalities in any of the following should be investigated:

1. Vital signs
2. Breasts
3. Uterine fundus
4. Lochia
5. Perineum
6. Bladder and bowel function
7. Extremities

Vital Signs

1. Pulse. Tachycardia in the sitting or standing position is frequently the first sign of excessive blood loss. It is also frequently secondary to fever.

2. Blood Pressure

a. Low blood pressure may reflect blood loss if the patient is experiencing dizziness or faintness, or if it is present with tachycardia. Otherwise, it is likely normal for a healthy young woman.

b. High blood pressure, if due to preeclampsia, may persist for several days or weeks postpartum and should be treated as described under "Preeclampsia." If not secondary to preeclampsia or to another preexistent condition, it should receive appropriate workup and management.

3. Temperature

a. Febrile morbidity is defined as a temperature greater than 100.4°F (38°C) on any 2 of the first 10 postpartum days after the first 24 hours.[1]

b. Any fever should be investigated with an eye toward:

(1) Endometritis
(2) Urinary tract infection
(3) Infected episiotomy
(4) Thrombophlebitis of extremities or pelvis
(5) Breast pathology
(6) Upper respiratory infection or pneumonia if general anesthesia was used during delivery

c. Appropriate workup should usually include examination of pelvic organs, lungs, breasts, and extremities, as well as a complete blood count and clean-catch urinalysis, and special studies as indicated.

4. Breasts

a. Lactation and milk let-down generally occur within 2 or 3 days after delivery.

---

[1] Joint Committee on Maternal Welfare.

(1) Lactation is the result of the action of prolactin after the fall of progesterone levels effected by delivery of the placenta.

(2) Milk let-down occurs secondary to oxytocin's contractile effect on the myoepithelial cells of the breast.

(3) These are accompanied by tremendous breast engorgement and perhaps by mild fevers. Temperature, however, should not be elevated above 101°F, nor last more than several hours on the basis of breast engorgement.

5. Breast-feeding Mothers

a. Most medications are secreted in breast milk and should be avoided as much as possible.

b. Nipple fissures secondary to overly aggressive suckling are painful as well as dangerous, because they provide a route for breast infection. If they occur, treatment should include:

(1) Nursing with a breast shield

(2) Topical emollient and antibiotic creams

(3) Careful gentle cleansing and drying

c. If these are ineffective:

(1) Stop nursing from the affected side.

(2) Maintain lactation with breast pumping until the fissure is healed.

d. Good support for lactating breasts will make them much more comfortable.

6. Non-Breast-Feeding Mothers

a. Hormonal suppression of lactation, as described under "Immediate Postpartum Care," above, may be attempted.

b. If hormonal suppression is not used or is not successful, symptomatic relief can be achieved with:

(1) Tight support

(2) Frequent use of ice packs

(3) Analgesia

(4) Explanation to the mother that this is a self-limited problem which only lasts several days

7. Uterine Fundus

a. Directly after delivery, the fundus contracts to level midway between the umbilicus and symphysis, then rises two or three fingerbreadths above that. Over the next several days, it involutes at the rate of one or two finger-breadths per day, so that by the tenth postpartum day, it is a pelvic organ.

b. Apparent delay in involution could suggest retained placenta but is more likely due to incomplete emptying of the bladder, which pushes the uterus upward.

c. Uterine tenderness after vaginal delivery suggests endomyometritis, and is usually accompanied by fever and abnormal lochia. (See "Lochia," below.)

d. Afterpains are the rhythmic contractions by which the uterus avoids atony. They are greater in multiparas and nursing mothers. Analgesia may be prescribed as needed.

8. Lochia

a. The vaginal discharge associated with involution of the uterus may persist and maintain a reddish color for several weeks after delivery, even until the first menstrual period.

b. The physician should be alert for lochia which is heavier and bloodier than normal, foul-smelling, or purulent. These suggest:

(1) Endometritis—usually associated with fever; lochia of streptococcal endometritis may be neither foul-smelling nor purulent.

(2) Retained secundines—usually associated with heavy bleeding and subinvolution of uterus.

(3) Retained vaginal sponge—odor is prominent.

c. Management consists of:

(1) Examination for foreign bodies and subinvolution

(2) Transcervical culture of the endometrial cavity

(3) Antibiotics after culture, if the patient is febrile. Ampicillin (500 mg. P.O. q.6h.) or a cephalosporin (same dose) is a good starting point in the not-too-ill patient while awaiting culture reports. If the patient is considered critically ill, treatment should be started with a combination of two or three parenteral antibiotics. This usually consists of an aminoglycoside (gentamicin 3 to 5 mg. per Kg. per day in 3 doses I.V. or kanamycin 500 mg. I.M.

b.i.d.) in combination with a penicillin derivative (ampicillin 1 g. I.V. q.6h.) or clindamycin (1,200 to 2,400 mg. per day in 3 or 4 divided doses I.V.) or both. Single-agent therapy using an I.V. second generation cephalosporin (e.g., cefotaxime 1 to 2 g. q.6h.) or semi-synthetic penicillin (e.g., piperacillin 1 to 2 g. q.6h.), may afford coverage almost as good with fewer side effects. Inappropriate antibiotics may then be discontinued when culture reports return.

(4) Curettage as needed for retained secundines

9. Perineum

a. It is normal for the perineum to be swollen and sore for a day or so after delivery, especially if episiotomy was performed. After the first day, this is best managed with local heat or topical anesthetics.

b. If the episiotomy is hot or red or purulent, it may be presumed to be infected. Management in this case consists of:

(1) Culture of discharge, if any

(2) Local heat

(3) Antibiotics (ampicillin or cephalosporin 500 mg. P.O. q.6h., pending culture and sensitivity reports)

(4) Drainage of any collection of pus

c. If it is necessary to open an episiotomy because of infection, healing should be by secondary intention. Cosmetic or functional repair may be done at a later date.

10. Bladder

a. Bladder function may be impaired for up to several days after delivery secondary to

(1) Traumatic delivery

(2) Conduction anesthesia

(3) Immediate postpartum urinary retention with distension

b. A distended bladder may be detected as a suprapubic cystic mass or, indirectly, by its elevating the fundus above the umbilicus. This should be checked several times daily in the first few days.

c. If the patient cannot void

(1) Catheterize every 6 to 8 hours

(2) If repeated catheterization is necessary or severe distension occurs, place an indwelling Foley catheter for 2 or 3 days.

d. If the patient has urinary incontinence in the first few days, catheterize for residual urine to rule out overflow incontinence.

11. Bowels

a. It is not unusual for the normal postpartum woman to go several days without a bowel movement, especially if she had enemas prior to delivery. This is not the medical emergency some patients think it is. It may be remedied with gentle laxatives (e.g., milk of magnesia, 30 ml. P.O. h.s.) for several days if necessary, or with a cathartic suppository (e.g., Dulcolax). Reassurance, however, is preferable.

b. Soreness of the episiotomy site may inhibit bowel movements. This may be treated with stool softeners, glycerin suppositories, and local or systemic analgesia.

c. If there has been a fourth-degree laceration with repair, many physicians use parts or all of the following regime for bowel regulation:

(1) Low residue diet for one or two days.

(2) Regular diet subsequently with stool softeners (e.g., Colace 100 mg. P.O. t.i.d. or Peri-colace, one capsule b.i.d., a mild cathartic).

(3) No rectal temperatures or enemas

(4) No mineral oil

(5) Systemic antibiotic (e.g., ampicillin 500 mg. P.O. q.6h. for several days)

d. Hemorrhoids regress several days after delivery. Symptomatic relief with seating cushions (doughnuts), topical analgesia (witch hazel, Anusol), and stool softeners usually suffices.

12. Extremities

a. The key to reducing postpartum phlebitis is early ambulation.

b. For patients who have varicose veins (which tend to improve after delivery), support stockings are helpful.

REMAINDER OF THE PUERPERIUM

Discharge from the Hospital

This occurs usually between the second and fourth postpartum days and is permitted if the patient has no signs of infection, retained secundines, or urinary retention.

Sexual Activity

1. Most physicians recommend against sexual activity until the lochia has completely disappeared and many until after the postpartum check (traditionally at 6 weeks).

2. When the puerperal woman resumes having sexual intercourse she should be warned of the following:

a. Perineal tenderness secondary to an episiotomy is likely to persist for weeks.

b. Vaginal dryness secondary to decreased estrogen levels is not uncommon and should not be a cause for concern. It will pass spontaneously within a few weeks, unless the mother is nursing, in which case suppressed ovarian function and hormone production may last for months. In these instances, lubrication and vaginal tone may be "menopausal" until resumption of normal cycles or cessation of breast-feeding. These can be overcome with patient foreplay and lubricating jellies if necessary.

c. Prior to the first menstruation, conception is less likely than normal but quite possible. Contraception should be used from first coitus.

Late Postpartum Complications

1. Mastitis

a. This may occur after the first postpartum week in a breast-feeding mother.

b. It is usually signaled by:

(1) Tender breasts, which are hot and engorged and may be locally reddened

(2) Fever and chills

(3) Possible breast abscess formation with fluctuance

c. It may be unilateral or bilateral.

d. Treatment consists of:

(1) *Discontinuation of breast-feeding.* This is controversial. Some pediatricians will allow the infant to nurse, even from the infected breast. Others will recommend cessation of breast-feeding until the infection is resolved. Emptying the breasts, however, is essential to rapid resolution of the problem. This may be done either by manual expression of the milk or via pump, if the mother does not continue to nurse.

(2) *Antibiotics.* Therapy should be begun immediately after obtaining a culture of the breast milk. Since the most common organisms are *Staphylococcus Aureus* and *Streptococcus*, one should start with either a semisynthetic penicillinase-resistant penicillin (dicloxacillin), a cephalosporin, (cephalexin), or erythromycin in a dosage of 250 to 500 mg. P.O. q.6h. for 7 to 10 days.

(3) *Drainage of abscess,* if present, should be performed.

2. Late Postpartum Hemorrhage

a. Hemorrhage after the first postpartum week is usually due to either retained secundines or subinvolution of the placental site. It is often accompanied by endomyometritis.

b. In addition to bleeding, one will often find:

(1) Fever and chills

(2) Uterine tenderness and bogginess

c. Treatment is usually begun with:

(1) Broad spectrum antibiotic coverage

(2) Perhaps ergot alkaloids for 24 hours

d. D&C is often necessary.

15 Forceps Delivery

David H. Fields

BASIC PRINCIPLES

1. Obstetrical forceps are used to effect vaginal delivery which might otherwise occur after a longer period of time.

2. They should not be used in situations where a more effective second stage would not produce vaginal delivery (cephalopelvic disproportion). Nor should they ever be applied to any part of the fetus other than the head.

3. Safe use of forceps also requires an understanding of their mechanics. The blades of the forceps have two curvatures: pelvic and cephalic. The pelvic curve allows the blades to reach into the pelvis and follow its curvature upward. Traction on the blades during delivery must be in a direction which allows the blades to follow the pelvis along this curve. The cephalic curve is the outward curve which allows the fetal head to nestle between the two blades.

4. Maximum force applied should not exceed 60 Kg. This crude number has little meaning to the obstetrician in the delivery room. Experience must guide him or her.

DEFINITIONS

1. Low Forceps (Outlet Forceps). The fetal head is on the perineum and the sagittal suture is the midline (occiput anterior [OA] or posterior [OP]). This usually amounts to little more than a last-minute assist to guide the head over the perineum or under the symphysis.

2. Midforceps. After engagement, until the head is on the perineum and in the direct OA or OP position, the delivery will be midforceps. An artificial category of low midforceps, with the head on the perineum but in an oblique position, is used by some obstetricians.

3. High Forceps. Use of blades prior to engagement of the fetal head. Although one never says "never" in medicine, one may never have better cause to say "never" than in reference to this practice.

INDICATIONS

1. To shorten the second stage of labor for maternal benefit in cases of:

- **a.** Severe cardiac disease
- **b.** Cerebrovascular disease
- **c.** Severe preeclampsia
- **d.** Maternal exhaustion

2. To shorten the second stage of labor for fetal benefit:

- **a.** Fetal distress
- **b.** Premature placental separation during second-stage labor
- **c.** Correction of abnormal fetal position (e.g., persistent OP, asynclitism)

3. To deliver the aftercoming head in a breech delivery

APPLICATION OF FORCEPS AND DELIVERY

Prerequisites for Application of Forceps

1. Cervix fully dilated
2. Membrane ruptured
3. Fetal head engaged
4. Position of fetal head known
5. Adequacy of pelvis known

Additional Precautions

1. Bladder empty
2. Rectum empty
3. Pelvis well anesthetized

Application and Delivery

1. The blades are applied, one at a time, to conform to the fetal head (cephalic application). One guides them with one's fingers so that they come to lie alongside the head with the tips just beyond the cheeks. One must remember that there is a pelvic curve as well, which must be honored during application and delivery.

2. If the left blade is always introduced first, crossing of the shanks will not be necessary. Some obstetricians prefer to apply the posterior blade first (when the head is in an oblique position). When the posterior blade is the right blade, the shanks must be crossed after application.

3. Once the blades have been applied, check their position. The following criteria should ALL be met:

a. Sagittal suture is midline between the blades and perpendicular to them.

b. Fenestrations (if any) admit one finger on each side.

c. Posterior fontanelle is one finger's breadth above handle of blades.

4. Once the blades have been appropriately placed and checked, they should be locked.

5. If rotation is necessary the handle of the blades should be swung in a wide arc, so that rotation occurs around the midpoint of the blades and the tips do not describe a wide arc. Rotation around the handles is a common cause of vaginal vault laceration.

6. Effect delivery by exerting traction in the axis of the pelvis. This may be accomplished by depressing the blades at their midpoint with one hand while exerting traction with the other.

7. Unless immediate delivery is necessary, pull rhythmically, mimicking uterine contractions and delivering gradually. The blades should be opened between contractions to relieve any pressure on the fetal skull.

8. Perform an adequate episiotomy and deliver the head slowly, to avoid perineal lacerations and fetal brain damage.

9. Remove the forceps either before or after delivery of the head. If before, there is less volume to be delivered through the vagina; if after, there is more control during the delivery.

Risks of Forceps Delivery

The three most common causes of injury during forceps deliveries are:

1. Failure to recognize the true station of the fetal head. Molding, caput, and the OP position, common in labors requiring the use of forceps, often give the impression that the head is significantly lower than it seems. **Accurate estimation of station is essential.**

2. Failure to recognize cephalopelvic disproportion (CPD). This is most common in transverse arrests, but is always a danger in midforceps applications. One avoids this not only by careful evaluation of the pelvis, but also by use of gentle traction and by not being committed to delivery (see "Trial and Failed Forceps," below).

3. Failure to honor the pelvic curve while rotating, or applying traction to, the forceps. Envisioning the blades within the pelvis and using the midportion of the blades as the center of motion will help one to avoid using their tips as a weapon.

Maternal

1. Perineal, vaginal, rectal, or bladder laceration. These are most common with midforceps rotations, but failure to apply traction in the axis of the pelvis will predispose to their occurrence.

2. Cervical laceration or ruptured uterus (lower segment), especially if cervical dilatation is not complete or the fetal head has not descended enough

3. Symphysis pubis separation, if outlet disproportion exists

Fetal

1. Bruises and cephalohematomas

2. Intracranial injury, especially tentorial tears and subdural hematomas

Specific Forceps Operations

1. Outlet Forceps

a. A low forceps delivery consisting of lifting the head over the perineum

b. Elliott or Tucker-McLean forceps for unmolded heads; Simpson forceps for molded heads

2. Rotations

Almost all midforceps deliveries are rotations, since the head does not rotate into the OA position until it reaches the pelvic floor.

a. From ROA or LOA to OA.

(1) These are the simplest rotations, involving simple placement of the blades and rotation through 45 degrees.

b. From posterior (OP, ROP, LOP) to OA with the head well descended

(1) Most commonly done by Scanzoni maneuver

(a) Apply forceps—preferably Tucker-McLean forceps, whose thin, unfenestrated blades tend to cause less vaginal trauma on rotation.

(b) Rotate from direct posterior or posterior oblique to anterior.

(c) Remove forceps, which are now inverted.

(d) Reapply forceps and deliver as for a low forceps.

(2) May be done using Kielland forceps for rotation (no pelvic curve), followed by application of blades with pelvic curve for delivery.

(3) May be delivered as posterior.

b. From transverse arrest

(1) May be done using Kielland rotation.

(2) The increasing tendency is to deliver by cesarean section, since the incidence of associated midpelvic CPD is high.

3. Delivery of Aftercoming Head

a. Although the head is backwards, the blades are applied as if for a vertex presentation.

b. Never hyperextend the fetal body—spinal cord injuries might result.

c. Use Piper long-handled forceps.

Trial and Failed Forceps

1. If the obstetrician suspects, but is not certain, that (s)he can accomplish a forceps delivery and the criteria for the application of the blades have been met then forceps may be applied. This must be done with the knowledge that the trial may not be successful and with willingness to stop and perform a cesarean section, if necessary, before damaging either mother or fetus.

2. *There are, unfortunately, no objective criteria for knowing when to stop.* CLINICAL JUDGMENT IS ESSENTIAL. Obviously, a failed forceps delivery indicates that delivery was not safely possible but was attempted. This should not occur too often.

16 Cesarean Section

David H. Fields

DEFINITION

Delivery of the infant by incision of the abdominal and uterine walls.

BASIC PRINCIPLES

1. Cesarean section (C/S) is a surgical procedure requiring anesthesia and postoperative recovery and carrying all their risks. Maternal mortality and morbidity are higher than for vaginal delivery, although rates are becoming lower with advances in technology. In past years, maternal mortality for C/S was quoted as 10 times higher than for vaginal delivery, but, recently, studies have shown markedly lower death rates, approaching those of mothers delivered vaginally.

Significant morbidity, however, remains considerably higher, and includes complications such as hemorrhage, uterine and wound infection, phlebitis, and intraoperative injury.

2. Cesarean section rates have increased tremendously over the last several years to rates of up to 25 per cent at some centers, and approximately 15 to 20 per cent in most areas.

3. The following factors have contributed to the increased incidence:

a. The increasing safety of C/S, due to:

(1) Extensive use of epidural rather than general anesthesia

(2) New antibiotics, offering better infection control

(3) Improved blood replacement techniques

(4) Better electrolyte management

b. An increase in the number and the liberalization of the indications for C/S, especially in the areas of:

(1) Fetal distress

(2) Abnormal presentation

(3) Use of midforceps

(4) Prematurity

(5) Genital herpes

c. Many repeat C/S

INDICATIONS FOR CESAREAN SECTION

A cesarean section is indicated when delivery is required and cannot be performed vaginally because it will take too long or because it will endanger the mother or the fetus.

1. Cephalopelvic Disproportion (CPD). This is the most common indication for cesarean section during labor. It is usually diagnosed by a trial of labor with careful fetal and maternal monitoring (vertex presentation only). In the past, x-ray pelvimetry played a significant role in diagnosing CPD, but it has been largely abandoned.

2. Fetal Distress. Diagnosed by intrapartum fetal monitoring, this is an indication for cesarean section when conservative measures (see Chap. 11, "Intrapartum Fetal

Monitoring") fail and vaginal delivery is not imminent. A true medical emergency, it is usually performed with general anesthesia for utmost speed.

3. Prolapsed Umbilical Cord. Another true emergency, this situation requires immediate delivery. This can be accomplished only by cesarean section unless full dilatation is present and the patient is multiparous.

4. Placenta Previa. If total, this is a mandatory indication for cesarean section. If marginal or partial, vaginal delivery may be attempted, but extreme watchfulness must be the rule, and immediate cesarean section must be available and should be prepared for in advance.

5. Placental Abruption. If attended by torrential hemorrhage, maternal shock, or fetal distress, this should be treated by immediate cesarean section. Otherwise, labor may be induced as long as there is careful fetal and maternal monitoring and cesarean section is immediately available if necessary.

6. Abnormal Presentation.

a. There is essentially no choice but cesarean section in cases of:

(1) Transverse lie or shoulder presentation

(2) Face presentation with posterior chin

(3) Footling breech or hyperextended breech

(4) Interlocking twins

b. In addition, cesarean section is increasingly used (although not mandatory) for the following situations related to abnormal presentation:

(1) Breech complicated by almost anything (prematurity, postmaturity, large fetus, mild pelvic abnormality, uterine dysfunction, maternal disease such as diabetes or preeclampsia, desire for sterilization)

(2) All face presentations

(3) Brow presentations

c. Finally, in some centers cesarean section is being used to deliver all breech presentations.

7. Extreme Prematurity. Increasingly, fetuses under 32 weeks are being delivered by C/S to avoid the neonatal morbidity and mortality associated with the trauma of labor and vaginal delivery of these infants.

8. Preeclampsia/Eclampsia. If this necessitates delivery prematurely and induction is unsuccessful or will take too long, cesarean section is indicated. Usually induction is possible.

9. Diabetes. Like preeclampsia, diabetes frequently requires early fetal delivery. Currently long inductions are out of favor, and cesarean section is becoming increasingly popular.

10. Genital Herpes Simplex. To avoid the risk of neonatal infection with herpes simplex virus, most obstetricians perform C/S on all mothers who have or have had evidence of active infection within 1 week of labor. Some use 10 to 14 days as a cutoff. In such circumstances, C/S should be done within 4 hours of ROM to minimize the chances of ascending infection.

11. Erythroblastosis Fetalis. This is another disease frequently requiring early delivery, although it is becoming increasingly rare. If induction is not possible, cesarean section should be performed.

12. Maternal Gynecological Malignancy. Carcinoma of the cervix or ovary discovered in the third trimester should indicate cesarean section followed by appropriate therapy. For carcinoma of the cervix, a classic incision should be made to avoid cutting through tumor.

13. Previous Surgery. If the patient has had previous surgery invading the endometrial cavity through the uterine wall, elective cesarean section is usually performed. This category includes previous cesarean section, transmural myomectomy, and correction of uterine abnormalities.

REPEAT CESAREAN SECTION vs. VAGINAL DELIVERY

1. Repeat cesarean section has become a major source of current cesarean section.

Because of the morbidity inherent in numerous surgical procedures, attempts have been made to delineate criteria under which repeat C/S might safely be avoided and vaginal delivery allowed. Current feeling is that labor may be safely undertaken if the following criteria are met:

a. The previous C/S was via a low transverse incision;

b. There was no postoperative infection after the previous C/S;

c. Intensive fetal and maternal surveillance are conducted during labor;

d. Labor spontaneously progresses well;

e. Blood replacement and C/S are immediately available.

2. Even under these circumstances, if the mother chooses, she has the option to elect for a repeat C/S, although official ACOG guidelines now call for the obstetrician to push for attempted vaginal delivery.

3. If repeated C/S is to be performed, the major risk, iatrogenic prematurity, is to the fetus. This may be avoided by:

a. Being sure of gestational age early in the pregnancy; OR

b. Verifying fetal growth by sonography before repeat C/S, and, if necessary, obtaining an L/S ratio; OR

c. Allowing labor to begin before performing C/S.

PREPARATION FOR CESAREAN SECTION

1. Informed consent

2. Nothing by mouth, preferably for at least 8 hours

3. Antacid, preferably sodium citrate, 30 ml. 30 to 45 minutes prior to surgery

4. Abdominal prep

5. Preoperative Foley catheterization

6. Preoperative CBC and urinalysis (and electrolytes if time permits)

7. Type and crossmatch (or screen, in many hospitals) 2 units packed RBC

8. Running I.V. line, preferably 18 gauge

ANESTHESIA

Epidural anesthesia is preferable for most cesarean sections because of its greater safety for the mother. Many, however, are still performed under general anesthesia. (See Chap. 10, "Anesthesia and Analgesia".)

TYPES OF INCISION

Abdominal Incision

1. Low Transverse. Also known as the Pfannenstiel incision, this is made transversely at or near the top of the pubic hairline. It offers the advantages of being cosmetically preferable (it is known as the bikini cut by patients) and less likely to undergo dehiscence. It does, however, require slightly more time to perform and more meticulous hemostasis, and it is more difficult to extend if not initially large enough.

2. Vertical Midline or Paramedian. This incision can be performed in a matter of seconds, with minimal blood loss, and is easily extendable. In spite of the fact that it is cosmetically less desirable and is, in fact, a weaker incision, it should be used if only a few minutes' delay will impose significant danger on either the mother or the fetus, or if operative exposure is likely to be a problem.

Uterine Incision

1. Transverse Lower Uterine Segment Incision (Intraperitoneal). This is the uterine incision of choice unless contraindicated (see "Classical Incision," below). It usually involves less blood loss, carries a lower risk of rupture during subsequent pregnancy, and lowers the risk of postoperative bowel adhesions when compared with the classical incision. The major disadvantage is a risk of extension laterally, tearing the major uterine vessels.

2. Vertical Lower Uterine Segment Incision. Used much less often, this incision requires extensive dissection of the bladder from the uterus. It does offer the option of extension upward, if necessary, but also carries the risk of tearing down into the vagina or bladder. Usually indicated in cases of transverse lie or extreme prematurity, which are likely to require extension of the incision, it is preferable to the high vertical (classical) incision because of the lower likelihood of catastrophic rupture.

3. Classical Incision. Beginning above the lower uterine segment and coursing upward to the fundus, this incision is usually only indicated in cases of placenta previa, transverse fetal lie, or carcinoma of the cervix, which may make lower segment surgery dangerous or difficult. It is rarely used because of its danger in subsequent pregnancy and because of the great blood loss that it usually involves.

TECHNIQUE

Low Transverse Abdominal Incision

1. Sterile prepping and draping of the abdominal wall is performed either after institution of anesthesia (if regional) or before (if general).

2. After anesthesia is effective, the skin incision is made. If a Pfannenstiel is to be performed, the skin incision should be at about the level of the pubic hair line and large enough to allow for easy delivery of the fetus.

3. Next, the subcutaneous tissue is incised down to the level of the rectus sheath, Large vessels are usually encountered. Whether they are clamped, clamped and tied, or just pressed upon at this point depends on how heavily they bleed and the urgency of the delivery.

4. The rectus sheath is next opened with a scalpel in the midline and incised (usually with scissors) transversely from the midline bilaterally. The two layers should be incised separately to minimize bleeding.

5. The sheath is then dissected free of its attachment to the rectus muscles in the midline as far up toward the umbilicus as possible and from the pyrimidalis muscles down to the pubic symphysis. Care must be taken here to avoid trauma to perforating blood vessels. If they are lacerated, they should be legated to avoid subsequent rectus sheath hematoma. The adequacy of the Pfannenstiel incision is usually determined by its fascial dimensions (fascia does not stretch well). Extending it as far laterally and as far upward as possible avoids difficult deliveries.

6. The rectus and pyramidalis muscles are separated vertically in the midline, and the posterior fascia and peritoneum are incised, also in the midline. This is done as high up as possible to avoid accidentally entering the bladder.

Vertical Midline or Paramedian Abdominal Incision

1. If the initial incision is to be vertical, it should be at or near the midline and of similar length.

2. The subcutaneous fat and underlying rectus sheath are also incised vertically.

3. The rest of the entry into the peritoneal cavity is the same as described above.

Transverse Lower Uterine Segment Incision

1. Upon entering the peritoneal cavity, a retractor (we use the lower blade of a Balfour retractor) is placed in the lower margin of the incision to aid visualization.

2. The junction of the bladder and anterior uterine serosal surfaces is identified (just below where the serosa becomes tightly adherent to the uterine surface), and a horizontal incision is made just above it, from the midline bilaterally.

3. The loosely adherent bladder is then separated from the lower uterine segment for 2 to 3 cm., using one's finger.

4. A horizontal incision is next made in the lower uterine segment through the exposed area. THERE ARE TWO CAVEATS HERE. Typically, the uterus bleeds a lot when one cuts into it, obscuring the surgeon's vision. Second, it is important to cut through the uterus (and perhaps membranes, if they are intact), but NOT TO CUT THE BABY. The best way to solve both these problems is to make a small midline incision all the way through, while applying pressure with a lap pad to the upper edge of the incision, tamponading the bleeding.

5. After identifying the uterine cavity, one extends the incision laterally (either with bandage scissors or manually), being careful to make it large enough WITHOUT extending it laterally into the large branches of the uterine arteries.

6. Recently, a new technique involving a stapler has become available. After making a stab wound in the desired area, one inserts a stapler and places two rows of hemostatic absorbable staples across the lower uterine segment. One then cuts between the rows, limiting the bleeding. This is most useful if the lower segment is somewhat thinned by labor.

Vertical Uterine Incisions

1. If one is performing a low vertical incision, one must "take down the bladder" further to allow as much of the incision as possible to be in the lower uterine segment.

2. For classic incisions, one begins above the vesicouterine junction and so does not take the bladder down at all.

Delivery of the Baby and Placenta

1. Upon entry into the uterine cavity, the surgeon inserts his hand, locates the part of the baby he intends to deliver and guides it toward the incision. Care must be taken, especially if the head is "down in the pelvis," to avoid extending the uterine incision. This is best accomplished by patience.

2. One delivers the infant by a combination of fundal pressure and traction, as if the opening were a vagina.

3. After briefly suctioning the infant, one cuts the cord and gives the infant to the pediatrician. The person carrying the baby changes gloves.

4. The delivery of the placenta is conducted under direct vision with care to be sure membranes are not left behind. The inner surface of the uterus is explored and patency of the cervix is verified.

Closure of the Incision

There are many acceptable techniques for uterine closure, usually using one or two layers of continuous or interrupted, large caliber absorbable sutures. All are designed to obtain hemostasis, reapproximation, and inversion of the uterine scar. The one I use is presented below.

1. The surgeon massages the uterus and the anesthesiologist rapidly infuses an oxytocin solution (20 u./1,000 ml. N.S. or R.L.), to assure uterine contraction and minimize bleeding.

2. Usually, at this point it is easiest to deliver the fundus of the uterus through the abdominal incision and complete its closure outside, since visualization is so much improved.

3. Both cut edges of the uterus are identified to the angles of the incision (and may be grasped with nontraumatic clamps), and angle sutures (chromic-1) are placed to guarantee hemostasis at the edges of the incision.

4. A running, locked suture (chromic-1) is next used to reapproximate the cut edges and obtain hemostasis. Care is taken to stay between the angle sutures, avoiding the large lateral vessels.

5. A second running suture (chromic-1), in the fashion of a Lembert imbrication stitch, inverts the incision line and secures additional hemostasis. At the end of this step, the uterine incision should be without bleeding. If it is not, separate sutures may be used on bleeding points.

6. One next reapproximates the "bladder flap" to the upper uterine serosa, using a running suture (chromic 2-0), covering over the uterine incision. This stitch should be superficial, and care should be exercised to avoid "advancing the bladder."

7. At this point, the surgeon, assistant, and scrub nurse change gloves.

8. The surgeon next inspects the pelvic viscera for abnormality or bleeding and then reinserts the uterus into the abdominal cavity, taking care not to trap bowel behind it. Some physicians suction spilled blood from the pelvic gutters.

9. Instrument and lap pad counts should now be completed before the abdominal incision is closed.

10. Abdominal closure is as for any laparotomy.

11. At the end of the procedure, one should express blood and clots from the vagina by downward pressure on the uterine fundus and verify that the uterus is well contracted.

12. Blood-tinged urine in the Foley catheter is not uncommon and is often due to blunt trauma to the bladder during the delivery. It should clear within several hours after surgery.

POSTOPERATIVE MANAGEMENT

Postoperative care of the cesarean section patient combines that of the postpartum patient with that of any postoperative patient.

Immediate Postoperative Care

1. Constant attendance until the patient has regained full consciousness, if general anesthesia was used

2. Vital signs q.15 minutes for 1 hour then q.1h. for 2 hours

3. Monitoring of urine output, vaginal bleeding and fundal firmness, q. 15 minutes for 1 hour

4. 1,000 ml. R.L. (D_5RL, 0.9 NaCl) plus 20 u.oxytocin at 200 ml. per h. for 1 to 2 hours

4) N.P.O.

5) Foley catheter

6) Pain relief. If general anesthesia was used, small doses of narcotic analgesia (morphine 2 to 5 mg. I.M., meperidine 25 to 50 mg. I.M.) may be used. If epidural blockade was performed, often nothing is necessary for the first few hours.

Subsequent Postoperative Management

1. Bed rest for 24 hours, followed by progressive ambulation

2. Vital signs every 15 minutes until stable, then every 4 hours.

3. Nothing by mouth for first 12 to 24 hours, then progressive increase in diet depending on patient's condition

4. Intravenous fluids providing 2,500 to 3,000 ml. of water, 70 to 140 mEq. of NaCl, and at least 100 g. of sugar per 24 hours. Continue until oral intake is adequate. Add 40 to 60 mEq. of potassium chloride on the second day. For the first 24 hours, 10 to 20 units of oxytocin should be added to each 1,000 ml. I.V. fluid.

5. Foley catheter discontinued within the first 24 hours after surgery unless there has been bladder trauma

6. Hemoglobin and hematocrit measurement on the first evening and following morning of the surgery

7. Pain relief as required, usually with narcotic analgesics (e.g., 50 to 100 mg. Demerol q.4h. p.r.n., meperidine 50 to 100 mg. or morphine 5 to 10 mg. I.M. q.3 to 4 hr. p.r.n. until the patient can take oral medication; then meperidine 50 to 100 mg., codeine 30 to 60 mg., Percocet or Percodan, P.O. q.3 to 4h. p.r.n.).

8. Sleeping medication as required

17 Abnormalities of Fetal Growth and Development Concerning both Antepartum and Intrapartum Care

David H. Fields

INCOMPETENT CERVIX

Definition

Painless effacement and dilatation of the cervix without detectable labor, usually after 16 weeks.

Basic Principles

1. If the cervix does not have sufficient integrity, as the intrauterine pressure increases after the thirteenth week it is forced to efface and dilate without detectable labor.

2. Usually, after significant dilatation, the membranes prolapse and eventually rupture.

3. Labor or amnionitis most often ensues.

Etiology

1. Structural or anatomic cervical defect, most often associated with diethylstilbestrol (DES) exposure

2. Previous cervical trauma, as from conization or late abortion

3. Idiopathic

Diagnosis

1. Suspect incompetent cervix in all patients at risk (see above).

2. Suspect incompetent cervix in any woman who has had second trimester rupture of membranes in the absence of labor.

3. Diagnose incompetent cervix if pelvic exam demonstrates cervical effacement or dilatation in the absence of labor.

4. Diagnose incompetent cervix in any woman who has had it in a previous pregnancy.

5. Since incompetent cervix is not associated with pain, cases occurring in women not in high-risk categories are usually diagnosed after significant dilatation has been followed by rupture of membranes. If vaginal examination were performed at every prenatal visit, some of these cases might be detected while still treatable.

Management

1. If there is a suspicion of incompetent cervix, perform weekly pelvic exams for cervical status from the thirteenth through the thirtieth week.

2. If incompetent cervix is diagnosed, either by history or by exam, treatment may be either surgical or nonsurgical, or a combination.

a. Cervical Cerclage

(1) Cervical cerclage (sewing the cervix closed) is frequently effective and much more so if significant effacement and dilatation have not yet occurred. If there is ballooning of the membranes into the vagina, most statistics on cerclage are dauntingly poor. (Goodlin et al., reported on several patients with ballooning membranes who were treated with a combination of amniocentesis for fluid removal to relieve the pressure, installation of intraamniotic antibiotics, repositioning of the membranes inside, cervical cerclage, and tocolysis. Their salvage rate was over 50 per cent. Prompted by their report, I similarly managed one such case involving hourglassed membranes at 18 weeks who subsequently delivered a healthy infant at 34 weeks)

(2) It may be done under spinal, epidural, or general anesthesia.

(3) The cerclage should be placed as close to the internal os as possible.

(4) Antibiotics and tocolytics are frequently used in the perioperative period. They may or may not be effective.

(5) Bed rest after surgery, until late in the third trimester, is advocated by some physicians.

(6) Two types of cerclage are commonly employed:

(a) Shirodkar procedure. By undermining the cervicovaginal mucosa, a Mersilene tape may be circumferentially sutured into place high on the cervix. If well placed this is extremely effective, but placement is difficult, and bleeding and infection are real risks.

(b) McDonald procedure. A simple nonabsorbable pursestring suture is sewn around the cervix as high up as possible without undermining the mucosa. This involves less blood loss than the Shirodkar procedure. It may, however, be less effective.

b. Bed Rest

(1) Some physicians say that removing the pressure from the cervix may be sufficient, by itself, to arrest the process and allow pregnancy to continue.

PRETERM LABOR

Definition

Onset of labor before the end of the thirty-seventh week of gestation.

Etiology

While a great percentage of preterm labors occur for no known reason, the following conditions predispose to prematurity:

1. Previous preterm labor or second trimester loss

2. Previous cervical conization (increased risk of incompetent cervix)

3. Preterm rupture of the membranes

4. Multiple gestation

5. Hydramnios

6. Uterine anomalies that decrease intrauterine capacity—especially if DES-related

7. Congenital anomalies

8. Maternal infection, especially pyelonephritis

9. Intrauterine infection, especially TORCH infections

10. Maternal age under 20 or over 35

11. Trauma, especially automobile accidents

Diagnosis

1. The diagnosis of premature labor is essentially the diagnosis of labor. Unfortunately, if treatment is likely to be successful it must be begun early, preferably before significant cervical dilatation has occurred.

2. When there are regular, painful contractions every 3 minutes and cervical effacement and dilatation are in progress, the diagnosis is indisputable. In such cases, the question is not *should* one stop labor, but *can* one stop labor. Therefore, the criteria become increasingly lax the earlier in the pregnancy one is making the diagnosis.

3. In the second and early third trimesters, contractions every 10 to 20 minutes, even if not painful, should be sufficient to arouse alarm; but by the thirty-fifth week they should be either more frequent than every 10 minutes or accompanied by some cervical change.

4. Any discharge that is even slightly bloody should arouse suspicion of cervical effacement or dilatation.

Risks

Prematurity is the number-one cause of perinatal mortality, principally on the basis of respiratory distress syndrome.

Management

1. Early in threatened preterm labor, bed rest and I.V. hydration in the lateral recumbent position are frequently helpful.

2. Active attempts to stop labor are indicated if:

a. The membranes are intact.

b. The cervix is less than 4 cm. dilated.

c. There is no evidence of fetal anomaly.

d. There is no evidence of fetal distress.

e. There is no suggestion of amnionitis.

f. The fetus is sufficiently premature that intervention is warranted. The usual guideline for intervention varies from 33 to 35 completed weeks.

g. There is no contraindication to use of a tocolytic agent.

3. Agents currently in general use for arresting premature labor are:

a. β-adrenergic agents

b. Magnesium sulfate ($MgSO_4$)

c. Prostaglandin inhibitors

d. Alcohol

4. *Beta-Adrenergic Agents*

a. These have become the mainstay of tocolysis. They bind to the β_2-adrenergic receptors in the myometrium and inhibit contraction.

b. They are epinephrine derivatives with preponderantly β_2-adrenergic effects, but significant residual β_1-adrenergic (cardiac) activity. Some are claimed to have fewer side effects, but the relative benefits of one compared to another have yet to be established.

c. Major side effects, which are dose-related, include:

(1) Tachycardia and other arrhythmias, usually experienced as palpitations

(2) Myocardial ischemia, experienced as chest pain or pressure, secondary to tachycardia

(3) Pulmonary edema

(4) Hypotension

(5) Hypokalemia

(6) Hyperglycemia

(7) Nausea and vomiting

(8) Headache

(9) Anxiety

d. They may be used I.V., I.M., subcutaneously, or orally. The most common regimes seem to begin with I.V. and progress to oral use.

e. Only ritodrine (Yutopar) is currently approved for the treatment of preterm labor, but other drugs in this group, such as albuterol, terbutaline sulfate, and fenoterol, have been used.

f. Use of ritodrine

(1) Prior to the beginning of therapy, the following should be performed:

(a) Complete history and exam

(b) EKG

(c) Serum potassium and glucose (SMA-8)

(d) Fetal heart rate (FHR) and contraction strip by electronic fetal monitoring (EFM)

(2) During I.V. therapy, constant monitoring of maternal and fetal vital signs is essential. Additionally, periodic assessment of maternal serum glucose and potassium should be performed. If long-term oral tocolytic therapy is planned, similar occasional testing is indicated.

(3) Prepare an I.V. solution of 150 mg./500 ml. 0.9% N.S. or R.L., yielding a concentration of 0.3 mg./ml.

(4) Administer by infusion pump, beginning at the rate of 0.1 mg./min. (20 ml./hr.)

(5) Increase by 0.05 mg./min. (10 ml/hr.) every 10 to 15 minutes until contractions cease, a maximal dose of 0.35 mg./min. is reached, or maternal side effects prevent further increases.

(6) Continue effective dose for 12 hours after contractions cease.

(7) Begin oral therapy with 10 mg. q.2h., 30 minutes before cessation of I.V. therapy.

(8) If oral therapy is well tolerated and effective, switch to 20 mg. q.4h. P.O. for maintenance. Effective maintenance doses may be between 10 and 20 mg. q.4h.

(9) Continue oral therapy as long as delivery is not desirable.

g. Contraindications to β-adrenergic agents include maternal heart disease, diabetes, and hypertension.

5. *Magnesium Sulfate*

a. Probably acting as a calcium antagonist to inhibit myometrial contraction by the same mechanism by which it prevents convulsions in preeclampsia, $MgSO_4$ is an alternative to β-adrenergics, especially in patients with hypertension, diabetes, and heart disease.

b. Use, monitoring, and risks for $MgSO_4$ therapy are described in Chap. 21, "Gestationally Induced Hypertension." These are the same for its use in stopping labor, except that after the initial loading dose of 4g. the infusion rate should be 2 g./hr. rather than the 1 g./hr. used for preeclampsia.

6. *Prostaglandin Inhibitors*

a. Since labor is a prostaglandin-mediated process, agents that block the synthesis and/or action of prostaglandins can inhibit labor.

b. Ibuprofen (Motrin), indomethacin (Indocin) and mefenamic acid (Ponstel), to name a few of these drugs, have been used to inhibit preterm labor. However, the widespread activity of these chemicals may have many side effects, not the least of which are maternal coagulation disorders and possible premature closure of the ductus arteriosus.

c. Their use, at the moment, is experimental.

7. *Alcohol*

a. Alcohol, commonly used to inhibit preterm labor before the advent of β-adrenergic agents and $MgSO_4$, is no longer used, because of its lesser effectiveness and unpleasant side effects.

Delivery

1. Should the above measures fail, one is faced with the delivery of a premature infant.

2. For the very premature (less than 32 weeks) cesarean section (C/S) may offer less traumatic delivery, perhaps decreasing the incidence of intraventricular hemorrhage and allowing a better neonatal course.

3. For vaginal deliveries, liberal episiotomy is essential.

4. For the premature breech, C/S is preferable.

5. A pediatrician skilled in resuscitation should be in attendance at the delivery of every premature infant.

PREMATURE RUPTURE OF MEMBRANES

Definition

Premature rupture of membranes (PROM) is defined as rupture of the membranes (ROM) at least 2 hours before the onset of labor. When this occurs before the thirty-seventh completed week, it is called preterm rupture of the membranes.

Etiology

Unknown

Diagnosis

1. Identification of amniotic fluid leaking from the vagina is frequently possible by:

a. Observing fluid leaking from the cervix by sterile speculum exam. Some physicians object to this on the grounds that there is no such thing as a sterile speculum exam.

b. Testing *p*H, using Nitrazine paper. Amniotic fluid is alkaline, whereas the normal vaginal discharge and urine are usually acidic.

c. Testing fluid for ferning by allowing it to dry on a slide

d. Staining it for fetal cells

2. Pitfalls in diagnosis include alkaline vaginal discharges and the loss of alkaline urine, especially with infection.

Risks

1. If PROM occurs at term, the major risks are:

a. Amnionitis, if spontaneous or induced labor does not follow shortly thereafter

b. Increased likelihood of cord complications during labor

2. If PROM occurs before term, the major risks are:

a. Amnionitis, if delivery is delayed.

(1) The risk of amnionitis increases sharply after 24 hours and tends to level off after several days.

(2) If intrauterine infection does occur, perinatal mortality may be 25 per cent.

b. Prematurity, with varying degrees of respiratory distress syndrome (RDS) and other neonatal complications (depending on how premature the baby is and how good the neonatal intensive care unit [NICU] is), if immediate delivery is performed.

(1) Immediate delivery of the preterm infant may result in minimal morbidity and mortality if the gestational age is over 35 weeks.

(2) Before 35 weeks, increasingly severe RDS and associated complications are likely.

(3) In many centers, physicians feel more comfortable dealing with prematurity than with the increased risk of infection (from delayed delivery) as early as 32 to 33 weeks.

(4) The incidence of RDS may be reduced by postponing delivery after PROM for 24 to 48 hours. Many studies have considered the acceleration of pulmonary maturation that may be prompted by postponement of delivery after PROM, but have been unable to resolve the question.

Management

1. Determine fetal maturity, if possible.

a. If PROM has occurred in a term pregnancy, pulmonary maturity may be presumed.

b. If PROM has occurred preterm, obtain ultrasonography (USG) and correlate with dates.

c. If there is a question about maturity, obtain amniotic fluid, if possible, either vaginally or by USG-directed amniocentesis, for L/S ratio and PG.

2. If the pregnancy is beyond 36 weeks or the L/S ratio is mature, perform a vaginal exam to verify membrane rupture and rule out cord prolapse; then induce labor. (Spontaneous labor may be awaited for a few hours, but as a rule delivery should be accomplished within approximately 24 hours of membrane rupture.)

3. If the pregnancy is under 36 weeks gestation or the L/S ratio is immature, the risks of prematurity must be weighted against those of amnionitis. These are assessed differently at different centers and depend upon patient population and the skill of the NICU.

4. If waiting is the choice, the following precautions must be taken:

a. No vaginal exams, except, perhaps, for the one "sterile speculum" exam to establish the diagnosis and obtain an amniotic fluid culture

b. Observation in the hospital for signs of labor or amnionitis

c. Bed rest until fluid leakage stops

d. Vital signs, including oral temperatures, every 4 hours

e. White blood cell counts daily

f. External fetal monitoring to rule out symptomatic cord prolapse

g. Antibiotics before delivery are of questionable value in forestalling amnionitis or fetal infection. If, however, the mother becomes febrile, broad-spectrum antibiotic therapy should be started after cultures are obtained. Delivery at this point is indicated, preferably by induction of labor, but by C/S if necessary.

5. In some centers, an attempt to induce pulmonary maturity (see below) followed by delivery in 24 to 48 hours is the preferred course of action.

6. Birth After Prolonged Rupture of Membranes

a. Infants born after prolonged rupture should be cultured at birth, especially from the gastric fluid and ear. The decision whether to begin antibiotics at birth should depend on the pediatric service.

b. Cultures of the fetal side of the placenta, the inside of the uterus, and the amniotic fluid should be obtained. If the mother is afebrile and there is no suspicion of infection, antibiotics may be withheld.

7. Enhancement of Lung Function

a. It has been shown that treatment of the mother with corticosteroids (betamethasone, 12 mg.) at least 24 hours (but less than 7 days) before delivery will significantly reduce the incidence of RDS in infants between 28 and 32 weeks gestation.

b. Since the results are transient, wearing off within several days, if one attempts to induce pulmonary maturation, one should probably be prepared to effect delivery within 1 to 3 days.

c. Before 28 weeks and after 32 weeks, the effectiveness of corticosteroids seems to be limited and their use is more controversial.

d. Potential side effects include:

(1) Sepsis due to the effect of steroids on the immune system

(2) Preexistent diabetes or preeclampsia may be considerably worsened.

(3) Long-term effects on the fetus. These are unknown; there are none demonstrated in humans to date.

TWINS

Definitions

1. Monozygotic (Identical) Twins. Cleavage of one zygote to form two embryos. Depending on the age of the zygote at cleavage, these exhibit various degrees of separation between the fetuses and chorioamnionic units. The earlier the cleavage, the greater the degree of separation. These are always same sex twins, unless there has been chromosomal dropping.

2. Dizygotic (Fraternal) Twins. Separate fertilization of two ova

3. Dichorionic, Diamnionic Twins. Separate chorions, amnions, and placentas. May be either dizygotic or monozygotic. If monozygotic, they represent separation before the third day after fertilization.

4. Monochorionic, Diamnionic Twins. Two fetuses with one chorion and one placenta, but separate amnions. Always monozygotic. Separation of the zygotes has occurred between the fourth and eighth postconceptual days.

5. Monochorionic, Monoamnionic Twins. Two fetuses with one amnion and, therefore, one chorion and one placenta. Always monozygotic. Separation after the eighth day, but before formation of the embryonic disc (ninth to eleventh day).

6. Conjoined twins. Separation at any time after the ninth day results in incomplete twinning. The degree of separation depends on the timing and may result in fetuses joined at the head (craniopagus), the chest (thoracopagus), the pelvis (ischiopagus), or the back (pyopagus).

Etiology

1. Dizygotic twinning accounts for most cases, and is increased in frequency in women who

a. Are black

b. Are over 35 years old

c. Have a family history of twins

d. Have received clomiphene citrate (5–7-per-cent incidence) or menopausal gonadotropins (20- to 40-per-cent incidence)

2. Monozygotic twinning is invariable in incidence, at approximately one case per 250 pregnancies.

Diagnosis

1. It used to be said that the diagnosis of twins was made more than 50 per cent of the time in the delivery room. Fortunately (since many of the complications are antenatal) this is no longer true.

2. Suspect twins if any of the following are found:

a. Higher-than-normal alpha-fetoprotein (AFP)

b. Larger-than-dates uterus

c. Many fetal parts

d. Two fetal hearts, at least 10 b.p.m. different from each other

3. Confirm diagnosis by USG

4. Rarely, twins may be diagnosed in the delivery room. This will never be missed if exploration of the uterus is routine.

Risks

1. Perinatal morbidity and mortality rates are many times higher than for singleton pregnancy (up to 15 per cent mortality).

2. Monozygotic twins have higher complication rates than dizygotic twins, and monoamnionic twins higher than diamnionic.

3. Major causes of morbidity and mortality are:

a. Prematurity—the major cause of morbidity and mortality. Usually attributed to increased intrauterine volume, from two fetuses or hydramnions, predisposing to premature labor.

b. Growth retardation.

c. Intertwin transfusion—resulting from vascular communications between fetal circulations in monochorionic twinning. This causes one fetus to become anemic while the other is plethoric. Most commonly associated with artery-vein communications. The result is one growth-retarded twin and one with cardiac hypertrophy and hypertension.

d. Congenital anomalies. More common among monozygotic than among dizygotic twins, and 2 to 3 times more likely than in singleton pregnancies.

e. Hyperemesis gravidarum

f. Preeclampsia—probably due to increased placental mass. This occurs earlier, more often, and with greater severity than in singleton pregnancies.

g. Labor complications, including:

(1) Hypotonic dysfunction
(2) Cord prolapse
(3) Premature placental separation
(4) Abnormal presentation
(5) Postpartum hemorrhage

Management

1. Antepartum. The aim of management is to prevent premature delivery and be alert for maternal complications. The only effective method to date for decreasing the ill effects of prematurity is strictly enforced bed rest, preferably from mid-second trimester until time of delivery. (While there is some controversy about whether bed rest actually prolongs pregnancy, it is clear that it does increase placental perfusion and enhance fetal growth, improving morbidity and mortality statistics.)

2. Labor. Once labor has begun, the following steps should be taken:

a. If labor is premature, attempt to stop it (see "Preterm Labor," above).

b. If labor is to continue:

(1) Institute fetal monitoring of both fetuses.

(2) Start a running intravenous system.

(3) Type and crossmatch 2 units of packed red blood cells.

(4) Keep analgesia and anesthesia during labor to a minimum. Conduction anesthesia carries a greater risk of precipitating hypotension in women who are at risk for hypertension and hemorrhage.

(5) While the use of oxytocin in dysfunctional labor complicated by twin gestation is generally not advocated, many physicians use it cautiously.

3. Vaginal Delivery

a. *First Twin*

(1) If the first fetus is a vertex, deliver it as a normal single birth.

(2) DO NOT UNCLAMP THE CORD.

(3) Explore the uterus immediately to determine the status of the second twin, including the presence of another amniotic sac, presentation, and position.

(4) If the first twin is a breech, many physicians will treat it as a premature breech because of its likely smaller size. One has the option of C/S or breech delivery.

b. *Second Twin*

(1) If the presenting part of the second twin is directly over the pelvis, guide it into the pelvis; then rupture the membranes.

(2) Monitor the fetal heart carefully with a stethoscope, or with a fetal monitor if it is available in the delivery room.

(3) As long as the there is no bleeding from the uterus (placental separation) and the fetal heart remains good, a normal breech or vertex delivery may be conducted. Oxytocin may be used cautiously.

(4) If the presenting part of the second twin is not directly over the pelvis, the fetal parts must be identified.

(5) Then rupture the membranes, locate the feet, grasp them, and perform a breech extraction. This is best done under adequate anesthesia. Epidural anesthesia, if already in place, is safest, but general anesthesia is sometimes used.

(6) Double-clamp the cord of the second twin, for later identification.

c. *Placenta and After*

(1) Immediately after the delivery of the second twin, the placenta is delivered, frequently by manual removal.

(2) Explore the uterus and cervix for lacerations.

(3) Begin oxytocin infusion to ensure contraction of the uterus, combined with uterine massage.

(4) After repair of the episiotomy, inspect the placentas and membranes for evidence of monozygosity.

Indications for Cesarean Section

1. Interlocking twins are an absolute indication for abdominal delivery. This diagnosis may be made when X-ray flat plate or USG reveals the presenting twin to be a breech, while the second presents a vertex with its head below the head of the first.

2. As with breech deliveries, many physicians now opt for C/S unless everything is perfect. Indications for abdominal delivery frequently include:

a. Either fetus presenting as other than vertex. The incidence of C/S is much higher if twin A is not vertex, but many physicians now prefer C/S even for a twin-B breech.

b. Growth retardation

c. Labor complications

3. Conjoined twins usually are delivered by C/S.

MULTIPLE GESTATION

Triplet, or greater, gestation poses all the risks and problems of twin gestation, except more so. Antepartum management is essentially the same as for twins. If the fetuses are large enough at the time of delivery to be reasonably sure of survival, C/S is probably the best method of delivery.

HYDRAMNIOS

Definition

Collection of amniotic fluid in volumes greater than 2,000 ml. is defined as *hydramnios*. Clinically significant hydramnios, however, usually involves volumes over 3,000 and 4,000 ml.

Etiology

Excess fluid is associated with a number of conditions and may result from various disturbances of amniotic fluid circulation:

1. Esophageal atresia of the fetus results in impaired swallowing, with a very high incidence of hydramnios.

2. Anencephaly, spina bifida, and omphalocele result in transudation of fluid across the meninges secondary to direct exposure of cerebrospinal membranes to amniotic fluid.

3. Twin gestation (monoamniotic) may result in greater placental mass and greater urine output into the amnion.

4. Diabetes and erythroblastosis fetalis are frequently associated with hydramnios. This may be related to a large placenta, but this is uncertain.

5. Pulmonary hypoplasia, by inhibiting fetal respiratory imbibing of amniotic fluid, may predispose to hydramnios.

Diagnosis

1. Suspect hydramnios when the uterus is larger than dates and the fetus is difficult to palpate. Fetal heart sounds may also be distant.

2. Document it by USG. At the same time, evaluate the fetus for abnormalities.

3. Be alert to the fact that "hydramnios" may be a large cyst.

Risks

The risks of hydramnios may not be generally recognized. Perinatal mortality may approach 50 per cent, because of the following factors:

1. Fetal

a. Clinically evident hydramnios is associated with congenital anomalies in up to 20 per cent of cases. Most commonly these are:

(1) Anencephalus
(2) Esophageal atresia
(3) Pulmonary hypoplasia

b. Premature labor secondary to uterine distension is frequent. In acute-onset hydramnios, labor commonly occurs before 28 weeks gestation.

c. Prolapse of the umbilical cord with rupture of the membranes is not uncommon.

2. Maternal

a. Extreme uterine distension leads to an increased risk of placental abruption, dysfunctional labor, and postpartum hemorrhage due to uterine atony.

b. Because of uterine enlargement, dyspnea and venous-compression symptoms of the lower extremities may be severe.

c. There is also a risk of other maternal disease, most notably diabetes.

Management

1. Determine, if possible, the presence of fetal abnormalities by USG.

2. Treat underlying maternal disease such as diabetes, if any.

3. If necessary, for maternal dyspnea or pain relief, perform amniocentesis with removal of several hundred ml. at a time. This may precipitate labor and is used only for maternal necessity, not to prolong pregnancy.

4. If labor begins and seems to be dysfunctional, amniocentesis with removal of several liters of fluid may help in more severe cases.

5. Gradual transcervical removal of fluid through a small-gauge needle between contractions may also be useful. However, rupture of the membranes is associated with a high risk of cord prolapse.

6. Diuretics and salt restriction are generally ineffective.

OLIGOHYDRAMNIOS

Definition

Oligohydramnios is defined, somewhat vaguely, as a less-than-normal amount of amniotic fluid. No clear volume-based definition of oligohydramnios has been made; but on biophysical profile (BPP) it corresponds to the absence of any pockets of fluid of a size of 1 cm. or larger.

Etiology

1. Renal agenesis and obstruction of the fetal urinary tract, resulting in failure to excrete urine into the amniotic fluid, are the two most common causally associated anomalies.

2. Postmaturity syndrome is commonly associated with oligohydramnios after term. The reason for this is unknown.

3. Most cases are of unknown origin.

Diagnosis

1. Antepartum: Oligohydramnios is usually suspected on abdominal palpation in the second or early third trimester because the uterus is not growing rapidly enough. Ultrasonography can be used to calculate total intrauterine volume and fetal size, allowing diagnosis by subtraction. Also, subjective evaluation of pockets of amniotic fluid may suggest oligohydramnios.

2. Intrapartum: Before rupture of the membranes, severe cord compression patterns may suggest oligohydramnios.

Risks

1. Antepartum

a. Fetal cutaneous and skeletal abnormalities may result from the lack of cushioning found with long-standing oligohydramnios.

b. Pulmonary hypoplasia, caused by the lack of sufficient fluid for fetal "breathing," is the most serious sequela of severe long-standing antepartum oligohydramnios.

c. Cord compression and antepartum fetal distress may occur, since the fluid normally cushions the cord. This is the major risk in postdates pregnancies.

2. Intrapartum

a. Fetal distress from severe cord compromise before rupture of the membranes is the major intrapartum risk.

Management

1. Antepartum

a. Evaluate fetus for cord compromise using BPPs and CSTs.

b. Evaluate fetal growth and relative degrees of oligohydramnios with serial USG.

c. If fetal jeopardy is diagnosed, the only option is delivery—usually by C/S, since cord compromise severe enough to endanger the antepartum fetus will preclude labor.

2. Intrapartum

a. Intensive EFM to detect cord compromise and therapy (see Chap. 11, "Intrapartum Fetal Monitoring").

b. After rupture of membranes, some physicians have attempted transcervical infusion of 200 to 300 ml. of sterile saline to provide cord cushioning during labor. This may be done through an intrauterine pressure catheter, and sometimes works.

POSTTERM (POSTDATES) PREGNANCY

Definition

This is pregnancy lasting beyond the end of the forty-second week of amenorrhea (two weeks beyond the EDC).

Etiology

The cause almost always is unknown, although cephalopelvic disproportion (CPD) is often a factor in postdates labors. This, however, may as likely be a result as a cause.

Diagnosis

The diagnosis of postterm pregnancy is made, most simply, by accurate dating, which is best done in the first trimester.

Risks

1. CPD. If the fetus continues to thrive and grow after term, it will gain approximately 200 g. per week, increasing the likelihood of CPD.

2. Postmaturity syndrome. If placental function begins to degenerate or the fetus begins to outgrow its placental supply,

postmaturity syndrome and fetal distress may occur.

a. This syndrome is characterized by long nails, desquamation, decreased subcutaneous fat, and oligohydramnios.

b. These fetuses generally tolerate labor poorly, due to both hypoxia and cord complications.

Management

1. Optimal management is to deliver safely as soon as possible after term to avoid postmaturity syndrome, placental insufficiency, and CPD, and to monitor the fetus carefully while waiting.

2. Beginning at term, perform some combination of NSTs, CSTs, and BPPs at intervals of at least 5 to 7 days, while awaiting spontaneous labor or inducibility.

3. Induce labor when the cervix becomes favorable, if the pregnancy has progressed beyond 41 completed weeks.

4. If the cervix remains unfavorable, continue careful observation of the fetus as described above. Unfortunately, the longer the pregnancy continues, the less the likelihood of successful vaginal delivery, because of either CPD or fetal distress in labor. The only alternative in these cases, however, is induction in the face of an unfavorable cervix, an unpleasant prospect at best.

5. If fetal monitoring suggests jeopardy (non-reactive NST combined with either +CST or poor BPP), end the pregnancy either by induction of labor under optimal conditions or by C/S.

6. EFM is mandatory in all postterm labors.

MACROSOMIA

Definition

Fetuses larger than 4000 g. are called *macrosomic.*

Etiology

1. Genetic and constitutional factors

2. Maternal diabetes without vascular disease

3. Excessive prenatal weight gain

4. Postdates pregnancy without placental compromise

Diagnosis

1. Prenatally, suspect macrosomia in all patients at risk and investigate with USG.

2. In labor, suspect macrosomia if labor does not proceed apace.

Risks

1. CPD and obstructed labor

2. Shoulder dystocia

Management

1. Ideally, one should attempt to prevent macrosomia by careful prenatal care.

2. If one suspects a macrosomic fetus, labor must be approached with caution and shoulder dystocia anticipated.

INTRAUTERINE GROWTH RETARDATION (IUGR)

Definition

1. Fetuses who weigh less than do 90 per cent of their gestational age peers (i.e., those below the tenth percentile) are Small for Gestational Age (SGA).

2. Except for those who are genetically or constitutionally small, these fetuses are growth retarded.

3. There are two patterns of IUGR: symmetric and asymmetric.

a. Symmetric IUGR is characterized by a uniformly small fetus, with head and body size both smaller than expected.

b. Asymmetric IUGR is characterized by sparing of head size (normal biparietal diameter [BPD]) in the face of decreased abdominal and thoracic circumferences.

Etiology

1. Symmetric IUGR usually results from:

a. Constitutional factors (small parents)

b. Genetic or chromosomal anomalies
c. Intrauterine infection:
(1) Congenital rubella
(2) Cytomegalovirus

2. Asymmetric IUGR is more likely due to nutritional or hypoxic insult. This may be a primary deficit or secondary to decreased blood supply.

a. Conditions resulting in hypoxia:
(1) Severe maternal anemia, especially hemoglobinopathies
(2) Cyanotic heart disease
(3) Severe pulmonary disease
(4) Pregnancy at very high altitude
(5) Maternal smoking

b. Conditions resulting in poor fetal nutrition:
(1) Maternal starvation or poor maternal weight gain
(2) Maternal drug use (heroin, cocaine)
(3) Maternal alcoholism

c. Conditions resulting in decreased placental perfusion:
(1) Preeclampsia
(2) Diabetes with microvascular disease
(3) Chronic renal disease
(4) Multiple gestation
(5) Placental anomalies and infarction
(6) Postterm pregnancy

Diagnosis

1. IUGR may diagnosed when:

a. The fetus is shown to be below the tenth percentile in size for its age by USG. This presumes an accurate knowledge of gestational age, which may be based on last menstrual period (LMP) correlated with either early exam or previous ultrasound.

b. The fetus has failed to grow sufficiently during a specific time interval. This requires two sonograms at an interval of 2 to 4 weeks.

c. Asymmetric IUGR is demonstrated by ultrasound.

2. Sonographic determination of size is subject to the limitations of ultrasound technology; its translation into gestational age depends on local growth curves and the age at which the measurements are made.

a. In the first 2 to 3 months, ultrasonography may date a pregnancy to within 2 to 3 days.

b. By the early third trimester, a given fetal size may correlate with fetal ages spanning 3 weeks.

Risks

1. Fetuses suffering from IUGR are at increased risk for morbidity and mortality, because something has interfered with their growth.

2. If the IUGR is of chromosomal or genetic origin, this is a risk in itself.

3. It is of nutritional or hypoxic origin, the major risks are:

a. Fetal distress or hypoxic brain damage, both antepartum and during labor

b. Prematurity, since, if the IUGR is diagnosed many weeks prior to term, the prospects for good intrauterine growth until term are extremely poor

Management

1. **Antepartum**

a. Extremely careful monitoring of fetal well-being and growth.

(1) NSTs, CSTs, and BPPs at least weekly, if not more often

(2) Ultrasonography for growth at least every third week.

(3) Amniotic fluid L/S ratio and PG if delivery is contemplated but not mandated. IUGR fetuses frequently tolerate early delivery very well because the hostile intrauterine environment seems to hasten pulmonary maturity.

b. Indications for delivery:

(1) Fetal distress. The combination of nonreactive NST with either a positive CST or a BPP score less than 7 is an absolute indication for delivery in the third trimester.

(2) Poor interval growth. In the absence of fetal distress this is a relative indi-

cation for delivery, depending on the state of pulmonary maturity.

(3) Oligohydramnios. This is an extremely poor sign, as it both reflects and compounds fetal jeopardy. Fetal nutrition is usually quite poor, and cord accidents resulting in fetal injury or death are much more likely.

2. Intrapartum

a. Labor. Fetuses suffering from IUGR do not generally tolerate labor well. BUT SOME DO. With optimization of fetal oxygenation (maternal hyperoxygenation, lateral recumbent positioning, and excellent hydration), up to 25 per cent of IUGR fetuses may be delivered vaginally. If this is attempted, the following guidelines should be observed:

(1) EFM during labor is mandatory.

(2) Fetal scalp *p*H and C/S should be immediately available.

(3) Epidural anesthesia should be used with great care, if at all.

b. Cesarean section (C/S)

(1) C/S should be immediately available if a trial of labor is undertaken, and will frequently be necessary. Oligohydramnios drastically increases the likelihood of this.

(2) C/S without labor is frequently chosen if:

(a) Fetal condition is poor.

(b) The fetus is very premature.

(c) The cervix is unripe, and labor is likely to be long and hard.

HYDROCEPHALUS

Definition

Internal hydrocephalus is the collection of excess fluid within the ventricles of the brain, resulting in a very large head filled with fluid, and very little brain tissue.

Etiology

This condition is usually due to a blockage in the cerebrospinal pathways at the level of the upper spinal cord. Hydrocephalus is frequently associated wih spina bifida.

Diagnosis

1. Suspect hydrocephalus when there is an unusually large fundal mass, or when widened fontanelles are felt through the dilated cervix.

2. If hydrocephalus is suspected antepartum, almost certain diagnosis may be made using ultrasonography.

3. If the diagnosis is suspected during labor, confirm it with an AP film of the abdomen. In vertex presentations this should make the diagnosis. In breech presentations, because of the magnification factor, even an AP film may not be diagnostic of hydrocephalus.

Risks

1. Cephalopelvic disproportion almost invariably accompanies clinically evident hydrocephalus.

2. If the condition is undiagnosed and labor is allowed to continue without drainage, or, even worse, if labor is stimulated, uterine rupture is a real risk.

3. There are essentially no additional fetal risks to decompression, since even in mild cases fetal mortality is well over 50 per cent.

Management

The key to management is drainage of the hydrocephalus using a large-bore (16 to 18 gauge) long needle. This may be accomplished:

1. Transcervically in vertices when the cervix is 3 to 4 cm. dilated

2. Transcervically in breeches when the body has been delivered

3. Transabdominally in vertices prior to induction

4. Transabdominally in breeches after the body has been delivered

In lesser degrees of hydrocephalus, C/S is also an option.

ANENCEPHALY

Definition

Anencephaly is the complete or partial absence of the brain and overlying skull, associated with adrenal and pituitary hypoplasia.

Etiology

Probably inherited as a polygenic predisposition, anencephaly may be precipitated by an environmental agent. Currently suspected as an etiologic agent is an enzyme produced by the potato blight organism. About 70 per cent of anencephalic fetuses are female.

Diagnosis

1. Maternal serum alpha-fetoprotein (AFP) screening. Most anencephalic fetuses may be detected by the presence of elevated maternal serum alpha-fetoprotein detected between 15 and 18 weeks. Confirmation is by level 3 ultrasonography and amniocentesis for amniotic fluid AFP and acetylcholinesterase. (See Chap. 8, "Antepartum Fetal Evaluation.")

2. Ultrasonography. If missed by AFP screening (a rare occurrence), or in mothers not screened, anencephaly is diagnosed initially when failure to feel the fetal skull prompts USG to determine fetal lie.

Risks

1. The recurrence rate for future pregnancies is currently accepted to be between 4 and 5 per cent.

2. Among those anencephalic fetuses that escape detection and abortion in the second trimester:

a. Prolonged gestation is the rule. This may be due to the hypoplastic or absent pituitary gland.

b. The presentation is usually breech, but this is actually a benefit since the breech is larger than the head. In vertex presentations, which are usually face, shoulder dystocia at the incompletely dilated cervix is not uncommon.

c. Hydramnios is a common complication. In fact, anencephalus is the most common cause of hydramnios.

d. The risk of a surviving child is very small. Most die within a few hours after birth.

Management

1. If anencephalus is diagnosed during the second trimester, the treatment is therapeutic abortion.

2. If it is diagnosed in the third trimester, pregnancy should be terminated by amniocentesis, to remove excess amniotic fluid, and subsequent oxytocin infusion or prostaglandin stimulation, to induce labor.

18 Complications of Labor

David H. Fields

DYSFUNCTIONAL LABOR

Definitions

1. Normal labor is divided into three stages.

a. *Stage I.* From beginning of labor to full cervical dilatation

b. *Stage II.* From full dilatation to birth

c. *Stage III.* From delivery of the child to delivery of the placenta

2. Stage I labor is also divided into several phases:

a. *Prodromal or Latent Phase.* Contractions are mild, irregular and short (less than 45 seconds); usual duration several hours; some cervical effacement, little dilatation.

b. *Active Phase.* Contractions are strong (greater than 25 mmHg pressure), regular (usually every 2 to 3 minutes) and last longer (more than 45 seconds); cervical dilatation progresses, after effacement, at the rate of at least 1.2 cm./hr. in nulliparas and 1.5 cm./hr. in multiparas; this phase usually lasts from 2 to 3-cm. dilatation until about 8-cm. dilatation, although it may begin earlier.

c. *Deceleration Phase.* Contractions are somewhat shorter, perhaps weaker, and less frequent; completes dilatation.

3. Dysfunctional labor is an abnormality in any of the stages or phases of labor (usually in either Stage I or Stage II). It is characterized by lack of appropriate progress, either in cervical dilatation or in descent of the presenting part.

4. Hypotonic dysfunction is characterized by contractions of less than normal intensity, frequency, or duration.

5. Hypertonic dysfunction (much rarer) is characterized by strong, painful contractions which are uncoordinated.

Hypotonic Dysfunction

When due to contractions of less than normal intensity, prolongation of any stage or phase of labor is hypotonic dysfunction. The following categories have been created:

1. Prolonged Latent Phase

a. *Definition.* Duration of latent phase greater than 20 hours in a "primip" or greater than 14 hours in a "multip." Occurs very early in labor.

b. *Etiology*

(1) Excess sedation

(2) Patient not actually in labor

c. *Risks to Mother/Fetus.* These are essentially created by aggressive intervention. If the membranes are intact, prolonged latent phase is not associated with fetal or maternal risk, only discomfort.

d. *Management.* Most important is to determine that the patient is actually in labor. This can be done by:

(1) *Sedation* for the mother, either a barbiturate (Seconal or Nembutal 100 mg. I.M.) or a narcotic (Demerol 50 mg. I.M.). This will usually result in several hours of good rest after which the patient will awaken either out of labor or in active labor.

(2) *Oxytocin stimulation.* If the mother awakens from sedation and her condition is unchanged, she is most likely in labor. Augmentation with oxytocin infusion then becomes the treatment of choice.

2. Prolonged Active Phase

a. *Definition.* Dilatation of the cervix at less than 1.2 cm. per hour in a primipara and at less than 1.5 cm per hour in a multipara, after the active phase of labor has begun.

b. *Etiology*

(1) Cephalopelvic disproportion (CPD)

(2) Fetal malposition

(3) Conduction anesthesia applied too early

(4) Overdistension of the uterus with twins or hydramnios

c. *Risks to Mother/Fetus*

(1) If membranes are ruptured, prolonged labor with risk of amnionitis and fetal distress

(2) Iatrogenic fetal distress with intervention

(3) Slow steady progress, even if below the usual limits, is not dangerous and need not be treated.

d. *Management*

(1) *Oxytocin* if CPD is ruled out. Oxytocin stimulation, with all precautions as for augmented or induced labor, is indicated.

(2) *Amniotomy,* if membranes are intact and the head is not high.

(3) *Cesarean Section.* If oxytocin and amniotomy fail to effect dilation in an effaced cervix over 2 to 3 hours, or if fetal distress occurs, cesarean section should be performed since unsuspected CPD is likely.

3. Prolonged Deceleration Phase

a. *Definition.* Failure of the cervix to reach full dilatation after approximately 8 cm. Also known as an *arrest disorder.*

b. *Etiology*

(1) CPD

(2) Uterine exhaustion

c. *Risks.* CPD is much more likely here than it is in the presence of a steady prolonged first stage. Oxytocin must be used with care.

d. *Management.* Same as for prolonged active phase

4. Prolonged Second Stage

a. *Definition.* Second-stage labor lasting longer than 1 hour in multiparas or 2 hours in a primipara.

b. *Etiology*

(1) CPD

(2) Malposition, especially occiput posteriors

(3) Maternal exhaustion with poor expulsive efforts

(4) Conduction anesthesia with expulsive efforts

(5) Uterine exhaustion

c. *Risks.* Most of the risks of prolonged second stage are incurred when the physician makes heroic attempts to deliver the baby "from below."

(1) *Fetal Injury.* Overzealous use of oxytocin or forceps may cause fetal distress or physical injury.

(2) *Maternal Injury*

(a) Uterine rupture—secondary to either oxytocin or untended second stage for many hours. This rarely occurs today.

(b) Lower uterine segment, vaginal bladder injury secondary to forceps deliveries

(c) Amnionitis secondary to prolonged labor; since second stage prolongation is evident after an hour or two, this is usually not much of a problem.

d. *Management*

(1) If the mother is not pushing well, instruct in proper technique and actively encourage. This is surprisingly helpful.

(2) *Epidural Anesthesia.* If recently reinforced, allow to wear off. If fetal condition is closely monitored and good, a delay of an hour or so is not dangerous.

(3) *Oxytocin.* If there is no CPD and the fetal vertex is beyond easy reach of forceps, oxytocin infusion done cautiously is the treatment of choice.

(4) *Forceps.* If there is no CPD and the vertex is at +2 or +3 station, forceps delivery may be chosen. Must be done with care. Second stage arrests are often due to CPD.

(5) *Cesarean Section.* In cases of oxytocin failure, high vertex, fetal distress, or CPD, transabdominal delivery is the method of choice.

Hypertonic Dysfunction

1. Definition. Uterine contractions which seem to cause pain out of proportion to their strength or effect; contractions are more frequent than every 2 minutes, last longer than 75 seconds, or uterine tonus does not completely relax between. Usually occurs early in labor.

2. Etiology. The uterine musculature contracts in a discoordinated fashion, with midsegment predominance. The result is painful contractions with poor or no cervical dilatation.

3. Risks

a. *Fetal Distress.* Since placental supply is cut off by contractions, if it happens too often or for too long, the fetus is jeopardized.

b. *Precipitate Labor.* If hypertonic contractions are coordinated and occur in the presence of a well-effaced cervix, extremely rapid dilatation and descent of the fetus may occur. This may result in:

(1) Fetal distress
(2) Cervical or vaginal lacerations
(3) "Delivery in bed"
(4) Postpartum hemorrhage

4. Management

a. If there is hypertonic discoordinated labor with no fetal distress:

(1) Sedation with meperidine 75 to 100 mg. I.M. or Nembutal 100 mg. I.M. often solves this problem.

(2) In rare cases, careful use of oxytocin will organize the contractions into useful labor.

b. If there is precipitate labor with fetal distress:

(1) Tocolysis with a beta-mimetic may be useful, but is rarely resorted to.

(2) C/S is the more usual option.

c. If there is precipitate labor with no fetal distress

(1) Careful attendance during and after labor is required.

CEPHALOPELVIC DISPROPORTION

Definition

Whenever the fetal head is too large to fit through the maternal pelvis without danger, this is termed *cephalopelvic disproportion (CPD).* It may be of either maternal or fetal origin.

Etiology

1. Larger-than-normal fetus

(a) Constitutional

(b) Gestational diabetes and/or excessive maternal weight gain

(c) Postdates pregnancy without placental compromise

2. Smaller-than-necessary maternal pelvis

(a) *Inlet Contraction.* Associated with small women (especially those less than 5 feet tall) and android pelves.

(b) *Midpelvic Contraction.* Associated with android pelves.

(c) *Outlet Contraction.* Rarely a cause of CPD.

Diagnosis

1. CPD is usually diagnosed in labor. The following are suggestive:

(a) Unengaged head at term, especially after rupture of membranes, suggests inlet disproportion.

(b) Hypotonic labor or slower-than-normal cervical dilatation suggests CPD.

(c) Transverse arrest or arrest of descent during the second stage suggests midpelvic disproportion.

(d) Prolonged second stage, especially with good contractions, suggests CPD.

Risks

1. The only major risk of CPD is an inappropriate attempt at vaginal delivery resulting from a failure to recognize the problem. Maternal and fetal morbidity and mortality are all increased with midforceps deliveries attempted in the face of CPD.

Management

1. When CPD is suspected, *occasionally,* a careful trial of augmentation of labor with oxytocin, with appropriate fetal and maternal monitoring, may be attempted.
2. If this is not fruitful, C/S should be done.

SHOULDER DYSTOCIA

Definition

Inability to deliver the shoulders after the delivery of the fetal head

Etiology

A large fetus, especially over 4,000 g., predisposes to dystocia. This is especially to be suspected in pregnancies complicated by diabetes.

Diagnosis

1. Suspect shoulder dystocia if the estimated fetal weight is 4,000 g. or more.
2. Final diagnosis is made as the shoulders resist delivery.

Risks

Perinatal mortality ranges up to approximately 15 per cent.

1. **Hypoxia.** As the head is delivered, the umbilical cord is placed on traction and compressed in the birth canal. If delivery of the shoulders takes too long, hypoxia results.

2. **Fetal Injury**

a. Attempts to deliver the shoulders may result in spinal cord injury to the fetus.

b. Fracture of the clavicle is sometimes necessary for delivery.

Management

1. Optimal management of shoulder dystocia is to avoid it by diagnosis of the macrosomic fetus and careful use of C/S. In reality, one will never know if shoulder dystocia would have occurred if C/S is done.
2. If shoulder dystocia is diagnosed after the head is delivered, management should be as follows:

a. Clear the infant's nose and mouth by aspiration.

b. Prevent impaction of the anterior shoulder under the symphysis by rotating the fetus to an oblique position.

c. Perform or extend the episiotomy to generous proportions.

d. With the fetus still oblique, attempt delivery by combined cephalic traction and fundal pressure.

e. If this does not succeed, sweep the posterior arm out and repeat.

f. If this does not succeed, rotate the opposite shoulder to the posterior oblique position, remove that arm, and repeat *d.*

g. As a last resort, fracture a clavicle by pressure with a finger from the supraclavicular fossa OUTWARD. This helps avoid pleural puncture by the fractured clavicle.

While fractured clavicles are undesirable, they usually heal with no permanent injury if properly splinted.

h. If none of this is successful, some have advocated pushing the head back into the pelvis and then delivering the baby by C/S.

ABNORMAL PRESENTATIONS

Breech Presentation

1. **Definitions**

a. *Frank Breech.* Buttocks presenting, flexed hips, extended knees.

b. *Full Breech.* Buttocks presenting, flexed hips, flexed knees.

c. *Footling Breech.* One or both feet presenting

2. Etiology

a. Although more than half of all breeches occur without any predisposing pathology, factors which seem to predispose to breech presentation are those which create either more room in the fundus or less room in the pelvis, so that the larger fetal pole resides in the fundus. These include:

(1) Multiparity
(2) Prematurity
(3) Hydramnios
(4) Hydrocephalus
(5) Placenta previa
(6) Low uterine fibroids
(7) Uterine anomalies
(8) Twins

3. Incidence. While at 28 weeks up to 40 per cent of all fetuses are breech, at term only 3 to 4 per cent have not converted to vertex.

4. Diagnosis

a. *Before Labor.* The head may be felt as a hard rounded mass in the fundus. Significantly, the head is NOT felt on vaginal exam. If the cervix is dilated, the irregular breech may be palpated through it. Definitive diagnosis is by ultrasound.

b. *During Labor.* Same as before labor, except that, if ultrasound is not available, x-ray flat plate may be used. If vaginal delivery is considered, x-ray to verify flexion of the fetal head and adequacy of the maternal pelvis may be indicated.

5. Risks

a. *Maternal.* There is no appreciable increase in risk for the mother.

b. *Fetal.* There is considerably increased risk for the fetus.

(1) Overall mortality in several series of breech deliveries has ranged up to 25 per cent.

(2) Even when corrected for prematurity and congenital anomalies, (increased twofold), the mortality rate for breech deliveries is still at least two to five times that for vertex deliveries.

(3) The major causes of fetal mortality and morbidity include:

(a) Traumatic delivery, with injury to:

1. The brain—intracranial hemorrhage, tentorial tears

2. Spinal cord

3. Brachial plexus—Erb's palsy

4. Abdominal viscera—liver, spleen, adrenals

(b) Cord prolapse, especially with footling breeches

(c) Associated congenital anomalies—twice as likely with breeches

(d) Prematurity

6. Management

a. *Cesarean Section.* Increasingly, breech presentation has become an indication for abdominal delivery. Some physicians advocate cesarean section for all breech deliveries, since for all practical purposes, the morbidity and mortality which seems to be inherent in breech vaginal delivery can be essentially eliminated by cesarean section. This is an argument which cannot be refuted. It can only be weighed against the increased maternal morbidity and mortality attendant to cesarean section and possibly repeat cesarean section. Below is a generally accepted list of indications for abdominal delivery of a breech fetus, according to Pritchard and MacDonald:

(1) Fetus with estimated weight over 8 pounds

(2) Premature breech with estimated weight 1,000 to 2,500 g.

(3) Any contracture of the maternal pelvis

(4) Hyperextension of the fetal spine or head

(5) Breech not in labor or not engaged

(6) Footling breech

(7) Dysfunctional labor

(8) Previous perinatal death

(9) Concurrent desire for tubal sterilization

(10) Nulliparous breech

b. *Vaginal Delivery.* If the fetus weighs between 2,500 g. and 4,000 g., is a frank or full breech with a flexed head and an older sibling, has chosen a mother with a good pelvis, and the physician opts for vaginal delivery, there are several measures that should be taken:

(1) Perform x-ray pelvimetry to verify an adequate pelvis, if the first child was not as large as or larger than the current one

(2) Monitor labor carefully, with external fetal monitoring until rupture of membranes and internal monitoring thereafter

(3) Maintain intact membranes as long as possible to effect a good dilating wedge

(4) Perform a very generous episiotomy (mediolateral, if necessary) under good anesthesia (epidural is most preferable).

(5) Allow spontaneous delivery to the umbilicus, if possible. The sooner one converts a *spontaneous* delivery to an *extraction*, the higher the neonatal morbidity.

(6) Most often, however, traction on the hips is necessary to deliver the legs. This must be applied to the hips, not the legs. If this is not successful, *decomposition* is performed by drawing the legs down one at a time.

(7) From this point, the fetus may be grasped by the hips or high on the thighs (held in flexed position), but never around the abdomen, as this is how the viscera are traumatized.

(8) Traction with the fetus now in the AP position accomplishes the delivery of the chest to the axillae.

(9) The arms are delivered by rotating the fetus back to the transverse and delivering either the anterior or posterior arm first. Usually this can be achieved spontaneously by raising or lowering the infant's body. If this does not work, the arms must each be extracted by traction on the elbow joint (not on the humerus—it will fracture).

(10) After delivery of the arms, maintain flexion of the head by continuous suprapubic pressure provided by an assistant.

(11) Deliver the head by raising the fetal body above the midline until the chin becomes visible. The Mauriceau maneuver may be used to aid flexion but should not be used for traction, since it may result in serious injury to the fetus.

(12) Continue the delivery of the head by *slowly* easing out the rest of the fetal skull to avoid tentorial tears and intracranial injury.

(13) If the delivery of the head is not accomplished easily, one should use Piper forceps. The application and use of Pipers is the same as for any other forceps, except for verification of their placement. They should be on the delivery table, unwrapped and ready for use, in every breech delivery.

c. ALWAYS TREAT A BREECH DELIVERY WITH THE RESPECT ACCORDED A CESAREAN SECTION. It should always be attended by

(1) Someone skilled in breech delivery

(2) A competent anesthesiologist, and

(3) Someone skilled in neonatal resuscitation

(4) Immediate cesarean section should always be available.

d. *External Version.* In an attempt to avoid the neonatal risks of breech vaginal delivery and the maternal morbidity of cesarean section, many obstetricians are turning increasingly to external version.

(1) Several considerations apply in deciding whether and when to perform version.

(a) The advantage of external version is avoidance of cesarean section.

(b) The risks of external version are disruption of the placenta and cord trauma, necessitating immediate delivery.

(c) Earlier versions (32 to 36 weeks) are more likely to be successful but also more likely to be unnecessary, as the fetus might turn by itself. Also, immediate delivery resulting from trauma during version is a more serious complication in the more premature.

(d) Later versions (37+ weeks) are less likely to be successful but more likely to be necessary. It is also of less consequence if immediate delivery is necessary.

(e) Versions can only be done if the breech is not engaged. The higher the presenting part, the better.

(2) Technique.

(a) Monitor the fetus with EFM for 20 minutes.

(b) Have mother N.P.O. in case immediate delivery is necessary.

(c) Most physicians use oral tocolysis (ritodrine, etc.).

(d) Identify fetal back and head, placenta, and cord (if possible) with real-time ultrasound.

(e) Rotate fetus as if in head-first roll (cord entanglement may be less likely to occur this way).

(f) Fix head in pelvis.

(g) Monitor fetus with real-time ultrasound and then with EFM for 20 minutes.

(h) Continue oral tocolysis.

Face Presentation

1. Definition. Extreme extension of the fetal head so that facial organs present against the cervix

2. Etiology. Anything that prevents flexion of the head predisposes to face presentation. This includes:

a. Pelvic inlet contraction

b. Pendulous abdomen

c. Anencephaly

d. Multiple loops of cord around the neck

e. Fetal cervical ligament contracture

f. Low pelvic tumors

3. Risks

a. Usually all major risks are from traumatic intervention.

b. If the chin rotates posteriorly, vaginal delivery is impossible.

4. Management

a. Rule out contracted pelvis.

b. If no pelvic contraction exists and the chin is anterior, spontaneous vaginal delivery may be allowed.

c. If there is any pelvic contraction, if the chin rotates posteriorly, or if operative intervention is contemplated, perform cesarean section.

d. Forceps should not be used.

Brow Presentation

1. Definition. The fetal vertex is midway between full extension (face) and full flexion (occiput). The presenting part at the inlet is essentially the forehead.

2. Etiology. Usually pelvic contraction

3. Risks

a. Engagement cannot occur as long as the brow presentation persists.

b. Rupture of membranes with an unengaged head predisposes to cord prolapse.

4. Management

a. If the fetus can be monitored, labor may be observed to see if the brow spontaneously converts to an occiput or to a face presentation.

b. If it converts to an occiput, vaginal delivery is anticipated.

c. If it converts to a face presentation, management is as described in the preceding section.

d. If conversion does not occur, or if fetal distress or dysfunctional labor occurs, perform cesarean section.

Transverse Lie (Shoulder Presentation)

1. Definition. The fetus lies perpendicular to the long axis of the uterus. The presenting part may be either a shoulder or the back. A slight variation of this is the *oblique* lie, with the fetus not quite perpendicular.

2. Etiology

a. Contracted pelvis

b. Pendulous abdomen in a grand multipara

c. Placenta previa

d. Prematurity

e. Hydramnios

3. Risks.

a. Vaginal delivery is impossible with a transverse lie. Maternal and fetal death may result from attempts at version during labor.

b. Rupture of the membranes in such cases carries a high risk of cord or arm prolapse.

c. Immediate cesarean section should be performed if one is certain of a transverse lie.

4. Management

a. If it is a true transverse lie, no presenting part is felt on vaginal exam. If a shoulder, the head is usually palpable in one of the iliac fossae. Ultrasound confirms the diagnosis. if ultrasound is unavailable, a single x-ray flat plate is obtained.

Compound Presentation

1. Definition. A combination of an extremity (usually a hand) and either the vertex (usually) or the breech presenting together

2. Etiology. Prematurity is most commonly identified.

3. Risks

a. Prolapsed cord from failure to occlude the inlet

b. If prolapsed cord does not occur, there is no inherent risk in a compound presentation since labor usually proceeds normally.

4. Management

a. Treat as normal labor until full dilatation.

b. If the prolapsed extremity is not withdrawn by full dilatation, it may be pushed upwards. It is sometimes more effective to pinch the hand or foot so that the fetus retracts it by itself.

Persistent Occiput Posterior (OP)

1. Definition. Vertex presentation which remains in the occiput posterior position after full dilatation. This occurs in bout 5 per cent of vertex labors.

2. Etiology

a. Persistent OP with an unengaged vertex is usually due to inlet contraction.

b. OP with an engaged vertex is most likely due to midpelvic dystocia, usually with an anthropoid or android pelvis.

3. Risks

a. If engagement occurs and satisfactory descent follows, the only major risk of an OP delivery is the likelihood of an episiotomy extension because of the greater excursion of the vertex.

b. If descent is impaired or labor dysfunctional, the risk of performing an unintentionally high forceps delivery is also present. This is because in the OP position, unusual elongation of the fetal skull with formation of tremendous caput may occur. In extreme cases, fetal hair may protrude at the vagina with an unengaged head.

4. Management

a. *Spontaneous rotation* to occiput anterior (OA) or *spontaneous delivery* as an OP may occur, especially if labor is aided with oxytocin, and if there is no CPD.

b. *Manual rotation* to OA followed by spontaneous or forceps delivery may be attempted.

c. *Forceps delivery* as an OP or forceps rotation to OA may be performed if there is no CPD. Be sure of the station of the vertex before applying forceps.

d. If any of the above is not easily feasible, cesarean section becomes the preferred method of delivery.

Persistent Occiput Transverse

1. Definition. Arrest of the fetal vertex with the sagittal suture in the transverse position after full cervical dilatation

2. Etiology. Transverse arrest may be divided into two categories: with and without CPD.

a. When complicated by pelvic dystocia, transverse arrest is commonly associated with android or platypelloid pelves.

b. When occurring without CPD, transverse arrest is usually due to hypotonic labor and conduction anesthesia.

3. Risks. The major risk of transverse arrest is an attempted forceps delivery in the face of unsuspected CPD.

4. Management

a. Determine presence or absence of CPD.

b. If CPD is not apparent and labor is not of good quality, an attempt to rotate the head with oxytocin infusion is warranted. If this is not successful, the physician should recheck for the presence of CPD.

c. If the physician is still confident that there is no disproportion, and the head is at plus 2 station or lower, a cautious attempt at forceps delivery may be made.

d. If at any time there is a suspicion of CPD, or measures *b.* and *c.* fail, cesarean section should be performed.

PROLAPSE OF THE UMBILICAL CORD

Definitions

1. Occult Prolapse. The umbilical cord falls into the pelvis next to the presenting part but not beyond it and cannot be reached by the examining finger.

2. Forelying Cord. The cord is in front of the presenting part but the membranes are intact.

3. True Prolapsed Cord. The membranes are ruptured, and the umbilical cord is in front of the presenting part, usually compressed by it.

Etiology

All conditions which interfere with engagement predispose to cord prolapse. These include:

1. Transverse lie, footling breech

2. Premature rupture of the membranes with a floating presenting part or with a very premature infant

3. Inlet contraction

4. Twins

5. Hydramnios

Diagnosis

1. Occult cord prolapse is detected by variable decelerations on fetal heart rate monitoring during labor.

2. Forelying cords and true prolapses are suspected by monitoring and can be confirmed by vaginal examination.

Management

1. Occult Prolapse. See "Variable Deceleration," Chap. 11, "Intrapartum Fetal Monitoring."

2. Forelying Cord. Cesarean section

3. True Prolapse

a. If vaginal delivery can be anticipated within 5 minutes, either spontaneously or by forceps, it may be attempted.

b. If vaginal delivery is not imminent:

(1) Position patient in deep Trendelenburg or knee-chest position.

(2) Elevate presenting part out of the pelvis and hold it there until cesarean section is performed.

(3) Prepare for immediate cesarean section.

AMNIOTIC FLUID EMBOLISM (AFE)

Definition

Infusion of amniotic-fluid particulate matter (vernix, lanugo, meconium) into the maternal circulation through the uterine veins

Etiology

Requiring simultaneous openings in the amnion and the uterine veins, AFE is most often associated with placental abruption.

Diagnosis

1. This relatively rare syndrome should be suspected when a woman in labor develops severe dyspnea, cyanosis, tachycardia, hypotension, and tachypnea.

2. Signs of disseminated intravascular coagulopathy (DIC) follow rapidly if death does not occur.

3. Definitive diagnosis is usually postmortem, with the demonstration of AF debris in the maternal circulation.

Risks

1. Cardiovascular Collapse. Particulate matter (lanugo, meconium, vernix) lodges within the pulmonary vasculature to cause acute cor pulmonale and right heart failure.

2. DIC. Thromboplastic substances, found in great quantities in AF, initiate DIC, usually manifested by bleeding from puncture sites and from the uterus.

3. Death. Most physicians question the diagnosis of AFE if the patient SURVIVES. Pulmonary vascular obstruction and systemic vascular collapse are usually rapidly fatal. Perhaps less serious cases escape our notice.

Management

Therapy is usually not successful but is directed at improving oxygenation, maintaining blood pressure and cardiac output, and combating coagulation defects. This is as much an emergency as cardiac or respiratory arrest. Resuscitation should involve the cardiac arrest team.

INVERSION OF THE UTERUS

Definition

The fundus of the uterus is prolapsed, inside out, through the cervix.

Etiology

This rare occurrence is almost always the result of traction placed upon a fundally implanted placenta directly after delivery.

Diagnosis

Manual exploration of the vagina and uterus after every delivery will identify inversion when it occurs.

Risks

Hemorrhage and shock secondary to blood loss are the major immediate risks.

Management

1. Immediate replacement of the fundus tremendously decreases morbidity by cutting down on blood loss.

2. If the placenta has separated in the process of inverting the uterus:

a. Use a fist to push the fundus back through the cervix immediately, while applying countertraction to the cervix with multiple ring clamps.

b. Provide oxytocin stimulation.

3. If the placenta is intact, try the same maneuver.

4. If not immediately successful:

a. Start a large-bore I.V., if none is in place already.

b. Begin fluid replacement, including blood if necessary.

c. Anesthetize the mother.

d. Remove the placenta manually.

e. Try again to replace the fundus through the cervix, as above.

f. Provide oxytocin stimulation.

5. If bimanual replacement is not possible because the cervix has constricted, immediate laparotomy should be performed.

PLACENTA ACCRETA

Definition

Placenta accreta is used as a generic term for abnormal implantation of the placenta. While the term *placenta accreta* strictly refers to only one degree of this abnormality, it is commonly used to refer to any penetration of the placenta into the uterus interfering with separation during the third stage of labor. There are three degrees of abnormal penetration:

1. Placenta accreta. Superficial penetration of the myometrium

2. Placenta increta. Deep penetration of the myometrium

3. Placenta percreta. Penetration totally through the myometrium

Etiology

1. The placenta normally implants into the decidua, which serves as a barrier to myometrial penetration. When something interferes with decidual formation, this barrier fails and some degree of placental penetration into the uterus itself occurs.

2. Interfering factors include

a. Endometrial trauma from previous curettage, C/S scar, or grand multiparity

b. Poor decidual response in the lower uterine segment, as seen with placenta previa.

Diagnosis

1. Most accretas and incretas are diagnosed after failure of the placenta to separate during an attempt at manual removal.

2. Percretas and previas often cause antepartum hemorrhage and so may be diagnosed earlier.

Risk

Maternal hemorrhage

Management

1. Appropriate therapy is obvious only after the fact, since it depends on the degree of penetration and the area of involvement. If the area of adherence is large, attempts at manual removal always result in massive blood loss.

2. Therefore, if the placenta does not separate and a plane of cleavage is not present, the following steps should be taken before proceeding:

a. Start a large-bore I.V.

b. Obtain blood for possible transfusion.

3. Attempt manual removal.

4. Sometimes curettage followed by uterine packing is effective.

5. More often in major accretas hysterectomy is necessary.

6. The real problem is deciding whether to attempt less drastic solutions or to go directly to hysterectomy.

7. If one knows there is a total accreta, one may leave the placenta in place and allow spontaneous involution in situ or treat with methotrexate. This has occasionally worked but cannot be attempted after partial removal has provoked bleeding.

19 Hemorrhage in Pregnancy

David H. Fields

DEFINITIONS

1. Vaginal bleeding during pregnancy is usually classified by the time of its occurrence. For practical purposes, it may be divided into bleeding during:

- **a.** First trimester
- **b.** Second trimester
- **c.** Third trimester
- **d.** Postpartum period

2. The bleeding may vary in quantity from a few drops, which may be of little or no meaning or may presage an impending problem, up to torrential hemorrhage.

BASIC PRINCIPLES

1. The first priority in antepartum vaginal bleeding is to ensure the safety of the mother, followed by the safety of the fetus. If the bleeding is not of life-threatening intensity this is best accomplished by establishing the etiology, from which prognostic and therapeutic decisions may be made.

2. Hemorrhage threatens pregnancy in two ways:

a. If the bleeding is of maternal origin, excessive loss will put the mother in danger of either shock or coagulatory dysfunction, and consequently will endanger the fetus.

b. If the bleeding is of placental origin, the fetus may be directly threatened by its own blood loss as well as by the consequences of maternal shock.

3. In the first 24 to 28 weeks of pregnancy, immediate delivery almost always means the death of the baby; so if there is an otherwise healthy fetus, maternal risk is what one weighs against delay in delivery.

4. In the third trimester, one weighs the risks of delay against those of immediate delivery for both mother and fetus.

FIRST TRIMESTER BLEEDING

Definition

Bleeding during the first thirteen weeks after the last menstrual period (LMP)

Basic Principles

1. One-third of all pregnant women bleed in the first trimester. Approximately half of these abort spontaneously. Among the rest there is a slightly higher incidence of congenital anomalies and of later pregnancy complications, such as premature labor.

2. If the bleeding is heavy enough to endanger the mother, then stopping it is the first priority, even if this requires immediate termination of the pregnancy.

3. If the bleeding reflects an ectopic pregnancy (almost all ectopic pregnancies bleed within the first 8 weeks), concerns for the pregnancy are irrelevant and management is as described in Chap. 5.

4. If the bleeding is associated with intrauterine pregnancy (IUP), management depends on whether there is a live embryo/ fetus or not.

Etiology

1. Threatened abortion
2. Incomplete abortion
3. Ectopic pregnancy
4. Loss of a twin
5. Placental consolidation
6. Cervicitis or vaginitis
7. Cervical or vaginal neoplasia
8. Molar pregnancy

Management

1. Perform pelvic exam to determine if bleeding is of intrauterine, cervical, or vaginal origin.

2. If the bleeding arises from the cervix or vagina, treat appropriately for vaginitis, cervicitis, laceration, etc.

3. If the bleeding is coming from inside the uterus and is heavy enough to endanger the mother or is associated with cervical dilatation or passage of tissue, stopping it is the first priority. Perform D&C and obtain pathology on intrauterine contents.

4. If the bleeding is from inside the uterus, but maternal condition does not mandate immediate therapy, attempt to determine fetal status and location:

a. If gestation is less than 6 to 7 weeks:

(1) Obtain quantitative human chorionic gonadotropin (HCG).

(2) If HCG is greater than 6,500 mIu/ ml., IUP should be demonstrable with ultrasonography (USG).

(a) If USG shows a living IUP, bed rest and proscription of sex for 1 week after the last bleeding are standard recommendations. They may or may not be of value.

(b) If USG does not reveal a living IUP, perform D&C and, if suspicion is high for ectopic pregnancy, laparoscopy as well.

(3) If HCG is less than 6,500 mIu/ml. the pregnancy may not be large enough to find reliably with USG transabdominal. With newer endovaginal probe, fetal viability may be demonstrated at HCG levels as low as 700–1,000 mIu/ml. Repeat HCG in 2 to 3 days. (If the new vaginal USG transducer is available, IUP may be demonstrable at HCG concentration lower than 1,000 mIu/ml.).

(a) If the trend is upward, continue to repeat at 2- to 3-day intervals and perform sonography when levels are higher than 6,500 mIu/ml (1,000–2,000 mIu/ml if endovaginal probe is available). N.b.: Most healthy IUPs are associated with HCG levels that double every 48 to 72 hours. If the rate of increase is less than this, suspect blighted ovum or ectopic pregnancy.

(b) If the trend is not upward, perform D&C.

b. If gestation is of more than 7 weeks, USG should be able to demonstrate a living embryo/fetus with fetal heart activity. If it does, recommend bed rest, abstinence from sex, and observation. If it does not, perform D&C.

SECOND TRIMESTER BLEEDING

Definition

Bleeding between the fourteenth and twenty-seventh weeks of pregnancy

Basic Principles

1. In the past, the second trimester was supposed to correlate with a period after embryogenesis, but before fetal viability. However, as medical care for the very premature infant has improved, extrauterine survival has become possible for babies delivered as early as 24 to 25 weeks in some centers. Consequently, management in this "gray area" must be tempered by the varying likelihood of fetal survival at individual hospitals.

2. Usually, second trimester bleeding is associated with a living fetus that will die if delivered. Therefore, the desired approach is to prolong the pregnancy if this can be done without significantly endangering the mother.

Etiology

1. Late spontaneous abortion
2. Hydatidiform mole

3. Incompetent cervix
4. Placenta previa
5. Premature placental separation
6. Abnormally formed placenta
7. Premature labor
8. Cervical or vaginal lesions

Management

1. Perform speculum exam to determine site of bleeding.

2. If the bleeding is of vaginal or exocervical origin, treat appropriately.

3. If the bleeding is of uterine origin, perform sonography to determine fetal status and placental location, and digital cervical exam to determine dilatation and effacement.

4. Manage as discussed under specific diseases. Since most causes of second trimester bleeding are treated in the same fashion as either first or third trimester causes, depending on fetal viability, they are discussed under headings found in those sections. Incompetent cervix is considered in Chap. 17, and hydatidiform mole in Chapter 5.

THIRD TRIMESTER BLEEDING

Definition

Bleeding after the twenty-seventh week of pregnancy

Basic Principles

1. In the third trimester one usually has the opton of terminating the pregnancy if necessary and still obtaining a living infant, albeit a sick one.

2. Therefore, issues of fetal as well as maternal health enter into decisions about whether to prolong the pregnancy or to terminate it.

Etiology

1. Placenta previa
2. Vasa previa
3. Premature placental separation
4. Abnormally formed placenta
5. Labor
6. Cervical and vaginal lesions

Management

1. Establish fetal well-being by verification of fetal heart tones and electronic fetal monitoring (EFM), if necessary.

2. If the bleeding occurs in the absence of active labor or pain, placenta previa is highly likely. Therefore, vaginal exam is not done until placental localization via sonography has ruled out this cause. Exceptions to this may be made if one can feel the head well applied to the lower uterine segment or cervix.

3. If the bleeding is accompanied by either contractions (suggesting labor) or pain (suggesting placental separation), abdominal exam and vaginal exam for cervical assessment should be the first steps.

4. Management for specific conditions is discussed below.

PLACENTA PREVIA

Definition

Implantation of the placenta in such a position that part or all of the placenta overlies the internal os of the cervix

1. **Total Placenta Previa.** The internal os is completely covered.

2. **Partial Placenta Previa.** The internal os is partially covered.

3. **Marginal Placenta Previa.** The placenta may be touched through the cervix, but does not extend beyond its edge.

4. **Low-lying Placenta.** The placenta lies in the lower uterine segment but is not a true previa.

It is important to realize that the placental-uterine relationship appears to be dynamic. A placenta previa sonographically documented early in pregnancy may migrate fundally and be "non-previa" near term. Additionally, what is not a previa early in labor may become so later as the cervix dilates.

Etiology

While there is no specific etiology, placenta previa seems to be more common in:

1. Multiparas of older age

2. Diseases complicated by large placentas, such as diabetes and hemolytic Rh disease

3. Previous lower segment scarring, as from C/S and perhaps curettage

Diagnosis

1. Ultrasonography (USG)

a. The key to diagnosis of placenta previa is ultrasonographic investigation of all painless, bright-red bleeding before the onset of labor.

b. An added benefit of ultrasonographic investigation is that fetal biparietal diameter and an estimation of fetal age can be obtained at the same time.

2. Double Set-up Examination. If bleeding is heavy enough to require immediate delivery, or the patient is in labor, a sterile vaginal exam may be performed under double set-up conditions. This means that the patient is on the operating room table, prepped and draped, ready for immediate C/S if necessary, at the time of the examination.

Risks

1. Maternal

a. *Hemorrhage with shock* is the major risk for the mother.

b. The initial bleeding episode is almost always self-limited and not fatal. However, with repeated episodes of bleeding, the mother may be brought to the "edge of shock," and pushed over by the next occurrence.

2. Fetal

a. *Premature delivery,* forced by repeated bleeding episodes, accounts for most of the fetal mortality associated with placenta previa.

b. Since the blood loss is usually maternal rather than fetal, fetal shock if present is usually due to asphyxia secondary to maternal shock and decreased uteroplacental blood flow.

General Management

1. Once the diagnosis is made, the physician must decide whether to deliver the fetus immediately or allow continued pregnancy. The rationale for allowing pregnancy to continue is only to await fetal maturity. Either way, hospitalization is mandatory.

2. Continuation of pregnancy is preferable if all of the following conditions are met:

a. Gestational age less than 37 weeks

b. Bleeding stopped, or slow enough not to threaten mother

c. No labor or abdominal pain

d. No fetal distress as demonstrated by nonstress fetal monitoring

3. Immediate delivery is preferable if any of the following occur:

a. Fetal maturity—gestational age 37 weeks or greater

b. Labor

c. Deteriorating maternal condition as evidenced by tachycardia, hypotension, or severe hemorrhage

d. Fetal distress

Hospital Orders for Conservative Management

1. Bed rest until there has been no bleeding for 24 hours

2. Vital signs q.1h. until bleeding has stopped; then q.4h.

3. N.P.O. until bleeding has been stopped for 24 hours

4. Running I.V. (D_5 W or salt solution at 100 to 150 ml. per hour) as long as patient is N.P.O.

5. Hematocrit/hemoglobin (H/H) on admission and as necessary

6. Type and crossmatch for 2 units of packed red blood cells.

7. Transfusion for H/H under 10/30 or as clinical condition warrants

8. Tocolytics are not approved for use in placenta previa. However, since the cause of the bleeding is effacement of the underlying cervix or lower segment, it would seem that their use might be beneficial. There is the theoretical objection that since they increase uterine blood flow and inhibit contractions, they might increase blood loss in the event of hemorrhage.

9. Similarly, although cervical cerclage is not generally used to treat placenta previa, there is at least one report of successful management of several cases in this fashion.

Method of Delivery

1. Cesarean Section (C/S)

a. Since the hemorrhage in labor may be life-threatening and in most cases of placenta previa the placenta obstructs the birth canal, cesarean section is almost always the method of delivery.

b. The uterine incision will depend on the location of the placenta. If it extends over the anterior wall of the uterus, a vertical incision above the placenta is necessary. Otherwise, a transverse low segment incision may be made.

c. If placental implantation is low enough that lower segment bleeding cannot be stopped after delivery, hysterectomy may be required.

2. Vaginal Delivery

a. If the diagnosis is made by double set-up examination and the placenta can be documented as partial or marginal, amniotomy may allow the fetal head to descend and stop the bleeding.

b. If this does not occur, or if maternal shock or fetal distress occurs, immediate C/S should be performed.

c. Intensive fetal heart rate (FHR) monitoring is mandatory in these labors.

LOW LYING PLACENTA

Basic Principles

1. If diagnosed when placenta previa is suspected, this condition should be treated in almost the same manner as a partial or marginal placenta previa, but with expectations for successful vaginal delivery.

2. What this means is that the causes of bleeding and dangers to the mother and fetus are of the same origin as in placenta previa, but usually are less severe.

Management

1. If the criteria for conservative management of placenta previa are met, observation is justified.

2. When there is labor, amniotomy generally suffices to control bleeding. Labor is conducted with careful maternal and fetal monitoring.

3. If amniotomy does not control the bleeding and maternal or fetal condition deteriorates, C/S is indicated.

MARGINAL SINUS RUPTURE

Definition

Minimal premature separation of the edge of the placenta

Etiology

Unknown

Diagnosis

1. Clinically, this is indistinguishable from placenta previa, being characterized by painless antepartum bleeding, although it is, in fact, a mild form of placental abruption.

2. The diagnosis is one of presumption when USG reveals a normally placed placenta and subsequent vaginal examination reveals no lesions.

Risks

Marginal sinus rupture may progress to more severe placental abruption, although there is no way to predict this. If it does not, risks are minimal and related to total maternal blood loss.

Management

1. As long as the bleeding continues, the patient should be maintained on bed rest.

2. If the bleeding remains mild, one should pursue expectant management, awaiting spontaneous labor or attainment of fetal maturity, while performing frequent assessment of fetal well-being with EFM and biophysical profile (BPP) as necessary.

3. When delivery is planned, because of either spontaneous labor or attainment of fetal maturity, amniotomy allows for better labor and a more accurate assessment of blood loss.

PLACENTAL ABRUPTION

Definition

1. Premature separation of an otherwise normally implanted placenta after the twentieth week of gestation is called *placental abruption.*

2. The degree of separation may vary from minimal, as in marginal sinus ruptures, to total.

3. Separations may be at the periphery of the placenta, in which case they tend not to extend because the blood can escape; or they may be central and progressive, with bleeding causing further dissection of the placenta from its bed, causing further bleeding, and so on.

Etiology

While no single cause of placental abruption is known, several maternal conditions seem to predispose to its occurrence:

1. Hypertension is the most commonly found predisposing factor, being found in almost 50 per cent of cases.

2. Multiparity

3. Rapid reduction of intrauterine volume, simulating delivery, as in rupture of membranes in the presence of hydramnios and delivery of the first twin

4. Trauma

5. History of placental abruption in previous pregnancy carries an extremely high risk of repetition.

Diagnosis

1. Suspect placental abruption whenever there is antepartum vaginal bleeding in combination with abdominal pain.

2. Localized or, in more severe cases, generalized uterine tenderness and rigidity strengthen the diagnosis.

3. Signs of maternal shock (hypotension, tachycardia) accompany major abruption.

4. EFM should be instituted in all cases of antepartum bleeding to detect fetal distress.

5. If the diagnosis is in doubt and maternal and fetal conditions do not mandate immediate delivery, perform USG for placental localization and perform cervical exam if there is no evidence of placenta previa.

If either the fetus or the mother is in sufficient distress to require delivery, perform double set-up exam.

Risks (Maternal)

1. Shock secondary to blood loss is the major risk for the mother with placental abruption. This often occurs in the face of apparently minor blood loss, because of retroplacental pooling of blood.

2. Defibrination with secondary coagulopathy may occur. This is most likely due to disseminated intravascular coagulation precipitated by release of placental thromboplastins; however, with central abruption, the formation of a large retroplacental clot may result in hypofibrinogenemia.

3. Disseminated Intravascular Coagulation is probably secondary to release of tremendous amounts of placental thromboplastin. Characterized by hypofibrinogenemia (fibrinogen level less than 100 mg. per 100 ml.), prolonged prothrombin time (PT) and activated partial thromboplastin time (APTT), elevated fibrin split products, and thrombocytopenia, it results in generalized bleeding from puncture and wound sites. Spontaneous hemorrhage may accompany platelet counts below 20,000 per cu. mm. Occasionally, a large retroplacental clot may consume enough fibrinogen to cause isolated hypofibrinogenemia.

4. Renal shutdown has classically been described with severe placental abruption. This is almost certainly secondary to hypovolemic shock.

5. The classically described Couvelaire uterus, secondary to extravasation of blood through the myometrium to below the uterine serosa, may result in functional impairment.

Risks (Fetal)

Fetal Distress occurs with all but the mildest abruptions. An otherwise healthy fetus may tolerate up to a 50-per-cent loss of placental function. However, when caused by abruption, this is usually compounded by decreased perfusion of the remaining placenta secondary to maternal blood loss. If abruption occurs to any significant degree outside the hospital, fetal death is likely.

Management

Once the diagnosis of placental abruption has been established, the need for delivery is apparent, unless the fetus is very immature or the symptomatology so mild that only a marginal separation is suspected.

The following plan of treatment optimizes fetal salvage and minimizes maternal morbidity.

1. Evaluation

a. Vital signs every 30 minutes

b. Frequent palpation of the uterus for signs of rigidity or increase in the height of the fundus

c. Frequent evaluation of the amount of uterine bleeding

d. Careful monitoring of urine output

e. Continuous FHR and contraction mointoring by EFM

f. Complete blood count (CBC), including platelet count

g. Electrolytes

h. Coagulation workup consisting of fibrinogen levels, PT, APTT, thrombin time (TT) and fibrin split product measurement. If a plain tube of blood is taken and observed for clot formation, coagulatory status can be roughly gauged in a matter of minutes. If a good clot is formed within several minutes, fibrinogen levels are almost certainly higher than 100 mg. per 100 ml. If not, all the above tests will most likely be abnormal.

i. Urinalysis, espcially for specific gravity and protein

j. Type and crossmatch for 4 units of packed cells with fresh frozen plasma if needed for coagulopathy. If fresh frozen plasma is not available, fresh whole blood should be used.

2. Therapy

a. Begin fluid replacement with intravenous Ringer's lactate or normal saline solution AND blood as necessary. It is far better to stay ahead than to get behind on blood replacement.

b. Definitive therapy for placental abruption is delivery. This stops the bleeding and disseminated intravascular coagulation and ends the danger to the fetus. However, if the abruption seems to be minor and the fetus is very premature, careful observation of both mother and child in the hospital, with the knowledge that the situation can worsen at any moment, may be preferable.

c. When delivery is undertaken, avoiding C/S is especially desirable for two reasons: Maternal blood loss may be greater and coagulopathy, if present, will significantly increase any operative risks. Furthermore, labor often occurs spontaneously and progresses quite well in cases of abruption, probably due to prostaglandin release by the injured placenta. This is true even if induction is necessary.

d. Labor and vaginal delivery may be attempted under the following conditions:

(1) Maternal vital signs are acceptable and measured frequently.

(2) Ongoing maternal blood loss is limited.

(3) Continuous EFM, preferably by internal electrode, verifies fetal well-being.

(4) Labor progresses well, as defined by a good contraction pattern and progressive cervical dilatation.

(5) Coagulation status is not severely abnormal.

(6) Blood and coagulation factor (fresh frozen plasma, platelets) replacements in sufficient quantity are IMMEDIATELY available.

(7) C/S is IMMEDIATELY available in case of worsening maternal or fetal condition.

e. If the above conditions are met and spontaneous labor has not occured, begin induction by oxytocin infusion and amniotomy.

f. Indications for C/S are a worsening in maternal or fetal condition as evidenced by any of the parameters directly above. Whereas it used to be a "rule" to perform abdominal delivery after 6 to 8 hours of labor, this is not necessary as long as maternal and fetal condition can be adequately monitored.

g. Coagulopathy should be treated only when:

(1) There are signs of abnormal bleeding, as from puncture sites

(2) C/S is imminent, or

(3) Platelet counts are less than 20,000/cu. mm.

h. Treat such cases as follows:

(1) Hypofibrinogenemia (<100 mg. per 100 ml.) or clinically evident bleeding calls for administration of fibrinogen, 4 g., or several units of fresh frozen plasma. Both of these carry considerable risk of non-A, non-B hepatitis.

(2) Thrombocytopenia (<50,000/cu. mm.)—Packed platelets. Since antibodies to these are formed rapidly, limiting their life span and invalidating future platelet transfusions, they should be given within minutes before beginning surgery.

i. If there is laboratory evidence of coagulopathy, but no evidence of active maternal hemorrhage, delivery itself will usually result in correction of these within one or two days.

j. If the fetus is dead on arrival at the hospital, the management should be as in sections (d) and (e) above, without fetal monitoring. Cesarean section may still be necessary if maternal condition necessitates immediate delivery.

CIRCUMVALLATE PLACENTA

Definition

1. A placenta in which a thickened ring consisting of a double fold of amnion and chorion surrounds the fetal portion of the placenta

2. When this ring is at the placental edge rather than on the fetal surface, the placenta is called *circummarginate.*

Etiology

Unknown

Risks

Painless antepartum hemorrhage may occur with this rare condition.

Management

1. Distinguish from placenta previa via USG.

2. Conduct labor and/or C/S as described under "Marginal Sinus Rupture," above.

PLACENTA MEMBRANACEA

Definition

When the chorion laeve fails to degenerate, chorionic villi develop all around the ovisac. This results in a very thin layer of functioning placenta all around the uterine cavity.

Etiology

Unknown

Risks

Since there is placenta in contact with the entire lower uterine segment (including over the os), placenta membranacea may behave as a total placenta previa, with increasing bleeding during the second half of pregnancy.

Management

As for placenta previa

VASA PREVIA

Definition

Vasa previa is the abnormal implantation of the fetal vessels into the placenta in such a fashion that some of them traverse the amnion overlying the cervical os.

Etiology

Unknown

Risks

Rupture of a vessel, especially at the time of rupture of the membranes, may result in fetal exsanguination.

Diagnosis

If amniotomy is accompanied by the onset of excess vaginal bleeding, test the blood for the presence of fetal cells. The Kleihauer-Betke acid elution test (Apt test) is suitable for this.

Management

1. Vaginal delivery may be performed if it can be accomplished in less time than it takes to arrange a C/S.

2. Prepare for a shocky baby at birth. The blood loss from vasa previa has been fetal.

VAGINAL AND CERVICAL LESIONS

A multitude of vaginal and cervical lesions may cause bleeding during pregnancy. The list is essentially the same as for vaginal and cervical lesions which may cause non-pregnant bleeding, and the diagnosis and workup are essentially the same: speculum exam followed by microbiologic, cytologic, and histological studies as necessary.

POSTPARTUM HEMORRHAGE

Early Postpartum Hemorrhage

1. Definition. Blood loss greater than 500 ml. in the first 24 hours after delivery

2. Etiology

a. Approximately 90 per cent of early postpartum hemorrhage is due to uterine atony after delivery. Common conditions predisposing are: general anesthesia, overdistended uterus (twins, hydramnios), prolonged labor, oxytocin-stimulated labor, multiparity, precipitate labor.

b. Cervical or vaginal lacerations which are unrecognized at delivery may continue to ooze blood.

c. Retained placental tissue may prevent uterine contraction and result in hemorrhage after delivery.

d. Coagulation abnormalities rarely cause postpartum hemorrhage in and of themselves. They may, however, exacerbate other bleeding.

3. Diagnosis

a. Uterine atony is diagnosed by feeling the fundus. Since it is so common, if the fundus is softer or higher than it should be, postpartum atony is presumed.

b. Sometimes repeated episodes of atony are caused by retained placental fragments. This may be diagnosed in the delivery room by manual exploration of the uterus; but after any significant interval this condition requires curettage, since the cervix usually "contracts down."

c. If the uterus is well contracted, another cause for the bleeding must be sought. Inspection of the cervix and vagina will detect any lacerations that are present.

d. Bleeding may occur in the presence of a well-contracted uterus, from uterine rupture or laceration secondary to trauma of labor or delivery. This is diagnosed by manual exploration of the uterus after suspect deliveries. Many physicians advocate routine exploration of the uterus after every delivery.

e. Sometimes, in the presence of a well-contracted uterus, blood will ooze from the cervix. Especially if it was not effaced well before dilatation (as in multiparas), the cervix may bleed within the canal from torn vessels. This may be diagnosed by excluding uterine rupture.

4. Management

a. The best management of postpartum hemorrhage is prevention. Two strategies are commonly employed toward this end:

(1) Routine manual exploration of the uterus after every delivery will detect retained placenta and uterine lacerations.

(2) Routine infusion of oxytocin (1,000 ml. of 0.9% NaCl or R.L. containing 20 units of oxytocin at 200 to 300 ml. per hour) for the first postpartum hour will prevent most atony. Most patients easily tolerate the fluid load.

b. If it occurs, atony is best treated by a combination of immediate bimanual uterine massage and oxytocin stimulation, using either oxytocin (20 units per 100 ml. Ringer's lactate at 200 to 300 ml. per hour) or an ergot alkaloid (Methergine or Ergotrate 0.2 mg. I.V. or I.M.) or both. If these are not successful, prostaglandin $F_{2\alpha}$ (I.V. or intramyometrially) should be tried. If these fail, another careful search of the uterine cavity should be performed to rule out retained placenta and rupture. As a last resort, surgical intervention (hypogastric artery ligation, hysterectomy) is available.

c. Lacerations of the genital tract obviously require suturing. Good exposure is critical for this. If an assistant is not present, get help.

d. Bleeding from torn vessels within the cervical canal, without frank cervical laceration, may sometimes be controlled by clamping with a sponge forceps for a few minutes.

e. Uterine rupture requires laparotomy with either repair of the laceration or hysterectomy.

f. If examination reveals retained placenta, remove it manually. If this is not possible, resort to curettage.

g. Adequate fluid replacement and transfusion when necessary are central to proper therapy.

Late Postpartum Hemorrhage

1. Definition. Blood loss greater than 500 ml. after the first postpartum day but within the first postpartum month

2. Etiology

a. Retained placental tissue or fetal membranes is the most common cause of late postpartum hemorrhage.

b. Subinvolution of the placental site is a second major reason for abnormal bleeding and may be due to endomyometritis.

3. Diagnosis. The diagnosis of late postpartum bleeding is best made by a therapeutic trial. (See directly below.)

4. Management

a. Begin by attempting therapy with oxytocin infusion (20 units in 500 to 1,000 ml. D_5W).

b. If this results in a decrease in the bleeding, continue with an ergot alkaloid (Ergotrate, Methergine 0.2 mg P.O., or I.M. q.4h. × 6 doses). This is frequently combined with systemic antibiotic administration (broad spectrum coverage, such as is provided by cefoxitin, piperacillin, or ampicillin/gentamicin/cleocin, is the usual initial choice), on the theory that local infection of the placental site predisposes to late hemorrhage.

c. If the above regime does not control the bleeding, or if the bleeding recurs, curettage is indicated.

PHILOSOPHY OF BLOOD REPLACEMENT

Basic Principles

1. Blood replacement therapy may be used for three general purposes:

a. Replacement of red cell mass
b. Replacement of volume
c. Replacement of clotting factors

2. Since all three are rarely necessary simultaneously, the art has changed its name to "Blood Component Replacement Therapy."

3. The implication of this is that one does not replace "blood" any longer, except in unusual circumstances; rather one replaces what is needed with the appropriate blood component.

4. Although it seems so obvious as not to require saying, blood replacement has become increasingly dangerous in the last few years because of the risk of transmission of viral diseases, which include:

a. Hepatitis B—largely eliminated by screening

b. Human Immunodeficiency Virus (HIV)—the most spectacular and frightening risk, which has been largely eliminated by ELISA screening.

c. Non-A, non-B hepatitis—undetectable. It may occur after 5 per cent of all transfusions, often causing serious disease.

d. Cytomegalovirus

Definition of Blood Components

1. Packed Red Blood Cells. One unit of "packed cells" is 250 ml. It contains the red cell mass of one unit (500 ml.) of blood with a hematocrit of 50 per cent.

2. Plasma The liquid portion of blood, before it clots, is plasma. If frozen before it has a chance to stagnate, it contains all the fibrinogen and clotting factors of blood. One unit of fresh frozen plasma (250 ml.) contains approximately 2 g. of fibrinogen.

3. Platelets. Platelets are centrifuged off, and stored as a separate component for specific use in cases of severe thrombocytopenia.

4. Fibrinogen. Pooled from the plasma of many donors, fibrinogen may be used specifically for correction of defibrination syndromes in obstetrics. However, because it is pooled, its use carries an unacceptably high risk of hepatitis. The use of cryoprecipitate is preferable if it is available, or of fresh frozen plasma if there is associated hypovolemia.

Correction of Loss in Specific Situations

1. Chronic Blood Loss. If transfusion is necessary, chronic blood loss is best corrected with packed red blood cells. Because in chronic situations intravascular volume is slowly replaced, volume-supplying blood components are not necessary.

2. Acute Blood Loss. In this situation both red-cell mass and volume need replacement. This can be accomplished with packed red blood cells and either crystalloid solutions (normal saline, Ringer's lactate) or fresh frozen plasma. The reasons for avoiding whole blood, when one can, are twofold:

a. To reduce the risk of hepatitis

b. To enable the whole blood to be fractionated for components (e.g., platelets, cryoprecipitate)

If blood loss is greater than 6 units, coagulation factors need replacement as well. Frozen plasma or FRESH whole blood is necessary, instead of crystalloids.

3. Coagulopathies. In obstetrics these can usually be corrected by delivery of the fetus. However, if necessary,

a. Platelets may be transfused separately.

b. Cryoprecipitate, frozen plasma, and fibrinogen are available for hypofibrinogenemia.

c. Frozen plasma is the therapy of choice for deficits of other coagulation factors, except factor VIII, which is usually corrected with cryoprecipitate.

20 Sepsis and Septic Shock

Hugh R. K. Barber

DEFINITION

Endotoxic or bacteremic shock: Gram-negative septicemia is a severe circulatory failure due to the toxins of bacteria. Although the original description was a gram-negative septicemia, it is a more complex problem, particularly in the field of obstetrics and gynecology.

In obstetrics and gynecology, infection is usually polymicrobial rather than monomicrobial. This makes it a more difficult problem to treat.

The toxins of bacteria cause vascular damage leading to increased capillary permeability or widespread arteriolar and capillary thrombosis (disseminated intravascular coagulation; DIC).

The condition has a mortality of over 60 per cent and may be a sequel of any operative procedure as well as of septic abortion.

A rare gynecological form is associated with the use of vaginal tampons. It is called the *toxic shock syndrome.*

1. *Septic shock* is defined as that condition seen in a patient with an apparent infection, a temperature either elevated or depressed above or below normal, a thready pulse of 110 or over, hypotension (usually systolic 80 mm. Hg or below), and a decrease in urinary output below 20 ml. per hour.

2. *Shock* is defined as a state in which capillary perfusion is inadequate to sustain life. Vital cells are starving for lack of oxygen and other nutrients and metabolic products are not being removed from tissues because capillary flow is too slow or does not exist at all.

3. Shock is an emergency situation no matter whether it is due to a severe injury with blood loss, a severe infection, heart failure, or other causes. The situation must be dealt with immediately or cellular injury and death will soon progress to organ failure and the death of the patient.

INFECTING BACTERIA

1. **Gram-Positive**
   - **a.** *Staphylococcus*
   - **b.** *Streptococcus*
   - **c.** *Clostridium*
2. **Gram-Negative**
   - **a.** *Escherichia coli*
   - **b.** *Bacteroides fragilis*
   - **c.** *Pseudomonas pyocyanea*

Any organism, including viruses and fungi, can cause shock. They release foreign polysaccharides or proteins into the bloodstream, either as specific exotoxins or by release of endotoxins after breakdown (as in the case of gram-negative bacteria), which activate the immune system. This leads to the release of vaso-active agents such as serotonin, prostaglandins, histamine, and some kinins (polypeptides).

BASIC PRINCIPLES

1. Bacteremic shock is one of the emergencies of medicine. It carries a mortality rate of 80 per cent, which is higher when

Proteus or *Cl. welchii* is the infecting organism.

2. The gram-negative organisms most frequently seen in this group are: *E. coli* (most common), *Proteus mirabilis, Pseudomonas aerogenes,* and *Aerobacter aerogenes.*

3. Among the most frequent gram-positive bacteria cultured are enterococcus, anaerobic streptococci, *Bacteroides, B. welchii* and *Clostridium perfringens. B. welchii* and *Clostridium* secrete exotoxins. Infections due to *Bacteroides* are now being reported frequently.

4. Shock is noted especially in conjunction with infected abortion, premature rupture of the membranes (chorioamnionitis), pyelonephritis (especially in pregnancy), and diffuse peritonitis. It may be associated with gynecological cancer or following extensive radical surgery. Sepsis and septic shock may follow chemotherapy for pelvic malignancy or trophoblastic disease.

5. Although the entire mechanism has not been completely elucidated, most physicians accept the theory that the basic physiopathology is generalized intravascular clotting initiated by the release of endotoxin (lipopolysaccharide) by the above-named gram-negative bacteria.

6. Currently, two main mechanisms have been invoked to explain the findings in endotoxic shock: selective vasospasm and DIC. The pathophysiology can be attributed to both these mechanisms as well as to reduced myocardial response to sympathetic stimuli.

7. *Clostridium perfringens (B. welchii* and *Clostridium*) secretes exotoxins. These are probably the most serious of all infections. The exotoxins become irreversibly bound to tissue soon after they are liberated from the infecting organism.

8. Since toxin is fixed to tissue, specific antitoxins are therefore of questionable value. The exotoxin contains the enzyme lecithinase (which causes necrosis of tissue as well as rapid lysis of red and white blood cells) as well as collagenase (a proteolytic enzyme that causes necrosis of muscle tissue).

9. There is lack of oxygen to vital organs, owing to compensatory generalized vasoconstriction which gives rise to impaired tissue perfusion.

The clinical syndrome is characterized by:

a. A change in the sensorium

b. A sudden drop in blood pressure below 70 systolic

c. A weak thready pulse

d. Respiratory disturbance (respiratory alkalosis)

e. Electrolyte deficits and urine suppression

10. The usual laboratory findings are a rise in the hematocrit, SGOT, SGPT, LDH, catecholamines, BUN, blood amylase, and blood sugar.

11. Metabolic acidosis occurs later.

PATHOLOGY

1. Ischemia of Organs. This is caused, at first, by a protective spasm as a means of preserving circulatory volume, and then by DIC.

2. Low Cardiac Output. First, there is an acute fall in the circulating blood volume due to peripheral vasodilatation, and myocardial failure follows as a result of endotoxins.

3. Cerebral Damage. Hypoxia increases vasospasm and leads to anxiety, confusion, and coma.

4. Lungs. Low tissue perfusion follows the fall in circulatory volume, but even after this is corrected, the capillary damage may lead to pulmonary edema (shock lung). This pulmonary insufficiency is currently called adult respiratory distress syndrome (ARDS).

5. Liver and Spleen. Endotoxins inhibit the phagocytic (Kupffer) cells of the liver and the reticuloendothelial system generally, which is important in disposing of microthrombi.

6. Kidney. Low perfusion leads to renal failure, metabolic acidosis, and further hypoxia.

DIFFERENTIATION OF SEPTIC ABORTION AND SEPTIC SHOCK

1. There is some confusion between these two terms. *Septic abortion* is defined as one associated with an elevation of temperature to 100.4°F (38°C) or more, of two days duration, not necessarily consecutive, or a single elevation to 102°F (38.9°C) or more caused by uterine infection. Only about 1 to 5 per cent of septic abortions develop septic shock. All cases of septic abortion are potential candidates for this dreaded complication. Only by exercising constant vigilance and instituting prophylactic measures can one prevent this.

2. Septic shock can occur at any time, but the infected abortion with a 12-plus-week size uterus that is tender with a closed cervix and a pus-like discharge exuding from the cavity is an especially likely candidate.

Diagnosis

1. Delay in diagnosis and delay in early institution of therapy are the most important factors in the production of mortality in septic shock. Although the diagnosis and management will be considered separately, the urgency of the time factor makes it necessary that these two overlap. The emergency nature of this condition is not unlike the diabetic presenting with hypoglycemic shock.

2. At the time that the initial blood is drawn for laboratory evaluation, the treatment is started.

3. Hyperventilation and respiratory alkalosis are helpful aids in making an early diagnosis of gram-negative bacteremia.

4. One of the earliest signs of impending shock is mental confusion and inappropriate behavior. When these occur in a patient with infection and fever, it usually indicates that the next step, hypotension, is about to occur. The importance of this triad in early diagnosis cannot be overemphasized: hyperventilation, mental confusion, and fever. Awareness of this may permit the diagnosis of shock at its very inception.

5. It must be stressed that the adrenergic effect is not prominent at this stage. The patient is warm, skin is dry, cardiac output and tissue perfusion are adequate.

6. It is only as the case progresses that the classic signs and symptoms of severe septic shock supervene, and here the adrenergic component takes over (vasoconstriction).

7. In the early hyperdynamic phase, the body's first reactions to sepsis are pyrexia and local vasodilatation to improve perfusion of the affected area. The fall in peripheral resistance is countered by an increased heart rate, and there may even be polyuria. At this stage, the patient, although mildly hypotensive, is usually warm, alert, and anxious.

In the next phase, which is the circulatory failure phase, the onset may be very sudden, simulating amniotic fluid embolism or myocardial infarction. The patient becomes comatose and extreme vasoconstriction produces cold cyanotic hands and feet. Blood pressure and pulse become almost unrecordable. Blood tests for DIC become positive and signs of failure of the different organs gradually make their appearance.

8. Signs of advancing septic shock are as follows:

a. Hypotension associated with fever or a subnormal temperature

b. Chills

c. Tachypnea and respiratory distress

d. Tachycardia (110 to 180 beats per min. with narrow pulse pressure)

e. Progressive oliguria (usually less than 20 ml./hr.). The urinary output is one of the best clinical indicators of tissue perfusion!

f. Cold, moist skin

g. Drop in temperature of extremities with peripheral cyanosis

h. Mental obtundity, primarily marked anxiety and inappropriate behavior

i. Unexplained ileus

j. Unexplained petechia with occasional bleeding

k. Jaundice

9. Laboratory findings that help confirm the diagnosis are as follows:

a. Drop in blood *p*H

b. Drop in serum bicarbonate

c. Blood gas determination indicating drop in pO_2 and rise in pCO_2

d. Rise in blood urea nitrogen and phosphate

e. Drop in serum sodium, potassium, and calcium levels

f. Positive toxicology studies

g. Positive cultures—from any site—for organisms that usually cause bacteremic shock (only about 25 to 30 per cent have positive blood cultures)

h. Rising hematocrit

i. Drop in platelet count, serum fibrinogen, or prothrombin

j. Elevation of SGOT, SGPT, LDH, and serum amylase

10. There is probably no specific laboratory test that absolutely confirms the diagnosis, but several positive tests lend credence to the supposition.

11. As usual, the clinical manifestations are paramount. The laboratory results merely reinforce the physician's clinical judgment.

OMINOUS SIGNS

Signs Usually Indicating a Lethal Outcome

Any of these should be disturbing, but the patient has a good chance of recovery. With two or three in combination, the prognosis must be guarded since these are usually lethal.

1. Coma

2. Increasing oliguria or anuria that does not respond to therapy, combined with a significant rise in BUN

3. Respiratory difficulty with a pCO_2 of 55 mm. Hg or more

4. Marked drop in fibrinogen or platelets

5. Severe sepsis that does not respond to antibiotics

6. Jaundice (hemolysis)

7. Marked acidosis with blood *p*H of 7.29 or less and a bicarbonate of less than 9.9 mEq./L.

8. Impaired liver function with jaundice

9. Cardiac failure or marked arrhythmia

10. Old age and/or debilitation from cancer, etc.

11. Any combination of the above suggests a grave prognosis.

12. Disseminated intravascular coagulopathy is discussed elsewhere.

Treatment

Any septic focus must, if possible, be dealt with surgically. Thus, if the shock is a consequence of septic abortion, the uterus must be emptied without delay. Hysterectomy, in some instances, is indicated.

Until bacteriologic guidance is available, the antibiotic cover must be empirical. That is, lincomycin 600 mg. q.8h. I.M., gentamycin 80 mg. q.6h. I.V., and metronidazole 500 mg. q.8h. I.V.

Time is the keystone of therapy in treating septic shock. An outline of treatment for the first 12 hours is given as follows:

1. Careful monitoring is essential.

2. The clinical measurements most useful are pulse rate, blood pressure, pulse pressure (reflecting stroke volume), central venous pressure (or pulmonary wedge pressure or pulmonary artery pressure), blood volume estimation (early shock only), and hourly urinary output. These factors also designate the type and volume of fluid replacement.

3. Thorough and complete history and physical examination, including pelvic and speculum examination.

4. I.V. fluids to augment fluid and electrolyte intake, but especially to keep a vein open in case of emergency. Use an 18-gauge needle.

5. Keep a catheter in the bladder so that hourly output of urine can be monitored. Record hourly intake and output.

6. Order gram-stained smears and cultures of blood, urine, cervix, draining wounds, and secretions from areas in which drains are inserted.

7. Get baseline complete blood count, hematocrit, and platelet count.

8. Order baseline serum electrolytes (sodium, potassium, chloride, carbon dioxide, calcium, phosphates) and *p*H.

9. Serum fibrinogen, prothrombin, and clotting time

10. Blood urea nitrogen and toxicological studies when indicated

11. Routine examination and culture of urine, plus bilirubin and toxicological studies when indicated

12. Radiograph of chest and abdomen for pathology, foreign bodies, or gas under the diaphragm

13. Baseline blood gas studies

14. Check the following hourly:

a. Blood pressure

b. Pulse

c. Respiratory rate

d. Rectal temperature

e. Urinary output

f. Urinary specific gravity

g. Any inappropriate mental aberrations

15. After the initial orders are instituted, additional procedures are indicated:

a. Where a removable septic focus is present, surgery is the keynote of treatment.

b. Where the septic nidus cannot be removed, therapy is medical by necessity.

c. Treatment is tailored to the needs of the patient.

d. An adequate airway should be ensured.

e. Fluid and blood replacement should be guided by central venous pressure, urinary output, and blood volume estimation.

f. Blood, plasma, or 5-per-cent dextrose in saline should be given as indicated.

g. Low-molecular-weight dextran provides volume replacement and reduces sludging in the microcirculation.

h. Metabolic acidosis is common, becoming progressive if not corrected; 0.45-per-cent saline with one or two ampules of sodium bicarbonate added is useful in this case.

i. Lactate should not be used to correct acidosis in these patients because conversion to carbon dioxide requires aerobic metabolism. Sodium bicarbonate, however, acts rapidly and provides good buffering action.

Antibiotic Therapy

1. Garamycin (gentamycin sulfate) 1.5 to 3 mg./Kg./day I.M. in divided doses, or Coly-Mycin (colistin) 120 to 300 mg. I.M. in 2 to 4 divided doses o.d. plus kanamycin 1 g. I.M. initially, followed by 0.5 g. q.12h., or Keflin 2 g. initially and then 1 g. I.M. initially, followed by 0.5 g. q.12h. In some instances all three may be required.

2. Metronidazole hydrochloride is a very valuable drug in treating severe infections. It can be effectively substituted for clindamycin and triple therapy.

a. In specific instances, metronidazole may afford selective advantages due to its ability to penetrate into virtually all body compartments.

b. The problem of bioavailability associated with abscesses argues for the selective use of metronidazole over clindamycin in this clinical setting. It can penetrate the wall of an abscess.

c. Intravenous metronidazole should be preferentially used when there is underlying gastrointestinal disease or a prior history of the development of diarrhea on antibiotic therapy.

d. Metronidazole does not afford totally comparable coverage to clindamycin owing to its inability to cover for the aerobic bacteria.

e. The beta-hemolytic streptococci, *Listeria monocytogenes, Neisseria gonorrhoeae, Hemophilus influenzae,* and the virulent exogenous aerobic pathogens are too important bacteria to be left uncovered in terms of two-drug therapy. The best potential combination for obstetrics and gynecology appears to be metronidazole hydrochloride and uriedopenicillin or possibly a selected third generation cephalosporin.

f. Metronidazole can effectively dismantle the effector-arm of the anaerobic progression and, consequently, is an effective drug in the area of prophylactic antibody administration for gynecological patients.

3. If these drugs fail to control the infection, chloramphenicol is given as an I.V. bolus, 1 g. every 8 hours. Penicillin or ampicillin should also be given as crystalline penicillin G in dosage of 10 million units every 4 hours in intravenous fluids. As an alternative to penicillin, ampicillin 500 mg., or cephalothin, 2 g. every 4 hours I.V. may be used. Nephrotoxic drugs should be avoided in the presence of oliguria.

4. Before instituting antibiotic therapy, it is good to consult the literature. There is a constant flow of new drugs and combinations for the treatment of infections.

Corticosteroids (If Indicated)

1. Solu-Medro (methylprednisolone) 240 mg. I.V. as a bolus and then q.4 to 6 h. or

2. Hydrocortisone 1 to 2 g. I.V. as an initial bolus and then 1 g. I.V. q.4 to 6 h.

3. Corticosteroids combat vasoconstriction and acidosis, but they also depress inflammatory responses, including vagocytosis.

4. Their use in shock conditions is debated.

Vasomotor Drugs (If Indicated)

1. In the warm-hypotensive phase, a vasopressor rather than a vasodilator is indicated.

a. The most potent vasopressor, metaraminol (Aramine), is given only in the smallest amount that will keep the systolic pressure just high enough to ensure adequate urinary output, and for as short a time as possible.

b. Aramine (metaraminol) is best administered in 500 ml. 5-per-cent glucose to which 100 to 200 mg. of the drug is added.

c. In critical cases where vasoconstrictors have failed, Isuprel (isoproterenol) in doses of 5 ml. (5 mg.) in 500 ml. of glucose may be administered.

Currently the best catecholamine to begin treatment of shock is dopamine. Dopamine is essentially three drugs in one, depending on the dosage used and the patient's response. Very small dosages (2–5 μg./kg./min.) produce a specific dilation of gut and kidney vessels to increase blood flow to essential viscera. Moderate doses (5–30 μg./kg./min.) have, in addition, an inotropic effect (increased heart forces) that increases cardiac output. Very high doses (more than 30 μg./kg./min.) cause vasoconstriction that is just as powerful as that of norepinephrine or epinephrine. In other words, very high doses of dopamine have the same pressor effects as norepinephrine.

2. In the cold-hypotensive phase, however, there is generalized vasoconstriction and usually hypovolemia.

a. Volume replacement plus vasodilator drugs in small doses is the treatment of choice at this phase.

b. Chlorpromazine (Thorazine) in a dose of 5 to 10 mg. I.V. every half hour, as needed, up to four times, is one of the best vasodilators in septic shock.

3. When the central venous, wedge, or pulmonary artery pressure is elevated and the pulse rate is in the normal range, isoproterenol (Isuprel) may be used for its inotropic and vasodilator (beta-receptor) effects. Because of its tendency to produce cardiac arrhythmia, proterenol should not be used when the pulse rate is above 120 beats per minute.

4. It is usual to measure right ventricular filling pressures as central venous pressure (CVP). This is a useful guide to fluid management in most patients.

a. In healthy patients bleeding 15 per cent of their blood volume, only a small change in mean arterial pressure would result. CVP would fall dramatically.

b. Thus, right ventricular filling pressures are especially useful in hypovolemia.

c. In disorders affecting only the left or right ventricle (lung disease, myocardial infarction), there is poor correlation between the right atrial pressure and the left ventricular end-diastolic pressure.

d. Even in these patients, changing blood volume causes similar changes in right and left ventricular filling pressures.

e. The ingenious Swan-Ganz catheter is a simple means of estimating left ventricular end-diastolic pressure without direct left heart catheterization.

f. In most patients without intrinsic lung disease, pulmonary arterial diastolic pressure, and especially pulmonary wedge pressure, are useful estimates of left ventricular end-diastolic pressure.

g. There are four advantages for the shock patient when the Swan-Ganz catheter is used rather than a central venous catheter. These include:

(1) First,it permits measurement of pulmonary arterial diastolic and wedge pressures that estimate left ventricular filling pressures.

(2) Second, continuous monitoring of pulmonary arterial systolic and mean pressures reflects changes in pulmonary vascular resistance secondary to hypoxemia, pulmonary edema, and pulmonary emboli.

(3) Third, it allows sampling of mixed venous blood for measurement of arterial venous oxygen differences, cardiac output, and venoarterial admixture.

(4) Fourth, it permits estimation by thermodilution of cardiac output from the right heart alone.

5. Digitalization should be carried out when the central venous pressure is above 12 cm. of water and tachycardia is present. Cedilanid (lanatoside C) should be given in 2 or 3 divided doses I.V. until 1.6 mg. to 3.5 mg. is given to produce digitalization.

6. With evidence of intravascular clotting, heparin sodium may be administered by I.V. bolus q.4 h., the initial dose being 10,000 units; subsequent doses usually are 5,000 units. The total daily dose of 25,000 to 35,000 units may be divided into four doses q.6 h.

Treatment for Specific Infections

1. Welchii Infections

a. Same regimen as for gram-negative bacterial infections plus penicillin 50 million units I.V. in 24 hours or ampicillin 8 g. I.V. in 24 hours

b. Although it is controversial for the protection it provides, some give polyvalent gas gangrene antitoxin, 60,000 to 100,000 I.U. I.V., with doses repeated every 2 to 4 hours depending upon the clinical situation.

c. Early D and C to be followed by hysterectomy at once if there is more than minimal uterine involvement or if there is spread outside of the uterus

d. In the absence of severe kidney involvement with oliguria or anuria, dialysis is indicated.

e. Hyperbaric oxygen, if available, might be efficacious.

2. Gram-Positive Cocci Infections

a. Same regimen as listed under gram-negative

b. Use of vasoconstrictors early (see previous dosage)

c. More liberal use of plasma and fluids

Clinical Evaluation

Although electronic gadgets and sophisticated laboratory procedures are helpful, the patient can be managed successfully without them. A clinical evaluation is summarized as follows:

1. Peripheral Resistance. Examine the patient—if cold and clammy, the peripheral resistance is increased.

2. Blood Volume. Observe the central venous pressure. Circulating blood volume is more important than the findings of the peripheral blood volume.

3. Cardiac Output. A narrowed pulse pressure correlates with a decreased cardiac output. A fast thready pulse indicates that there is incomplete filling of the heart with a diminished output.

4. Visceral Organ Blood Flow. Measure the output of urine. The urine output is proportional to renal blood flow. Since the kidney is the target-sensitive organ and the renovascular bed is particularly sensitive as far as response to endotoxin is concerned, it is obvious that if the kidney is responding, as evidenced by an adequate urinary output, the other organs are being adequately perfused.

Surgical Treatment

1. In the presence of chorioamnionitis, if vaginal delivery is not accomplished within 12 hours, abdominal delivery should be seriously considered. For the patient with severe infection or endotoxic shock, cesarean hysterectomy should be performed, together with ligation of the inferior vena cava and ovarian veins as indicated.

2. In an occasional patient with persistent anuria, dialysis may be required. Consultation with a nephrologist is indicated.

3. An infected abortion should be removed with adequate supportive measures, within 12 hours.

4. Usually, dilatation of the cervix and evacuation of the uterus with ring forceps followed by digital and sharp curettage are adequate to remove the septic focus.

5. Suction curettage is probably more effective than sharp curettage up to the fourteenth week of pregnancy.

6. When the disease has advanced to the stage of microabscess formation in the myometrium, hysterectomy is the only logical surgical treatment. Hysterectomy should be considered in the following situations:

a. The patient continues in shock after curettage and adequate supportive measures.

b. The uterus is over 14 weeks size.

c. The uterus is perforated.

d. The patient is oliguric.

e. Intrauterine *Clostridium welchii* infection is diagnosed.

f. The technique should be tailored to the problem.

g. In the presence of clostridial infection, a minimum of devitalized tissue should be left behind.

Thrombotic Complications

1. Septic pelvic thrombophlebitis involving both ovarian and hypogastric vessels is not uncommon in patients with longstanding septic abortion, postpartum endometritis, chorioamnionitis, pelvic inflammatory disease, and peritonitis.

2. Septic pulmonary embolization may occur.

3. Sepsis complicated by embolization is the basic problem. Therefore, ligation of the inferior vena cava and ovarian veins is the treatment of choice.

4. Vena caval plication is not adequate because the infected thrombi are small.

5. Heparinization is indicated as outlined earlier.

SHOCK LUNG SYNDROME—ADULT RESPIRATORY DISTRESS SYNDROME (ARDS)

Basic Principles

1. The syndrome is often referred to as adult respiratory distress syndrome, congestive atelectasis, shock lung, respiratory lung, or postperfusion lung.

2. The term *adult respiratory distress syndrome* is attractive because it does not attribute the pathologic changes of the lung to one mechanism.

3. Shock lung is not a new disease, but it is being seen more frequently as progressively more sophisticated means of combatting profound hypotension and other perfusion problems save more severely ill patients.

4. Pulmonary complications are one of the leading causes of death in hemorrhagic or endotoxic shock successfully treated for the initial insult.

Basic Mechanism

1. Complications Predisposing to Shock Lung

a. Hypotension

b. Sepsis

c. Rapid blood volume restoration

2. Four Phases

a. First is the initial phase of injury and usual resuscitation: respiratory alkalosis commonly occurs.

b. Second is that of circulatory stabilization. The patient is often lucid and oriented but may show early signs of respiratory difficulty, such as tachypnea.

c. Third is one of progressive pulmonary failure that responds poorly to an increase of oxygen to the alveoli.

d. Fourth is characterized by severe hypoxia, hypercarbia, acidosis, and cardiac arrest.

Pathology

1. Shock lung has been confused with such pathologic diagnoses as bronchopneumonia, patchy atelectasis, and agonal changes.

2. In the acute stage the lung grossly shows edema, congestion, hemorrhage, heaviness, and relative airlessness.

3. Microscopically, there is patchy atelectasis, intra-alveolar edema, inter-alveolar edema, congestion, and hemorrhage. There may or may not be microthrombi.

Treatment

1. As outlined earlier for the treatment of septic shock. However, there are additional cautions to be used in these critically ill patients.

2. Initial fluid replacement is important. Early, one unit of plasma or plasmanate should be given for each L. of crystalloid solution.

3. All fluids infused or perfused in the patient with shock lung should be multiple-filtered to remove microemboli and to eliminate aggregation of colloids.

4. Serum salt-poor albumin (50 g. over a 1-hour period) or low-molecular-weight dextran enhances the colloidal osmotic pressure of the pulmonary perfusate. This helps to prevent pulmonary edema.

5. Fluid therapy is monitored by urine output.

6. Central venous pressure (CVP) is not an infallible indicator of myocardial efficiency. Its use should be accompanied by frequent auscultation of the lungs to determine the presence of moist rales and of the heart to determine the presence of protodiastolic gallop sounds. CVP monitoring measures only the function of the right side of the heart.

7. Pulmonary artery pressure (PAP) and pulmonary wedge pressure (PWP) monitoring by means of a Swan-Ganz catheter give an index of left ventricular competence.

8. In the critically ill, the auscultation of blood pressure by the cuff method is inaccurate, and it is better to cannulize a peripheral artery and connect it to a strain-gauge transducer measuring device. It also affords easy access for sequential arterial blood gas determinations and other laboratory blood samples.

9. Fluid replacement is adequate when either urine output returns to adequate levels (more than 40 ml./h.) or CVP or PWP rises rapidly.

10. If urine output is not reestablished by fluid loading, furosemide (80 mg.) is given.

11. In most patients, arterial blood pressure, CVP, PWP, urine output, and pulse rate will be restored to normal or near normal levels with the measures above. If, however, urine output does not return to adequate levels, indicating adequate perfusion, the patient should be rapidly digitalized.

12. Regulation of breathing with a machine that can maintain a positive end-expiratory pressure (PEEP) is perhaps the most important treatment that can be given to the patient when the shock lung syndrome develops.

a. The end-expiratory pressure is first set at 8 cm. H_2O and gradually increased to 18 to 20 cm. H_2O, a level that maintains arterial pO_2 at the desired level of 60 to 90 mm. Hg on a minimum percentage of inspired oxygen.

b. A volume-cycled respirator is more useful in these patients than the traditional pressure-cycled ventilators.

DISSEMINATED INTRAVASCULAR COAGULATION (DIC) SYNDROME

1. There are two forms of the DIC syndrome that are recognizable:

a. The acute form, which is often associated with spontaneous hemorrhage and shock. This form frequently requires therapy.

b. The subacute form in which hemorrhagic manifestations rarely occur unless the patient's hemostatic defense mechanism is stressed by either surgery or trauma. This form rarely requires specific therapy.

2. Thus, the syndrome of DIC is not a defined disease entity but rather an intermediary mechanism in a host of totally unrelated disease states.

3. The therapy of DIC should, therefore, be directed toward therapy of the underlying disorder whenever this is possible.

4. A useful coagulation profile for DIC should include the following tests:

Test	*Acute DIC*	*Subacute DIC*
Prothrombin time (PT)	Prolonged	Variable
Partial thromboplastin time (PTT)	Prolonged	Variable
Thrombin or creptylase time	Prolonged	Prolonged
Fibrinogen level	Decreased	Decreased
Fibrin degradation products (FDP)	Increased	Increased
Platelet count	Decreased	Variable

5. Since fibrin degradation products interfere with either fibrin polymerization or the action of thrombin, the thrombin time can serve as a rapid screening test for gross elevations of fibrinogen degradation products.

6. The fibrinogen time, however, is relatively insensitive and valid results can be obtained only if the fibrinogen level is greater than 75 mg.

7. Sensitive and specific methods are available for detecting fibrin degradation products.

a. The best of these at present is the tanned red cell hemagglutination inhibition immunoassay, which is sensitive to both early and later split products.

b. The Fi and the staph clumping tests are relatively insensitive to late products, that is, fragments D and E.

c. The euglobulin clot lysis time, an index of plasma fibrinolycin, is relatively insensitive and difficult to perform.

8. Some degree of DIC is inevitable in severe shock, and if there is an inadequate response to whole blood, fresh frozen plasma must be given.

TOXIC SHOCK SYNDROME

Toxic shock syndrome is a very rare complication usually associated with the use of tampons.

It can occur in women wearing internal tampons during menstruation but can also develop from infection in any tissue following trauma, insect bites, abscess, childbirth, or abortion.

Definition

1. There is usually a high fever, syncope, and an erythematous skin rash.

2. Desquamation of palms and soles occur after 7 to 14 days.

3. The blood pressure is usually below 90 mm. Hg systolic.

4. There is involvement of at least three other organ systems, which can include: diarrhea and vomiting, myalgia, blood urea twice upper normal, and liver tests twice upper normal.

5. There is disorientation and varying consciousness.

Clinical Features

1. Fever and malaise develop about the second day of the menstrual period with headache, sore throat, and muscle pains.

2. By the fourth day the diagnostic signs should appear (except for desquamation).

3. If treatment is ineffective, signs of shock appear, including vasoconstriction, oliguira, and respiratory distress.

4. The mortality rate is said to be about 7 per cent.

Pathogenesis

1. The syndrome has been attributed to proliferation of a strain of *Staphylococcus aureus* that produces an enterotoxin. It is a recently described toxin of *S. aureus* (enterotoxin F or exotoxin C).

2. Organisms are introduced into the vagina during insertion of the tampon; the menstrual blood acts as a culture.

Treatment

1. Vaginal swabs, used tampons, and blood samples should be sent for culture.

2. Antibiotic drugs are given, particularly erythromycin and those that are not penicillin A–resistant.

3. One or more of these antibiotics deals with the *S. aureus*, but a broad spectrum antibiotic should be given.

Prophylaxis

1. Women should be advised to change their tampons frequently and to wash their hands before insertion.

2. Patients who have multiple sexual partners should exert extra caution when they use tampons and must change them frequently and observe good perineal hygiene.

21 Gestationally Induced Hypertension

David H. Fields

DEFINITIONS[1]

1. Hypertension

a. Systolic blood pressure greater than 140 mm. Hg, or a rise greater than 30 mm. Hg over first trimester levels

b. Diastolic blood pressure greater than 90 mm. Hg, or a rise greater than 15 mm. Hg over first trimester levels

2. Proteinuria. More than 0.3 g. excreted per 24 hours

3. Edema. Persistent edema of lower extremities after overnight bed rest, or edema of hands or face

4. Preeclampsia. The development of hypertension with proteinuria or edema, or both, after the twentieth week of gestation or during the first 24 hours postpartum

a. Mild preeclampsia: The occurrence of preeclampsia uncomplicated by any of the signs that characterize severe preeclampsia.

b. Severe preeclampsia: Preeclampsia complicated by the occurrence of any of the following:

(1) Systolic blood pressure greater than 160 mm. Hg or diastolic blood pressure greater than 110 mm. Hg at bed rest

(2) Proteinuria of 5 g. or greater per 24 hours

(3) Oliguria (urine output less than 500 ml. per 24 hours)

(4) Cerebral or visual disturbances or hyperreflexia

(5) Right upper quadrant or epigastric pain

(6) Pulmonary edema or cyanosis

(7) Thrombocytopenia or other evidence of disseminated intravascular coagulation (DIC)

5. Eclampsia. When convulsions occur in a preeclamptic woman, the condition is upgraded to eclampsia.

6. Gestational Hypertension. The development of hypertension in the second half of pregnancy without either proteinuria or edema

7. Gestational Edema. The isolated accumulation of 5 pounds of edema fluid in one week

8. Chronic Hypertension. Hypertension existing before the twentieth week of pregnancy or persisting after the puerperal period

9. Superimposed Preeclampsia. Preeclampsia occurring in a woman who has pre-existing hypertension

PREECLAMPSIA

Basic Principles

1. Preeclampsia is a disease whose etiology is still unknown. However, much of the underlying pathology is beginning to be understood. Central to the condition is generalized vasospasm. This results in many of the symptoms and signs of preeclampsia:

---

1. Committee on Terminology of the American College of Obstetrics and Gynecology.

a. Hypertension secondary to increased arterial constriction

b. Edema, probably secondary to increased transudation of fluid out of the vascular system

c. Multiple organ symptomatology secondary to spasm in the vessels supplying the involved organs, with associated decreases in blood flow

d. Fetal malnutrition and distress secondary to decreased uterine and placental blood flow and functional placental insufficiency

2. Although the cause of the vasospasm is unknown, it has been determined that preeclamptic women exhibit an increased sensitivity to infused angiotensin II.

a. This is the most potent vasopressor identified in the body. It is an end product of the reaction initiated by renin acting on renin substrate to produce angiotension I, a decapeptide, which is further cleaved by angiotensinase to angiotensin II, an octapeptide.

b. Angiotensin, renin, and aldosterone levels all increase during normal pregnancy, but sensitivity to them apparently decreases, so that a drop in blood pressure occurs during much of normal gestation. In preeclamptic women, although these hormones are, in fact, present in lower concentration, vascular reactivity to them seems increased. As stated above, this happens for unknown reasons.

3. Secondary to vasospasm, the preeclamptic woman has a decreased intravascular volume. The more severe the preeclampsia, the lower the circulating blood volume is likely to be. *Understanding this is of key importance to the management of preeclampsia.*

4. Preeclampsia threatens pregnancy in three ways:

a. At any time it may progress to eclampsia. Eclamptic convulsions carry a significant risk of death for both mother and fetus.

b. With progressively worse vasospasm and decreased uteroplacental blood flow, the fetus is in danger of intrauterine growth retardation and fetal distress.

c. With progressively worse vasospasm, various maternal organ systems may be compromised to the point that delivery is necessary for the health of the mother. The most common indications for this are oliguria and coagulation disturbances.

5. All therapy for preeclampsia currently available is ameliorative. The only cure for the disease is termination of pregnancy.

6. Eclampsia is an immediate threat to the life of both mother and fetus and requires termination of the pregnancy as soon as possible.

7. All the changes of preeclampsia and eclampsia are reversible with termination of the pregnancy, except for infarction in specific organs.

SPECIFIC ALTERATIONS IN PREECLAMPSIA AND ECLAMPSIA

Renal

These have been most extensively studied and are primarily related to two factors:

1. **Decreased Glomerular Filtration Rate (GFR)** proportional to the severity of the disease

a. Because of decreased renal blood flow secondary to decreased intravascular volume, GFR also decreases. In very severe preeclampsia, it may even fall to, or below, nonpregnant levels.

b. This lowered GFR results in a fall in clearance by the kidney of substances such as creatinine, urea nitrogen, and uric acid and accounts for increased serum levels of these substances found in preeclampsia.

c. In very severe preeclampsia, renal blood flow and GFR are lowered to the point of creating oliguria or anuria (usually due to acute tubular necrosis). This requires aggressive therapy.

d. Renal blood flow may occasionally be lowered so far that renal cortical necrosis develops. This is rare and is thought to be caused by renal artery spasm.

2. Glomerular Capillary Endotheliosis

a. The deposition of fibrin monomer, a fibrin split-product, within the endothelial cells of the glomerular capillaries is considered to be the pathognomonic lesion of preeclampsia.

b. Damage to the glomerular capillary endothelium is probably responsible for the proteinuria characteristic of the later stages of preeclampsia.

Uterus and Placenta

1. Uteroplacental blood flow is typically compromised in the more severe cases of preeclampsia. It has been posited in the past that uterine ischemia might well "fuel the fire" of preeclampsia by resulting in release of a toxin. This has not been demonstrated.

2. Decreased uteroplacental blood flow is detrimental to the fetus by decreasing nutritional and oxygen supply.

3. The uterus seems to be more irritable in preeclamptic and eclamptic pregnancy, accounting for the ease with which induction is frequently performed. Whether this is related to decreased blood supply is unknown.

Liver

1. Hepatic blood flow is somewhat decreased in severe preeclampsia, as are tests of liver function such as BSP excretion. Elevation of hepatic enzymes (SGOT, SGPT, GGT, and alkaline phosphatase) is not uncommon.

2. Pathological changes in the liver, such as periportal necrosis and hemorrhage, seem to be results of eclampsia.

3. Edema of the liver and/or subcapsular hemorrhage, resulting in stretching of Glisson's capsule and right upper quadrant pain, are considered grave prognostic signs.

Brain

1. Cerebral edema as documented by funduscopic examination may occur in severe preeclampsia. It is usually attended by blurred vision and unrelenting headache, and is a grave sign.

2. Cerebral lesions, including thrombosis and cerebrovascular hemorrhage, have been documented on postmortem examination of eclamptic women. Their occurrence may be either a result or a cause of eclamptic convulsions and death.

Cardiopulmonary Changes

1. With the exception of decreased cardiac output secondary to decreased circulating blood volume, all the cardiopulmonary alterations are related to eclampsia.

2. During a convulsion, lack of respiration results in carbon dioxide retention and respiratory acidosis, with subsequent compensatory hyperventilation.

3. Pulmonary edema and congestive heart failure are rarely seen except on postmortem examination, where they are common findings.

Hematologic Changes

1. Hemoconcentration results from the decrease in intravascular volume. A progressively rising hematocrit is a sign of worsening preeclampsia.

2. Coagulation abnormalities have been among the most extensively studied hematologic changes of preeclampsia and eclampsia, partly on the premise that these diseases might be due to a chronic form of disseminated intravascular coagulation (DIC).

a. Thrombocytopenia may be found in a significant percentage of severely preeclamptic women, with or without other clotting abnormalities. It is generally taken as an indication for delivery. Hemorrhage on the basis of thrombocytopenia is not common and does not occur until the count falls below 20,000 per cu. mm.

b. Evidence of intravascular coagulation consisting of elevated fibrin degradation products, prolonged thrombin time, and less often elevated prothrombin and partial thromboplastin times and hypofibrinogenemia, have been identified in severe preeclampsia and eclampsia with varying frequency. Current feeling is that they are more likely to be results of the disease process than causes of it.

c. Microangiopathic hemolysis may occur in severe preeclampsia and eclampsia. It is probably secondary to intravascular fibrin deposition.

Eyes

1. Visual changes are usually secondary to retinal edema and ischemia, and are transient.

2. Rarely, retinal detachment will occur. This usually reattaches spontaneously within a few weeks.

Fluid and Electrolyte Changes

1. Vasoconstriction, decreased intravascular volume, and decreased glomerular filtration rate, all of which have been discussed, are the major changes.

2. Although total-body sodium may be somewhat low, serum concentrations of sodium and other electrolytes are unchanged.

Diagnosis

1. The key to diagnosis of preeclampsia is suspicion. Careful watching for early signs is indicated in cases of:

a. First pregnancy

b. Previously existing hypertension, renal disease, or vascular disease

c. Diabetes

d. Multiple gestation

2. Be alert for:

a. "Transient" increases of blood pressure, especially diastolic pressures approaching 90 mm. Hg

b. Edema of the lower extremities upon rising in the morning

c. Rapid weight gain (more than 2 pounds in any week)

d. All the later signs, such as proteinuria, visual disturbances, headaches, epigastric or right upper quadrant abdominal pain

3. Perform the roll-over test on all suspect nulliparas between 28 and 32 weeks gestation. This test is performed by measuring blood pressure in the lateral recumbent position, then repeating the measurement after rolling-over to the supine position. A rise of 20 mm. Hg or more in the diastolic pressure is indicative of an exaggerated pressor response to aortocaval compression and is an excellent predictor for the development of preeclampsia.

Management of Preeclampsia

The management of preeclampsia is directed to two objectives:

1. Prevention of maternal injury, especially convulsion

2. Delivery of a healthy, mature infant, if possible

3. Once the diagnosis of preeclampsia is made, subsequent care should be in the hospital. Orders on hospital admissions for mild preeclampsia should be:

Maternal Management

1. Bed Rest. Rest in quiet surroundings, preferably in a lateral recumbent position. This serves both to lower maternal blood pressure and to increase uterine blood flow. Bathroom privileges should be allowed.

2. Vital Signs. Especially blood pressure q.4h. except 4 A.M.

3. Diet. Should provide ample protein and at least 2,400 calories daily. Salt should not be restricted in uncomplicated cases of preeclampsia, nor should fluids.

4. Weight. On admission and daily throughout

5. Fluid Intake. Fluid sufficient to maintain an *output* of at least 1,000 ml. per 24 hours

6. Complete Urinalysis, urine culture and 24-hour urine for protein and creatinine on admission, and urine for protein at least twice daily

7. CBC

8. Electrolytes, BUN, creatinine, uric acid, liver, enzymes, serum total proteins and albumin, glucose (SMA6–SMA12)

9. Baseline Coagulation Studies. Fibrinogen, fibrin degradation products, thrombin time (TT), prothrombin time (PT), and activated partial thromboplastin time (APTT)

10. Mild Sedation. Phenobarbital, 30 to 60 mg. q.i.d., is traditional but of questionable efficacy.

11. Diuretics. Once popular, these are not indicated in the treatment of preeclampsia. While they may lower blood pressure, they do not lessen the risk of convulsion and may even make fetal condition worse because of further decreases in uterine blood flow.

12. Eclamptic Precautions. Airway, anticonvulsant, and tracheostomy set in the room

Fetal Studies

Preeclampsia threatens the fetus by progressively decreasing uteroplacental blood flow. If delay in delivery is anticipated because of prematurity, the following studies should be performed to ensure fetal well-being while the mother's condition is being controlled.

1. NST and, if necessary, CST and BPP should be performed on admission and at minimum intervals of twice weekly until delivery.

2. Ultrasonography (USG) for determination of fetal size and possible intrauterine growth retardation (IUGR) should be obtained on admission and at 2- to 3-week intervals until delivery.

3. Amniocentesis for L/S ratio and PG are useful after 34 to 35 weeks if delivery is contemplated.

4. Estriol and human placental lactogen (HPL) measurements are rarely done because of their inaccuracy and the delay in obtaining meaningful results.

Management of Severe Preeclampsia

If the blood pressure is greater than 160 systolic over 105 MHg diastolic, or the mother has neurologic signs such as hyperreflexia or visual disturbance or epigastric pain, the following additions are made to the above orders:

1. Magnesium Sulfate

a. Magnesium sulfate blocks the myoneural junction and, in adequate doses (to achieve serum levels of 4 to 7 mEq. per L.), prevents convulsions. Overdose may result in cardiorespiratory arrest.

b. Administration: This may be given either I.V. or I.M. and is the cornerstone of management.

(1) I.V. solution is made with 10 g. $MgSO_4 \cdot 7H_2O$ in 1,000 ml. D_5 W. This is infused at 1 g. (100 ml.) per hour after an initial loading dose with 4 g. (20 ml. of 20-per-cent solution).

(2) I.M. initial dosage of 10 g. (20 ml. of 50-per-cent solution) injected into buttocks (one-half on each side), followed by 5 g. (10 ml. of 50-per-cent solution) every 4 hours on alternating sides.

c. Magnesium sulfate therapy must be carefully monitored to avoid hypermagnesemia. The following guidelines should be observed:

(1) A patellar knee jerk is obtainable

(2) Urine output is at least 25 to 30 ml. per hour

(3) Respiratory rate is greater than 8 per minute

d. Signs of magnesium toxicity of increasing severity which should be watched for are:

(1) Loss of patellar reflex (8 to 10 mEq. per L.)

(2) Respiratory depression (12 mEq. per L.)

(3) Cardiorespiratory arrest (15+ mEq. per L.)

e. Serum magnesium levels are commonly measured today. These are especially useful if standard doses do not accomplish sufficient suppression of hyperreflexia.

f. If necessary, the antidote for magnesium toxicity is calcium gluconate I.V., 10 ml. of a 10-per-cent solution.

g. Magnesium sulfate therapy should not be continued beyond 2 or 3 days; so once it is begun, preparations for delivery should not be far behind.

2. Antihypertensive Therapy

a. Specific control of blood pressure is indicated if levels are such that the physician fears the risk of cerebral hemorrhage. Therapy is begun for systolic levels greater than 180 mm. Hg and diastolic levels above 110 mm. Hg.

b. Hydralazine (Apresoline) is the agent of choice as it not only lowers pressure by direct vasodilatation, but also increases cardiac output. The preferred method of administration is I.V., 5 to 10 mg. every 20 minutes until desired control is achieved. Maintenance may be with I.V., I.M., or P.O. doses t.i.d. or q.i.d.

c. Diazoxide (Hyperstat) has been used. It has the advantages of long duration of action and no need for titration. However, its disadvantages include rapid drops in blood pressure with fetal compromise, occasional thrombocytopenia, and circulatory overload due to sodium retention. A dose of 300 mg. by rapid I.V. push is given. Blood pressure usually drops within several minutes and remains lowered for several hours. It should be given with a dose of furosemide, 40 mg., to prevent salt retention and circulatory overload. It also causes uterine muscle relaxation and may stop labor.

3. Coagulopathy

a. Thrombocytopenia (less than 100,000/cu. mm.), hypofibrinogenemia (less than 150 mg. per 100 ml.) and abnormalities of prothrombin time (PT) and activated partial thromboplastin time (APTT) are now considered evidence of severe preeclampsia and are best treated by delivery rather than "medical management."

b. Hemostasis is likely to be impaired if:

(1) The platelet count falls below 50,000/cu. mm. (Spontaneous hemorrhage, especially cerebrovascular accident, is likely at counts lower than 20,000/cu. mm.)

(2) The fibrinogen level falls below 100 mg. per 100 ml.

(3) A red-topped tube of blood does not clot within 5 minutes.

c. Vaginal delivery may be attempted in the absence of clinically evident coagulopathy, but for cesarean section (C/S) laboratory parameters should be at least as above. The following may be used to achieve surgical hemostasis:

(1) Platelet transfusions. Indicated for C/S if counts are less than 50,000/cu. mm. Since antibodies form rapidly and repeat transfusions are ineffective, they must be given immediately prior to C/S.

(2) Fresh frozen plasma. Indicated for fibrinogen lower than 100 mg. per 100 ml. or abnormal PT or APTT.

(3) Both of the above carry high risks (up to 4 to 5 per cent per transfusion) of non-A, non-B hepatitis, so they must be used with discretion.

Termination of Pregnancy

1. Indications

a. Development of severe preeclampsia unresponsive to therapy as described above

b. Development of eclampsia, regardless of response to therapy

c. Fetal jeopardy as determined by whichever tests are being used

d. Development of fetal maturity

e. Spontaneous labor may be awaited if preeclampsia remains mild and fetal distress does not supervene.

2. Method

a. The preferred method is induction of labor via oxytocin infusion. This is usually quite successful because of uterine irritability, but special attention should be paid to the likelihood of uterine hypertonus. Continuous fetal heart rate (FHR) monitoring should be performed during labor, with scalp *p*H determinations used as necessary.

b. If induction is not successful or if fetal distress in labor occurs, C/S should be performed.

3. Conduct of Labor

a. All precautions as for routine labor

b. Vital signs every 30 minutes

c. Check patellar reflexes hourly.

d. If magnesium sulfate has been begun, continue through labor. If not, consider its use during labor in all but the mildest cases, as preeclampsia may progress rapidly during labor.

e. Running I.V. throughout labor

f. Continuous fetal monitoring

g. Epidural anesthesia must be used with great care, since volume-depleted preeclamptics are especially sensitive to the precipitous drops in blood pressure that may occur. Volume loading is especially important for these patients.

h. Outlet forceps may be used to shorten the second stage.

4. Conduct of Cesarean Section (C/S)

a. Make all normal preparations for C/S as outlined in Chap. 16.

b. As stated above, epidural anesthesia must be used with care. Balanced general anesthesia may be preferable.

Postpartum Management

1. The risk of convulsion remains during the first 24 hours postpartum. Therefore, careful observation beyond normal postpartum care should be maintained at least that long. After the first day, convulsions are extremely rare and may not be eclampsia.

2. If magnesium sulfate has been previously begun, continue for 24 hours postpartum. If not, mild sedation in the form of phenobarbital 30 mg. q.6h. may be used.

3. Avoid ergot alkaloids in the postpartum patient as these may precipitate a hypertensive episode.

4. Check for persistence of proteinuria daily until it subsides.

5. All other routines are as for normal postpartum management.

ECLAMPSIA

The occurrence of convulsions in a preeclamptic woman is a true emergency. It must be prevented if possible (see "Management of Preeclampsia," above) or treated immediately. The foregoing precautions for preeclampsia are designed to prevent convulsions. If they fail and eclampsia occurs, the following steps should be taken:

Termination of the Convulsion

1. This may effectively be done using parenteral magnesium sulfate as described above (the loading dose of 4 g. I.V. is essential).

2. If this fails, diazepam (Valium) 10 mg. I.V. or amobarbital 250 mg. I.V. should promptly arrest the convulsion.

Prevention of Further Convulsions

This is most effectively done by continuing magnesium sulfate therapy until delivery and 24 hours into the postpartum period.

Maternal Support Pending Delivery

1. Complete bed rest

2. Vital signs every 30 minutes

3. N.P.O.

4. I.V. fluids (D_5W) to keep vein open and maintain urinary output at a minimum of 30 ml. per hour

5. Foley catheter to monitor urine output

6. Continuous oxygen by mask at 5 L. per minute

7. Frequent observation to detect congestive heart failure or impending pulmonary edema. Digitalis therapy for these conditions as indicated.

Fetal Monitoring

Continuous monitoring should be instituted and continued until delivery.

Delivery

Termination of pregnancy should be begun by induction of labor as soon as the above measures have been instituted. The old arbitrary rule of waiting 12 to 24 hours after a convulsion should be disregarded, as the best way to prevent a second or third or fourth convulsion is to end the pregnancy.

1. Most physicians avoid epidural anesthesia.

2. Indications for C/S are the same as in severe preeclampsia.

Postpartum Management

Same as for severe preclampsia

Prognosis

1. After delivery, the disease remits with no known permanent sequelae, unless there has been specific organ infarction or hemorrhage.

2. Subsequent pregnancies in women who have had preeclampsia or eclampsia are likely to be similarly affected in 15 to 20 per cent of cases.

3. Nonpregnancy hypertension does not appear to occur more commonly in women who have had preeclampsia or eclampsia.

22 Chronic Hypertension in Pregnancy

David H. Fields

DEFINITION

The presence of hypertension (blood pressure greater than 140/90) before the onset of pregnancy or occurring before the twentieth week in pregnancy not complicated by multiple gestation or molar disease is termed *preexistent* or *chronic hypertension.*

BASIC PRINCIPLES

1. This is essentially hypertension unrelated to pregnancy which happens to be present. As such it occurs more often in women at increased risk for hypertension:

a. Black females

b. Gravidas over the age of 35

c. Obese women

d. Diabetics

2. Its cause may be any of the causes of hypertension. Most commonly this is essential hypertension, but it may also be:

a. Renal disease (either acute or chronic)

b. Hormonal abnormality (e.g., hyperaldosteronism)

c. Tumor (e.g., pheochromocytoma)

d. Renovascular disease

e. Collagen vascular disease (e.g., systemic lupus or periarteritis nodosa)

f. Diabetic nephropathy

3. Since blood pressure tends to drop during the second trimester, a pregnant hypertensive woman first seen at this time may have a pressure within the normal range. Blood pressures at the upper end of normal during the second trimester should be suspect. They may be pushed out of the normal range by the expected third-trimester rise.

4. Hypertension may be grouped into mild and severe cases and used to predict outcome:

a. Mild hypertension—blood pressure remains below 160/105. There is no associated renal or cardiovascular disease.

b. Severe hypertension—blood pressure is above 160/105. There may be associated renal, hypertensive cardiovascular, or retinal disease.

5. The diagnostic workup for chronic hypertension during pregnancy should be the same as outside of pregnancy except for the radiographic studies.

a. A particular search for pheochromocytoma should be made since this rare tumor carries a 50 per cent maternal mortality in pregnancy if not treated. The major symptoms are: headache, sweats, palpitations, nausea, vomiting, tachycardia, blurred vision, vertigo, and tremulousness.

b. If the hypertension persists after pregnancy, x-ray studies, including a hypertensive IVP, should be done at that time.

RISKS OF HYPERTENSION DURING PREGNANCY

1. Preeclampsia. There is an increased risk of preeclampsia superimposed on the pregnant woman with chronic hypertensive vascular disease. This may vary from

15 to 50 per cent depending on the study and criteria used. It is usually a very severe disease with poor prognosis.

2. Fetal Jeopardy and Growth Retardation. If maternal blood pressure remains below 160/105 and there is no evidence of vascular disease, there is no measurable increase in perinatal complications. If the hypertension is severe or associated with vascular disease, IUGR, placental insufficiency, and placental abruption contribute to an increased incidence of fetal compromise.

3. Placental Abruption. Chronic hypertension is one of the only conditions that has been well documented as predisposing to premature separation of the placenta.

4. If pheochromocytoma is the cause of the hypertension, maternal mortality may approach 50 per cent.

5. Prognosis. Pregnancy does not worsen the course of hypertension after the end of gestation.

ANTEPARTUM MANAGEMENT

Diagnostic Studies

1. Upon diagnosis the following maternal studies should be obtained. If normal, they should be repeated as the need arises.

a. Urinalysis

b. SMA-6 electrolytes, BUN, glucose

c. Serum creatinine and creatinine clearance

d. Funduscopic exam

e. Oral glucose tolerance test

2. The following studies of fetal well-being should also be done:

a. *Ultrasonography.* Initially between 20 and 24 weeks gestation and then every 3 to 6 weeks, if there is any evidence of maternal hypertensive vascular disease

b. *EFM Testing.* NST and, if necessary, CST and BPP, should be initiated at 30 to 32 weeks and repeated at least weekly. After 35 weeks, they may be repeated as often as every 3 to 5 days.

c. *Amniocentesis* for fetal maturity, when elective delivery is contemplated

3. Early termination of pregnancy may be necessary for preeclampsia, if it occurs, or for fetal distress. Otherwise, spontaneous labor is awaited.

Therapy

1. Biweekly visits until the thirtieth week and then weekly until delivery should be the rule.

2. Salt restriction is unnecessary unless the mother has heart disease.

3. Antihypertensive Medication. Therapy is only indicated for pressures above 160/105. The risk of decreasing placental blood flow must be weighed against the benefits of lowered blood pressure. Pressures should be maintained at the upper limits of normal to minimize this risk. The following agents may be used:

a. *Hydralazine* (Apresoline) is the drug of choice because it is a direct vasodilator which simultaneously increases cardiac output and tends to maintain placental blood flow. It may be used orally in doses ranging from 10 to 50 mg. q.i.d.

b. *Methyldopa* (Aldomet) is also an excellent drug. Acting as a false transmitter, it lowers blood pressure without decreasing cardiac output. Starting in its lower range, the dosage may vary from 250 mg. P.O. t.i.d. up to several g. per day.

c. *Diuretics* are *not* indicated for the treatment of hypertension during pregnancy.

MANAGEMENT OF LABOR

Labor is conducted normally, with the following exceptions:

1. Electronic fetal monitoring is mandatory.

2. Blood pressure should be checked frequently to detect intrapartum preeclampsia.

POSTPARTUM MANAGEMENT

The postpartum orders are essentially unchanged from those of normal pregnancy, except for:

1. Frequent blood pressure checks

2. Avoiding the use of ergot alkaloids

23 Diabetes and Pregnancy

David H. Fields

DEFINITION

1. Diabetes is an endocrine disorder characterized by higher-than-normal plasma glucose levels resulting from inadequate insulin secretion to meet metabolic needs. This results in an inability to move sugar from the plasma into the cells. "Intracellular starvation," in the face of high blood sugar (with a switch to fatty acid metabolism and the formation of ketone bodies), results in the typical picture of hyperglycemic ketoacidosis of the "out of control" diabetic.

2. While the metabolic effects are most dramatic, in the long run changes in the vascular system may be more significant. This is also true for complications of pregnancy in the severely diabetic woman.

BASIC PRINCIPLES

Effects of Pregnancy on Diabetes

1. During normal pregnancy insulin levels are higher in both fasting and postprandial states. However, its effects are lessened by placental insulinase, which shortens its half-life, and by peripheral resistance, tending to raise plasma glucose levels. Counterbalancing this, the fetus serves as a constant glucose drain (which becomes significant during fasts). Therefore, normal plasma glucose concentrations are higher during pregnancy at all times except during the (overnight) fasting state.

2. If insulin production is borderline or decreased (diabetes), not only are postprandial blood sugars elevated even more but fasting levels also rise. In addition, because of peripheral insulin resistance and a corresponding inability to get glucose into cells, ketosis is more likely to occur. Therefore, women who are borderline or chemical diabetics before pregnancy may become overtly diabetic while pregnant. This condition reverts in the postpartum period and tends to recur with the next pregnancy.

3. Six to 10 per cent of otherwise normal women develop chemical diabetes while pregnant (gestational diabetes, Class A diabetes) which reverts to normal after delivery. While up to 30 per cent of these women may later become diabetic, there is no evidence that pregnancy increases this tendency (only that it unmasks it).

4. Overt or insulin-dependent diabetics who become pregnant tend to become more severely diabetic with increases in insulin needs averaging between 50 and 100 per cent.

Effects of Diabetes on Pregnancy

1. Three factors seem responsible for the adverse effects of diabetes on pregnancy:

a. Glucose freely crosses the placenta, while insulin does not. This may affect the fetus in several ways:

(1) The fetus is subjected to hyperglycemia, which results in antepartum fetal hyperinsulinemia. Since insulin is an important growth hormone for the fetus, the combination causes increased fat deposition and protein synthesis (macrosomia).

(2) Antepartum hyperinsulinemia also predisposes to neonatal hypoglycemia when the sugar supply is cut off by the clamping of the cord.

(3) Hyperglycemia in the first trimester may be an important cause of congenital anomalies.

b. The fetus may be adversely affected by ketosis. Congenital anomalies may result from either hyperglycemia or ketosis.

c. Maternal vasculopathy, seen frequently in severe diabetes, may lead to placental insufficiency.

2. Specific risks:

a. Increased perinatal mortality. Prior to careful blood sugar control and antepartum fetal evaluation, perinatal mortality varied from 4 per cent in the mildest (Class A) diabetics to upwards of 50 per cent in the most severe cases. These figures are being revised sharply downward as modern management begins to be widely used; perinatal mortality for Class A diabetics is approaching that of the population at large, and for the rest of diabetic mothers it is between 3 and 10 per cent. Major causes are:

(1) Sudden intrauterine death (cause unknown); probably not truly "sudden," since it can be prevented by careful maternal glucose control and scrupulous antepartum fetal monitoring.

(2) Prematurity—secondary to fetal distress, hydramnios, preeclampsia

(3) Hydramnios—occurs in up to 25 percent of cases

(4) Congenital anomalies—most often cardiovascular or neurologic

(5) Preeclampsia/eclampsia (risk increased 2 to 4 times)

b. Other fetal complications:

(1) Macrosomia—usually in diabetics without vascular disease

(2) Intrauterine growth retardation (IUGR)—usually in diabetics with vascular disease

(3) Increased risk of respiratory distress syndrome (RDS) even in the face of L/S ratio greater than 2. However, the presence of phosphatidylglycerol indicates little risk of RDS.

(4) Neonatal hypoglycemia

(5) Neonatal hypocalcemia

c. Maternal complications include increased risks of:

(1) Ketoacidosis

(2) Postpartum hemorrhage

(3) Preeclampsia

(4) Urinary tract infection

CLASSIFICATION OF DIABETES

White System

The most widely used classification is the White system, upon which a rigid delivery schedule was superimposed.

1. Class A—chemical diabetes or an abnormal glucose tolerance test (GTT).

2. Class B—adult-onset diabetes of less than 10 years' duration; no vascular disease.

3. Class C—onset of diabetes between ages 10 and 19 (C_1) or diabetes of 10 to 19 years' duration (C_2); no vascular disease.

4. Class D—onset of diabetes before age 10 (D_1), diabetes present for more than 20 years (D_2), or complicated by benign retinopathy (D_3), calcified leg vessels (D_4), or hypertension (D_5).

5. Class E—calcified uterine or iliac vessels (no longer considered significant).

6. Class F—diabetic nephropathy.

7. Class G—recurrent reproductive failure (new category).

8. Class H—cardiomyopathy (new category).

9. Class R—proliferating (as opposed to benign) retinopathy.

10. Class T—renal transplant (new category).

Functional Classification

For purposes of modern management with intrauterine surveillance and careful blood sugar control, a simpler, more functional classification might be made:

1. Gestational Diabetes. Onset during pregnancy.

2. Pre-existing Diabetes. Onset before pregnancy.

3. Diet-Controlled (Non-Insulin Dependent) Diabetes. Diabetes that can be controlled with diet. This group roughly correlates with Class A, including only patients with normal fasting blood sugars. These patients are mostly gestational diabetics.

4. Insulin-Dependent Diabetes. Diabetes that requires insulin for blood sugar control (as in all patients with elevated fasting blood sugars). For prognostic significance, this group may be broken down into two subgroups.

a. No evidence of renal or retinal vascular disease—this group will usually present no problems beyond sugar control; for the fetus, the risk of growth retardation is small, although macrosomia may occur if blood sugars are high.

b. Evidence of renal or retinal vascular disease—likely to have additional problems beyond sugar control (retinal hemorrhage, renal failure, and intrauterine growth retardation).

DETECTION OF DIABETES

1. Basic Parameters. The cornerstone of the detection of diabetes is blood sugar measurement. If the patient has an elevated fasting blood sugar (more than 90 mg. per 100 ml. in whole blood or 105 mg. per 100 ml. in plasma), she is overtly diabetic. If the fasting blood sugar is normal, the condition of gestational diabetes may be diagnosed by the 3-hour oral glucose tolerance test (OGTT).

2. Indications for OGTT

a. Family history of diabetes

b. Glucosuria

c. Maternal age over 35

d. Obesity

e. Excessive weight gain during any stage of pregnancy

f. Previous macrosomic fetus

g. Previous stillbirth

h. Grand multiparity

i. Recurrent urinary infection

3. Performance of OGTT

a. Load the patient's diet with carbohydrate for 3 days preceding the test.

b. Test in the morning after an overnight fast.

c. Draw a fasting blood sugar.

d. Administer a 100-g. glucose load.

e. Obtain blood specimens at 1, 2, and 3 hours after glucose load.

4. Interpretation of OGTT

a. Normal values (mg. per 100 ml.):

Fasting	90 whole blood
	105 serum
One hour	165 whole blood
	185 serum
Two hours	145 whole blood
	165 serum
Three hours	125 whole blood
	145 serum

b. Chemical diabetes may be diagnosed if at least two values are exceeded other than the fasting blood sugar. If the fasting sugar is elevated, the patient may be considered to be an overt diabetic in need of insulin. A patient with a normal OGTT at 13 weeks may have an abnormal test at 28 to 32 weeks. The test, therefore, should be repeated early in the third trimester.

5. Mini-Glucose Tolerance Test (MGTT)

a. Many cases of gestational diabetes will be missed by the screening of only those with risk factors. Most obstetricians now employ the 1-hour OGTT or MGTT to screen all pregnant women.

b. This consists of:

(1) Measurement of fasting blood sugar

(2) Administration of 50 g. glucose in water solution

(3) Measurement of 1-hour postprandial blood sugar

c. Various standards place normal 1-hour levels below 135 to 150 mg. per 100 ml. plasma.

d. If the test is normal, diabetes is extremely unlikely. If it is abnormal, a 3-hour OGTT should be performed for definitive diagnosis.

e. Most physicians perform the test at 28 to 32 weeks gestation. Many are performing it more often, in an attempt to avoid the complications of mild diabetes by early detection.

MANAGEMENT OF OBSTETRICAL PATIENTS WITH DIET-CONTROLLED DIABETES

1. With careful management, perinatal mortality should be within the normal range for intrauterine pregnancy.

2. Once identified by OGTT, these patients are placed on a diet designed to maintain normal blood sugars (2-hour postprandial levels at no more than 140 mg. per 100 ml. and fasting levels below 100 mg. per 100 ml.). If this cannot be accomplished with a diet providing at least 1,800 to 2,000 calories per day, the physician should recognize the need for insulin and treat the patient accordingly. For specific diets a nutritionist should be consulted, or the ADA diets may be used.

3. In addition to the routine antepartum laboratory testing, obtain:

a. Fasting and 2-hour postprandial blood sugars at 2-week intervals until delivery

b. Glycosolated hemoglobin (hemoglobin A_{1C}) levels monthly

c. Urine culture and sensitivity upon diagnosis

4. If blood sugars are within the acceptable range, no special attention is given to glycosuria.

Testing of Fetal Condition

1. Ultrasonography (USG). Obtain initial measurements as early as possible (preferably by 20 weeks gestation) for accuracy of dating the pregnancy. Repeat every 3 to 6 weeks to assess fetal growth and detect macrosomia.

2. Electronic Fetal Monitoring (EFM). NSTs should be begun at 35 weeks and repeated at 5- to 7-day intervals. CSTs and BPPs are added if NST is nonreactive. After term, many will do CST and BPP as a matter of course until delivery.

3. Amniocentesis. For L/S ratio or other fetal maturity studies, before anticipated elective delivery

Timing of Delivery

1. If blood sugar control is good and fetal parameters indicate no jeopardy, the physician may await spontaneous delivery, even beyond 40 weeks gestation.

2. Induced delivery should be preceded by amniocentesis with L/S ratio or other fetal maturity studies.

Planned Delivery

1. If delivery is easy (ripe cervix or repeat cesarean section), and all fetal indicators are favorable, deliver, by induction or by repeat cesarean section, when the L/S ratio is more than 2 and phosphatidyl glycerol is present.

2. If delivery is not easy (unripe cervix, no cesarean section planned) but the fetus appears healthy, continue monitoring until labor begins or the cervix becomes favorable.

3. If fetal jeopardy is demonstrated by fetal testing, attempt careful induction under optimal conditions with cesarean section readily available.

Conduct of Labor or Cesarean Section for the Diet-Controlled Diabetic

With the exception of mandatory EFM in labor, these may be conducted in the same fashion as for normal patients.

MANAGEMENT OF OBSTETRICAL PATIENTS WITH INSULIN-DEPENDENT DIABETES

As will be obvious from protocols below, pregnant insulin-dependent diabetics should be managed by physicians skilled in the management of diabetes mellitus, and at hospital centers familiar with their problems.

1. Prenatal Visit Schedule. Unlike nondiabetic prenatal patients, diabetics should be seen at least biweekly during the first half of pregnancy and weekly during the second half.

2. Diet and Insulin. Strict control of blood sugar (fasting blood sugar below 100 mg. per 100 ml. and 2-hour postprandial less than 140 mg. per 100 ml.) should be attempted through careful regulation of diet and a mixture of short- and long-acting insulins. Ideally, blood sugar monitoring should be done by the patient herself at least 4 times each day, either with glucose strips or with a glucometer. This should include FBS and one- or two-hour postprandial sugars after each meal. Much less desirable, but sometimes necessary, is weekly fasting blood sugar, postprandial blood sugar, and hemoglobin A_{1C} testing, with occasional glucose panels. Weight gain should be as for a normal pregnancy. Acetonuria and ketosis should be avoided.

3. Laboratory Testing

a. Routine prenatal tests

b. Blood sugar testing as above

c. Creatinine clearance should be done early in pregnancy and at least once, preferably twice, in each trimester subsequently.

d. Urine culture and sensitivity early in pregnancy and again in the third trimester

e. Retinal exam—for baseline early in pregnancy and again in the third trimester

Fetal Status Testing

1. Ultrasonography. Obtain by 20 weeks gestation and at 3- to 6-week intervals thereafter to detect IUGR or macrosomia. If there is evidence of vascular disease secondary to diabetes, do ultrasonography at 3-week intervals.

2. EFM. Begin with weekly NSTs as early as 28 weeks and supplement with CST and BPP as necessary. By 32 weeks, depending on the severity of the diabetes, increase the frequency to every 3 to 5 days.

3. Amniocentesis. Obtain amniotic fluid for L/S ratio and PG when considering elective or semi-elective delivery. Unless there is IUGR, fetal lung maturity is not likely before 36 or 37 weeks.

Timing of Delivery

1. Spontaneous Delivery. This may be awaited until 38 or even 40 weeks if all parameters of fetal well-being (USG, NST, CST, BPP) are reassuring, especially if the L/S ratio is less than 2.0 and PG is not present.

2. Planned Delivery

a. If tests of fetal well-being are all within normal limits, planned delivery may be attempted when the L/S ratio is more than 2.0 or preferably 2.5, PG is present, and delivery will be easy (cervix favorable for induction or repeat cesarean section planned).

b. If any one test of fetal well-being is ominous, but all the other tests indicate that the fetus is in no jeopardy, delivery may be postponed until the L/S ratio is more than 2.0. Under these circumstances, extremely careful surveillance in the form of daily NST, CST, and BPP must be maintained.

c. If both NST and CST indicate fetal jeopardy, immediate delivery should be performed, by whatever route is obstetrically indicated. A sudden drop in insulin requirements of 50 per cent or more is generally accepted as an ominous sign and an indication for delivery.

Conduct of Labor and Cesarean Section

1. With the advent of at-home glucose testing, well-controlled diabetics with

healthy fetuses may remain as outpatients until they go into labor. Patients managed less aggressively during the prenatal course should be admitted several days to several weeks before delivery for careful surveillance. Less well-controlled patients may need earlier hospitalization.

2. During Labor

a. Glucose levels between 60 and 120 mg. per 100 ml. are desirable and are best maintained by a combined infusion of D_5 W at 125 ml./hr. and regular insulin, 1 to 3 u./hr. Insulin may also be given subcutaneously. Blood glucose should be measured every 1 to 2 hours.

b. Continuous EFM during labor is essential.

3. For Elective Cesarean Section

a. Various regimens have been used successfully. No insulin on the morning of surgery, with cesarean section by what would normally be breakfast time, is quite effective, as is administering one-half to one-third the normal morning dose and D_5 W as above.

Common Indications for Cesarean Section in Diabetes

1. Fetal macrosomia, especially in milder cases of diabetes

2. The need for early delivery in the face of a virtually uninducible cervix. Long inductions, with their metabolic drain on the diabetic mother and fetus, are currently in some disfavor.

Anesthesia for Delivery

1. Diabetes itself should not affect the choice of anesthesia for labor. However, because of the high incidence of IUGR and fetal distress in diabetic pregnancies complicated by vascular disease, epidural anesthesia should be used only with great care.

2. For cesarean section, either general or nonemergency conduction anesthesia is appropriate.

Postpartum Management

1. Because of the removal of the placental hormones and the fetus as metabolic stresses upon the mother, diabetes of any class tends to become much less severe immediately after delivery.

2. Chemical diabetics usually revert to normal in the postpartum period and remain so, requiring no further care.

3. Insulin requirements for other diabetics decrease markedly and may remain low for several weeks. For this reason, the mother should be managed on a reduced dosage of long-acting insulin (one-half to two-thirds the prepregnancy dose), or with no long-acting insulin until urine testing reveals a need for it.

4. In place of a fixed insulin dose, urine sugar and acetone should be checked q.i.d. for several days to weeks until stabilization occurs. Urinary glucose should be covered with short-acting insulin, usually according to the standard scale:

4 + sugar—15 units of insulin
3 + sugar—10 units of insulin
2 + sugar— 5 units of insulin
0–1 + sugar—no insulin

Five units of insulin should be added for 3+ acetonuria.

5. As the need for insulin stabilizes during this period, fixed combinations of long- and short-acting insulins are gradually reinstituted.

24 Pregnancy Complicated by Medical Illnesses

David H. Fields

BASIC PRINCIPLES

1. Almost any disease that can occur in a nonpregnant woman may also affect a pregnant woman.

2. When disease is concurrent with pregnancy, it is important to consider several things:

a. How does pregnancy affect the diagnosis of the disease?

b. How does pregnancy affect the course of the disease?

c. How does the disease affect the pregnancy?

d. How does the treatment affect the pregnancy and vice versa?

3. Many medical illnesses in pregnancy should be handled jointly by an internist (or subspecialist) expert in the particular disease and an obstetrician alert to the needs of pregnancy.

HEART DISEASE

Effects of Pregnancy on Diagnosis

1. As detailed in Chap. 2, many of the normal cardiovascular accommodations to pregnancy would be suggestive of heart disease in a nonpregnant woman. These include the following signs and symptoms:

a. Tachycardia

b. Apparent enlargement of the heart with displacement of the PMI outward

c. Systolic murmurs, present in up to 90 per cent of normal gravidas

d. Diastolic and continuous murmurs, present in up to 10 to 15 per cent of normal gravidas

e. Third heart sounds

f. Dyspnea

g. Dependent edema

2. Because these "abnormal" findings are normal, the diagnosis of heart disease during pregnancy must be made before pregnancy or must be based on different criteria. Suggested criteria[1] from 20 years ago have essentially not changed.

a. A diastolic or continuous murmur, although often normal, is presumptive of disease until proven normal.

b. Unquestionable cardiac enlargement

c. A loud, harsh systolic murmur

d. Severe arrhythmia (atrial fibrillation or flutter or advanced heart block)

Effects of Pregnancy on Disease

1. Pregnancy tends to worsen heart disease, since it places an increased strain on an already stressed system.

2. Most of the physiologic studies determining risks at various stages of pregnancy

1. Burrell, C. S., Metcalfe J., *Heart Disease and Pregnancy,* Boston, Little & Brown, 1958.

(by measuring cardiac output) failed to account for aortocaval compression by the growing uterus and falsely predicted that cardiovascular volume and strain peaked in the early third trimester and then declined.

a. In fact, they continue to rise until the end of pregnancy, although more slowly after about 32 weeks.

b. There is an additional strain immediately postpartum, precipitated by contraction of the postpartum uterus with injection of several hundred ml. of blood into the vascular tree.

3. The degree of worsening which is likely is adequately predicted by the New York Heart Association classification (see below).

Effects of Disease on Pregnancy

1. Maternal prognosis is roughly proportional to the severity of congestive failure and will be discussed individually for each type of heart disease.

2. Fetal prognosis is proportional to the severity of both hypoxia and congestive failure, increasing the risks of

a. Congenital anomalies

b. Intrauterine growth retardation (IUGR)

c. Fetal distress in labor

Therapy and Its Interaction with Pregnancy

1. The management of most heart disease during pregnancy is directed at:

a. Predicting and combating the development of congestive heart failure

b. Protecting the mother against progression of her heart disease, especially valvular problems

c. Protecting the fetus against hypoxic insult

2. Most therapies are not changed during pregnancy but will be discussed individually.

Functional Classification of Heart Disease

The New York Heart Association has formulated a widely accepted classification for heart disease (outside of pregnancy) based on functional capacity rather than etiology or physical findings. It serves well, however, for prognostication during pregnancy. "Symptoms" as used below refers to angina, dyspnea, palpitations, or severe fatigue.

1. Class I. Patients with no symptoms of heart disease on ordinary activity

2. Class II. Patients who are comfortable at rest but have symptoms on ordinary activity

3. Class III. Patients who are comfortable at rest but have symptoms on minimal activity

4. Class IV. Patients who have symptoms at rest

Management of Heart Disease

1. In general, a plan of management for the pregnant woman with heart disease may be based on her functional classification in the nonpregnant state, since this will likely predict her ability to withstand the increase in cardiovascular work required by pregnancy.

2. All pregnant cardiacs should be managed in conjunction with a cardiologist.

Antepartum Management

1. Class I and Class II Cardiac Disease

a. These patients will generally tolerate pregnancy but may find themselves on the edge of decompensation at the slightest complication.

b. Patients should be seen at least biweekly in the first 6 months of pregnancy by both obstetrician and internist and weekly thereafter.

c. Adequate rest, usually at least 10 hours of sleep at night and a midafternoon nap, as well as a nap after meals, should be encouraged.

d. Work should be limited to light housework or employment as tolerated WITHOUT symptoms.

e. Dietary restriction may be minimal, with exhortation to avoid excessive amounts of salt. If the patient is without symptoms on an unrestricted diet and on no medications, this regime may continue.

f. Since even mild respiratory infections are likely to provoke decompensation, they should be avoided, even to the point of not seeing people who have colds. Symptoms such as cough, shortness of breath, or increasing fatigue should be reported immediately and thoroughly investigated by the physician.

g. Since anemia increases cardiac work and is so common in pregnancy, it should be avoided if possible.

h. Careful attention to avoid cardiac decompensation is essential. If symptoms or signs of congestive failure occur, immediate hospitalization with aggressive therapy is mandatory. (See "Treatment of Acute Cardiac Decompensation [Pulmonary Edema]," below.)

i. Antepartum fetal jeopardy is proportional to the degree of maternal congestive failure and/or hypoxia. If there is no evidence of these, no special testing is necessary.

2. Class III Cardiac Disease

a. Consider therapeutic termination of pregnancy. Patients who have symptoms on minimal exertion while not pregnant are at grave risk for decompensation during pregnancy, a complication associated with a maternal mortality rate of up to 15 per cent.

b. For Class III cardiacs who continue pregnancy, bed rest and close observation throughout pregnancy are preferred. Constant care by a cardiologist is necessary.

c. Salt-restricted (2 to 3 g. of sodium) diets help avoid congestive failure.

d. Continue all cardiac medications in appropriate dosage. These patients, who are in borderline failure before pregnancy, are usually already receiving various medications, which may include:

(1) digoxin (Lanoxin)

(2) a diuretic such as hydrochlorothiazide (Hydrodiuril) or furosemide (Lasix)

(3) an antiarrhythmic agent such as procainamide (Pronestyl) or quinidine

e. Hospitalize at the first signs of worsening condition and continue hospitalization until after delivery. Once congestive failure has occurred during pregnancy, it will almost inevitably recur unless exceedingly meticulous management is undertaken.

f. Institute antepartum fetal evaluation during the third trimester if the mother is hypoxic at all, since chronic hypoxia predisposes to IUGR.

(1) Ultrasonography for fetal growth: begin at 24 to 28 weeks and repeat every 3 to 6 weeks.

(2) NST, CST, BPP: begin NSTs at 28 weeks and repeat at least weekly. Add CST and BPP as necessary.

g. While early termination of pregnancy for fetal jeopardy may be necessary, it is usually not indicated for maternal disease. Long, hard, induced labors or cesarean section may be more strenuous for the mother than continuing pregnancy.

3. Class IV Cardiac Disease

a. Advise termination of pregnancy in the first trimester. These patients are in frank congestive failure before pregnancy. The strain of gestation and delivery carries a high mortality rate.

b. If the patient insists on continuing pregnancy, hospitalization for the entire pregnancy, with management using digoxin, diuretics, salt restriction, and other aids to cardiac control, is mandatory.

Management of Delivery

1. Admission to the hospital before the onset of labor for Class I and Class II cardiacs is encouraged, although patients who have tolerated the entire pregnancy without incident may not require this. Class III and Class IV cardiacs almost always find themselves hospitalized before delivery for management of congestive failure.

2. While labor does involve cardiovascular strain, abdominal delivery is far more stressful, both intraoperatively and postoperatively. Vaginal delivery should be the rule, with cesarean section only for obstetrical reasons in all classes of cardiac disease.

3. The following orders should be written for labor:

a. Vital signs every 15 min.

b. Bed rest, sitting or semi-Fowler's position

c. I.V. fluids—D_5W at 50 to 60 ml. per hour

d. N.P.O.

e. Continuous electronic fetal monitoring

f. Oxygen by mask or nasal catheter

g. A Fleet's enema may be given if necessary.

h. More intensive care with monitoring of digoxin, diuretics, and oxygen status may be necessary for Class III and Class IV cardiacs.

4. Analgesia and sedation should be kept mild. The usual combinations of a narcotic and a tranquilizer may be used in reduced dosage.

5. If necessary, epidural anesthesia may be used. Every effort must be made to avoid hypotension since this may precipitate cardiac decompensation. Spinal anesthesia should be avoided for this reason.

6. Prophylactic low forceps may be used to shorten the second stage. Unless cardiac decompensation occurs, second-stage labor is preferable to midforceps delivery.

7. Local or pudendal block anesthesia is preferred for vaginal delivery. If cesarean section becomes necessary, balanced general or well-performed epidural (be wary of hypotension) anesthesia is acceptable.

8. Avoid ergot alkaloids for management of the third stage as they may raise venous pressure.

9. Treat acute cardiac decompensation as it develops, although this is more likely postpartum.

Postpartum Management

1. While Class I and Class II cardiacs who have tolerated pregnancy well to this point usually encounter no problems, some may go into failure in the postpartum period. Therefore, the same careful surveillance is necessary for several days postpartum.

2. Class III and Class IV cardiacs frequently need intensive care and management of severe congestive failure in the postpartum period, especially during the first 48 to 72 hours.

3. In all cases, avoid the use of ergot alkaloids unless necessary for postpartum hemorrhage.

4. Hypotension and infection still represent serious threats, and careful attention for signs of either is mandatory in all cases.

Treatment of Acute Cardiac Decompensation (Pulmonary Edema)

1. Get help. A cardiologist should be available and aware of the patient's condition.

2. Elevate the patient's head; sitting upright is best.

3. Morphine, usually 10 to 15 mg. I.M. q.2–4h., decreases anxiety, tachypnea, and pulmonary congestion. In acute pulmonary edema, a smaller dose (4 mg.) may be given intravenously to begin.

4. Oxygen, 100 per cent by positive pressure if necessary, relieves hypoxia.

5. Perform rapid digitalization using digoxin 0.25 mg. stat and q.6h., up to a total dose of 1.0 mg., for the patient who has not previously received digoxin. For patients already digitalized, small additional doses of digoxin or ouabain may be required.

6. Furosemide (Lasix) in doses of 40 to 80 mg. by intravenous push may be life-saving.

7. Aminophylline, 500 mg. slowly I.V. and q.4h., relieves bronchospasm.

8. Rotating tourniquets will provide an immediate decrease in cardiac load by cutting down venous return.

9. Phlebotomy is rarely necessary but may be used in addition to rotating tourniquets. Not more than 500 ml. of blood should be withdrawn.

Additions to Management for Specific Diseases of the Heart

1. Rheumatic Heart Disease (RHD)

a. Antibiotic prophylaxis is indicated throughout pregnancy for all patients who have evidence of rheumatic valvular heart disease. This may be done with benzathine penicillin (Bicillin) 1,200,000 units I.M. monthly or penicillin V 250 mg. P.O. b.i.d. For the penicillin-allergic patient, erythromycin 250 mg. P.O. b.i.d. will suffice.

b. Wider coverage is indicated for delivery. Current recommendations are for broad-spectrum coverage with a combination of ampicillin and gentamicin, or, if one prefers a single agent, with a semisynthetic third-generation penicillin (e.g., pipericillin) or second-generation cephalosporin (e.g., cefoxitin). Broad-spectrum coverage should be begun during labor and continued for 1 to 2 days after delivery.

c. The following valvular lesions, seen in RHD, present special problems:

(1) *Mitral Stenosis*

(a) Decreased cardiac output, right heart failure, and pulmonary edema. Tend to worsen as pregnancy progresses, peaking during labor and immediately postpartum.

(b) Atrial fibrillation and clot formation with arterial embolization. Digitalization appears to be safe during pregnancy. Anticoagulation, if required, should be with heparin as the warfarin derivatives are associated with teratogenesis.

(c) Definitive treatment for severe mitral stenosis is commissurotomy or valve replacement, preferably before pregnancy, but during if absolutely necessary.

(2) *Aortic Stenosis*

(a) If mild, usually benign; if severe, resultant hypoxia greatly increases risk of IUGR, fetal distress, and congenital anomalies (mostly cardiac).

(b) Left ventricular hypertrophy with increased cardiac oxygen requirements makes angina common.

(c) Syncope and/or dyspnea on slight exercise (and durng labor), due to inadequate output through a severely stenotic valve, pose grave dangers for both mother and fetus.

(d) Definitive therapy is commissurotomy or valve replacement, preferably before conception. Anticoagulation through the pregnancy is necessary only if artifical valves are used.

(3) *Mitral Insufficiency*

(a) Rarely severe; usually occurs with other more severe valvular disease and rarely requires additional special management.

(b) See *Prolapsed Mitral Valve* under "Congenital Heart Diseases," below.

(4) *Aortic Insufficiency*

(a) Most often occurs in tandem with mitral damage. Usually causes only minor problems during pregnancy, unless combined with mitral disease.

(b) In severe cases, cardiac oxygenation is compromised, and then the prognosis is poor.

2. Congenital Heart Diseases
Increasingly common in women of childbearing age, this category includes a number of discrete lesions. Most are recognized during childhood and corrected, and, therefore, pose no danger during pregnancy. If they are not recognized and/or fixed, the risk during pregnancy is proportional to the degree of hypoxia or CHF. Those which result in pulmonary hypertension contraindicate pregnancy, since the maternal mortality rate may approach 50 per cent in such cases. Antibiotic prophylaxis is generally indicated at delivery.

a. *Prolapsed Mitral Valve*

(1) Present in as many as 10 per cent of women

(2) Usually hemodynamically insignificant

(3) Sometimes associated with conduction defects resulting in arrhythmias (mostly PAT)

(4) Requires no special attention except for antibiotic prophylaxis with delivery

b. *Atrial Septal Defect*

(1) Even if the defect is large, with a significant left-to-right shunt, pulmonary hypertension with reversal of the shunt and cyanosis does not usually occur until after the childbearing years.

(2) These patients usually tolerate pregnancy well. Fetal loss is not overwhelming unless the mother is cyanotic.

(3) Antibiotic coverage for delivery may not be necessary, but the benefits would seem to outweigh the risks.

c. *Patent Ductus Arteriosus*

(1) Usually diagnosed in childhood because of the "machinery murmur," patent ductus has usually been repaired before adulthood.

(2) If the defect is small, the left-to-right shunt will not reverse itself for years. If the defect is large, pulmonary hypertension may occur earlier, with reversal of the shunt and cyanosis.

(3) If there is no cyanosis, pregnancy is well tolerated. If, on the other hand, the mother is hypoxemic, fetal loss is very high. Early abortion, prematurity, and an increased incidence of fetal anomalies are results of chronic hypoxia.

(4) Sudden systemic hypotension may lead to acute reversal of the shunt with cardiovascular collapse. Avoid conduction anesthesia and be alert for postpartum hemorrhage.

(5) Prophylactic antibiotics are probably indicated for delivery.

d. *Ventricular Septal Defect (VSD)*

(1) Usually, patients who survive to childbearing age have small VSDs. These are associated with left-to-right shunts of varying degree and no particular problems during pregnancy.

(2) If the VSD is larger and a right-to-left shunt with pulmonary hypertension has developed, pregnancy is very poorly tolerated.

(3) Fetal loss in the face of pulmonary hypertension and cyanosis is high.

(4) The warnings about hypotension as given for patent ductus arteriosus apply as well to VSDs if pulmonary hypertension has resulted.

(5) Again, antibiotic coverage for delivery is probably desirable.

e. *Pulmonary Stenosis*

(1) A relatively common defect, this lesion causes symptoms proportional to the degree of stenosis.

(2) If it is severe with symptoms of dyspnea and syncope, surgical correction is indicated.

(3) If it is not severe, pregnancy is usually well tolerated.

(4) Antibiotic therapy is definitely indicated for coverage of delivery, even after surgery.

f. *Coarctation of the Aorta*

(1) Usually the lesion is near the ligamentum arteriosum, which may remain as a patent ductus arteriosus.

(2) It is usually asymptomatic and discovered during a workup for hypertension.

(3) Major complications in pregnancy are rupture, bacterial infection, and congestive heart failure. Rupture during pregnancy is most likely to occur in the late antepartum period or in the puerperium, not during labor.

(4) Surgical repair during pregnancy is controversial but probably not indicated, since maternal and fetal survival do not appear to be increased.

(5) Antibiotic prophylaxis is indicated throughout pregnancy and during delivery.

(6) Vaginal delivery is preferred, unless abdominal delivery is necessary for obstetrical reasons.

g. *Tetralogy of Fallot*

(1) The syndrome of ventricular septal defect, pulmonary stenosis, right ventricular hypertrophy, and overriding aorta is the most common cause of cyanotic heart disease beyond infancy.

(2) Because of cyanosis, the fetal loss rate is high, the rate depending on the degree of cyanosis. This has been roughly correlated with hematocrit. If the cyanosis is severe enough to result in hematocrit over 65 per cent, spontaneous abortion is a virtual certainty.

(3) Antibiotic coverage for delivery is indicated.

h. *Idiopathic Hypertrophic Subaortic Stenosis*

(1) This rare condition is characterized by hypertrophy of the ventricular system such that outflow obstruction occurs with increased cardiac output (exercise, labor), resulting in a rapid decrease in output with syncope, fetal distress, and, occasionally, sudden death.

(2) Treatment consists of a β-adrenergic blocking agent, propranolol (Inderd). Although several theoretical risks may be suggested, in practice only mild cases of IUGR have been noted. This risk must be weighed against the benefits.

(3) Pregnancy and vaginal delivery are well tolerated if vigorous exercise is limited.

i. *Marfan's Syndrome*

(1) Because of a collagen defect inherited as an autosomal dominant trait, these patients are likely to develop aortic aneurysms and rupture.

(2) Pregnancy greatly increases this risk and carries a maternal mortality up to 50 per cent.

(3) If pregnancy occurs and abortion is declined, bed rest in the hospital throughout is the wisest course.

Other Heart Diseases

1. Cardiomyopathy and Myocarditis

a. CHF is the prominent feature of both these diseases.

b. Because maternal mortality rates approach 50 per cent and fetal loss rates are almost equally high, pregnancy should be avoided.

c. If pregnancy does occur, and abortion is declined, management of CHF must be aggressive.

d. Steroidal and non-steroidal anti-inflammatory agents may be necessary. Their risks are small compared to the risks of unchecked disease.

2. Endocarditis

a. Seen in patients with valvular disease and in I.V. drug users.

b. Life-threatening during pregnancy, it must be aggressively treated with appropriate antibiotics.

THROMBOEMBOLIC DISEASE

THROMBOPHLEBITIS

Effects of Pregnancy on Diagnosis

1. Symptoms and signs of deep vein thrombophlebitis (DVT) are sometimes mimicked by pregnancy.

a. Pain, tenderness, and edema may be due to venous distension caused by the enlarged uterus.

b. Erythema, usually a later sign, is more suspect.

2. Laboratory testing is also complicated by pregnancy.

a. Doppler plethysmorrheography (PRG) and impedance plethysmography (IPG) are quite accurate if negative, since normal blood flow through the venous system makes phlebitis extremely unlikely. However, venous stasis during late pregnancy often creates false positives.

b. Venography is the definitive test but involves injection of radiopaque dye and exposure of the fetus to radiation. Sometimes essential, this may be done while attempting to shield the fetus.

c. ^{125}I-fibrinogen scanning is contraindicated.

Effects of Pregnancy on Disease

1. DVT does not affect pregnancy or the fetus directly. If it progresses to pulmonary embolism, however, the life of the mother is in grave danger.

2. Once it has occurred, it is equally dangerous in the pregnant and nonpregnant.

Therapy and Its Interaction With Pregnancy

1. The only effective treatment for DVT is anticoagulation. This carries extra risks during pregnancy (see below).

2. Because of the thrombogenicity of pregnancy, therapy must be continued until after the early puerperal period, regardless of when it is begun.

3. Anticoagulation is combined with strict bed rest (in a lateral recumbent position to avoid caval compression) for several days, until clot fixation, and then continued by itself for the remainder of the pregnancy.

4. Heparin

a. Because it does not cross the placenta, heparin is the agent of choice for anticoagulation of the pregnant woman.

b. It is not, however, completely safe. The risks of both maternal hemorrhage and hemorrhagic infarcts with compromise and abruption are considerable.

c. Method

(1) Begin with constant I.V. infusion after a loading dose, usually 3,000 to 6,000 units, followed by 1,000 to 2,000 units/hour.

(2) The actual rate is adjusted according to the APTT, which should be maintained at 1.5 to 2 times normal. It is not unusual for pregnant patients to require much greater doses of heparin to maintain adequate anticoagulation because of high Factor VIII and fibrinogen levels.

(3) Maintain I.V. heparin for 10 to 14 days and then switch to subcutaneous heparin q.12h. (doses range from 5,000 to 15,000), still sufficient to maintain the APTT at 1.5 to 2 times normal.

(4) During labor, I.V. heparinization is again instituted. This is terminated and reversed (with protamine sulfate) 1 hour before anticipated delivery, and restarted 1 to 2 hours postpartum.

(5) After several days of I.V. therapy postpartum, anticoagulation is maintained with either intermittent subcutaneous heparin (in nursing mothers) or oral warfarin for 1 to 3 months.

5. Warfarin Derivatives

a. These are usually not used during pregnancy. Use in the first trimester may result in a well-documented fetal syndrome, warfarin embryopathy, consisting of nasal hypoplasia and skeletal abnormalities, probably related to multiple small hemorrhagic infarcts. In later pregnancy, multiple anomalies have also been found to occur, again probably related to repeated episodes of fetal hemorrhage.

PULMONARY EMBOLISM

Effects of Pregnancy on Diagnosis

1. As with phlebitis, the diagnosis of pulmonary embolism is more difficult during pregnancy. The signs and symptoms are unchanged but, again, may be mimicked.

a. Shortness of breath, tachycardia, and tachypnea are quite common during normal pregnancy.

b. Wheezing, rales, fever, and pleuritic chest pain may be caused by asthma, pneumonia, or bronchitis.

c. Hemoptysis is slightly more suspect.

2. Laboratory testing, therefore, is of great importance.

a. The ECG, which often only confirms sinus tachycardia, is not affected by pregnancy.

b. Arterial blood gases typically show hypoxia ($pO_2<80$ mm. Hg), hypocarbia ($pCO_2<30$ mm. Hg), and a metabolic alkalosis ($pH<7.35$). However, during normal pregnancy, hypocarbia and metabolic alkalosis are not unusual.

c. Chest x-ray may be safely done during pregnancy with adequate shielding. It may show an infiltrate, an effusion, or atelectasis but usually is not specific and is more difficult to read than in the nonpregnant, because of elevation of the diaphragms.

d. The ventilation-perfusion scan is the usual procedure which makes the diagnosis. Although it involves a radioisotope, ^{125}Tc, it has such a short half-life that it is considered safe for use in pregnancy. Its interpretation is not influenced by pregnancy. Normal scans virtually rule out significant pulmonary embolism.

Effects of Pregnancy on Disease

1. Pulmonary embolism is life-threatening in both the pregnant and the nonpregnant.

Effects of Disease on Pregnancy

1. The obvious risk is that of maternal cardiovascular collapse, which will endanger the fetus as well.

2. There is the added risk of hypoxia for the fetus, secondary to degrees of maternal hypoxia which may not directly threaten the mother.

Therapy and Its Interaction with Pregnancy

1. The therapy for pulmonary embolism in pregnancy is the same as that for DVT: anticoagulation, which, as above, is associated with extra risk in the pregnant patient.

2. Additionally, maternal pO_2 levels must be maintained in order to avoid fetal hypoxia.

3. If the embolic event has been severe enough to cause cardiovascular compromise, various degrees of cardiopulmonary support will be necessary.

PULMONARY DISEASE

Basic Principles

1. The diagnosis and treatment of the most commonly occurring pulmonary diseases of young women are largely unaffected by the presence of pregnancy.

2. With a few exceptions, pregnancy is largely unaffected by the course or treatment of most pulmonary diseases of young women.

PNEUMONIA

Basic Principles

1. In or out of pregnancy, by far the most common cause of pneumonia is *Diplococcus pneumoniae.*

2. Pregnant women, however, do seem to be somewhat more susceptible to viral pneumonia, developing it more often and more severely than nonpregnant women.

3. The diagnosis of pneumonia hinges upon clinical suspicion leading to the chest radiograph. This is unchanged by the presence of pregnancy. A chest radiograph may be performed with abdominal shielding without endangering the fetus at any stage of pregnancy.

4. The radiologic pictures of the various pneumonias are unchanged by pregnancy.

5. The major risks to pregnancy posed by pneumonia are:

a. A decrease in ventilatory capacity in more severe cases, and

b. High fevers

Management

1. Once the diagnosis of pneumonia is made, the management is essentially the same as out of pregnancy.

2. Hospitalization, followed by treatment with an appropriate antibiotic, most often penicillin (or erythromycin in penicillin-allergic patients) usually leads to rapid resolution of pneumococcal pneumonia.

3. The treatment for viral pneumonias, as in nonpregnant women, is largely supportive, with attention to the prevention of high fever and hypoxia.

Effects of Pregnancy on Diagnosis

1. The diagnosis of the various pneumonias is unchanged by pregnancy.

a. Chest x-rays, the diagnostic mainstay for all pneumonias, may be safely performed while shielding the fetus. Their interpretation is not influenced by pregnancy, except late in its course when the diaphragms may be elevated.

b. Sputum smears for the diagnosis of pneumococcal pneumonia are similarly reliable.

c. Cold agglutinins, useful in the diagnosis of mycoplasmal pneumonia, are unchanged during pregnancy.

Effects of Pregnancy on Disease

1. Pneumococcal pneumonia remains the most common pulmonary disease in or out of pregnancy. Its course is unchanged in the gravid woman.

2. Mycoplasmal pneumonia seems similarly unaffected.

3. Viral pneumonias may occur somewhat more frequently in pregnant women and seem to be more severe, with longer courses and higher fevers.

Effects of Disease on Pregnancy

1. Pneumonias commonly affect pregnancy in only two ways:

a. High fevers are not good for developing fetuses.

b. If the pneumonia is severe enough to cause maternal hypoxia, fetal hypoxia may also occur.

Therapy and Its Interaction with Pregnancy

1. The therapies of the various pneumonias are the same as in the nonpregnant state, except that more careful attention must be accorded to the prevention of high fevers and hypoxia to prevent fetal injury.

2. Penicillin (for pneumococcal pneumonia) and erythromycin (for the penicillin-allergic and for mycoplasmal and, possibly, viral pneumonias) both seem safe at all stages of gestation.

ASTHMA

Effects of Pregnancy on Diagnosis

Pregnancy, for practical purposes, has no effect on the diagnosis of asthma.

Effects of Pregnancy on Disease

1. Approximately 25 per cent of asthmatics who become pregnant will experience a worsening of their disease, while 25 per cent will improve. In the remaining 50 per cent, their disease will be unaffected by pregnancy.

2. Usually those with more severe disease are the ones who become worse.

3. Two factors contribute to this process:

a. The oxygen needs of the gravida are 25 per cent higher than before pregnancy, tending to worsen the disease, and

b. The high progesterone (and possibly corticosteroid) levels in pregnancy cause bronchiolar dilation, tending to improve the disease.

Effects of Disease on Pregnancy

Unless there is severe chronic hypoxia, asthma has no particular effect on pregnancy.

Therapy and Its Interaction with Pregnancy

1. The management of asthma during pregnancy is almost the same as in the nonpregnant. Major differences are:

a. Maternal pO_2 must be maintained at a higher level to avoid fetal hypoxia.

b. Iodide-containing bronchodilators should be avoided, lest they induce fetal goiter.

c. The (unknown) risks of other medications must be weighed against need. Most of the commonly used drugs in asthma are either Category B (no *known* risks for human fetuses or test animals) or Category C (no *known* risk for human fetuses, but teratogenic in test animals). There are no Category A drugs (*known* to be safe during human pregnancy).

2. Basics of Therapy

a. Hydration is critical during acute exacerbations.

b. Epinephrine and aminophylline are the mainstays of therapy of acute disease.

c. Methylxanthines (theophylline, aminophylline) and sympathomimetics (metaproterenol, terbutaline, and albuterol) are central to the chronic control of brochospasm.

d. Corticosteroids (prednisone) have no known ill effects on the fetus, except during the first trimester, when their use may be associated with a slight increase in the incidence of cleft palate.

e. Cromolyn sodium, which blocks mast cell release and prevents bronchospasm, appears to be safe during pregnancy, although its use is not officially approved.

TUBERCULOSIS (TB)

Effects of Pregnancy on Diagnosis

1. Screening for tuberculosis using the Tine or Mantoux test should be part of every prenatal evaluation.

2. If the test is positive, indicating previous exposure to TB, a chest radiograph should be taken to rule out disease.

3. If the chest radiograph shows evidence of disease, a full diagnostic workup, including sputum cultures, should be obtained to distinguish old from active disease.

4. A patient whose Tine or Mantoux test has converted from negative to positive within the last year, but who has no evidence of active disease, is termed a "converter."

Effects of Pregnancy on Disease

1. The above elaborate screening program has been devised because there is a definite tendency for inactive TB to become active during pregnancy.

2. Although the reservoir of latent TB was decreasing over the last 2 decades, it has again begun to increase.

Effects of Disease on Pregnancy

1. Pulmonary tuberculosis has no effect on pregnancy unless the mother has far-advanced lung disease with respiratory decompensation, or unless there is hematogenous spread of the organism.

2. Congenital tuberculosis is rare, but neonatal infection is a real possibility if the mother has positive sputum.

Therapy and Its Interaction with Pregnancy

1. Active Disease

a. If active TB is diagnosed in a pregnant patient, therapy is initiated immediately. This consists of:

(1) Hospital isolation until sputum cultures turn negative

(2) Isoniazid (INH) 300 mg. daily

(3) Para-aminosalycylic acid (PAS) 12 g. daily

(4) Streptomycin 1 g. daily

(5) Two other drugs, ethambutol (15 mg./Kg. O.D.), and rifampin (600 mg. O.D.), have been shown to be highly effective and safe for treating nonpregnant patients. In fact, the combinations of INH and ethambutol and INH and rifampin have replaced PAS and streptomycin regimes in nonpregnant patients. Both of these drugs are currently recommended for treatment of resistant cases in pregnancy and are under investigation for safety for the fetus. Their use should be initiated in the postpartum period.

b. Therapy should be continued as follows:

(1) INH—for 18 months (24 months in far advanced disease)

(2) PAS—until delivery, then switch to ethambutol

(3) Streptomycin—until sputum cultures turn negative and sensitivity of the organism to both of the other drugs is demonstrated. No longer than 3 months.

(4) If the mother has active disease at the time of delivery, the infant should be isolated from her until she has received at least 3 weeks of therapy. The infant should be treated prophylactically under these circumstances with INH.

(5) Ethambutol—there is a small risk of maternal optic neuritis.

(6) Rifampin is extremely effective but may be teratogenic (limb reduction defects).

(7) Streptomycin, 1 g. daily, may be used for the first 3 months of treatment but carries a risk (not measurable) of fetal ototoxicity.

c. Therapy with INH and ethambutol should be continued for 1 year.

2. Inactive Disease Which Has Never Been Treated and Converters

a. Until very recently, women in both of these categories were treated with INH therapy alone, treatment begun during the pregnancy and continued for one year. However, recent recommendations of the Centers for Disease Control have altered this because of reports of teratogenicity from INH.

b. Therapy is now withheld from pregnant women without active disease and begun in the postpartum period.

RENAL DISEASE

INFECTION

Basic Principles

1. There are three levels of urinary tract infection:

a. Asymptomatic bacteriuria—urinary colony count 100,000 per ml., no symptoms.

b. Cystitis—infection of the bladder with dysuria but with no upper tract involvement.

c. Pyelonephritis—infection of the kidney.

2. Since the route of infection seems to be ascending, the above infections occur in the population with decreasing frequency (a>b>c).

3. By similar reasoning, treating asymptomatic bacteriuria decreases the risk of cystitis and pyelonephritis.

Effects of Pregnancy on Diagnosis

1. With the exception of increased urinary frequency, pregnancy does not confound the diagnosis of urinary tract infection.

2. The major symptoms, dysuria (cystitis), hematuria (cystitis), and flank pain (pyelonephritis), are not affected.

3. Nor are the signs, bladder and urethral tenderness (cystitis) or fever and flank tenderness (pyelonephritis).

4. Similarly, lab tests, such as urinalysis (WBC, casts, proteinuria, hematuria) and urine culture, remain equally reliable.

Effects of Pregnancy on Disease

1. During pregnancy there is a tendency toward mild hydroureter and hydronephrosis with increased urinary stasis.

2. In addition, asymptomatic bacteriuria (a urinary colony count of 100,000 per ml. with no symptoms of infection) is present in up to 7 per cent of pregnant women.

3. Overt infection in the form of pyelonephritis or cystitis will occur in 20 to 40 per cent of women with asymptomatic bacteriuria, while its incidence in women without asymptomatic bacteriuria is under 2 per cent.

Effects of Disease on Pregnancy

1. Acute pyelonephritis carries an increased risk of prematurity.

2. Asymptomatic bacteriuria and cystitis do not adversely affect the pregnancy.

Therapy and Its Interaction with Pregnancy

1. The best therapy for urinary tract infection in pregnancy is treatment of asymptomatic bacteriuria.

a. To this end, a complete urinalysis (including microscopic exam) at the first visit, followed by culture in all cases of abnormality, should be performed.

b. In the eyes of many, screening urine culture at the first prenatal visit is worthwhile.

c. All cases of asymptomatic bacteriuria should be treated.

2. In symptomatic disease, urine culture should always be obtained before beginning treatment.

3. Antibiotic therapy. See Table 24-1.

4. Hospitalization for pyelonephritis is desirable, because of both the risk of premature labor and the preferability of parenteral antibiotics.

ACUTE GLOMERULONEPHRITIS

Effects of Pregnancy on Diagnosis

1. This condition is extremely rare, with an incidence of approximately one per 40,000 pregnancies.

2. The diagnosis is based on the occurrence of hematuria, proteinuria, oliguria, and hypertension 2 weeks after Group A β-hemolytic streptococcal infection, and it is confirmed by elevated antistreptolysin O (ASLO) titers and low serum complements. Renal biopsy is not indicated in pregnancy.

3. During the third trimester, it may be virtually clinically indistinguishable from preeclampsia; ASLO titers and serum complement levels will aid in diagnosis if there is persistent hematuria.

Effects of Pregnancy on Disease

1. The disease is self-limited and usually runs its course in 2 weeks, unless chronic disease occurs.

Effects of Disease on Pregnancy

1. Reported fetal loss varies from very high to normal.

Therapy and Its Interaction with Pregnancy

1. Therapy is exactly the same for pregnant and nonpregnant women: supportive.

a. Control blood pressure using diazoxide, hydralazine, or α-methyldopa.

b. Restrict fluid to output plus insensible loss.

c. Restrict salt.

d. Treat presumed streptococcal infection with penicillin.

2. If the disease persists beyond 3 to 4 weeks, termination of pregnancy may be advisable.

CHRONIC RENAL DISEASE WITH IMPAIRED FUNCTION

Effects of Pregnancy on Diagnosis

1. Chronic renal disease may result from any of a number of diseases, including chronic pyelonephritis, glomerulonephritis, or diabetic nephropathy.

2. Primary symptoms are varying degrees of proteinuria, impaired renal function, and hypertension.

Effects of Pregnancy on Disease

1. Gestation may worsen the expression of chronic renal disease since it places increased demands on the kidney.

2. In general, if renal function is more than half lost, it will become worse during pregnancy.

Table 24-1. Preferred Antibodies for Urinary Tract Infection

	Agent	Dosage	Possible Pregnancy-Related Effects
For asymptomatic bacteriuria	Sulfasoxizole (Gantrisin)	1 g. P.O. q.i.d.	When used late in pregnancy competes with bilirubin for binding by albumin and glucuronyl transferase
	Nitrofurantoin (Macrodantin)	50–100 mg. P.O. q.i.d.	May precipitate hemolytic anemia in presence of G-6-PD deficiency
	Ampicillin	500 mg. P.O. q.6h.	No significant effects known
	Oral cephalosporin (any)	500 mg. P.O. q.6h.	No significant effects known
For pyelonephritis	Ampicillin	1–2 g. I.V. q.6h.	No significant effects known
	Parenteral cephalosporin	500 mg.–2 g. q.6–8h. (depending on specific agents)	No significant effects known
For infection resistant to above agents	Gentamicin (Garamycin)	3–5 mg./Kg./day I.V. in 3 doses 60–80 mg. I.V. q.8h.	May be ototoxic or nephrotoxic to both mother and fetus
	Kanamycin (Kantrex)	500 mg. I.M. q.12h.	May be ototoxic or nephrotoxic

Other agents, according to culture and sensitivity results.

Sulfa/trimethoprim combinations (septra, bactrim) are the agents of choice in the nonpregnant and have been used by some during pregnancy. They may be safe but seem objectionable on theoretical grounds, since trimethoprim is a folate antagonist.

Avoid tetracyclines and chloramphenicol during pregnancy because of severe fetal side effects.

Effects of Disease on Pregnancy

1. The prognosis for pregnancy depends on the severity of the disease:

a. If there is severe hypertension (greater than 160/100) or severely impaired renal function (creatinine clearance under 60 ml./min., BUN greater than 25 mg. per 100 ml., creatinine greater than 1.5 mg. per 100 ml.), the prognosis for pregnancy is poor with a high incidence of fetal loss.

b. If renal function is normal and hypertension is absent or mild, the prognosis for pregnancy is good.

2. The maternal danger from chronic glomerulonephritis is primarily related to the high incidence of superimposed preeclampsia, the risk of degenerating renal function, and the severe anemia which frequently coexists.

Therapy and Its Interaction with Pregnancy

1. Manage jointly with a nephrologist.

2. Test renal function frequently, using creatinine clearance as the yardstick.

3. If renal function begins to decrease, terminate pregnancy.

4. Control hypertension using antihypertensive agents and diuretics if necessary.

5. Restrict dietary salt and protein in proportion to the kidney's ability to excrete them, as measured by BUN, serum creatinine, and urinary sodium and protein levels.

6. Correct severe anemia with packed-cell transfusions. Iron and folate therapy are generally unrewarding.

7. Severe electrolyte, *p*H, and azotemic abnormalities may require dialysis.

8. Monitor fetal growth (USG q.3 to 4 weeks) throughout pregnancy and fetal well-being (NST, CST, BPP q.5 to 7 days) in the third trimester.

ACUTE RENAL FAILURE

Basic Principles

1. Acute renal failure may be secondary to anything that acutely decreases renal blood flow to the point of ischemia.

2. In pregnancy, inciting incidents are usually:

a. *Hemorrhage*—placenta previa, placental abruption, postpartum hemorrhage, uterine rupture

b. *Severe preeclampsia/eclampsia* resulting in intravascular spasm

c. *Septic shock*—septic abortion, pyelonephritis (rarely), chorioamnionitis

d. *Intravascular hemolysis*—disseminated intravascular coagulation, mismatched transfusion

3. Most renal failure is acute tubular necrosis. If the patient survives the oliguric phase, a diuresis occurs and the disease reverses itself, usually without residual damage.

4. Renal cortical necrosis resulting from more severe and prolonged ischemia is less common and is irreversible.

ACUTE TUBULAR NECROSIS

Effects of Pregnancy on Diagnosis

1. Suspect acute tubular necrosis when oliguria (urine volume less than 500 ml./24 hrs.) occurs after one of the insults mentioned above.

2. Distinguish it from hypovolemia by determining urine concentration, osmolality, and sodium concentration.

a. In hypovolemic oliguria, the urine is:

(1) *Concentrated*—specific gravity greater than 1.015.

(2) *Hyperosmolar*—greater than 300 mOsm./L.

(3) *Salt-poor*—sodium less than 10 mEq./L.

b. In renal failure, the urine is:

(1) *Dilute*—specific gravity 1.010 or less.

(2) *Isosmotic with plasma*—280 to 300 mOsm./L.

(3) *Rich in sodium*—sodium greater than 30 mEq./L.

None of the above are altered by pregnancy.

Effects of Pregnancy on Disease

1. Most acute renal failure during pregnancy results from a pregnancy-related disease (see "Basic Principles," above).

2. Once the process has begun, pregnancy does not seem to affect its course, other than to change the fluid and electrolyte needs of the mother.

3. If the patient survives the oliguric phase, recovery of most, if not all, renal function is the rule.

Effects of Disease on Pregnancy

1. Maternal mortality rates in acute renal failure may be as high as 20 per cent.

2. Since the inciting events (hypovolemic episodes) all threaten the fetus, fetal loss rates are considerable. If the fetus survives the initial insult, subsequent jeopardy will depend on the quality of fluid and electrolyte management.

Therapy and Its Interaction with Pregnancy

4. Immediate

a. Immediate volume correction at the time of the insult with plasma expanders (Ringer's lactate) and blood is the first step.

b. After shock, hypovolemia, or other precipitating cause has been corrected, if oliguria persists, attempt to increase urine flow with a diuretic. Furosemide (Lasix) 40 mg. I.V. q.4h. is the best agent for this.

c. If this fails to maintain urine flow and no hypovolemia exists, oliguric renal failure may be presumed.

d. In the third trimester, immediate assessment of fetal condition and appropriate responses are indicated.

5. Oliguric Phase

a. Obtain daily BUN, creatinine, sodium, and potassium levels.

(1) BUN will rise approximately 15 mg. per 100 ml. daily and creatinine 1 to 2 mg. per 100 ml. daily until equilibrium is reached at levels dependent on ultimate renal function.

(2) Serum potassium levels may quickly rise above 7 mEq./L. The rate will depend on intake.

b. Measure input and output of fluid daily.

c. Weigh daily.

d. Replace urine water and sodium output daily, with an extra 500 ml. water for insensible loss in the absence of fever.

e. Avoid renal infection by not using indwelling catheters, if possible.

f. Avoid potassium intake.

g. Restrict dietary protein to 20 g. daily.

h. Provide adequate carbohydrates to avoid catabolism of body protein.

i. Treat hyperkalemia with exchange resins (Kayexalate) and correction of acidosis.

j. Consider hemodialysis if there is:

(1) Resistant hyperkalemia

(2) Life-threatening hypervolemia

(3) BUN greater than 120 mg. per 100 ml., or neurologic symptoms felt to be due to uremia.

b. Perform frequent assessment of fetal well-being by NST, CST, and BPP.

6. Diuretic Phase. After approximately 2 weeks, urine output begins to gradually increase and may reach several L. per day. Management at this point should include:

a. Replacement of fluid loss, now in much larger amounts.

b. Daily measurement of BUN, serum creatinine, and sodium and potassium in both the urine and serum.

c. Replacement of sodium loss.

d. Replacement of potassium loss beginning as soon as levels fall into the normal range.

e. Liberalization of protein intake when BUN falls below 80 mg. per 100 ml.

CORTICAL NECROSIS

1. If the oliguric phase persists beyond 2 weeks, cortical necrosis should be suspected.

2. Diagnosis may be verified by renal biopsy.

3. Cortical necrosis is largely irreversible. It is usually fatal unless dialysis is instituted early.

HEMATOLOGIC DISEASES

ANEMIAS

Definitions

1. The presence of a hemoglobin concentration less than 10 g. per 100 ml. or a hematocrit less than 30 per cent is evidence of anemia during pregnancy.

2. Hemoglobin concentrations from 10 to 12 g. per 100 ml. may be dilutional, or the so-called physiologic anemia of pregnancy.

3. Lower levels or abnormalities of RBC shape or size should arouse suspicion of another cause of anemia.

Basic Principles

1. Anything that may cause anemia in a nonpregnant woman may also cause anemia in a pregnant woman.

2. The diagnostic workup of anemia is the same in and out of pregnancy, with one basic exception: since iron deficiency is the most common cause of anemia in pregnancy and since pregnancy itself is the most common cause of iron deficiency, any microcytic hypochromic anemia in pregnancy is presumed to be secondary to nutritional iron deficiency until it fails to respond to iron supplements.

Effects of Pregnancy on Disease

1. All pathologic anemias tend to be exacerbated by pregnancy since hemodilution reduces the effective hemoglobin concentration, regardless of the underlying pathology.

2. Additionally, specific anemias may be adversely or positively affected. These will be discussed individually below.

Effects of Disease on Pregnancy

1. All anemia threatens pregnancy by reducing hemoglobin concentration, thus decreasing the oxygen-carrying capacity of maternal blood and, at low-enough levels, interfering with fetal oxygenation and growth.

2. Typically, the babies of severely anemic mothers are at increased risk for prematurity, low birth weight, and perinatal mortality.

3. Some anemias, especially the sickling anemias, also precipitate acute events which may injure the fetus.

Therapy and Its Interaction with Pregnancy

For the most part, the therapy of anemias is unaffected by and does not affect pregnancy. Specifics will be discussed below.

IRON DEFICIENCY ANEMIA

Basic Principles

1. The normal menstruating woman frequently lives on the edge of iron deficiency, although she is not frankly anemic.

2. Although menstruation ceases with pregnancy, the tremendous iron requirement of a normal term pregnancy (300 mg. for the fetus and 500 mg. for expanded red cell mass) virtually guarantees clinical iron deficiency in a woman not receiving supplementation.

3. This results in progressively decreasing bone marrow stores of iron.

4. A shortage of iron in the marrow leads to decreased synthesis of the heme molecule.

5. Decreased hemoglobin production leads to the formation of smaller erythrocytes.

6. Eventually, as iron stores are used up, the number of cells produced, as well as their size, decreases.

Effects of Pregnancy on Diagnosis

1. A complete blood count done once in each trimester as part of routine prenatal care will identify the presence of anemia. Microcytosis and hypochromia will be detected by CBC. Their meaning is unchanged by pregnancy.

2. Overwhelmingly the most common cause of anemia during pregnancy, iron deficiency is presumed (until proven otherwise) to be the cause of any microcytic hypochromic anemia in a pregnant woman.

3. If adequate iron therapy (see below) fails to correct the anemia, further workup is indicated. This may consist of measurement of serum iron and total iron-binding capacity, bone marrow aspiration with

***Table 24-2.* Iron Studies in Other Microcytic Anemias**

Disease	*Serum Iron*	*Iron-Binding Capacity*	*Iron in Bone Marrow*	*Type Hemoglobin*
Chronic Disease	Low	Low	Present	A
Sideroblastic Anemia	Low	Low	Present in ring sideroblasts	A
Beta-Thalassemia	High	Low	Present	A_2 greater than 5%

staining for iron stores, and, finally, hemoglobin electrophoresis, to rule out these other causes of microcytic hypochromic anemia (see Table 24-2):

a. Chronic disease anemia

b. Beta-thalassemia minor

c. Sideroblastic anemia

4. Findings suggestive of iron deficiency are:

a. Low serum iron which may be low based on hemodilution

b. High iron-binding capacity which may be artefactually high

c. Absence of iron stores in the bone marrow

d. Hemoglobin A on electrophoresis

5. Findings suggestive of other disease are listed below.

Effects of Pregnancy on Disease

1. As stated above, pregnancy is the major cause of iron deficiency anemia.

Effects of Disease on Pregnancy

1. Unless hemoglobin levels fall to less than 8 g. per 100 ml., there is little effect on either the mother or the fetus.

2. Below this level, maternal high-output congestive failure may occur.

3. Also, fetal oxygenation may suffer. However, the fetus itself is almost never anemic because the placenta actively transports iron from the maternal circulation.

Therapy and Its Interaction with Pregnancy

1. Iron deficiency anemia is best treated *before* it occurs by prophylactic administration of ferrous sulfate 325 mg. O.D. throughout the pregnancy.

2. Once anemia is diagnosed, supply iron supplementation—ferrous sulfate 325 mg. P.O. t.i.d., ferrous gluconate 450 mg. P.O. t.i.d., ferrous fumarate 325 mg. P.O. t.i.d.

a. Many feel that iron is better absorbed on an empty stomach and when taken with 250 mg. vitamin C. This may cause more nausea and cramping but results in less constipation.

b. Usually, a prenatal vitamin with 0.8 to 1 mg. of folic acid, if not already prescribed, is added.

3. Check the response in 10 to 14 days with a reticulocyte count. If the count is not over 3 to 5 per cent, pursue further workup as outlined above.

4. If further workup still suggests iron deficiency and rectal exam suggests that the patient is, indeed, taking her iron, consider the possibility of an absorption defect.

5. Parenteral iron in the form of intravenous or intramuscular iron dextran (Imferon) over several days to weekly is indicated if the patient cannot tolerate oral iron or appears to have an absorption defect. Total doses are calculated according to the patient's weight and hemoglobin concentration.

6. Transfusion is only indicated for anemia when it is discovered in labor and hemorrhage or surgery is anticipated.

7. If another cause for the anemia is discovered, treat that.

MEGALOBLASTIC ANEMIA

Basic Principles

1. Folic acid, present in the blood as tetrahydrofolic acid, participates in many reactions, including DNA synthesis, as a coenzyme. In this capacity it is an essential participant in the production of nuclear material in red-cell synthesis. Folate deficiency results in an inability of the red cell to undergo fission within the marrow, with retarded development and persistence of megaloblasts. Similar effects occur in the maturation of neutrophils and platelets, and folic acid deficiency is characterized by a pancytopenia.

2. Adequate intake of folic acid is supplied by a diet rich in eggs, milk products, and leafy vegetables. Absence of these items, combined with the increased daily needs of pregnancy, frequently results in folate deficiency.

3. Within 3 weeks, on a folate-deficient diet, blood levels begin to drop. In 5 weeks, hypersegmented neutrophils are seen in the marrow. By 18 weeks, the marrow is frankly megaloblastic and the patient is anemic.

4. Except in cases of severe long-term deprivation or tremendously increased needs (especially in twin gestation, epileptics taking diphenylhydantoin, and chronic hemolytic anemia), clinical evidence of folate deficiency does not occur until the third trimester.

5. It also commonly occurs in the postpartum period in nursing mothers, precipitated by the production of breast milk, which is extremely high in folic acid content.

Effects of Pregnancy on Diagnosis

1. Most commonly megaloblastic anemia is first detected by low hemoglobin levels or high-mean corpuscular volumes found on routine blood counts.

2. Further confirmation is obtained by a peripheral smear showing macrocytosis and hypersegmented polymorphonuclear leukocytes.

3. Bone marrow aspiration reveals a megaloblastic marrow, with red cells in arrested development.

4. Although vitamin B_{12} deficiency is rare, folic acid and vitamin B_{12} deficiency anemia are clinically indistinguishable. Since therapy is different, blood should be drawn for determination of serum folic acid and B_{12} levels before the therapy is begun for presumed folic acid deficiency.

5. Diagnosis may be complicated by the concurrent presence of iron deficiency. In such cases, a biphasic population of red blood cells is formed, some being macrocytic and some microcytic. Red cell indices by automated counters may average out to normal, but the situation becomes clear upon seeing the peripheral smear.

Effects of Pregnancy on Disease

Pregnancy increases the likelihood of folic acid deficiency because of increased metabolic demands.

Effects of Disease on Pregnancy

1. As in iron deficiency anemia, sufficiently low hemoglobin levels will endanger the mother (CHF) and the fetus (hypoxia).

2. Also as in iron deficiency anemia, the placenta actively transports folic acid, so that the fetus is rarely anemic.

3. In addition, many have suggested that folic acid deficiency may be a cause of fetal anomalies, placental abruption, and preeclampsia. These associations have not been proven.

Therapy and Its Interaction with Pregnancy

1. Folic acid deficiency is best treated by avoiding it.

2. Provide a diet rich in folic acid–containing foods for the average gravida.

3. Supply all patients at high risk for folic acid deficiency with some supplemental folate. Most prenatal vitamins contain 0.8 mg. folic acid, an amount adequate for almost all needs. If uncertainty still exists, folic acid tablets, 1 mg. daily will eliminate any question of deficiency. Conditions which expose the pregnant woman to a greater likelihood of folate depletion include:

a. Twin gestation

b. Chronic hemolytic anemia, especially sickling disease

c. Epilepsy with diphenylhydantoin (Dilantin) therapy

d. Malabsorption states

e. Acute infection

4. Consider the possibility of concurrent iron deficiency anemia, and supply iron supplements.

5. Reticulocyte counts will rise within 1 week, and the anemia will begin to respond within 2 to 3 weeks.

6. If the source of the megaloblastic anemia is B_{12} deficiency, this is almost never on a dietary basis but is usually due to a lack of intrinsic factor. The therapy, therefore, is usually B_{12}, 1 mg. I.M., monthly.

OTHER ANEMIAS IN PREGNANCY

HEMOLYTIC ANEMIAS

Basic Principles

1. Any of the causes of hemolytic anemia may occur in a pregnant woman.

2. Primary causes include:

a. Glucose-6-phosphate dehydrogenase (G-6-PD) deficiency

b. Hereditary spherocytosis

3. Other disease processes which frequently cause hemolytic anemia include:

a. Preeclampsia

b. DIC from any cause

c. Autoimmune diseases, especially lupus and thrombotic thrombocytopenic purpura

d. Valvular heart disease

Effects of Pregnancy on Diagnosis

1. The diagnosis of these diseases and of the hemolysis itself is largely unchanged by pregnancy.

2. Once anemia has been diagnosed, examination of the peripheral smear reveals fragmented RBCs or, in the case of spherocytosis, microcytic spherocytes and a high reticulocyte count.

3. Urinary studies will reveal hemosiderin-laden macrophages.

4. Decreased serum haptoglobin and increased bilirubin levels complete the picture, although haptoglobins may be spuriously elevated since they are alpha-2 globulins, which are increased during pregnancy.

5. A search for specific etiology should be performed.

a. In autoimmune hemolytic anemias, either the direct or indirect Coombs' test will be positive. Identification of the antibodies should be performed.

b. RBC G-6-PD levels may be measured if this deficiency is suspected, but they are often normal after an acute hemolytic event, since it is the older RBCs which are more deficient, and, once they are lysed, the remaining younger cells may be normal.

Effects of Pregnancy on Disease

1. In some cases, pregnancy is the cause of the hemolytic anemia, e.g., preeclampsia.

2. In other cases it may exacerbate the process. This is especially true for autoimmune hemolytic anemias such as thrombotic thrombocytopenic purpura (TTP).

3. In still others, such as G-6-PD deficiency and spherocytosis, the pregnancy often has no particular effect.

Effects of Disease on Pregnancy

1. In addition to the previously mentioned effects of anemia (CHF, fetal hypoxia), in cases of autoimmune hemolytic anemia, IgG antibodies may cross the placenta and cause anemia, thrombocytopenia, and congestive failure in the fetus.

2. In other cases, such as G-6-PD deficiency, there is minimal or no effect on the pregnancy. When an oxidizing agent such as aspirin, sulfa, or nitrofurantoin causes acute hemolysis, the older RBCs, which have lower levels of G-6-PD, lyse, leaving a younger population which has higher levels and is resistant to further hemolysis. The "crises," therefore, are self-limited and rarely result in maternal or fetal compromise.

Therapy and Its Interaction with Pregnancy

1. The treatment of hemolytic anemias in pregnancy is essentially no different than in its absence.

a. In cases of autoimmune disease, prednisone or other corticosteroids may be used.

b. Splenectomy may be necessary to control the hemolysis associated with spherocytosis.

c. Folate supplementation and probably iron as well should be provided, to compensate for the rapid cell turnover.

d. Transfusion, if necessary, may be performed.

2. Underlying diseases must be treated appropriately.

3. The fetus should be monitored with NSTs, CSTs and BPPs in the third trimester. If fetal hemolysis is suspected, the fetus should be followed as described below under "Rh Isoimmunization."

4. A standard hematologic workup is necessary to identify the cause of hemolysis, followed by specific treatment.

HEMOGLOBINOPATHIES

Basic Principles

1. Hemoglobinopathies are hereditary disorders of hemoglobin production, resulting in the formation of abnormal hemoglobin (e.g., S, C, A_2).

2. They fall into two major categories:

a. *The sickling diseases,* which are characterized by the formation of abnormal hemoglobin (S, C) which changes shape under low oxygen tension, causing sickling of the red cell, and

b. *The thalassemias,* which result from a decreased rate of production of one of the peptide chains (alpha, beta) that form the globin molecule.

3. When present in heterozygous forms (sickle trait, minor thalassemias), there is usually enough normal hemoglobin produced that pregnancy is well tolerated.

4. Homozygous hemoglobin abnormalities are usually either fatal in childhood (major thalassemias) or severely debilitating in adulthood (SS disease and SC disease) and associated with an increase in maternal and perinatal morbidity and mortality.

5. Diagnosis is by hemoglobin electrophoresis for identification of abnormal hemoglobins.

SICKLE CELL ANEMIA (SS DISEASE)

Basic Principles

1. Production of hemoglobin S as the sole hemoglobin results in sickle cell anemia, which occurs in approximately 1 in 500 blacks.

2. This results in hemoglobin levels that usually vary from 7 to 10 g. per 100 ml., and in red blood cells which sickle under hypoxic conditions, causing sludging in capillaries in all organ systems. These "sickle crises" result in intense pain and sometimes infarction in affected organs.

Effects of Pregnancy on Diagnosis

1. Sickle cell anemia is invariably diagnosed in childhood or early adulthood because of the repetitive crises.

2. Additionally, all black women who are pregnant or considering pregnancy should be screened for sickle trait.

Effects of Pregnancy on Disease

1. SS disease is excerbated by pregnancy. The metabolic and cardiovascular stresses tend to increase the likelihood of a sickling crisis.

2. The major maternal complications of SS disease in pregnancy are:

a. Severe anemia, frequently in the 7 to 8 g. per 100 ml. range

b. Frequent crises, with a high incidence of drug addiction because of pain

c. Folate deficiency anemia

d. Frequent pulmonary and urinary infections, especially pyelonephritis

Effects of Disease on Pregnancy

1. Maternal mortality may be as high as 2 to 5 per cent, resulting from infarcts caused by sickling cells obstructing the circulation of various organs and from congestive failure.

2. Fetal loss may be up to 40 per cent (half as miscarriage, half as perinatal mortality). Fetal damage usually follows crisis, resulting in acute hypoxia.

3. SS patients are often drug-dependent because of the necessity for frequent narcotics to combat the pain of crises. All the problems attendant on narcotic addiction are, in these cases, added to the pregnancy.

Therapy and Its Interaction with Pregnancy

1. Antepartum Management

a. The ideal therapy for SS disease is to avoid crisis. This may be accomplished by prophylactic exchange transfusion, which aims to maintain hemoglobin S levels below a certain level, usually about 50 per cent. Beginning at various times during pregnancy, from the late first to the late second trimester, and continuing until delivery, this definitely decreases maternal and perinatal mortality. However, there are several important complications:

(1) The incidence of transfusion reactions increases with each exchange (multiple transfusions are necessary).

(2) Non-A, non-B hepatitis is a common complication.

(3) The risk of AIDS, while less of a concern than it was several years ago, is a consideration as well.

b. Because of these risks, prophylactic transfusion is not universal therapy. For patients not so managed, the following course is indicated:

(1) Supplement the diet with up to 5 g. of folic acid and 0.5 g. of iron per day.

(2) Carefully screen for increasing anemia, urinary tract infection, and pulmonary complications.

(3) Avoid the tendency to attribute all symptoms to "crises" and seek other causes for pain or fever.

(4) Transfuse with packed red cells for signs of congestive failure secondary to anemia or for hemoglobin levels below 6 g. per 100 ml.

(5) Treat crises aggressively with hydration, antibiotics, oxygenation, and pain relief. The value of transfusion after a crisis has occurred is unproven.

(6) Monitor fetal growth and well-being with USG and EFM throughout pregnancy.

2. Management of Labor

a. Maintain intensive fetal and maternal monitoring.

b. Administer continuous oxygen by nasal cannula or mask during labor and delivery. Consider hypoxia as something to be avoided at all costs.

c. Avoid general anesthesia if possible.

d. Be alert for crises during labor and immediately postpartum.

SICKLE CELL–HEMOGLOBIN C DISEASE (HEMOGLOBIN SC)

Basic Principles

1. This rare condition is characterized by production of types S and C hemoglobin instead of the normal A hemoglobin.

2. Having a tendency to both anemia and sickle crises, these patients have basically the same risks in the antepartum period as do those with SS disease.

3. Management during all stages of pregnancy is essentially the same as for sickle cell anemia.

SICKLE CELL TRAIT

Basic Principles

1. When the mother is heterozygous for the production of hemoglobin S, half of her hemoglobin is type A. This is sufficient to prevent sickling under all conditions except severe hypoxia. Sickle cell trait occurs in approximately 8 per cent of the American black population.

Effects of Pregnancy on Diagnosis

1. Diagnosis of sickle trait is begun by performance of the "sickle prep." This identifies all those who have any hemoglobin S.

2. Discrimination between sicklers (SS, SC) and sickle trait (SA) is by hemoglobin electrophoresis.

3. Neither of these tests is affected by pregnancy.

Effects of Pregnancy on Disease

1. Since SA hemoglobin does not sickle except under extreme hypoxia, pregnancy does not usually affect sickle trait adversely.

Effects of Disease on Pregnancy

1. Mothers carrying the sickle trait are at increased risk for asymptomatic bacteriuria and symptomatic UTI. This seems to be the only ill effect on most pregnancies.

Therapy and Its Interaction with Pregnancy

1. Strict avoidance of UTI is the only special management required.

THE THALASSEMIAS

Basic Principles

1. The thalassemias may be either alpha or beta chain. They are all diagnosed by hemoglobin electrophoresis.

2. The alpha-thalassemias result from gene deletions which cause defects in one, two, three or all of the four alpha chains. They occur mostly in Chinese and to a much lesser extent among blacks. The severity of the disease is proportional to the number of chains affected.

a. Deletion of all four genes results in alpha-thalassemia major. It is incompatible with extrauterine life.

b. Deletion of three causes hemoglobin H disease (associated with severe hemolytic anemia).

c. If only two chains are abnormal, the result is alpha-thalassemia minor (clinically insignificant microcytic anemia).

d. Abnormality in only a single chain results in an asymptomatic carrier state (clinical normalcy).

3. The beta-thalassemias occur when there is defective beta chain production and may be present in either homozygous or heterozygous forms. This genetic abnormality is clustered among groups originating in the Mediterranean area.

a. Homozygous disease, beta-thalassemia major (Cooley's anemia), is usually not associated with survival past early childhood.

b. Heterozygous disease, beta-thalassemia minor (Mediterranean anemia), results in mild, often clinically insignificant anemia.

4. Because they cause extreme microcytosis, the thalassemias are often confused with iron deficiency anemia, which may be excluded by finding adequate iron stores in the bone marrow.

Effects of Pregnancy on Diagnosis

1. The diagnosis of the thalassemias is suggested by extreme microcytosis found on CBC or by failure of a microcytic anemia to respond to iron supplementation.

2. Definitive diagnosis is by hemoglobin electrophoresis.

3. Neither of these tests is affected by pregnancy.

Effects of Pregnancy on Disease

1. The minor thalassemias are largely unaffected by pregnancy, except that the already present anemia is exaggerated by hemodilution.

2. Pregnancy frequently exacerbates the hemolytic anemia of hemoglobin H disease.

Effects of Disease on Pregnancy

1. As with sickle trait, the minor thalassemias seem to predispose to UTI.

2. Occasionally the anemia will become severe enough to cause CHF in the mother or hypoxia in the fetus.

Therapy and Its Interaction with Pregnancy

1. No special management, other than a vigilance for infection, is necessary.

THROMBOCYTOPENIA

Basic Principles

1. Thrombocytopenia in pregnancy may occur as a manifestation of many diseases, most commonly:

a. Preeclampsia (probably increased consumption)

b. DIC (increased consumption)

c. Severe folic acid deficiency (decreased production)

d. Idiopathic thrombocytopenic purpura (ITP) (destruction)

2. Since it has already been considered in the context of each of the above except ITP, a discussion of this disease follows.

IDIOPATHIC THROMBOCYTOPENIC PURPURA (ITP)

Basic Principles

1. This is an autoimmune disease characterized by anti-platelet antibodies which stimulate reticuloendothelial destruction of platelets.

2. The cause of antibody production is not known.

3. Antibody-coated platelets are destroyed by the spleen, causing thrombocytopenia.

Effects of Pregnancy on Diagnosis

1. Pregnancy does not change the laboratory parameters:

a. Peripheral platelet counts below 100,000/cu. mm.

b. Abnormal clot retraction

c. Prolonged bleeding time

d. Normal or hyperactive bone marrow production of megakaryocytes

e. The presence of an IgG anti-platelet antibody. This is not diagnostic as it may be found in other thrombocytopenic diseases.

2. Ultimately, diagnosis is by exclusion of other causes of thrombocytopenia. This has often been made before the onset of pregnancy.

Effects of Pregnancy on Disease

1. Pregnancy usually worsens this disease, even if the mother is in a state of relative remission, for unknown reasons.

2. Additionally, the disease usually becomes worse, as evidenced by falling platelet counts, as the pregnancy progresses.

Effects of Disease on Pregnancy

1. The maternal risk is hemorrhage.

a. If platelet counts fall below 20,000/cu. mm., hemorrhage may occur spontaneously at any time.

b. Between 20,000 and 50,000/cu. mm., surgical hemostasis is definitely impaired, so hemorrhage may occur from C/S, episiotomy, and vaginal or cervical lacerations. Uterine hemorrhage usually does not occur because the contracting myometrium "ligates" the open vessels of the placental site after separation.

c. Between 50,000 and 100,000/cu. mm., hemostasis may be sufficient for uncomplicated vaginal delivery, but levels above 100,000 are desirable, especially for C/S.

2. Fetal thrombocytopenia results from transplacental passage of antibodies in approximately 25 per cent of cases.

a. Unfortunately, without sampling fetal blood there is no way to identify these fetuses, since maternal levels or responses to therapy do not parallel events in the fetus.

b. Thrombocytopenic fetuses are at significant risk for intracranial hemorrhage during vaginal delivery.

Therapy and Its Interaction with Pregnancy

1. Maternal

a. Initial therapy is instituted if platelet counts fall below 50,000/cu. mm.

b. Prednisone, beginning with a large dose (40 to 60 mg./day) and tapered after several days to a maintenance dose of 10 to 20 mg./day, is usually sufficient to raise the platelet count enough to prevent hemorrhage.

(1) The small risk of teratogenesis with corticosteroids is outweighed by risks of non-treatment to the mother.

c. Splenectomy may be necessary if steroids do not produce an adequate response.

(1) Splenectomy during pregnancy is not benign. Fetal and maternal morbidity and mortality are not inconsequential.

(2) If ITP has been diagnosed before the onset of pregnancy, some advise splenectomy before conception.

d. Platelet transfusions may be performed, as a last resort, if platelet counts are too low at time of delivery. This is a one-time alternative which should be reserved for the last minute as platelets are destroyed within hours and stimulate the formation of still more antibodies, negating the value of future transfusions.

e. Intravenous infusion of high doses of IgG, which seems to inhibit reticuloendothelial destruction of antibody-coated platelets, is a relatively new therapy which shows promise.

2. Fetal

a. There is no good way to determine which fetuses are thrombocytopenic before labor since a good platelet count in the mother, in response to steroid therapy, does not guarantee a similar response in the fetus, and, similarly, a poor maternal count does not necessarily imply fetal thrombocytopenia.

b. To avoid unnecessary C/S in mothers at risk for hemorrhage and dangerous vaginal delivery in thrombocytopenic fetuses, one should obtain fetal scalp blood for a platelet count (technique is as for *p*H in suspected fetal distress) as early as possible in labor. If the fetus is severely thrombocytopenic, C/S should be done.

ENDOCRINOPATHIES

HYPERTHYROIDISM

Basic Principles

1. After diabetes, hyperthyroidism is the most common endocrinopathy associated with pregnancy.

2. Most thyrotoxicosis during pregnancy is due to Graves' disease (rather than toxic nodular goiter), which is a diffuse condition resulting from production of long-acting thyroid stimulator (LATS), a 7s-immunoglobulin.

Effects of Pregnancy on Diagnosis

1. Clinical signs of hyperthyroidism may be confused by pregnancy:

a. Weight loss of hyperthyroidism may be offset by the weight gain of pregnancy.

b. Mild tachycardia may result from the increased cardiac demands of pregnancy.

c. Pretibial edema may result from hydrostatic changes of normal pregnancy.

d. Exophthalmos and extremity tremors are rarely the result of pregnancy.

2. Hyperthyroidism should be suspected in pregnant women who:

a. Fail to gain weight during pregnancy while consuming an adequate diet.

b. Have an elevated pulse rate.

c. Are extremely "high-strung," especially those with a fine tremor of the hands or feet.

d. Have exophthalmos. Exophthalmos, the most familiar sign of thyroid disease, is not medically reversible.

3. Laboratory diagnosis of hyperthyroidism was similarly confounded in pregnancy until the easy determination of free thyroxine (T_4) became available. This was because the hyperestrogenism of pregnancy causes excess production of alpha-2 globulins, which bind most of the T_4 and T_3. So even though the free levels of these hormones are unchanged, total amounts of each are increased. This results in the following alterations of thyroid testing during pregnancy:

a. Total T_4, increased up to 25 per cent (FREE T_4 NOT CHANGED)

b. Total T_3, increased up to 25 per cent (FREE T_3 NOT CHANGED)

c. T_3RU, decreased

3. Thyroid scanning and radioactive iodine uptake studies are contraindicated during pregnancy.

Effects of Pregnancy on Disease

Pregnancy does not alter the course of thyroid disease.

Effects of Disease on Pregnancy

1. Mild hyperthyroidism seems not to affect the course of pregnancy, either for the mother or for the fetus.

2. More severe disease may predispose to

a. Thyroid storm (see below)

b. Preeclampsia

c. Spontaneous abortion

d. Premature labor

e. Fetal hyperthyroidism (in Graves' disease), secondary to transplacental passage of LATS

Therapy and Its Interaction with Pregnancy

The treatment for hyperthyroidism may be medical or surgical or both.

1. Medical management is indicated especially during the first and third trimesters when surgery poses the threat of inciting abortion or premature delivery. It is also indicated to control disease and shrink the gland prior to surgical procedure.

2. Surgical management is preferred when medical control is difficult or inconstant, and should be performed during the late first, second, or early third trimester.

Medical Management

1. Propylthiouracil (PTU) is the agent of choice for medical therapy. It blocks the synthesis of thyroxine and is therefore without effect for one to several weeks until stores of the hormone have been exhausted.

a. Initial dose of PTU is 100 mg. P.O. t.i.d. (as above, for several weeks).

b. Continue until the patient becomes clinically normal (no tachycardia, no tremor), then decrease to 50 mg. P.O. t.i.d. over 1 to 2 weeks.

c. When chemical euthyroidism is achieved, decrease dose further, to as little as 50 mg. per day.

d. Maintain on the smallest dose which achieves high-normal or even slightly elevated T_4 levels, to minimize fetal effects.

e. Maternal complications of PTU include skin rashes and agranulocytosis, so therapy should be monitored with periodic WBC counts. A falling WBC count mandates immediate termination of therapy.

f. Fetal complications reduce, essentially, to one: fetal hypothyroidism. Since PTU crosses the placenta, if maternal function and fetal function are sufficiently suppressed, cretinism may result. There are two possible solutions to this:

(1) Keep the dose of PTU as low as possible to minimize maternal and fetal suppression of thyroid function. Some also taper or discontinue the PTU in the last few weeks to allow recovery of the fetal thyroid.

(2) Administer thyroid replacement to the mother while suppressing her own endogenous production. Although this would seem to have obvious advantages, it does not reliably supply the fetus, since thyroxine crosses the placenta poorly and the higher doses of PTU required create greater suppression of fetal thyroid function.

2. Propranolol (Inderal), a β-adrenergic blocking agent, has been suggested as alternate therapy for hyperthyroidism in pregnancy.

a. It blocks such "hyper" actions of thyroxine as tachycardia and decreases the likelihood of thyroid storm. It does not affect the production of thyroxine.

b. If used, the initial dose is 40 mg. t.i.d., increased 10 mg. t.i.d. every 2 to 3 days until adequate control of side effects occurs.

c. Although not common, IUGR has been reported in fetuses chronically exposed to propranolol, so sonographic and biophysical fetal monitoring should be performed.

d. Propranolol is the drug of choice for the treatment of thyroid storm. See below.

3. Management of Thyroid Storm. This is a medical emergency. Therapy, designed to control the extreme β-adrenergic symptoms until hyperthyroidism can be treated, is as follows:

a. Propranolol 1 to 2 mg. I.V. then 40 mg. P.O. q.6h. to control tachycardia

b. Institution of high doses of PTU therapy to prevent further thyroxine production

c. Massive immediate fluid replacement to combat dehydration

d. Hypothermia blankets and other cooling agents to reduce fever

Surgical Management

1. Partial thyroidectomy is the preferred treatment for patients who respond poorly to medical therapy.

2. While surgery is suggested by some as the therapy of choice, the morbidity and mortality risks are such that medical therapy, if effective, is preferable.

3. If performed, surgery is best done toward the middle of pregnancy, when uterine irritability is least.

4. The major complications of thyroid surgery, other than the actual risks of surgery and anesthesia, are subsequent hypoparathyroidism and recurrent laryngeal nerve paralysis. Both are extremely difficult to treat.

5. Thyroid replacement is necessary postoperatively.

HYPOTHYROIDISM

Basic Principles

1. Hypothyroidism, due to any one of many etiologies, is relatively rare in pregnant women.

2. Severely depressed thyroid function results in a high incidence of infertility and early abortion.

3. Diagnosis during pregnancy is complicated by the changes in thyroid function discussed under "hyperthyroidism."

4. Management consists of thyroid replacement with either USP thyroid, thyroxine (Synthroid), or triiodothyronine (Cytomel).

HYPOPARATHYROIDISM

Basic Principles

1. Hypoparathyroidism is extremely rare during pregnancy. It is found almost exclusively in patients who have undergone thyroid ablation by surgery or radiotherapy, which often results in simultaneous parathyroid destruction.

Effects of Pregnancy on Diagnosis

1. Diagnosis is accomplished by screening at-risk patients for decreased serum calcium and elevated serum phosphate. Except for a slight decrease in serum calcium secondary to dilutional hypoalbuminemia, pregnancy does not affect diagnosis.

Effects of Pregnancy on Disease

None.

Effects of Disease on Pregnancy

1. If the mother becomes sufficiently hypocalcemic, tetany may suggest severe preeclampsia or eclampsia.
2. Fetal or neonatal hypocalcemia may result in heart block.
3. If calcium and phosphate levels are well controlled, there are no ill effects on the pregnancy.

Therapy and Its Interaction with Pregnancy

1. The usual therapy is large doses of vitamin D and adequate calcium supplementation to maintain serum calcium levels in the normal range. Calcium needs are increased somewhat during pregnancy.

HYPERPARATHYROIDISM

Basic Principles

1. Hyperparathyroidism may be the result of an adenoma, a carcinoma, or hyperplasia.

Effects of Pregnancy on Diagnosis

1. The finding of hypercalcemia and hypophasphatemia suggests hyperparathyroidism in or out of pregnancy.

Effects of Pregnancy on Disease

None.

Effects of Disease on Pregnancy

1. The major risk of hyperparathyroidism is the development of hypocalcemic tetany in the neonate.

Therapy and Its Interaction with Pregnancy

1. Effective therapy is usually surgical ablation of the parathyroids, which may be done safely during pregnancy.
2. Oral phosphate supplementation may be successful in lowering serum calcium sufficiently to allow postponement of surgery until after delivery, in some cases.

PITUITARY ADENOMA

Basic Principles

1. The most common pituitary disease in pregnancy is prolactin-producing adenoma.

Effects of Pregnancy on Diagnosis

1. Usually, pituitary adenoma has been diagnosed before conception while investigating oligo- or amenorrhea.
2. If not, the normal hypertrophy occurring during pregnancy may be exaggerated, resulting in sudden loss of vision.
3. Diagnosis by neurological exam is unchanged in the gravida.
4. CT scan and hypocycloidal tomography are usually not done but may be if necessary.

Effects of Pregnancy on Disease

1. As above, pregnancy serves as a stimulus to pituitary hypertrophy and tends to increase the growth of adenomas.

Effects of Disease on Pregnancy

None.

Therapy and Its Interaction with Pregnancy

1. Bromocriptine (Parlodel) is the therapy of choice. This has been used during pregnancy but usually only in cases in which active pituitary growth is evidenced by headaches or compromise of vision. The long-term fetal effects of bromocriptine are not known.

2. Trans-sphenoidal hypophysectomy may be necessary.

3. Late in the pregnancy, delivery is advisable.

HYPERADRENALISM (CUSHING'S SYNDROME)

Basic Principles

1. Adrenal hyperfunction during pregnancy is uncommon.

2. It may be due to adrenal carcinoma, adenoma, or hyperplasia, or it may be secondary to pituitary disease.

Effects of Pregnancy on Diagnosis

1. The physical diagnosis of hyperadrenalism is obscured by pregnancy.

a. Weight gain, edema, hyperpigmentation, and striae all are common in normal gestation.

b. Hypertension is more often a sign of preeclampsia than of Cushing's syndrome.

c. Increasing hirsutism, moon facies, and purple striae, however, suggest hyperadrenalism.

2. Laboratory testing is also affected by pregnancy.

a. Cortisol levels are elevated in normal pregnancy.

b. Similarly, the dexamethasone suppression test must be interpreted with care.

c. Elevated serum ACTH levels may help to diagnose Cushing's syndrome of pituitary origin, which may be confirmed on CT scan of the pituitary.

d. Since CT of the abdomen involves much radiation to the fetus, if there is strong suspicion of an adrenal tumor and diagnosis during pregnancy is critical, exploratory surgery may be preferable.

Effects of Pregnancy on Disease

Pregnancy does not seem to affect the course of Cushing's disease.

Effects of Disease on Pregnancy

1. Florid Cushing's syndrome with hypertension is associated with a high incidence of preeclampsia, gestational diabetes, and fetal loss of up to 50 per cent.

2. Neonates whose mothers have untreated disease are also at considerable risk for Addisonian crisis in the first 1 to 2 days after birth, because their own pituitary function has been suppressed.

Therapy and Its Interaction with Pregnancy

1. For most cases, the therapy is resection. Pituitary surgery may be safely done during pregnancy (for secondary Cushing's syndrome), but adrenal resection carries significant risk and may be best postponed until after delivery, if possible.

2. After surgery, steroid replacement is essential.

ADRENAL INSUFFICIENCY (ADDISON'S DISEASE)

Basic Principles

1. Adrenal insufficiency may be secondary to chronic disease (most commonly in the past, tuberculosis), or it may be the result of previous adrenalectomy for hyperfunction.

2. Before the use of replacement steroids, Addison's disease resulted in infertility. With adequate replacement, however, a woman with adrenal hypofunction may become pregnant and carry to term.

Effects of Pregnancy on Diagnosis

1. The diagnosis during pregnancy is complicated by the fact that the major symptoms, fatigue, nausea and vomiting, weight loss, and increased skin pigmentation, may either be mimicked or masked by pregnancy.

2. Laboratory diagnosis, when the disease is suspected, is by measurement of plasma cortisol levels, which should be low, even during pregnancy.

Effects of Pregnancy on Disease

1. Pregnancy does not significantly alter the course of Addison's disease.

Effects of Disease on Pregnancy

1. The major danger associated with adrenal insufficiency in pregnancy is the development of acute Addisonian crisis at times of severe stress, especially soon after delivery. This is a risk in the previously diagnosed patient who receives inadequate replacement to cope with the puerperium, and it may be the presenting episode in a previously undiagnosed patient.

2. Addisonian crisis is a medical emergency whose symptoms are: fever, nausea and vomiting, and shock. It may be due either to the stress of the puerperium combined with the withdrawal of placental steroidogenesis or to superimposed infection. It should always be in the back of one's mind as a possible cause, in cases of puerperal shock, especially in those which do not respond immediately to adequate blood and fluid replacement.

Therapy and Its Interaction with Pregnancy

1. For previously diagnosed Addison's disease, therapy during pregnancy is relatively straightforward. One need not alter the normal replacement therapy for nonpregnant individuals. This consists of:

  a. A glucocorticoid, either hydrocortisone acetate, 37.5 mg., or prednisone, 7.5 mg., daily, and

  b. A mineralocorticoid, desoxycorticosterone acetate (DOCA), available as an injectable oil, implantable subcutaneous pellets (Percorten), or a depot injection (also Percorten). This dose must be titrated.

2. During labor and delivery, supplemental steroids are necessary (e.g., hydrocortisone 100 mg. I.V. q.8h. for the length of labor) to avoid adrenal crisis.

3. Additional doses of cortisone should be continued until the third day of the puerperium or if puerperal infection occurs.

4. *Management of Adrenal Addisonian Crisis*

  a. Hydrocortisone 100 mg. I.V. immediately followed by an additional 100 mg. in 1,000 ml. normal saline over 4 hours

  b. Fluid replacement with 2 to 3 L. of normal saline over the first 12 to 14 hours, since decreased intravascular and extravascular volumes may approach 20 per cent of normal

  c. Potassium replacement as necessary

  d. Broad-spectrum antibiotic coverage, instituted immediately even if a source of infection cannot be found

  e. Blood replacement with packed red cells, if hemorrhage has precipitated the crisis

  f. Vasopressors as necessary, after (*a*) through (*e*) have been performed

CONGENITAL ADRENAL HYPERPLASIA

Basic Principles

1. Congenital adrenal hyperplasia (CAH) is perhaps the most common adrenal disorder that occurs concurrently with pregnancy.

2. The adult form, usually due to a partial 21-hydroxylase deficiency, results in elevated levels of 17-hydroxyprogesterone, androstenedione, and DHEAS, with associated virilization.

Effects of Pregnancy on Diagnosis

1. Most cases of CAH are diagnosed long before pregnancy.

2. Elevated androstenedione and DHEAS levels may be masked to some extent by placental hormone production.

Effects of Pregnancy on Disease

None.

Effects of Disease on Pregnancy

1. Fetal virilization is usually due to *fetal* CAH. CAH in the mother severe enough to threaten a fetus most often results in anovulation. In those cases, however, in which the fetus is affected:

a. The female fetus will be subject to varying degrees of masculinized genitalia.

b. The male fetus will usually exhibit larger genitalia.

Therapy and Its Interaction with Pregnancy

1. The treatment is corticosteroid replacement (cortisone acetate, 20 mg. per day or prednisone, 5 mg. per day) to block feedback. It is unchanged by pregnancy.

2. Often, these virilized women have android pelves, so labor complications are more frequent.

DISEASES OF THE GI TRACT

ESOPHAGITIS

Basic Principles

1. Esophagitis is the most common GI disease during pregnancy.

2. The mildest form of this, heartburn, occurs in more than half of all pregnant women.

3. When there is more than superficial irritation of the esophageal mucosa, heartburn becomes esophagitis.

4. Even though the symptoms are most bothersome during the day, most of the irritation occurs at night.

Effects of Pregnancy on Diagnosis

1. The basic symptom, "heartburn," often accompanied by chest pain on swallowing as the food traverses the irritated esophagus, is unchanged by pregnancy.

2. Substernal chest pain radiating to the back, shoulders, or arms is not uncommon, suggesting pancreatic or gallbladder disease. The differential of cardiac disease is much less likely in women of childbearing age.

3. Definitive diagnosis is by esophagoscopy, which is rarely done in the pregnant woman. Instead, therapeutic trial with antacids is the approach of choice.

Effects of Pregnancy on Disease

1. Several factors contributing to esophagitis are worsened during pregnancy. Reflux of acid is increased by:

a. Decreased GI motility

b. Relaxation of the esophageal sphincter

c. Increased intra-abdominal pressure from the uterus

Effects of Disease on Pregnancy

None.

Therapy and Its Interaction with Pregnancy

1. Calcium- or aluminum-containing antacids serve to neutralize stomach acid. They should be taken after each meal and especially before bed. One in particular, Gaviscon, which creates a foam atop the stomach contents, may be useful.

2. These should be combined with a bland diet and cool, nonacidic liquids.

3. Since most of the irritation occurs at night, steps to decrease this, such as not eating for several hours before bedtime, taking an antacid upon retiring, and sleeping in the right lateral recumbent position, may be quite helpful.

4. Cimetidine (Tagamet), 300 mg. q.i.d., and related drugs are most useful in nonpregnant patients, but experience with them during pregnancy is limited. A single bedtime dose may suffice.

PEPTIC ULCERS

Basic Principles

1. Ulcers are rare during pregnancy since gastric acid secretion is decreased.

2. Their diagnosis and management are unchanged, except that the GI series is avoided and cimetidine (Tagamet) and similar drugs, which have become mainstays of therapy in nonpregnant patients, are used in extreme cases only.

INFLAMMATORY BOWEL DISEASE

Basic Principles

1. Ulcerative colitis and Crohn's disease (regional enteritis) are now often grouped together as inflammatory bowel disease (IBD).
2. Their diagnosis and treatment often overlap.

Effects of Pregnancy on Diagnosis

1. The diagnosis of these diseases requires radiologic studies, endoscopy, and biopsy. This is unchanged during pregnancy, except that one avoids the barium enema and small bowel series and goes directly to endoscopy.

Effects of Pregnancy on Disease

1. Approximately half the patients with IBD will improve during pregnancy, while the other half will experience exacerbation. There are no markers to determine who is likely to do which.

Effects of Disease on Pregnancy

1. If IBD is quiet before conception, the prognosis for the pregnancy is good.
2. If it is active, flare-ups during pregnancy are likely. These are associated with elevated miscarriage rates as well as premature labor.

Therapy and Its Interaction with Pregnancy

1. Prednisone and sulfasalazine, both of which may be used during pregnancy, are the mainstays of therapy.
   a. As noted elsewhere, prednisone is loosely associated with a small risk of cleft palate in the first trimester. This, however, is outweighed by the benefits of therapy.
   b. Sulfasalazine, being a sulfa drug, should be discontinued a week before delivery to avoid binding to bilirubin receptor sites on fetal albumin, which would put the newborn at risk for hyperbilirubinemia.
2. Mercaptopurine and azathioprine, otherwise used often, are usually avoided during pregnancy.

DISEASES OF THE LIVER

CHOLESTATIC JAUNDICE OF PREGNANCY

Basic Principles

1. Cholestatic jaundice of pregnancy usually occurs during the third trimester.
2. Due to the effect of high estrogen levels on the liver, which result in decreased conjugation of bilirubin, cholestatic jaundice often recurs in subsequent pregnancies and in patients who take oral contraceptives.
3. The disease resolves spontaneously shortly after delivery.

Effects of Pregnancy on Diagnosis

1. Typically, this disease presents with mild jaundice and intense pruritus.
2. These reflect a mild hyperbilirubinemia and a marked elevation of bile acids. SGOT and alkaline phosphatase are usually somewhat elevated. Other liver function tests are frequently abnormal.
3. Diagnosis is usually suspected because of the intense itching and requires excluding gallstones and hepatitis.

Effects of Pregnancy on Disease

This is essentially a disease found only during pregnancy.

Effects of Disease on Pregnancy

1. For reasons unknown, there may be a significant incidence of fetal distress and prematurity and even fetal demise.

Therapy and Its Interaction with Pregnancy

1. The itching may be relieved by binding bile salts using cholestyramine (Questran). Since it is not absorbed, it has no direct fetal effects. It does interfere with the absorption of fat-soluble vitamins, however, and may result in depletion of vitamin K-dependent coagulation factors.

2. Intensive fetal monitoring must be begun from the time of diagnosis.

ACUTE FATTY LIVER OF PREGNANCY

Basic Principles

1. Of unknown origin, acute fatty liver presents as progressive degeneration of liver function in the mid-to-late third trimester.

2. Potentially fatal, it necessitates rapid diagnosis and appropriate action.

Effects of Pregnancy on Diagnosis

1. Malaise, nausea, and vomiting are the first symptoms. Occurring in the third trimester, they are often ignored as "part of pregnancy" in their early stages, until there is progression to jaundice and right upper quadrant abdominal pain.

2. Soon after coagulopathy, hepatic encephalopathy and death from liver failure may occur, suggesting fulminant hepatitis. This may usually be distinguished by serological testing for hepatitis antigens.

3. Hypertension is not an uncommon concomitant, which forces one to consider severe preeclampsia in the differential diagnosis.

4. Laboratory abnormalities include a general derangement of all liver function and coagulation tests.

5. Definitive diagnosis may be made on liver biopsy, but this is usually contraindicated by the coagulopathy.

Effects of Pregnancy on Disease

1. Like cholestatic jaundice, this is a disease which occurs only in pregnancy.

Effects of Disease on Pregnancy

1. Maternal mortality in unchecked cases may approach 90 per cent.

2. In properly managed cases, it may still be as high as 30 per cent.

3. Fetal mortality rates are usually higher than those of the mother.

Therapy and Its Interaction with Pregnancy

1. Therapy is delivery. In this sense, the distinction between acute fatty liver and severe preeclampsia is unimportant, since the therapy is the same.

2. All necessary supportive measures before either induction or C/S are appropriate.

3. Most cases resolve promptly and completely upon termination of the pregnancy, unless there has been permanent damage from encephalopathy or intraorgan hemorrhage.

VIRAL HEPATITIS

Basic Principles

1. There are three varieties of viral hepatitis: A, B, and non-A, non-B.

2. Each is caused by a different infectious particle. Hepatitis A is transmitted orally, while B and non-A, non-B are both spread via body fluids (transfusion, needle-sharing among drug users, and sexual intercourse).

3. Pregnancy has no effect on the transmission of any of the three.

Effects of Pregnancy on Diagnosis

1. Hepatitis is initially suspected because of symptoms of malaise or lassitude, sometimes associated with arthralgia. These may be associated with normal pregnancy.

2. The appearance of jaundice, however, is not obscured.

3. Laboratory tests usually show hyperbilirubinemia and markedly elevated alkaline phosphatase, SGOT, SGPT, and GGT.

a. In severe cases, coagulation tests may also be disturbed.

4. Distinction among the three types is made serologically.

a. Hepatitis A antigen (IgM) becomes positive early in the course of the disease.

b. In cases of hepatitis B, the B surface antigen, "e" antigen (this is actually whole virus), and B core antibody are present. After several weeks, as the infection resolves, these are replaced with hepatitis B surface antibody.

c. Non-A, non-B hepatitis is diagnosed when the serologic criteria for neither hepatitis A nor hepatitis B are fulfilled.

5. None of these tests is affected by pregnancy.

6. Fulminant hepatitis is usually fatal. Distinction from acute fatty liver of pregnancy and from cholestatic jaundice of pregnancy may be difficult (see above) but is often academic, since delivery of the fetus is necessary in most cases anyway (in the first two, for the health of the mother; in fulminant hepatitis, to save the baby).

Effects of Pregnancy on Disease

1. Pregnancy does not affect the course of any of the forms of viral hepatitis. Hepatitis A remains a benign disease; hepatitis B remains a serious one. It does, however, accentuate the symptoms.

Effects of Disease on Pregnancy

1. Hepatitis A has little effect on pregnancy. The fetus is almost never infected in utero. Fulminance is rare.

2. The effects of hepatitis B are different:

a. If the disease occurs in the third trimester, there is a significant risk of transmission to the fetus during the pregnancy, delivery, and postpartum period (nursing).

b. Those most likely to transmit the disease are those who have "e" and surface antigens.

3. Non-A, non-B hepatitis seems to act more like B than like A.

Therapy and Its Interaction with Pregnancy

1. Treatment for all three consists of bed rest and a good diet. Obviously, pregnancy does not influence this.

2. Extra measures are indicated for mothers who have hepatitis B:

a. Their infants should receive hepatitis B immune globulin and vaccine at birth. This is highly protective.

b. These mothers should not breastfeed.

c. Delivery room personnel must exercise great care in dealing with these patients, as all their body fluids are highly infectious.

3. Non-A, non-B patients should be handled as if they had hepatitis B, but there are no vaccines or hyperimmune globulins.

4. As stressed above, if the hepatitis becomes fulminant, immediate delivery is essential.

NEUROLOGIC DISEASES

EPILEPSY

Effects of Pregnancy on Diagnosis

1. If a woman has seizures for the first time during pregnancy, the diagnosis of epilepsy becomes more difficult, especially during the last trimester, when eclampsia must be considered.

2. Most epilepsy, however, has been diagnosed before conception.

Effects of Pregnancy on Disease

1. Women who have been seizure-free for more than 1 year tolerate pregnancy well, with only a small risk of recurrent seizures.

2. Those who have been poorly controlled, however, often become even worse during pregnancy.

3. There are several ways in which pregnancy affects the control of epilepsy:

a. Expanded blood volume and increased renal clearance tend to lower serum levels of anticonvulsants.

b. Estrogen increases seizure threshold, while progesterone decreases it.

c. The mild respiratory alkalosis of pregnancy may also predispose to seizure activity.

d. Patients fearful of congenital anomalies from their medicines tend not to take them.

Effects of Disease on Pregnancy

1. Epilepsy has no direct effect on pregnancy, if the seizures are controlled. The danger of grand mal seizures is that the mother does not breathe during them.

Therapy and Its Interaction with Pregnancy

1. There are no anticonvulsants known to be completely safe for use in pregnancy. The question, therefore, is whether to continue anticonvulsant medication. The risk of stopping is that the mother may convulse, endangering both herself and her fetus. This risk must be balanced against the possible ill effects of the various drugs on the fetus.

2. The most commonly used drug, diphenylhydantoin (Dilantin) has several possible effects.

a. It has been linked to a teratogenic syndrome, consisting of craniofacial and limb defects and mental retardation, which may affect as many as 10 per cent of exposed fetuses.

b. Cleft palate and cleft lip may also occur with increased frequency in these infants.

c. It also may cause depletion of vitamin K-dependent clotting factors in the fetus and thereby predispose to hemorrhagic disease of the newborn. This can usually be avoided by prompt administration of vitamin K to the infant at birth or even to the mother in labor.

3. Phenobarbital, which has been weakly associated with cleft lip and palate, is the drug of second choice.

4. Trimethadione (Tridione), carbamazepine (Tegretol) and valproic acid (Depakine) are known teratogens. Trimethadione is strictly contraindicated; carbamazepine has been associated with mild microcephaly and valproic acid with neural tube and skeletal defects.

HEADACHE

Basic Principles

1. Headaches are the most common of all neurological conditions complicating pregnancy.

2. Most are merely inconvenient, although some are disabling and some represent serious disease.

3. The two most common are the tension headache and the migraine.

Effects of Pregnancy on Diagnosis

1. Most headaches are adequately diagnosed by history and examination. This is not altered by pregnancy.

2. The major diagnostic concern during pregnancy is the possibility that the headache represents a manifestation of preeclampsia. This is especially true with migraines, which are often accompanied by auras.

Effects of Pregnancy on Disease

1. Migraine headaches seem to improve about as as often as they worsen during pregnancy.

2. Tension headaches are frequently exacerbated by the physical and emotional strains of pregnancy.

Effects of Disease on Pregnancy

None.

Therapy and Its Interaction with Pregnancy

1. Acetaminophen (650 to 1000 mg.q.4h.) is usually sufficient for minor headache and seems to be without risk.

2. Ergot alkaloids, the most common therapy for migraines, are not used during pregnancy. If analgesia with acetaminophen, aspirin, a narcotic, or a barbiturate is not sufficient, propranolol (Inderal), 40 mg. t.i.d., may be effective. It seems to be safe for the fetus for short-term use.

SYSTEMIC LUPUS ERYTHEMATOSUS (SLE)

Basic Principles

1. Affecting as many as 1 out of every 1,000 people, primarily women between the ages of 20 and 40, systemic lupus erythematosus is the most common of the serious autoimmune diseases to coexist with pregnancy.

2. Consisting of a complex of inflammatory reactions in various organ systems, manifested most commonly as arthritis, dermatitis, serositis, and renal and neurological diseases, it causes major morbidity during pregnancy.

Effects of Pregnancy on Diagnosis

1. In the nonpregnant, one suspects the diagnosis of lupus when a patient manifests any 4 of the 11 criteria (below) listed by the American Rheumatism Association:

a. Malar butterfly rash

b. Discoid rash

c. Photosensitivity

d. Oral ulcers

e. Arthritis

f. Serositis

g. Renal disease, consisting of proteinuria or casts

h. Neurologic disease, consisting of seizures or psychosis

i. Hematologic disease, consisting of hemolytic anemia, leukopenia, lymphopenia, or thrombocytopenia

j. Immunologic disease, consisting of positive LE prep, positive anti-DNA or anti-Sm antibodies, or false-positive VDRL

k. Positive antinuclear antibody (ANA)

2. During pregnancy, especially during the second half, many of these symptoms and signs are suggestive of preeclampsia, with which the diagnosis may be confused.

3. Pregnancy also has considerable effects on a number of the tests used to gauge the activity of the disease:

a. Serum C3 and C4 complement levels. During pregnancy falling levels are ominous. *Falling* is the key word, as opposed to low, because baseline complement levels are elevated during pregnancy and may be spuriously high.

b. The sedimentation rate, employed extensively in nonpregnant patients, is of little use during pregnancy, since it is markedly elevated in all gravidas.

c. Anti-DNA antibody, which correlates closely with flare-ups of SLE and renal disease, is unaffected by pregnancy.

4. Lupus flare-ups, involving hypertension, acute worsening of renal disease, convulsions, thrombocytopenia, and hemolysis, and may be extremely difficult to distinguish from severe preeclampsia/eclampsia, which is also more common in SLE patients.

Effects of Pregnancy on Disease

1. If lupus has been quiet for at least several months before conception, pregnancy apparently does not seem to exacerbate it.

2. Similarly, well-controlled lupus without renal involvement which remains under therapy usually remains quiet during pregnancy.

3. Patients who are poorly controlled, discontinue their steroids, or have severe renal disease at the start of the pregnancy are likely to experience a worsening of their disease.

Effects of Disease on Pregnancy

1. SLE is a vasculitis. As such, it can be expected to imperil the fetus, which depends on an intact vascular supply for growth. In fact, there is danger in all three trimesters.

a. Spontaneous abortion rates may be as high as 25 per cent.

b. Rates of IUGR, prematurity, and perinatal mortality may each be as high as 30 per cent even in cases without severe renal disease, which further worsens the prognosis.

2. SLE also has effects directly on the fetus.

a. Congenital heart block is so common among babies born to mothers with SLE that the mothers of all infants born with heart block should be evaluated for lupus.

b. Neonatal lupus may also occur, apparently from transplacental transfer of a circulating antibody, anti-Ro. This is a self-limiting disease lasting less than 1 year.

Therapy and Its Interaction with Pregnancy

1. The primary therapy for SLE is corticosteroid administration. This should not be discontinued during pregnancy. The small risk of teratogenesis is greatly outweighed by the risk of exacerbation of the disease. Flare-ups are treated with increased doses.

2. Recent investigations have shown decreased fetal loss in all trimesters with daily low-dose (75 mg. per day) aspirin administration.

3. Azathioprine (Imuran) is teratogenic in animals and may be in humans as well, but some consider it worth the risk in cases unresponsive to cortocosteroids.

4. Therapeutic abortion is no longer commonly performed and may not be beneficial.

5. Careful fetal surveillance with serial sonography, EFM, and BPPs is mandatory. In addition, measurement of umbilical vessel waveforms by Doppler shows promise for early detection of fetal jeopardy.

SEXUALLY TRANSMITTED DISEASES

SYPHILIS

Basic Principles

1. Syphilis is an STD which has its major effect on systems other than the genital. Spread around the body hematogenously, if active during pregnancy it almost always affects the fetus.

2. It is easy to diagnose (if one is properly suspicious), easy to safely treat, and extremely dangerous for the fetus if unchecked.

Effects of Pregnancy on Diagnosis

1. Because of the above, screening for syphilis (VDRL, STS) is a basic part of prenatal care.

a. The interpretation of serological screening and its confirmation with the FTA-abs (fluorescent treponemal antibody absorption) test is unchanged by pregnancy.

2. Similarly, the diagnosis of newly acquired syphilis is made the same way as in the nonpregnant state.

a. A chancre occurs several weeks after infection and its syphilitic origin may be confirmed by dark-field identification of treponemes.

b. The VDRL (or its equivalent) should be obtained immediately upon suspicion of the disease but may not become positive for several weeks after infection.

(1) If initially negative it should be repeated a maximum of 6 weeks later.

(2) Since it is very accurate if negative (high sensitivity) but less so if positive (low specificity), a positive VDRL should be verified with the FTA-abs, which is extremely specific.

3. If the infection escapes early detection, the condylomata lata of secondary syphilis occur but may be transitory and often pass unnoticed.

4. Since syphilis is so easily missed during so much of its course and potentially so serious for the fetus if untreated, screening with the VDRL during each trimester is considered routine.

Effects of Pregnancy on Disease

None.

Effects of Disease on Pregnancy

1. Since the short-term damage from syphilis is usually minor, the major ill effects of infection are fetal.

a. Early infection may cause abortion. It was previously thought that the spirochete did not cross the placenta during the first trimester. In fact, tissue reaction to it is minimal, making detection difficult.

b. Infection which is less severe or later may result in stillbirth or in congenital syphilis in a surviving neonate. Typical pathology includes invasion by the spirochete of the liver and spleen, and of the lymphatic, skeletal, and neurologic systems.

2. All infants born to mothers known to have had syphilis should be thoroughly evaluated at birth.

Therapy and Its Interaction with Pregnancy

1. The treatment for syphilis during pregnancy is penicillin or, in the penicillin-allergic, erythromycin, both of which seem to be safe for the fetus.

2. Dosages established by the Centers for Disease Control depend on the duration and extent of disease:

a. *Duration less than 1 year:* Benzathine penicillin G, 2.4 million units I.M. (1 dose) *or* aqueous procaine penicillin G, 600,000 units/day I.M. for 8 days *or* erythromycin 500 mg. q.i.d. for 15 days.

b. *Duration more than 1 year (latent or tertiary, except neurosyphilis):* Benzathine penicillin G, 2.4 millions units I.M. per week for 3 weeks *or* procaine penicillin G, 600,000 units per day I.M. for 15 days *or* erythromycin 500 mg. q.i.d. for 30 days.

c. *Neurosyphilis:* I.V. penicillin G up to 20 million units per day for up to 2 weeks, followed by benzathine penicillin weekly for 3 weeks.

3. As above, all infants born to mothers known to have had syphilis should be thoroughly evaluated at birth.

GONORRHEA (GC)

Basic Principles

1. Unlike syphilis, gonorrhea is primarily a disease of the genital system. Most cases do not progress to hematogenous spread or systemic involvement.

2. Like syphilis, it is fairly easy to detect and treat during pregnancy.

Effects of Pregnancy on Diagnosis

1. Screening for GC, as for syphilis, is considered standard prenatal care. It is typically performed at the first prenatal visit. In high-risk populations, third trimester screening is also not unusual.

2. Good transport media (eg., Transgro) and immunologic slide tests (eg., Gonozyme) have made this process much more accurate, cheaper, and easier.

3. The symptomatology of GC (purulent discharge or symptoms of salpingitis) is not altered by pregnancy.

Effects of Pregnancy on Disease

1. Pregnancy, by obliterating the uterine cavity as a pathway to the fallopian tubes after the twelfth week, may ameliorate the course of gonorrhea, by protecting the mother against salpingitis.

2. Conversely, delivery frequently causes a flare-up of active disease in a mother who has silent cervical carriage.

Effects of Disease on Pregnancy

1. Gonorrheal cervicitis does not alter the course of pregnancy, nor does it threaten the fetus before rupture of the membranes.

2. The fetus may, however, become infected at birth, the most common sequela of which is gonococcal ophthalmitis.

Therapy and Its Interaction with Pregnancy

1. The CDC-recommended treatment for gonorrheal cervicitis is procaine penicillin G, 4.8 million units I.M. (or ampicillin 3.5 g. P.O. or amoxicillin 3 g. P.O.) and probenecid 1 g. P.O. to prolong high tissue levels. The oral therapies are not effective against pharyngitis, so throat cultures should be performed.

2. For the penicillin-allergic or for GC which is penicillin-resistant, spectinomycin (Trobicin), 2 g. I.M. or 1 to 2 g. I.M. of one of the newer cephalosporins (cefoxitin or cefoxatime) may be substituted.

3. Tetracycline and doxycycline, which are alternatives in nonpregnant patients, should not be used during pregnancy.

4. Needless to say, sexual partners must be treated to prevent recurrent disease.

CHLAMYDIA TRACHOMATIS

Basic Principles

1. Chlamydial infection, now much more common than gonorrhea (with a prevalence of up to 15 per cent in some U.S. populations), may be considered an analogous disease.

2. Although prenatal screening is not part of the classic repertoire, it should be.

Effects of Pregnancy on Diagnosis

1. As with GC, the symptomatology of either cervicitis or salpingitis is unaltered in the pregnant patient.

2. None of the laboratory tests for Chlamydia is affected by pregnancy.

a. Definitive diagnosis by tissue culture of infected cervical cells is difficult and expensive and therefore carries significant false-negative rates in many labs.

b. The immunologic slide tests (Chlamydiazyme, Microtrak) detect both living and dead organisms and are considerably cheaper. Their sensitivity and specificity approach those of culture.

Effects of Pregnancy on Disease

Same as for gonorrhea.

Effects of Disease on Pregnancy

Same as for gonorrhea.

Therapy and Its Interaction with Pregnancy

1. During pregnancy, erythromycin, 500 mg. q.6h. P.O. is used for a period varying from 10 days to 3 weeks. Longer periods of treatment are associated with lower rates of recurrence.

2. Follow-up testing should be performed after therapy.

3. As with all STDs, treatment of the partner is essential to prevent recurrence.

HERPES SIMPLEX VIRUS (HSV)

Basic Principles

1. There are two major groups of Herpes simplex virus, types I and II. Traditionally, type II has been associated with genital lesions and type I with disease above the umbilicus, especially in the oropharynx. As sexual practices have changed, a significant proportion of genital herpes has become type I and a significant proportion of oral herpes, Type II. EITHER TYPE MAY INFECT ANY SKIN SURFACE, INCLUDING THE FETUS.

2. Since Herpes simplex is, for the most part, a lifelong infection with periodic recurrence, the prevalence in the population is constantly increasing. Some studies estimate that as much as 35 per cent of the sexually active population carries the virus.

3. Initial Infection. The disease is spread by direct contact with virus shed from an active lesion and has an incubation period of from 3 days to perhaps 2 weeks. It first manifests as clusters of vesicles which then ulcerate. If they are on dry skin, they usually crust within 1 day or so and then heal over 1 week to 10 days. On mucous membrane, they remain ulcers until healed. Minor secondary infection with skin organisms is not rare. Local lymph nodes are frequently enlarged and sometimes tender. Typically, because there is no preexisting immunity, the clusters appear in several generations over a 2- to 3-week period. Viremia is not rare with primary infection, often resulting in a flu-like syndrome and occasionally in disseminated Herpes, the most serious form of which is encephalitis.

4. Recurrence. During the course of the initial infection, the virus takes up residence in the nerve cells supplying the area of exposure. A variety of stimuli, which have not been clearly delineated but which include local irritation and, possibly, systemic disease and stress, may, at any time in the future, cause recurrence by "awakening" the dormant virus in the nerve cell. It then somehow travels to the skin and causes new lesions to be formed. Unlike primary infection, recurrences usually last only 7 to 10 days and involve only a single outbreak. However, RECURRENCES MAY BE EXTREMELY MINOR, EVEN CLINICALLY INAPPARENT, AND STILL RESULT IN SHEDDING OF THE VIRUS AND TRANSMISSION. Up to 70 per cent of those infected may experience recurrent disease. The frequency of recurrence may vary from every few weeks to less often than yearly.

Effects of Pregnancy on Diagnosis

1. The clinical events of HSV are unchanged by pregnancy.

2. Laboratory diagnosis of herpes, also unchanged during pregnancy, is, ideally, by viral culture from the lesion. Slide and tube tests using monoclonal antibodies may soon be clinically available.

Effects of Pregnancy on Disease

None.

Effects of Disease on Pregnancy

1. Primary infection during pregnancy, with viremia, may infect the fetus. Transplacental transmission in the first trimester may result in abortion.

2. Since there is no associated viremia, recurrences during the antepartum period are of no danger. They do, however, endanger the fetus during passage through the birth canal at delivery or by ascending infection after rupture of the membranes.

3. If the fetus is infected, a spectrum of disease ranging from localized pustules to generalized herpes with brain damage and death may result. In the pre-acyclovir era, as many as 80 to 90 per cent of infected fetuses were severely damaged.

Therapy and Its Interaction with Pregnancy

1. Primary HSV

a. Initial infection during pregnancy may be treated with acyclovir (Zovirax), 200 mg. q.4h. (5 doses/day) for 14 days.

b. Whether this offers significant benefits or poses long-term dangers to the fetus is not known. There are no known short-term adverse fetal effects.

2. Recurrent HSV. Since recurrent disease is of no danger to the mother or to the unborn fetus, management is designed to avoid transmission of the virus to the fetus at birth. To this end:

a. The mother is counseled to avoid genital irritation (especially sex) in the last few weeks before anticipated delivery, in the hope of avoiding a recurrence, and to be alert for symptoms of recurrence.

b. Additionally, since viral shedding may occur in the absence of symptoms, careful weekly examination and viral cultures from the external genitalia, cervix, and vagina (and, obviously, from any suspect lesions) should be performed.

c. Positive cultures are often repeated at 3- to 5-day intervals to determine the earliest time at which cultures become negative.

d. If neither the mother nor the obstetrician has any suspicion of recurrence within 10 to 14 days of delivery, labor and vaginal delivery are allowed. Internal electrodes for FHR monitoring should be eschewed, if possible, since scalp puncture may be a portal of entry for the virus.

e. If lesions are evident or positive cultures are obtained within this period, C/S is usually performed. If abdominal delivery is opted for, it should be done as soon as possible in early labor, certainly no later than 4 to 6 hours after rupture of the membranes.

3. Newborns who are inadvertently exposed (positive culture returns after delivery) may be watched very carefully for the potential incubation period or prophylactically treated with acyclovir.

4. The mother who has her initial HSV infection during pregnancy may not benefit from the above management, since transplacental infection of the fetus may have occurred with viremia.

ACQUIRED IMMUNODEFICIENCY SYNDROME (AIDS)

Basic Principles

1. AIDS is the result of infection with human immunodeficiency virus (HIV), which selectively destroys parts of the immune system, most notably T4 lymphocytes, resulting in opportunistic infections and malignancies which kill their victims.

2. Approximately 50 per cent of people infected with HIV develop full-blown AIDs (which is, to date, uniformly fatal within 3 years); 30 per cent develop the less serious AIDS-related complex (ARC); and 20 per cent remain asymptomatic carriers of the virus. However, the longer the follow-ups, the more these numbers shift to the left (more AIDS, fewer carriers). Why some remain asymptomatic carriers and what may precipitate clinical disease are not known. Infection with HIV seems to be for life.

3. Transmitted through body fluids (blood, semen, vaginal secretions), AIDS has spread most rapidly through the groups with the greatest exposure. These are termed *high-risk categories:*

a. Homosexuals (extreme promiscuity was a significant part of much homosexual behavior until recently)

b. I.V. drug abusers (through needle sharing)

c. Hemophiliacs (through multiple cryoprecipitate transfusions)

4. Also at high risk are sexual partners of infected people and heterosexuals with multiple sex partners.

5. Most pregnant women with HIV are either I.V. drug users or partners of men in high-risk groups, although as HIV is spread throughout the population by sexual intercourse (transmission in either direction between men and women during penile-vaginal intercourse is definitely possible, although it may be more efficient from men to women) and needle sharing, the infection will gradually spread into low-risk groups.

6. Until the recent advent of effective screening of the blood supply, transfusion was similarly dangerous.

7. Estimates of the number carrying the virus in the U.S. today range from 500,000 to 2,000,000, most in the so-called high-risk categories above. However, these numbers have at least doubled yearly since AIDS was first described 8 years ago, and there is no evidence this rate of increase will change significantly in the near future.

8. There is significant risk (although not 100 per cent) of transplacental transmission to the fetus, which, if infected, seems to have a more fulminant course than adults.

Effects of Pregnancy on Diagnosis

1. AIDS and ARC are suspected on clinical criteria, including the presence of a number of opportunistic infections, wasting diseases, and Kaposi's sarcoma (see CDC guidelines). Some of these infections, e.g., recurrent candidiasis, occur with increased frequency in pregnant women.

2. Definitive diagnosis is by identification of antibody to HIV.

a. Initial screening is via an ELISA test, which is easy, cheap, and extremely sensitive (very few false negatives). False positives, however, may occur up to 5 per cent of the time, especially in women on oral contraceptives, perhaps those in pregnancy, and among certain HLA types.

b. All positive ELISA tests are then checked with another more specific assay, usually the Southern blot. False positives using the Southern blot are rare. False negatives are slightly less so. A positive Southern blot is currently considered proof of infection. This test is not affected by pregnancy.

Effects of Pregnancy on Disease

1. Not enough is known at this point to say whether pregnancy worsens the prognosis of women infected with HIV, whether clinically ill or not.

Effects of Disease on Pregnancy

1. The risk is transplancental infection of the fetus. These babies most often

a. Are growth-retarded

b. Are born prematurely

c. Have abnormal reticuloendothelial and immune function, manifested as hepatosplenomegaly, generalized lymphadenopathy, decreased numbers of T4 lymphocytes, and liability to the same constellation of opportunistic infections as their mothers, especially oral candidiasis and pneumonias

d. Fail to thrive and die within 1 to 2 years

Therapy and Its Interaction with Pregnancy

1. There is no known cure for either AIDS or infection with HIV, although multiple drug trials are underway both in the U.S. and worldwide. In this country, zidovudine (AZT, Retrovir) seems to be promising in halting progress of the disease. By the time this book is actually published, much more information will be available regarding various therapies.

2. Efforts, at the moment, must be directed at identifying those who carry the virus and advising them against becoming pregnant. At the very least, HIV screening for all women who are I.V. drug users or whose partners are in high-risk categories (hemophiliacs, bisexuals, or I.V. drug users) is currently advisable. With time, screening will probably become more the rule than the exception for all women considering pregnancy.

3. If a woman known to be positive for HIV becomes pregnant, therapeutic termination may be considered. For those who will deliver, meticulous attention to monitoring fetal growth and maternal health is necessary.

4. Obviously, delivery room personnel must exercise great care to avoid exposure to the body fluids of these women and their infants.

HUMAN PAPILLOMAVIRUS (HPV)

Basic Principles

1. HPV is a group of 55 viral subtypes, with new ones being discovered every year, which cause the skin lesions known variously as warts, condylomas, flat condylomas, and papillomas.

2. These lesions may occur on all skin surfaces, including the cervix, vagina, vulva, penis, hands, feet, and larynx (and perhaps others, such as the esophagus). Conventional wisdom is that certain viral types infect certain skin surfaces, although this may be a parallel to the belief, 20 years ago, that Herpes types I and II were specific for nongenital and genital lesions, respectively. More likely, as with Herpes, the distribution of subtypes reflects past patterns of exposure.

3. Similarly, HPV infection may take various morphological forms, including flattish but slightly raised, papilliform, pedunculated, and invisible except after staining with acetic acid. This may depend on the skin surface infected as much as, or more than, on the viral type.

4. In addition, certain serotypes (6, 11, 16, 18, 31, 33, 35, 51–55) are now clearly linked to the development of genital malignancy (cervix, vagina, vulva, and penis). Using sophisticated DNA hybridization techniques, HPV can be isolated from virtually all cervical neoplasia.

5. They are transmitted by skin-to-skin contact, being "venereal" when the contact involves genital skin. Theoretically, however, one should be able to infect genital skin from non-genital skin (as from a wart on one's finger or hand).

6. Like HSV, HIV, and Chlamydia, genital condylomatosis is a disease which has been spreading rapidly through the population during the last few years and becoming more important in pregnant women.

Effects of Pregnancy on Diagnosis

1. Most genital HPV infections during pregnancy are diagnosed by seeing the characteristic lesions of the vulva or vagina, although a significant number of HPV infections are now also being detected by abnormal cervical cytology. A normal Pap smear, however, does not preclude the presence of HPV, especially before the onset of CIN.

2. Biopsy of lesions demonstrating koilocytosis and nuclear atypia is definitive. All suspected cases should be investigated by colposcopy of the vulva, vagina, and cervix, with biopsy if necessary. These procedures are essentially unchanged in the gravid woman, although cervical biopsies tend to bleed more.

3. A newly available immunological test for the identification of HPV types 6, 11, 16, 18, 31, 33, and 35 (Vira-Pap) now enables physicians to screen for these types. This test is unaffected by pregnancy.

Effects of Pregnancy on Disease

1. There is much anecdotal evidence suggesting that many cases of HPV infection, especially the cauliflower-like lesions of the vulva and introitus, seem to progress markedly during pregnancy.

2. There is no evidence that pregnancy adversely affects the course of either cervical HPV or CIN.

Effects of Disease on Pregnancy

1. Lesions of the vulva and labia may grow enough to obstruct delivery. This is not common. More often the intravaginal lesions, noticeable as papillary or cobblestone type lesions, do not pose significant problems for the mother.

2. More important, maternal genital HPV infection may be transmitted to the fetus at delivery. The most serious consequence of this is the development of giant laryngeal papillomas in the neonate. Although past statistics indicate that this seems to happen once in several thousand deliveries, the risk of transmission to the neonate is not known.

3. There have been several reports of isolation of HPV from amniotic fluid and cases of neonates born with anogenital lesions. The significance of these rare occurrences is not known.

Therapy and Its Interaction with Pregnancy

1. In the nonpregnant, there are many treatments, none wholly acceptable.

a. Recurrence rates are very high, mostly because eradication of the lesions does not extend to asymptomatically infected adjacent areas (in the vagina, this probably includes the entire intravaginal surface) or to infected partners.

b. Almost all methods involve destruction of the infected skin. They include application of podophyllin, trichloracetic and bichloracetic acids, electrocautery, cryosurgery, laser evaporation, 5-fluorouracil cream (Efudex 5%), and various interferons.

2. In the pregnant woman, all of the above methods except podophyllin, 5-FU, and interferon may be used. The obliteration of vulvar and vaginal lesions by various methods can be done safely during pregnancy. Cryotherapy and laser have been used, apparently safely, to treat cervical disease.

3. Common sense would seem to dictate against first trimester therapy, given the high spontaneous abortion rate.

4. Since the risk of transmission to the neonate during vaginal delivery is not known, sensible recommendations regarding the advisability of C/S to avoid it cannot be made. At the time of this writing, the ACOG has no currently stated policy, so each M.D. and his or her patient must jointly decide on the route of delivery. Obviously, in cases where the lesions are large enough to cause outlet obstruction, C/S should be performed.

OTHER INFECTIONS AFFECTING PREGNANCY

RUBELLA

Basic Principles

1. Rubella (German measles) is a minor disease for most adults and a potential disaster if it infects a fetus.

2. Since infection and/or vaccination usually confers life-long immunity, the ideal is to assure the immune status of all women of childbearing age.

Effects of Pregnancy on Diagnosis

1. The clinical diagnosis of rubella is not affected by pregnancy but must be confirmed by serology. Since the infection may be minor, a high degree of suspicion of all "viral syndromes" is appropriate.

Effects of Pregnancy on Disease

None.

Effects of Disease on Pregnancy

1. The fetus can only be infected by transplacental passage of the virus during the viremia which occurs with initial infection.

2. The severity and likelihood of intrauterine infection vary with the stage of pregnancy.

a. In the first month, 50 per cent of fetuses are severely damaged; in the second, only 25 per cent; and in the third month, 15 per cent.

b. Infants with congenital rubella most commonly suffer from blindness, deafness, multiple cardiac abnormalities, hepatosplenomegaly, and neurologic deficits. Other systemic involvement may also occur.

Therapy and Its Interaction with Pregnancy

1. There is no treatment for rubella infection.

2. If maternal infection occurs during the first trimester, the family should be counseled regarding potential fetal sequelae and offered the option of therapeutic abortion.

3. If the already-pregnant woman is found to be susceptible, she must be counseled to avoid exposure during the pregnancy and should be vaccinated immediately postpartum.

4. Maternal vaccination poses no threat to the newborn.

CYTOMEGALOVIRUS (CMV)

Basic Principles

1. CMV is the cause of the most common congenital infection in the U.S.

2. Up to 50 per cent of the population may carry the virus and as many as 2 per cent of all neonates are infected.

3. Most infections are minor (often subclinical), but life-long carriage with potential reactivation and viral shedding is the rule.

4. More severe consequences of infection occur in the immunosuppressed and in fetuses.

5. It may be transmitted orally, sexually, transplacentally, at birth, via breast-feeding, or through transfusion. The urine and oral secretions of those infected frequently contain live virus.

Effects of Pregnancy on Diagnosis

1. The clinical and serological diagnosis of CMV is unchanged by pregnancy.

2. In fact, many include CMV (as part of a TORCH panel) in their prenatal screening.

Effects of Pregnancy on Disease

1. Pregnancy seems to cause reactivation of viral shedding.

2. Although clinical disease does not usually recur, cervical shedding of the virus may be demonstrated with increasing frequency as pregnancy progresses.

Effects of Disease on Pregnancy

1. The fetus may be infected transplacentally (only during primary infection) or by direct transmission during birth, the neonate from breast milk.

2. Up to 2 per cent of all babies born in this country are infected. However, only a small percentage of these become ill, so that the incidence of congenital cytomegalic inclusion *Disease* is probably only 1/1,000 live births.

a. Such clinically ill babies are often severely damaged. Up to 30 per cent die, with over 50 per cent of the survivors being severely mentally retarded or neurologically impaired. Most of the rest suffer lesser degrees of permanent impairment.

b. Those who are normal at age 2, however, are likely to remain so.

Therapy and Its Interaction with Pregnancy

1. There is no therapy for CMV, nor is there a vaccine.

2. Most primary infection is undetectable at the time of its occurrence and most cervical shedding does not result in symptomatic infection of the fetus delivered vaginally.

3. Therefore, C/S is not indicated for CMV infection.

TOXOPLASMOSIS

Basic Principles

1. Caused by the parasite *Toxoplasma gondii*, it may be contracted by eating inadequately cooked infected beef, lamb, or pork, or from the stool (hand-to-mouth) of an infected cat.

2. As in rubella, toxoplasmosis

a. Is dangerous to the fetus only if the initial infection occurs during pregnancy

b. Infection confers lasting immunity.

Effects of Pregnancy on Diagnosis

1. The diagnosis of toxoplasmosis should begin before conception.

a. If immunity is demonstrated prior to pregnancy, there is no risk of future infection.

b. If antibody screening indicates susceptibility, advice concerning transmission is in order since there is no vaccine. This should include advice regarding international travel, since although infected meat is quite rare in the U.S., this is not the case elsewhere.

2. If a susceptible gravida develops suspicious illness, *Toxoplasma* titers determine if she has been infected.

a. IgM will appear within 2 to 3 weeks, IgG several weeks later.

b. If no preconceptual titers are available, the presence of IgM is suggestive but not diagnostic, as low levels may persist for long periods of time. In these cases, serial titers demonstrating a four fold increase in IgG titers, over a 3 to 4 week interval, are highly suggestive of recent infection. High levels of IgM by the ELISA method are also extremely suggestive of recent infection.

3. If maternal infection is confirmed, fetal infection may be diagnosed by obtaining amniotic fluid and fetal cord blood via fetoscopy and testing it for IgM and the presence of the organism.

a. This is usually performed between the twentieth and the twenty-second weeks.

b. Positive results are diagnostic; negative results are less reliable.

c. All pregnancies during which maternal infection has occurred, even if fetal infection has not been demonstrated, should be followed with serial ultrasound to detect hydrocephalus.

Effects of Pregnancy on Disease

None.

Effects of Disease on Pregnancy

1. As above, the fetus is at risk only if the mother becomes infected during pregnancy, when transplacental transmission of the organism may occur.

2. The earlier in the pregnancy the infection, the more likely fetal damage.

a. In the first trimester, this may include spontaneous abortion.

b. Among fetuses who survive, chorioretinitis, microcephaly, hydrocephaly, intracranial calcifications, hepatosplenomegaly, anemia, and low birth weight are common.

c. Some infants infected are clinically normal at birth, but evidence disease later on. Therefore, careful observation of the exposed neonate for several years is indicated.

Therapy and Its Interaction with Pregnancy

1. Intrauterine infection may be treated with a combination of pyrimethamine (Daraprim) and a sulfonamide. Since this therapy may be teratogenic in animals and the untreated fetus may not be severely damaged, this is often not an easy choice.

2. In cases of first trimester infection, termination of the pregnancy is an option.

VARICELLA

Basic Principles

1. Chickenpox is an extremely common childhood illness, so that most adults have had the disease and are immune.

2. For the minority who have not, however, varicella can be dangerous, especially if complicated by pneumonia, which sometimes even results in death. This is at least as true, and perhaps more so, during pregnancy.

Effects of Pregnancy on Diagnosis

1. Chickenpox is easily identified by its characteristic rash, unchanged by pregnancy.

2. More often, however, the question arises regarding mothers who are exposed to others with the disease. Although serology to identify the susceptible is not routinely done, varicella-zoster IgG levels are available to determine immunity for those exposed who are unsure.

Effects of Pregnancy on Disease

None.

Effects of Disease on Pregnancy

1. Some authors say varicella is more dangerous among the pregnant than among other adults, resulting in higher incidences and more severe cases of pneumonia.

2. First trimester infection may result in spontaneous abortion.

3. Later maternal infection is usually benign, UNLESS IT OCCURS WITHIN 4 DAYS BEFORE OR 2 DAYS AFTER BIRTH. These babies are in considerable danger, as generalized neonatal varicella, with neurologic damage and a high mortality rate, is likely.

Therapy and Its Interaction with Pregnancy

1. Infants born in the danger period described above should receive varicella-zoster immune globulin (VZIG), which is highly effective in preventing neonatal damage, at birth.

2. Whether therapy is indicated for susceptible pregnant women who have been exposed is not certain. Some treat them with VZIG.

FETOMATERNAL ISOIMMUNIZATION

Rh ISOIMMUNIZATION

Basic Principles

1. The Rh antigen system, found in all human blood, is composed of three antigens: C, D and E. Both C and E have alleles, termed c and e, but there is NO d allele. There is a weak D antigen (D^u) which is functionally the equivalent of D.

2. Each individual inherits either C or c, and E or e from each parent, but, in the case of D, inherits either D (or D^u) or nothing.

a. The possible genotypes are the combinations of (CC, Cc or cc), [DD, D(−) or (−)(−)] and (EE, Ee or ee).

b. Everyone possessing at least one D (or D^u) antigen [DD or D(−)] is termed *Rh positive* (Rh+). Those lacking D, i.e., (−)(−), are *Rh negative* (Rh−). In this country, approximately 15 per cent of the white population and 8 per cent of the black are Rh−.

c. Rh(−) mothers [(−)(−)] whose partners are Rh+, therefore, will have Rh+ fetuses either 100 per cent of the time (if the father is DD) or 50 per cent of the time [if the father is D(−)]. If both the mother and father are Rh(−) [(−)(−)], all the fetuses will also be Rh(−). If the mother is Rh+, all of this is irrelevant.

3. Unsensitized Rh(−) people may develop anti-D antibodies if exposed to the D antigen.

a. This may occur during improperly matched transfusion, abortion, pregnancy, or delivery of an Rh+ infant.

b. Typically, sensitization does not produce detectable anti-D antibody levels for several weeks or even, during pregnancy, for several months.

4. Sensitized Rh(−) people may carry low or even undetectable levels of anti-D but have an anamnestic response upon reexposure (as in pregnancy with an Rh+ fetus).

5. Anti-D antibodies are IgG, small enough to cross the placenta and attack the red cells of an Rh+ fetus, causing hemolysis.

6. Sensitization may be prevented by binding an anti-D antibody, Rh immune globulin (RHOgam), to Rh+ cells released into the maternal circulation before they are recognized (within 48 to 72 hours). While Rh isoimmunization used to be a significant cause of perinatal morbidity and mortality, it has been largely eliminated by the use of Rh immune globulin in susceptible women at times of exposure to Rh+ blood.

7. Once sensitization has occurred, Rh immune globulin is of no use.

Etiology

1. Since blood banking procedure has eliminated most cases of Rh-incompatible transfusion, most cases of initial sensitization are related to pregnancy. Introduction of fetal red cells into the maternal circulation may occur during:

a. Spontaneous or intentional abortion after formation of fetal blood

b. Amniocentesis

c. Spontaneous feto-maternal bleeds during uncomplicated pregnancy

d. Delivery

2. Clinical Rh disease almost never occurs during the same pregnancy as sensitization.

3. During subsequent pregnancy with an Rh+ fetus, if there is no feto-maternal transfusion, anti-D antibodies may remain low. However, even small amounts of Rh+ fetal blood will serve to engage a full-fledged anamnestic response with high-level anti-D production.

4. The anti-D then crosses the placenta and hemolyzes fetal blood cells.

a. If the hemolysis is severe enough, anemia, heart failure, and the other stigmata of hydrops fetalis in utero result, often killing the fetus if the process is not interrupted.

b. This hemolysis in the fetus also results in the production of much bilirubin, which is reflected in an increase in amniotic fluid bilirubin concentration. The rise in AF bilirubin parallels the severity of hemolysis and fetal anemia. This is the basis for estimation of fetal jeopardy (see below).

c. The fetus itself does not become severely hyperbilirubinemic until after birth, because the maternal circulation clears it.

Management of the Unsensitized Woman

1. The management of Rh disease begins with the identification of every pregnant woman as either Rh+ or Rh(−).

2. If she is Rh(−), her blood is screened for anti-D antibodies. If there are none, she is not sensitized and appropriate management is to prevent sensitization.

a. If the father of her child is also Rh(−), the fetus must similarly be Rh(−), so there is no risk of becoming sensitized from the pregnancy.

b. If the father is Rh+, the fetus may be as well, and may serve as a source of sensitizing blood at the time of a miscarriage, abortion, amniocentesis, placental abruption, or delivery. This can almost always be prevented by administering 300 μg. of Rh immune globulin (RHOgam), I.M., within 72 hours of the potentially sensitizing event. This is enough to cover 15 ml. of transfused fetal blood and will not harm the Rh+ fetus in utero.

c. There is also a small incidence (less than 1 per cent) of silent transplacental feto-maternal transfusion resulting in sensitization during otherwise untraumatized pregnancy. This can be largely prevented by giving the same dose of Rh immune globulin to all Rh(−) unsensitized women at 28 weeks gestation.

3. Occasionally, feto-maternal transfusion greater than 15 ml. is suspected. The degree should be estimated from a Kleihauer-Betke stain on maternal blood and the dosage of Rh immune globulin increased proportionately.

Management of the Sensitized Woman

1. If the mother has anti-D antibodies at any time before the twentieth week of gestation, she may be considered to have been previously sensitized and should be followed with serial antibody titers every 4 to 6 weeks.

2. If the titers remain below 1:16, the chances of a severely affected baby are very small and only continued surveillance is indicated.

3. If the titer is 1:16 or higher, the risk of a severely affected baby is considerable and further investigation is warranted as early in the pregnancy as effective therapy (see below) will be instituted based on the results.

a. Perform amniocentesis to obtain fluid for analysis of bilirubin levels by the delta-OD_{450} method.

(1) If one is capable of performing intrauterine transfusion (which may be begun as early as the twenty-second week), amniocentesis for should be begun then.

(2) If intrauterine transfusion is not available, amniocentesis should be begun as soon as delivery is a viable option (usually 26 to 28 weeks).

b. Plot the result on the Liley curve.

(1) If it falls into Zone 1, the fetus is unaffected or only mildly affected and is felt to be safe for 2 to 3 weeks. Repeat amniocentesis at 2- to 3-week intervals, but otherwise treat as a normal pregnancy, as long as the results remain in Zone 1.

(2) If it falls into Zone 2, the infant is moderately affected, with projected hemoglobin levels from 8 to 11 g. per 100 ml. (upper Zone 2) or 11 to 14 g. per 100 ml. (lower Zone 2). As long as results remain in Zone 2, repeat amniocentesis weekly (performing, in addition, L/S ratio and PG studies) until fetal maturity is obtained. Monitor with EFM and BPP at least weekly. Deliver as expeditiously as possible as soon as lung maturity occurs.

(3) A Zone 3 result indicates a fetus in danger of death who should be either transfused (if too premature to be viable) or delivered immediately.

c. In addition to following the delta-OD_{450}, the fetus threatened by Rh disease should be monitored with EFM and BPPs, as with any other fetus in jeopardy.

d. Very early delivery is usually by C/S.

OTHER BLOOD GROUP INCOMPATIBILITIES

There are numerous other blood group antigens which are quite rare, some of which may cause significant antenatal hemolytic disease of the Rh type. Kell, Duffy, and Kidd are among the more common of these less common antigens which may endanger the fetus. They are detected by the antibody screens of maternal blood, which should be a part of every Rh type and screen, and are managed in the same fashion as Rh incompatibility.

ABO INCOMPATIBILITY

Mothers of blood type O have circulating anti-A and anti-B antibodies, which may cause hemolysis in fetuses who are A, B, or AB. Unlike Rh disease, this is not truly isoimmunization and may occur in primigravidas. Since anti-A and anti-B titers are meaningless, there is no way to know antenatally if the process is happening, but it is rarely necessary because ABO incompatibility usually does not cause severe antenatal hemolysis. After delivery, however, significant hemolysis may occur, causing neonatal jaundice and possibly kernicterus if unobserved. All cord blood should be screened, if the mother is type O, for circulating antibodies.

25 Surgical Disease in Pregnancy

Hugh R. K. Barber

BASIC PRINCIPLES

1. In addition to obstetrical complications, the pregnant patient can have any surgical disease that occurs in the nonpregnant state. The obstetrician must make the decision on what constitutes the best management of the pregnancy. The surgeon should think as an obstetrician, and the obstetrician as a surgeon.

2. The plan of treatment is the same as for the nonpregnant patient.

3. If signs and symptoms indicate that a surgical emergency exists, especially if there is progressive deterioration, surgical exploration should be carried out even though a firm diagnosis has not been made.

4. An outline for differential diagnosis of the acute abdomen in the pregnant woman is:

a. Conditions requiring immediate operation

b. Conditions not requiring immediate operation

c. Nonsurgical conditions presenting as an acute abdomen

5. Physical appearance of the patient often provides valuable clues:

a. With peritonitis the patient lies quietly on her back with knees drawn up.

b. With appendicitis the patient pulls up the right hip and knee in order to relax the psoas muscle.

c. With pancreatitis the patient lies on her side with knees, hips, and back flexed.

d. With ureteral stone the patient rolls around in pain.

6. The abdomen should be divided into quadrants and the symptoms, signs, and physical findings evaluated by visualizing the structures in each quadrant as:

a. *Right Lower Quadrant.* Appendicitis, twisted ovarian cyst, Meckel's diverticulum with inflammation, regional enteritis, stone in the ureter

b. *Left Lower Quadrant.* Twisted ovarian cyst, stone in the ureter, regional enteritis, large-bowel obstruction

c. *Right Upper Quadrant.* Acute cholecystitis, acute pyelonephritis, pancreatitis

d. *Left Upper Quadrant.* Spleen, pancreatitis, appendicitis, diabetic crisis

CHANGES IN THE ALIMENTARY TRACT DURING PREGNANCY

1. The most striking change in the digestive function in pregnancy is nausea, or morning sickness, which occurs in greater or lesser degree in about a third of pregnancies. As a rule it begins at the sixth week and stops spontaneously before the fourteenth week.

2. Although it is generally limited to the early morning, it may occur at other times of day. Usually the symptoms are slight; excessive or prolonged vomiting is certainly pathological. The cause is uncertain.

3. As a rule the appetite is good during pregnancy, but minor digestive upsets are common. They are probably due to the relaxant effect of progesterone on smooth muscles.

4. Sometimes gastric or intestinal distension occurs. In early pregnancy especially, this causes a feeling of abdominal enlargement.

5. Heartburn is a common complaint and is caused by relaxation of the cardiac sphincter of the stomach. In a few of the more severe cases, this symptom is caused by a hiatus hernia.

6. The emptying time of the stomach is prolonged during pregnancy and even more so during labor (a fact of considerable importance in relation to the risk of vomiting during anesthesia).

7. The gastric acidity is often reduced. Peptic ulcers almost invariably become quiescent during pregnancy.

8. Constipation is not uncommon. This, together with the pelvic hyperemia and pressure of the enlarged uterus, may lead to formation, or increase in size, of hemorrhoids.

ACUTE APPENDICITIS

Basic Principles

1. Early in the course the patient may not look ill.

2. There is persistent pain in the right lower quadrant, aggravated by walking. The point of tenderness is usually higher than McBurney's point. In retrocecal appendicitis the point of tenderness may be lateral to McBurney's point.

3. A high retrocecal appendicitis may be difficult to differentiate from cholecystitis or kidney disease.

4. If the clinical picture points to appendicitis, a few white cells in the urine should not keep the responsible physician from making the diagnosis of appendicitis.

5. Clumps of white cells and a great number of white cells strongly suggest the presence of pyelonephritis either as a concurrent problem or as the main pathologic entity.

6. Most series have a 60- to 70-per-cent correct preoperative diagnosis.

7. The mortality from appendicitis is the mortality of delay.

Diagnostic Signs and Studies

1. Nausea and vomiting are present.

2. Moderate abdominal distension may be present with progression of the disease.

3. Temperature usually ranges from 100 to 101°F.

4. A progressive rise in the white blood cell count with a shift to the left is significant.

5. The pulse rises steadily.

6. There are no characteristic x-ray findings in appendicitis, but x-ray studies may be necessary in the differential diagnosis.

Helpful Adjunctive Procedures

1. Nasogastric tube
2. Indwelling urinary catheter
3. Coagulation studies
4. N.P.O.
5. Intravenous fluids

Management of Acute Appendicitis by Trimesters

1. First Trimester (Appendix in its Usual Position)

a. If possible and practical, remove the appendix.

b. If there is a generalized peritonitis, the appendix should be removed, provided that removal is possible and practical. Antibiotics and appropriate fluids, plasma, and electrolytes should be administered. Choice of appropriate antibiotics will depend upon the culture reports.

c. If an abscess makes it impossible or impractical to remove the appendix, it should be drained and antibiotics started.

2. Second Trimester (Appendix at the Iliac Crest)

a. In localized appendicitis, the appendix should be removed without drainage.

b. In the presence of generalized peritonitis, the appendix should be removed and antibiotics, fluids, plasma, and electrolytes instituted.

c. In the presence of a localized abscess, it is better to drain unless the area of the appendiceal-cecal junction is intact. If the appendix can be removed in toto, this should be done.

3. Third Trimester (Appendix between the Iliac Crest and the Liver)

a. In localized appendicitis, the appendix should be removed without drainage.

b. In the presence of generalized peritonitis, the appendix should be removed and antibiotics, fluids, plasma, and electrolytes instituted.

c. In the presence of a localized abscess, it is always better to drain. If the appendix can be removed in toto, this should be done. Antibiotics should be given.

d. If there is a large abscess, it should be drained. After the peritoneum has been closed, an extraperitoneal cesarean section should be carried out if further childbearing is desired. If the uterine wall is part of the abscess, a cesarean hysterectomy is indicated with drainage. Antibiotics should be given.

ACUTE CHOLECYSTITIS

Basic Principles

1. Acute cholecystitis is a rare complication of pregnancy.

2. Since the gallbladder is not displaced in pregnancy, the signs and symptoms are similar to those in the nonpregnant state. The diagnosis is usually made on clinical signs and symptoms, but a past history of gallbladder attacks is helpful in confirming the diagnosis.

3. In the third trimester the appendix is often displaced into the right upper quadrant and may make an accurate diagnosis difficult, if not impossible.

4. Onset is usually characterized by biliary colic accompanied by nausea, vomiting, and, less often, chills. Subcostal pain may radiate to the back, and fever up to 101°F may be present. Palpation of a tender gallbladder is a helpful diagnostic finding in acute cholecystitis.

5. Leukocytosis may increase progressively.

6. The disease may subside spontaneously.

7. Cholelithiasis may complicate pregnancy, but usually is not diagnosed until the postpartum period. The following factors predispose to the increased incidence of gallstones in the pregnant patient:

a. Increased bile stasis

b. Elevation of the amount of cholesterol in the bile

c. Biological changes within the bile salts and acids

8. Close observation of the patient's course is mandatory, with frequent reexamination and evaluation, since progressive infection, necrosis, gangrene, and perforation are not infrequent and demand surgical intervention.

9. Conservative therapy is initially followed. If the patient does not respond to conservative treatment within 12 to 36 hours—particularly if the white blood count continues to increase, fever is higher, and tenderness persists or gets worse—operation is indicated.

Diagnostic Signs and Studies

1. The clinical signs and symptoms are discussed above.

2. Oral cholecystogram. Nonvisualization may represent failure of the diseased gallbladder to concentrate.

3. The oral cholecystogram test is not valid in the presence of jaundice, vomiting, diarrhea, or associated liver disease.

4. Intravenous cholangiography may outline the bile ducts as well as the gallbladder.

Helpful Adjunctive Procedures

1. Nasogastric tube
2. Indwelling urinary catheter
3. Intravenous fluids
4. Antibiotics

Helpful Points in Evaluating the Patient

1. The liver usually functions normally in pregnancy.

2. Serum cholesterol may rise to 500 mg./dL in the last trimester.

3. In the third trimester, serum albumin and gamma globulin decrease, and alpha and beta globulins increase. This may account for the abnormal cephalin flocculation and thymol turbidity tests seen in the third trimester.

4. The serum alkaline phosphatase rises in pregnancy and peaks in the third trimester. The increase is due primarily to a heat-stable fraction which arises from the placenta, while the hepatic phosphatase remains normal.

5. Serum transaminase and lactic dehydrogenase remain normal in pregnancy, but may be elevated during labor and shortly thereafter.

6. Jaundice of pregnancy may represent bile stasis and is often hormonally mediated, primarily by estrogens. This type of jaundice is more common in the last trimester, disappears spontaneously in the postpartum period, and tends to recur in subsequent pregnancies.

7. Jaundice may also occur as the result of drug reaction (carbon tetrachloride, tetracycline, chloroform, phenothiazine, halothane) or of hemolytic anemia, or with liver damage resulting from pregnancy toxemia, idiopathic fatty liver, acute hepatitis, or transfusion reaction.

8. The bromosulphalein is elevated, and the serum glutamic oxaloacetic transaminase and alkaline phosphatase may be elevated too.

9. If the patient has had this problem in previous pregnancies, the diagnosis is highly probable.

PERFORATED GASTRIC ULCER

Basic Principles

1. The first signs of a problem relating to the intestinal tract during pregnancy are often delayed.

2. Since the acute abdominal problems complicating pregnancy are sometimes difficult to differentiate from exaggerated normal pregnancy symptoms, and because the classic signs are often changed by the enlarged uterus, one must be aware of the different clinical pictures produced by pregnancy.

3. Cardiospasm occurs in pregnancy with varying degrees of severity. It may have an insidious or a sudden onset. Cardiospasm is due to an imbalance of the parasympathetic innervation, resulting in an inability of the sphincter of the esophagus to relax, as well as decreased peristaltic activity.

4. Heartburn and epigastric distress are common in pregnancy, making the diagnosis of peptic ulcer difficult.

5. The gastric acid curves (both free and total) decrease considerably, with the low point in the 6-to-10-week group. This gradually increases to near normal at term.

6. There is an increase in gastro-esophageal reflux and a delay in gastric emptying time.

7. The digestion and absorption of the small bowel remain unchanged. There is a decrease in peristalsis of the large bowel.

8. In general, pregnancy has no direct effect on preexisting gastrointestinal disease. Most changes reported are psychologically oriented.

9. Perforation and hemorrhage may occur and cause serious complications. These complications occur almost exclusively in the third trimester.

10. The accepted treatment for peptic ulcer is medical management.

Diagnostic Signs and Studies

1. Previous history of ulcer disease

2. Typically, pain is of sudden onset and is severe. Pain may be referred to one or both shoulders—usually the right, because of subphrenic irritation.

3. There is nausea, but usually no vomiting.

4. Examination reveals a rigid, silent abdomen, although in some instances bowel sounds may be heard.

5. There may be diminished liver dullness due to escape of gas into the peritoneal cavity.

6. In delayed cases, after 12 hours or more, the features of peritonitis with paralytic ileus are present and the patient is extremely toxic and oliguric.

7. Other conditions with which perforated ulcer is confused are acute perforated appendicitis, acute pancreatitis, and myocardial infarction.

8. X-ray film of the abdomen in the upright position may show free gas below the diaphragm. This sign is absent in one-third of patients.

Helpful Adjunctive Procedures

1. Nasogastric tube
2. Intravenous fluids
3. Antibiotics
4. Semi-Fowler's position
5. Indwelling urinary catheter

Treatment

1. The treatment for either perforation or excessive bleeding is the same as for the nonpregnant patient, with surgery done immediately. The aim should be to attack the life-threatening complication first and to deal with the pregnancy after this is controlled. More than half of mothers will be lost after perforation or hemorrhage from a peptic ulcer.

2. Cesarean section is reserved for obstetrical indications, but occasionally it may be in the best interest of the patient to empty the uterus by cesarean section at the time of laparotomy in order to technically facilitate the control of bleeding from the ulcer.

3. The fetal survival is directly related to depth and length of shock, as well as to the degree of peritonitis.

INTESTINAL OBSTRUCTION

Basic Principles

1. Intestinal obstruction may occur in pregnancy and occasionally presents difficulty in diagnosis. Vomiting secondary to bowel obstruction in early pregnancy may be regarded as the usual emesis associated with gestation. The pain of obstruction coming on late in pregnancy may be mistaken for the onset of labor. A careful history and physical examination will avoid both these errors.

2. The usual case of intestinal obstruction is secondary to a volvulus or an adhesive band. Adhesions, in the pregnant as well as in the nonpregnant patient, constitute the single most frequent factor in producing intestinal obstruction.

3. Intestinal obstruction occurs more commonly in the third trimester than in the first. It may be related to the pulling of the growing uterus on adhesions, causing bands that can obstruct the bowel.

4. The presence of a scar on the abdomen, colicky abdominal pain which is intermittent, vomiting which is frequent and copious, distension, and obstipation indicate an intra-abdominal pathologic complication, especially an intestinal obstruction.

5. Auscultation at the time of pain reveals loud, metallic, high-pitched peristaltic rushes. The frequency and severity of the rushes decrease as the bowel gets quiet. This may take 6 to 8 hours, or more, after the start of obstruction. On auscultation there is a change from the high-pitched, frequent rushes to a subdued sound described as a tinkling or as sounding like water going down a drain.

6. X-ray studies that show air and fluid levels on an upright film serve to confirm the diagnosis. Ultrasonography is often employed as a diagnostic measure. Since the patient cannot be given any fluid by mouth, it must be given intravenously.

7. As the time interval of the obstruction lengthens, the clinical picture changes:

a. Fluids and electrolytes pour into the bowel. The circulating blood volume decreases. The hemoglobin and hematocrit increase due to the shift of fluid to the extracellular space.

b. The glomerular filtration rate (GFR) is decreased secondarily to the diminished extracellular fluid and the abdominal distension.

c. The urinary output drops, with an increase in the specific gravity of the urine. The urea nitrogen, sulfates, and phosphates increase in the plasma.

d. The diaphragm is elevated secondarily to abdominal distension. Carbon dioxide retention follows and a respiratory acidosis compounds the metabolic acidosis produced by the above mechanisms. Atelectasis complicates the problem.

Roentgenographic Studies

1. Fluid levels in the small bowel, or step-ladder effect of fluid levels, indicates obstruction of the small intestine.

2. The thickness of the wall of the intestine indicates fibrinous exudate.

3. A very large, ovoid, distended, isolated loop of bowel usually indicates a volvulus.

4. A distended cecum is a dangerous sign in bowel obstruction. The ileocecal valve is competent, causing it to distend. Perforation may occur if the obstruction is not rapidly relieved.

5. If the diagnosis remains uncertain after correction of the fluid and electrolyte imbalance and the passage of a nasogastric tube, further studies are indicated.

6. Contrast studies will clarify the diagnosis, using a contrast medium of one-half meglumine diatrizoate (Gastrografin) and one-half barium. A minimum of radiation exposure should be used and all efforts taken to protect the fetus. The mixture can be followed either to the point of obstruction or to its entrance into the large bowel. This mixture is liquid enough to identify an obstruction. If there is an obstruction, it will pass promptly when the obstruction is relieved surgically.

Helpful Adjunctive Procedures

1. Gastrointestinal decompression with a long tube

2. Intravenous fluids

3. Antibiotics

4. Sigmoidoscopy and barium studies in chronic obstruction

5. Enemas to remove feces and prepare the bowel for elective surgery when chronic obstruction of the large bowel is present

6. Indwelling urinary catheter

Management

1. The surgical management of intestinal obstruction is the same as in the nonpregnant state. Vascular impairment of the obstructed bowel must be avoided if the fetus is to be saved. Surgical intervention for intestinal obstruction should be performed earlier than might be done in a nonpregnant patient.

2. Necrotic bowel requires resection.

3. Obstruction of the colon may require colostomy. The obstructing mechanism must be identified and relieved.

LARGE BOWEL OBSTRUCTION ASSOCIATED WITH PREGNANCY

Basic Principles

1. There are three times when this complication occurs: between the fourth and sixth months, near term, and shortly after delivery.

2. It was first described following delivery, and was due to mechanical obstruction by the postpartum uterus.

3. In the postpartum period the patient may have a slow onset of lower abdominal pain followed by progressive increase in abdominal distension. The pain increases as the distension increases. If the ileocolic valve is incompetent, the small bowel may become distended.

4. It is important to rule out unrecognized carcinoma or volvulus.

5. A flat plate or ultrasound of the abdomen often shows a distended bowel from the cecum to the pelvic brim on the left side.

6. Examination usually reveals a palpable, slightly tender cecum and highpitched sounds on auscultation during the pain.

Management

1. If the patient is placed in the knee-chest position and the uterus pushed gently away from the bowel, considerable gas may escape, with relief of symptoms resulting. In this position a tube may be threaded up the bowel. If the patient improves after this type of management, it is acceptable to treat the patient conservatively.

2. The management is a Levin tube inserted in the stomach, a tube threaded up the sigmoid from below, and intravenous administration of fluids.

3. In about 48 to 72 hours the signs and symptoms regress and the patient improves. If the symptoms are not relieved, however, and deterioration progresses with a rising pulse, increase in the white blood count with a shift to the left, increasing distension, and localized tenderness, the diagnosis of volvulus with compromise must be considered and surgical intervention undertaken.

PARALYTIC ILEUS ASSOCIATED WITH PREGNANCY

Basic Principles

1. This is common.

2. The cause of the complication is not definitely known, but it may be due to the relaxed abdominal muscles, a decrease in the size of the uterus, and hormonal effects.

3. The abdomen is often markedly distended, with feeble or absent bowel sounds. There is no pain.

4. Vomiting is common. The patient looks well. The physical signs are minimal.

5. The condition clears within 24 to 48 hours without treatment.

MESENTERIC VASCULAR OCCLUSION

Basic Principles

1. This complication may affect either the venous or the arterial blood supply.

2. It often presents with acute colicky pain and is frequently associated with vomiting and diarrhea, which may be bloody.

3. Early in the course there may be no signs of peritoneal irritation, and tenderness on deep palpation may be the only finding. Bowel sounds may be present early in the development of the occlusion. Gradually the tenderness increases, and the infarcted bowel may be felt as a mass.

4. Mesenteric venous thrombosis results in loss of blood into the intestinal wall, lumen, and peritoneal cavity, with rapid onset of shock.

5. Mesenteric arterial occlusion, if massive, may also result in shock.

6. Arterial occlusion without infarction may produce symptoms of intestinal angina, in which abdominal pain follows meals, and steatorrhea.

7. The signs of peritonitis occur after gangrene and perforation of the bowel.

8. A rising pulse rate and leukocytosis indicate progression of disease.

9. A flat plate of the abdomen usually shows nonspecific dilated loops of small and large intestine.

Helpful Adjunctive Procedures

1. Nasogastric tube
2. Intravenous fluids
3. Antibiotics
4. Abdominal paracentesis (serosanguineous fluid)
5. Arteriograms
6. Indwelling urinary catheter

Management

1. Exploratory laparotomy
2. Bowel resection as determined on opening of the abdomen

PANCREATITIS

Basic Principles

1. Pancreatitis is a rare complication of pregnancy.
2. It is seen with increasing frequency among heavy users of diuretics such as chlorothiazides, as well as in patients with gallbladder disease, alcoholism, dietary indiscretion, chronic adrenal steroid therapy, trauma, and hyperparathyroidism.
3. Pain is severe, constant, and epigastric, and often radiates to the back. Vomiting may be profuse. The patient looks sick.
4. The abdomen reveals generalized tenderness and moderate distension. Bowel sounds are diminished or absent. The usual signs of tenderness between the stomach and the spleen, elevation of the diaphragm, and low-grade fever may be present.
5. Shock, rapid pulse, and cyanosis may be present.
6. Painful, unexplained erythematous subcutaneous nodules may be present.
7. The incidence is higher among primigravidas than among multiparas.
8. It occurs in all trimesters, but is most common in the third trimester and the postpartum period.
9. The diagnosis should be considered in any patient with acute abdomen accompanied by protracted vomiting, electrolyte imbalance, increased serum amylase, hypocalcemia, and elevated urinary diastase. Occasionally glycosuria is present.

Roentgenographic Studies

1. A flat plate of the abdomen may show nonspecific ileus.
2. Ultrasonography has been very helpful in identifying changes that occur in the pancreas. It can often detect the edematous and imflammatory responses that are present in the pancreas.
3. A chest film may show fluid at the base of the pleural cavity.

Helpful Adjunctive Procedures

1. Nasogastric tube
2. Intravenous fluids
3. Calcium given intravenously
4. Antibiotics
5. Indwelling catheter

Management

1. Treatment is medical.
2. Surgery is indicated if it is impossible to establish a firm diagnosis; with pseudocyst; with recurrent attacks; and, occasionally, when unexplained persistent diabetes is present.
3. The pancreatic bed should be carefully and adequately drained.
4. Dramatic recovery has been reported after the delivery of the baby. Therefore, after viability of the fetus, induction of labor or cesarean section has a place in the management of these patients.

ULCERATIVE COLITIS

Basic Principles

1. Ulcerative colitis is an unpredictable disease in pregnancy. In patients who are labile, with swings between exacerbation

and remission, the exacerbation rate in pregnancy is 50 to 60 per cent.

2. Most cases are diagnosed before pregnancy; the problem then is merely how to manage them during pregnancy. If the patient has been in remission for two or more years, there is an excellent chance that she will be symptom-free during her pregnancy.

3. Gastrointestinal symptoms in the presence of a history of ulcerative colitis should be suspect until reactivation of the disease has been ruled out.

4. In patients having the disease for the first time in pregnancy, the symptoms and signs are similar to those in nonpregnant patients. The symptoms are abdominal cramps accompanied by diarrhea that is often bloody. Fever and tachycardia are common. A monoarticular, migrating arthritis is often present.

Diagnostic Signs and Studies

1. The diagnosis can often be made on sigmoidoscopy, which demonstrates the beefy-red, edematous bowel with ulcerated areas in which grayish necrotic tissue and slough are seen.

2. X-ray studies are usually not needed to confirm the diagnosis, but should be done if considered necessary.

3. The diagnosis is often confirmed by response to medical treatment.

Management

1. The primary treatment is medical. It includes a low residue diet, antispasmodic drugs, and sulfa and steroid therapy.

2. Surgery is indicated if the medical regimen fails or if hemorrhage or peritonitis is present.

3. Total colectomy with terminal ileostomy is the treatment that must be carried out; the perineal removal of the rectum and anus may be delayed.

4. Bypassing ileostomies, various drainage procedures, and other halfway measures done to avoid colectomy or protocolectomy are to be condemned. These procedures are followed by a stormy postoperative course, and in more than two-thirds of reported cases have resulted in a stillborn fetus and a maternal death.

REGIONAL ILEITIS

Basic Principles

1. Regional ileitis may occur for the first time during pregnancy.

2. Most often the diagnosis has been made before pregnancy.

3. Symptoms developing during pregnancy are the same as those seen in the nonpregnant patient.

4. The disease is often present with a malabsorption syndrome including anemia, hypoproteinemia, and clotting defects due to malabsorption of vitamin K.

5. It may mimic an atypical appendicitis or inflamed Meckel's diverticulum.

6. The chronic form may be confirmed by x-ray studies.

7. The acute form often is not diagnosed until laparotomy has been carried out.

Management

1. Prompt surgery is indicated if there is intestinal obstruction, perforation with peritonitis, or localized abscess.

2. The surgery should consist of a short-circuiting operation or intestinal resection.

3. The pregnancy should be preserved, if possible.

DEGENERATING FIBROID (LEIOMYOMA UTERI)

Degeneration of a fibroid causes pain, vomiting, tenderness, and pyrexia. The diagnosis is difficult. The condition should subside with rest and sedation; operation is indicated only when there is torsion of a pedicle of a fibroid.

OVARIAN CYST

1. Torsion of the pedicle of an ovarian cyst causes acute pain, tenderness, vomiting, and often pyrexia. Under anesthesia a mass separate from the uterus may be distinguished. In this case a laparotomy must be performed.

2. Ultrasonography is very helpful in making a diagnosis, particularly in the pregnant patient. Since the patient has vomiting, it is important to fill the bladder by giving intravenous fluid.

URINARY CALCULUS

1. Although this is not generally considered a surgical disease in pregnancy, occasionally it may require surgery.

2. A urinary calculus causes acute pain radiating to the groin. Hematuria is present. Treatment is conservative unless hydronephrosis develops; then ureteric drainage is required.

3. Any surgical disease or acute abdominal condition in pregnancy that requires laparotomy may bring on labor or abortion. However, since morbidity and mortality in pregnancy are often due to inordinate delay in carrying out surgery when there is a strong indication that an acute surgical process is present, surgery should be undertaken and the possibility of labor or abortion accepted as a complication of the treatment.

26 Gestational Trophoblastic Neoplasms (GTN)

Hugh R. K. Barber

DEFINITION

Gestational trophoblastic neoplasms initiated a new concept of interconnection of such disease processes as choriocarcinoma, invasive mole, and hydatidiform mole. The term *gestational trophoblastic neoplasms* is used to define the spectrum of disease that has at one extreme benign hydatidiform mole and at the other highly malignant choriocarcinoma. Not only do these diseases form a spectrum, but to understand and adequately manage a patient with one of these conditions requires knowledge of the entire group.

BASIC PRINCIPLES

1. Hydatidiform moles occur in a ratio of 1 to 2,000 normal pregnancies in the United States, and 80 per cent are benign. In certain geographic areas such as Asia, the incidence may be as high as 1 in 60 to 1,000 normal pregnancies.

2. It is higher in patients of very low economic status, and poor diet has also been noted to be associated with an increased incidence.

3. Incidence of molar pregnancy rises steeply after the age of 40, and, over age 50, almost 50 per cent of pregnancies result in hydatidiform molar pregnancies.

The majority of molar pregnancies are XX due to replication of paternal X. Triploid chromosomal pattern may occur with partial moles. In spite of XX genotype, GTN may follow normal conceptions of either sex.

Risk of choriocarcinoma is 1 to 30 moles; it is 1 to 50,000 normal pregnancies.

4. Approximately half of the patients with metastatic trophoblastic disease and 75 per cent of patients with nonmetastatic trophoblastic disease develop these tumors as sequelae to molar pregnancy.

5. Approximately 20 per cent of patients with moles require additional treatment.

6. Recurrent molar pregnancy is four to five times higher than the risk of the first.

7. When a urinary HCG excretion greater than one million international units (I.U.) per 24 hours is encountered in association with an enlarged uterus and vaginal bleeding, the diagnosis is almost always molar pregnancy. However, a higher percentage of patients with molar pregnancy have urinary HCG levels in the normal range for a single fetus, which makes this test relatively nonspecific.

8. In addition, approximately one-half of hydatidiform moles will be found in uteri that are small for dates. Therefore, the diagnosis should not be disregarded if the uterus is small or normal-sized for dates.

9. Gestational trophoblastic neoplasm after any pregnancy other than a molar pregnancy is always choriocarcinoma. These cases usually present with symptoms caused by bleeding from metastases to the lung, brain, liver, or genital tract. When there is choriocarcinoma in the uterus, the presentation mimics threatened abortion or ectopic pregnancy.

HISTOPATHOLOGY

1. Recent information suggests that hydatidiform mole is caused by the deletion or inactivation of all the female chromosomes in the ova site and duplication of the male chromosomes from a fertilizing sperm.

a. Pathologically, it is important to distinguish between two different forms of hydatidiform mole. These have been called the *complete* and the *partial* or *incomplete* types.

b. The complete hydatidiform mole is the classic form of the disease that includes dilated avascular villi, the absence of membranes or fetal parts, and at least some degree of trophoblastic proliferation.

c. Occasionally, patients with hydropic placental villi are seen who also have an associated fetus (usually malformed) or membranes.

d. These patients do not have trophoblastic proliferation and they are classified as having a partial mole. This lesion is almost always benign.

e. The classic complete mole has a 46 XX chromosome complement, while partial moles usually demonstrate cytogenic abnormalities such as triploidy.

2. The classic complete mole is a conceptus most often lacking an intact fetus, showing swelling of the villi.

3. Three changes are found in the villi and are typically identified with hydatidiform mole. These are:

a. Trophoblastic proliferation of both the cytotrophoblast (Langhan's cells) and syncytiotrophoblast

b. Hydropic changes in the stroma

c. Absence of blood vessels

4. Several authors have studied the degree of trophoblastic proliferation associated with the villi of hydatidiform mole in an attempt to predict the likelihood that a patient will develop persistent malignant disease.

5. The conclusion is that the likelihood of malignant sequelae developing is increased in patients whose trophoblastic cells showed increased proliferation and anaplasia.

6. Unfortunately, metastatic choriocarcinoma has developed from the most benign-appearing mole. It is therefore imperative that serial gonadotropin assays be obtained in all patients who have had a hydatidiform mole.

CLINICAL FEATURES

1. There is a higher incidence of hydatidiform mole below the age of 20 and above the age of 40.

2. Vaginal bleeding occurs in virtually all patients and is generally noted at between 6 and 8 weeks following the missed period. The bleeding may range from dark brown ("prune juice") to bright red and may lead to marked anemia.

3. More than half of the patients have uterine enlargement beyond the expected gestational age. When the uterus enlarges it does so rapidly and at a nonuniform rate.

4. The uterus feels boggy and despite its size no fetal parts can be felt.

5. Amniotic fluid is absent and ballottement cannot be elicited.

6. Massive enlargement of the ovaries may occur because of theca-lutein cyst formation. Molar pregnancy should be suspected when these cysts are detected. The cysts regress after delivery of the mole.

7. Uterine size is consistent with gestational dates in approximately 35 per cent of the patients and smaller in 10 to 15 per cent.

8. About 20 per cent of patients with molar pregnancy develop signs of preeclampsia which include hypertension, edema, and/or albuminuria. Rarely does eclampsia occur in association with molar pregnancy. Since this occurs in the first or early second trimester at a much earlier time than toxemia is seen, it should alert the physician to the possibility of this diagnosis.

9. Hyperemesis occurs in approximately 30 per cent of the patients. Interestingly, urinary estrogen levels are not necessarily elevated in this group. Therefore, nausea and vomiting are apparently due to some other cause.

10. About 1 in 10 patients develops some clinical and laboratory evidence in the form of elevated serum-protein-bound iodine tests accompanied by tachycardia and enlarged thyroid glands.

11. Hyperthyroidism in molar pregnancy is due to the production of trophoblastic cells of molar thyrotropin, which is similar to the hormone isolated from the pituitary gland and the placenta.

12. When this clinical state occurs, the patient must be given antithyroid therapy prior to the institution of anesthesia in order to avoid thyroid storm. This condition may be subtle and not recognized until after the patient is given general anesthesia at the time of evacuation.

13. In summary, the clinical signs of hydatidiform molar pregnancy present as follows: vaginal bleeding 100 per cent, uterine enlargement 50 per cent, hyperemesis 30 per cent, toxemia 20 per cent, hyperthyroidism 10 per cent, and trophoblastic emboli 2 per cent.

DIAGNOSTIC STUDIES

1. CBC and hematocrit

2. Urinalysis

3. A quantitative HCG test that is sensitive and reliable is most important. Detailed discussion under laboratory tests (see Choriocarcinoma below).

4. Ultrasonography is playing a significant and increasingly valuable role in the diagnosis of molar pregnancy.

a. May be employed in uteri smaller than 14 weeks size.

b. Is employed if there is an equivocal amniogram as well as a method chosen before amniography.

c. The diagnosis can be made as early as 8 weeks apparent gestation.

d. At this time a gestational sac is not visualized and the pattern described as a snow storm is pathognomonic for molar pregnancy.

e. Currently multilayered ultrasound screening as well as the gray mode have made ultrasonography the best method of diagnosing a mole.

ROENTGENOGRAPHIC STUDIES

1. Flat plate of the abdomen

2. Amniography

a. If the uterus is above the symphysis, a radiopaque dye can be injected transabdominally into the uterine cavity.

b. A single flat plate of the abdomen and perhaps lateral or oblique films are obtained within 5 minutes of the time of injection.

c. The x-ray appearance of molar pregnancy is that of a moth-eaten or honeycomb pattern.

3. Arteriography is discussed under "Nonmetastatic Trophoblastic Disease," below.

4. Chest radiograph

5. Brain and liver scan as indicated

6. Transaminase studies including an SMA-12

7. Type and crossmatch for at least 1,000 ml. of blood.

TREATMENT

1. When a definitive diagnosis of a molar pregnancy is made, evacuation should be carried out without waiting for spontaneous passage of the mole. Evacuation is best accomplished by suction curettage, even though the uterus may be 20 weeks or more in size.

2. A Pitocin infusion should be running prior to the start of the evacuation. Accumulated old blood as well as fresh bright blood may gush out at first, but continued suction will remove the mole and control bleeding.

3. After the uterus is evacuated, sharp curettage should be carried out, and these curettings should be sent to the laboratory as a separate specimen.

4. In multiparous patients and in those with advanced age total hysterectomy with or without salpingo-oophorectomy (depending on age) is the procedure of choice for treatment of molar pregnancy, leaving the mole in situ.

5. Some advocate prophylactic chemotherapy prior to evacuation of the molar pregnancy. Since there is toxicity associated with chemotherapy, the prophylactic method is not universally accepted.

a. However, it should be considered in the high-risk group, in unreliable patients who may avoid follow-up, and in parts of the world where gonadotropin follow-up may not be available or where the incidence of trophoblastic complications following molar pregnancy may be greater than in the United States.

b. The regimen employed is a single 5-day course of dactinomycin, at a daily dosage of 12 μg./Kg., starting 2 to 3 days before evacuation. This reduces the 15- to 20-per-cent rate of persistent trophoblastic disease following a hydatidiform mole to 1 or 2 per cent.

c. Since hepatitis may occur in these patients because of increased use of blood, some prefer methotrexate, 15 to 25 mg. intramuscularly or intravenously per day for 5 days.

d. If hepatitis develops and additional therapy is required, dactinomycin can then be given.

e. Methotrexate should not be given in the presence of impaired hepatic or renal function, since the toxicity may be overwhelming.

COMPLICATIONS OF TREATMENT

1. It is noted that embolization may occur before, during, or after evacuation, regardless of the method used.

a. Typically, the patient develops cyanosis, tachypnea, tachycardia, dyspnea, and, in some severe cases, signs of right heart failure.

b. Supportive treatment should include oxygen, sedation, and digitalis for cases of right heart failure. These usually prove adequate.

c. Parenteral cortisone is helpful in severe cases of pulmonary edema.

d. Signs of embolization generally subside spontaneously within 72 hours. This complication is not associated with a higher incidence of pulmonary metastases.

2. Gynecologists who treat patients with hydatidiform mole need to be alert to the factors associated with the risk for embolization of molar tissue. A blood-oxygen tension may identify this phenomenon as a subclinical syndrome. Once the diagnosis is made, invasive monitoring of cardiopulmonary function is advisable. Adrenal steroids should be given early. Nonmetastatic trophoblastic sequelae are frequent, if not universal, following molar embolization and should be treated by adjunctive chemotherapy.

3. Disseminated intravascular coagulation may also arise and should be treated immediately.

FOLLOW-UP

1. The prime objective is detection of persistent malignant disease following molar pregnancy in the individual patient.

2. The protocol for postevacuation follow-up must be carefully observed to detect persistent or recurrent disease.

3. The HCG assay must be recorded at evacuation and then weekly thereafter. If the HCG level becomes normal on three consecutive assays it can be done at monthly intervals for 6 months. If the titer remains within normal limits after 6 months, it can be discontinued and repeated after 6 months. During this time pregnancy should be avoided.

4. A chest radiograph is taken at the time of evacuation and at 4 and 8 weeks.

5. A lesion may persist in the lung for several weeks, and no further treatment is needed if the HCG level continues to fall.

6. If the HCG level plateaus, or rises, or if metastases appear, treatment should be instituted without delay.

7. The Pill serves a twofold purpose in that it prevents pregnancy and suppresses the secretion of pituitary gonadotropins.

NONMETASTATIC TROPHOBLASTIC DISEASE (INVASIVE MOLE, CHORIOADENOMA DESTRUENS)

Basic Principles

1. The hydatidiform mole invades the myometrium.

2. It retains its villous structure and is usually confined to the uterus.

3. The villi may metastasize to the vagina, to the parametrium, and even to the lungs and brain.

4. The invasive mole may be of this form from the beginning or it may follow an apparently simple mole.

Clinical Features

1. After evacuation of a mole there may be no symptoms or signs for weeks or months. Then episodes of irregular bleeding occur, usually accompanied by pain.

2. On examination the uterus is enlarged and cystic ovaries may be felt.

3. The presenting symptoms may be dysuria from local extension, or dyspnea with or without pleuritic pain, or headache and visual disturbances due to cerebral metastases.

Diagnostic Signs and Studies

1. It may be impossible to differentiate from choriocarcinoma.

2. HCG is usually elevated.

3. Curettage reveals a friable, hemorrhagic growth with villi present.

4. The histologic structure is usually benign even in cases with metastases.

5. Arteriography has a role in diagnosis but it is limited. In those patients failing to achieve complete remission with systemic chemotherapy, arteriography may demonstrate a focus of trophoblastic disease deep in the myometrium.

Treatment

1. There are dangers which make it imperative that active therapy be instituted.

a. Hemorrhage may occur and be fatal.

b. There may be extension to the parametrium, resulting in intra-abdominal hemorrhage.

c. Extension of growth with embolization occasionally is a complication. The pulmonary and cerebral manifestations may be serious and require urgent treatment.

d. There may be progression to choriocarcinoma.

2. Chemotherapy should be employed as for choriocarcinoma.

3. In older women or with great parity, total hysterectomy is often chosen as the best therapy.

4. Since operative procedures in these patients may result in dissemination of viable tumor cells, surgery should be carried out on the third day of a 5-day course of chemotherapy.

5. The follow-up is essentially the same as outlined above for hydatidiform mole.

CHORIOCARCINOMA

Caution: Choriocarcinoma—A Diagnostic Problem

Gestational trophoblastic disease is a great masquerader. It is an enigma. The symptoms may appear as nongynecological. In patients in whom a diagnosis cannot be established or in whom the primary site of the tumor cannot be determined, an HCG should be obtained. Since choriocarcinoma has been reported in the postmenopausal years, it is no longer advisable to limit the HCG assay to those in the childbearing years. It is important that physicians who care for women consider the possibility of choriocarcinoma in a variety of medical conditions whose cause is not apparent, such as brain tumor, cerebrovascular accident, gastrointestinal bleeding, or a mass in the region of the liver.

Basic Principles

1. A rare disease. Incidence is roughly 1 in 14,000 pregnancies in the United States. In Hong Kong, it is 1 in 114.

2. It usually follows immediately after a mole, abortion, or normal pregnancy.

3. It may appear many years after the last pregnancy. Cases have been reported as occurring after the menopause.

4. Trophoblastic tissue is in the nature of an allograft, and one would expect an immunologic reaction between the host and the tumor.

5. In 90 per cent of cases, the tumor allows reactive signs, which consist of lymphocytes, plasma cells, and histiocytes. The more marked the immunologic reaction, the better the prognosis.

6. The ABO system also influences prognosis, which is worse in women of groups B and AB whose husbands are O or A.

Histopathology

1. Villus Formation. Villus formation is almost universally absent.

a. The tumor consists of masses of syncytium and cytotrophoblast.

b. It invades and destroys the surrounding tissues and causes gross hemorrhage owing to its ability to erode blood vessels.

c. The cells are irregular with hyperchromic nuclei.

d. Mitotic figures are frequent.

e. The syncytial masses are usually fenestrated.

Definition

1. High-Risk Metastatic Disease

a. Constitutes 20 per cent of all cases

b. Gonadotropin excretion (HCG) over 100,000 I.U./24 hours

c. Duration of disease over 4 months from the termination of the antecedent pregnancy or the onset of symptoms

d. Metastatic disease in multiple sites, including the liver or brain or both, as well as metastases to the small bowel

e. Failure of treatment to control the disease

2. Low-Risk Metastatic Disease

a. Constitutes 80 per cent of all cases

b. Gonadotropin excretion (HCG) under 100,000 I.U./24 hours

c. Duration of disease under 4 months from the termination of antecedent pregnancy or the onset of symptoms

d. Metastatic disease to the lung or vagina or both

Clinical Features

1. These are variable.

2. The primary uterine growth may cause hemorrhage or even cerebral symptoms.

3. Metastases may give rise to respiratory or cerebral symptoms.

4. Hemoptysis may occur.

5. Irregular uterine bleeding may be present.

6. There may be pulmonary shadows on x-ray examination.

7. HCG titer may be high.

Treatment

1. Method of single-agent chemotherapy for patients in the low-risk group (good prognosis). Metastatic trophoblastic disease as published include:

a. *Repetitive 5-day Courses.* Methotrexate, 15 to 20 mg. I.M. q.d., or actinomycin D, 10 μg. to 13 μg./Kg. I.V. q.d.

(1) Consider hysterectomy during first course of chemotherapy if further reproduction is not desired.

(2) Minimum interval between courses—7 days.

(3) Maximum interval between courses—14 days (unless laboratory values are too low)

(4) Consider oral contraception for pituitary suppression.

b. *Signs to Look For.* Continue repetitive 5-day courses of the same drug until

(1) HCG titer drops to normal pituitary range—cease treatment.

(2) HCG titer "plateaus" elevated,
(3) HCG titer rises tenfold,
(4) New metastases appear,
} Change to alternate drug.

c. *Oncolytic Effect.* Monitor oncolytic effect by weekly HCG titers, chest radiographs, and pelvic examinations.

d. *Treatment Safety Factors (Done Daily During Treatment, Less Frequently Between Courses).* Do not start, continue, or resume a dose of medication if:

(1) White blood count less than 3,000/cu. mm.

(2) Polymorphonuclear leukocytes less than 1,500/cu. mm.

(3) Platelets less than 100,000/cu. mm.

(3) Significant elevations of BUN, SGOT, or SGPT

e. *Duration of Course.* Treatment is terminated when HCG titer is within normal pituitary range. Three consecutive normal weekly HCG titers for diagnosis of remission.

f. *Follow-up*

(1) HCG titers monthly for 6 months, bimonthly for 6 months, then every 6 months thereafter

(2) Physical, pelvic exams, chest radiographs, blood survey every 3 months for 1 year, every 6 months thereafter

(3) No pregnancy for 1 year

g. *Success Rate.* Patients cured—98 per cent.

2. Method of triple-agent chemotherapy for patients in the high-risk group (poor prognosis). Metastatic trophoblastic disease as reported in the literature:

a. The management is similar to that outlined under the single-agent chemotherapy, but this includes three drugs and x-ray therapy.

b. The drug regimen is given in combination of methotrexate, 15 mg. I.M., actinomycin D, 10 μg/Kg. I.V., and chlorambucil, 10 mg. P.O.

c. Each drug is given daily for 5 days (triple therapy).

d. The interval between treatment should be longer than 10 days but shorter than 21 days.

e. After two or three courses of such combination chemotherapy, treatment is altered to single-agent therapy with actinomycin D at a dosage of 13 μg I.V. for 5 days.

f. This change is necessary because of cumulative toxicity from the combination chemotherapy.

g. If cerebral or hepatic metastases have been demonstrated, immediate institution of whole-brain or whole-liver irradiation of 2,000 rads (total dose) should be given simultaneously with combination chemotherapy. Cortisone should be given to reduce the cerebral edema secondary to the radiation therapy.

h. Patients cured—47 per cent.

i. Failure to cure patients with gestational trophoblastic disease is more frequently due to drug toxicity than to drug resistance, although the latter certainly occurs.

h. Recently, two regimes have proved to be useful in patients not tolerating MAC (methotrexate, actinomycin D, and cyclophosphamide). They may even produce cures after failure with MAC. These are the multi-drug Bagshawe regime and the Einhorn triple drug therapy (vinblastine, bleomycin, and cisplatin). Currently, these regimes are reserved for second line therapy.

Contraindications to Initiation and Continuation of Therapy

Laboratory Contraindications	
WBC	<2,500/mm³
Total poly count	<1,500/mm³
Platelet count	<100,000/mm³
SGOT level	>50 units
BUN	Rising

1. **Clinical**
   a. Leukopenia
   b. Thrombocytopenia
   c. Hepatocellular disease
2. **Judgment Decisions**
   a. Stomatitis
   b. Maculopapular rash
   c. GI disturbances
   d. Alopecia
   e. Vulvitis
   f. Conjunctivitis

3. Sequential chemotherapy is not without its toxic manifestations.

a. Leukopenia and thrombocytopenia are the main signs of marrow damage. Both are reversible if the danger is appreciated and precautions taken.

b. *Other Systemic Side Effects.* Stomatitis, skin rash, alopecia, gastrointestinal disturbances, and conjunctivitis may be treated symptomatically.

c. They rarely if ever determine whether a course is to be initiated or continued.

d. Life-threatening toxicity should be treated vigorously. Reverse isolation, infusions, antibiotics, fresh white cell and platelet transfusions, and supportive therapy as needed. All other therapy should be immediately discontinued.

Laboratory Tests

1. HCG is the best method to evaluate and follow the progress of a patient with gestational trophoblastic disease. Eleanor Delfs has asserted that between days 60 and 100 of normal pregnancy, there is no level of chorionic gonadotropin, however high, that could not be caused by a normal pregnancy or some variation thereof.

2. Higher HCG levels may also be associated with multiple gestation or toxemia of pregnancy. A continued rise in HCG levels after the fourteenth week of pregnancy is the best evidence of a molar pregnancy that can be obtained by using HCG assays.

3. Routine immunoassays available in most hospital laboratories are not sensitive enough to monitor the progress of the patient. The Pregnosticon tube test is capable of a minimal detectable level of HCG of 700 to 750 I.U./liter. The Gravindex is capable of a minimal detectable level of HCG of 3,500 I.U./liter.

4. Patients with gestational trophoblastic disease usually have gonadotropin titers initially in excess of 1,000 I.U./24-hour urine required to give a positive test.

5. Approximately 25 per cent of patients with malignant trophoblastic disease have gonadotropin titers in excess of pituitary level but below that required for a positive pregnancy test.

6. Radioimmunoassay is a hundred times more sensitive than either the immunoassay or bioassay methods, being able to detect approximately 0.01 I.U./ml.

a. β-subunit portion of the HCG molecule represents only HCG and only minimally crossreacts with human pituitary LH.

b. The β-subunit assay, since it is specific for HCG, enables those using it to measure HCG down to zero rather than down to levels consistent with normal pituitary LH.

7. Serum leucine aminopeptidase, human placental lactogen, and estrogens are of little assistance in differential diagnosis or monitoring the progress of treatment.

Indications for Surgery

1. Evacuation of molar pregnancy

2. Diagnostic D and C for persistent localized disease

3. Treatment of surgical emergencies

4. Total hysterectomy in the patient over 40 years of age or with high parity

PROPHYLACTIC CHEMOTHERAPY FOR ALL MOLAR PREGNANCIES

1. It has been proposed that all patients passing a hydatidiform mole or having one evacuated should be given chemotherapy. Although there is evidence that this is beneficial in decreasing the number of patients who have an elevation at 8 weeks or who subsequently develop metastatic disease, it is not clear that chemotherapy decreases these problems any more than does the careful follow-up of patients by chest radiographs and gonadotropin studies.

2. Because approximately three-fourths of patients having a molar pregnancy will be free of disease with 2 months, the potential dangers of chemotherapy can be avoided by waiting until that time to begin therapy.

3. The use of routine prophylactic chemotherapy has been shown to be useful in Asia, where careful follow-up and gonadotropin studies are impossible.

4. It is also chosen for those in the indigent population who may not return for their follow-up visits.

REASONS FOR GESTATIONAL TROPHOBLASTIC DISEASE RECEIVING ATTENTION DISPROPORTIONATE TO ITS INCIDENCE

1. Unique Responsiveness to Chemotherapy

a. Virtually all patients with nonmetastatic disease can be cured, with most retaining reproductive function.

b. Eighty to ninety per cent of the patients with metastatic trophoblastic neoplasms can be cured when appropriate treatment is given.

2. Consistent Production of Human Chorionic Gonadotropin (HCG)

a. Human placental chorionic tissue, whether normal, molar, or choriocarcinomatous in nature, produces HCG when viable and growing.

b. This consistent production by molar or choriocarcinomatous tissue of a "tumor marker" allows it to be useful in diagnosis, management, and follow-up of patients.

3. Origination in Fetal Tissue

a. Because the placenta is fetal in origin, one-half of its genetic material comes from the father and is therefore potentially foreign to the maternal host.

b. Since there is no other human malignancy in which the host of origin differs from that of the host, this unique characteristic has attracted much attention.

Gestational Trophoblastic Treatment Centers

1. Gestational trophoblastic disease is probably handled best in a center. HCG is available there and is accurate. The technique of chemotherapy and the management of side effects and toxicity are understood. Supporting consultative assistance and laboratory and ancillary services are available. Unless these services are locally available, the patient should be referred to a center. Resistant diseases should be referred without delay.

2. If there is any indecision or lack of confidence on the part of the responsible physician, the patient should be referred to a center. Inadequate treatment may convert a low-risk patient with an excellent chance for cure to a high-risk patient with a decreased chance for cure. All high-risk patients should be referred to a center. When drug toxicity reactions occur, the patient is a candidate for treatment at a trophoblastic center.

27 Gynecological Endocrinology

Sherwin A. Kaufman

Although gynecological patients can exhibit any endocrinopathy found in both men and women, the female patient possesses a unique, overtly responsive mechanism which readily informs the physician of the possible presence of an endocrine disorder. This is the alteration of the regular menstrual pattern.

ABNORMAL PATTERNS OF MENSTRUATION

1. Amenorrhea (absence of menses)

a. Primary. Menstruation has never occurred.

b. Secondary. Menstruation has occurred in the past, but has stopped.

2. Oligomenorrhea. Less frequent menstruation, occurring at intervals longer than 5 to 6 weeks.

3. Polymenorrhea. More frequent menstruation, occurring at intervals of less than 3 weeks.

4. Hypomenorrhea. Menses at regular intervals (approximately every 28 days) but with significantly reduced amount of flow. The duration of flow, in days, is equal to or shorter than that of the patient's usual menses.

5. Hypermenorrhea. Regular menses at approximately 28-day intervals that last the usual 4 to 6 days but are excessive in amount.

6. Menorrhagia. Menses may come at regular intervals, but bleeding is either profuse, excessive in duration (8 days or more), or both.

7. Metrorrhagia. Unexpected bleeding between menstrual periods which, if prolonged, may manifest itself as totally irregular menses. Normal menstrual function requires an intact hypothalamic-pituitary-ovarian axis and a normal uterus. These may be influenced in turn by the thyroid or adrenal glands or by another endocrine organ.

THYROID DYSFUNCTION IN GYNECOLOGY

HYPOTHYROIDISM

Basic Principles

1. Clinical Features

a. Loss of cephalic, pubic, axillary, and eyebrow (lateral aspect) hair. These changes may be subtle in patients with early or minimal diminution of thyroid function.

b. Dry skin. This occasionally can resemble hyperkeratosis and may be sallow in color.

c. Edema

d. Weight gain

e. Intolerance to cold and tolerance to heat

f. Tendencies toward lethargy, obesity, constipation, bradycardia, and hypothermia

g. Occasionally, psychiatric depression or psychosis occurs.

h. The thyroid gland may be normal in size or enlarged.

i. Deep tendon reflexes exhibit delayed return.

2. Laboratory Tests

a. *T_4 (Thyroxine) by Radioimmunoassay (RIA).* Low, rarely normal

b. *T_3 (Triiodothyronine) by RIA.* Low or normal

c. *Free T_4 Index (FT_4I).* Low (confirmation of T_4 RIA)

d. *TSH (Thyroid-Stimulating Hormone) by RIA (Radioimmunoassay) or IRMA (Immunoradiometric Assay).* High (except in the rare patient with pituitary or hypothalamic hypothyroidism)

Management

1. L-Thyroxine (T_4; Synthroid, Levothroid). Start with small doses and increase at 2-week intervals to an average maintenance dose of 0.1 to 0.15 mg. orally daily.

2. Liothyronine (T_3; Cytomel) or desiccated thyroid tablets are not generally indicated for replacement therapy.

3. If adrenal insufficiency is present or suspected, administer prednisone 5 to 7.5 mg. orally daily prior to thyroid hormone therapy. All patients with central (pituitary or hypothalamic) hypothyroidism must be tested for adrenal function (see below) prior to administration of thyroid hormone.

4. Measurement of thyroid-stimulating hormone (TSH), after therapy has been established, with a stable dose of L-thyroxine is the best means of determining the proper replacement dose.

HYPERTHYROIDISM

Basic Principles

1. Clinical Features

a. Weight change (usually loss), with increased appetite

b. Warm and moist skin

c. Thin and fine hair

d. Occasionally, psychiatric disturbances occur.

e. Palpitations and tachycardia

f. Nervousness is common. Occasionally, manic behavior occurs.

g. Intolerance to heat

h. Diarrhea and/or frequent bowel movements

i. Eye signs may include exophthalmos, conversion defect, and widening of palpable fissures (in Graves' disease), and lid lag.

j. The thyroid gland usually is palpable and enlarged (diffusely in Graves' disease) or nodular, unless substernal in position.

k. Pretibial myxedema appears occasionally (Graves' disease).

2. Laboratory Tests

a. *T_3 by RIA.* High

b. *T_4 by RIA.* High, rarely normal (esp. early)

c. *FT_4I.* High, rarely normal

d. *TSH by RIA.* Usually undetectable

e. *TSH by IRMA.* Decreased or undetectable

Management

1. Medical: Antithyroid drugs such as methimazole (MMI) and propylthiouracil (PTU) are commonly used, as follows:

a. *Methimazole.* Ten to thirty mg. orally q.d. generally provides adequate control of hyperthyroidism. Not for use in pregnant patients.

b. *Propylthiouracil.* Fifty to 150 mg. orally t.i.d. generally provides adequate control of hyperthyroidism. May be used in pregnant patients if needed.

c. *Cautions.* Drug reaction, including pruritus and urticaria, does not necessitate stopping therapy, inasmuch as these conditions may subside with continuous treatment. Depression of WBC below 3,500, however, requires immediate cessation of the drug. Arthralgia and significant and generalized malaise may be an expression of drug toxicity; in such cases, cessation of therapy may be necessary.

d. Medical management is appropriate for initial therapy and for management of hyperthyroidism for up to 2 years. If at the end of 1 to 2 years removal of antithyroid medication results in recurrent hyperthyroidsm, then definitive therapy (radioactive iodine or surgery) should be instituted. The likelihood of spontaneous remission of hyperthyroidism decreases with increasing size of the thyroid gland, degree of hyperthyroidism, and the patient's age.

2. Radioactive Iodine (RAI)

a. Destruction of the gland with radioactive iodine (RAI) is generally safe and effective therapy of hyperthyroidism. However, it is contraindicated in pregnant patients.

b. Two to three per cent per year of all patients treated with RAI become hypothyroid; thus permanent hypothyroidism may occur in a significant number of patients so treated. For these patients, lifelong replacement with thyroid hormone becomes necessary.

c. Unreliable patients or those exhibiting adverse effects of medical management may require RAI (or surgery).

3. Surgical

a. Ablation of overactive thyroid tissue by surgery is indicated in toxic nodular goiter and in some patients less than 40 years old who prefer this procedure to radioactive iodine due to the small potential risk of damage to reproductive function posed by ionizing radiation.

b. A small percentage of patients who are surgically treated may show some measure of decreased parathyroid function after a thyroidectomy, or may develop frank hypoparathyroidism. It is important to measure serum calcium before and after thyroid surgery to detect hypocalcemia. Hypoparathyroidism, which can lead to depression, atonia of the gut, and tetany, rarely is a permanent complication of thyroid surgery.

c. Many patients treated surgically for Graves' disease (subtotal thyroidectomy) become hypothyroid some months to years after surgery. This complication is somewhat less common in such patients than in those treated with radioactive iodine.

ADRENAL DYSFUNCTION IN GYNECOLOGY

HYPOADRENALISM

Basic Principles

1. Clinical Features

a. Weakness and general debilitation, with weight loss, anorexia, and diarrhea

b. Hypotension, including postural hypotension

c. Increasing pigmentation of exposed areas of the body and mucous membranes, except in secondary (pituitary) and early primary hypoadrenalism

d. Decreased or absent pubic and axillary hair

e. Occasional vitiligo (rare in secondary hypoadrenalism)

f. Occasional craving for salt (not in secondary hypoadrenalism)

2. Laboratory Tests

a. *Sodium.* Serum low, urine high

b. *Potassium.* Serum high, urine low (not in secondary hypoadrenalism)

c. *Plasma Cortisol.* Low; no diurnal variation

d. *Plasma Adrenocorticotropin Hormone (ACTH).* High in primary hypoadrenalism, low in secondary hypoadrenalism

e. *Urine Free Cortisol.* Low

f. *Urine 17-Ketosteroids.* Low; also decreased by ingestion of opiates, Dilantin, probenecid, and estrogens

g. *Urine 17-Hydroxysteroids.* Low; also decreased by ingestion of opiates, Dilantin, thiazides, and estrogens

h. *Cosyntropin (ACTH 1-24) Stimulation Test.* Primary adrenal insufficiency: no response. Secondary adrenal insufficiency: no response initially, but adrenal glands will respond with prolonged (48- to 72-hour) cosyntropin dosing

i. *Metyrapone Test (Only for Secondary Hypoadrenalism).* Depressed 11-deoxycortisol (compound "S") response

Management (Chronic)

1. Glucocorticoid: Hydrocortisone 20 to 30 mg. orally per day in divided doses (e.g., 20 mg. P.O. q.A.M. + 10 mg. P.O. q.P.M.) or prednisone 5 to 7.5 mg. P.O. q.d.

2. Mineralocorticoid (generally only for primary hypoadrenalism): Fludrocortisone, 0.1 mg. P.O. q.d. (Note: This steroid may produce excess sodium retention with increased body weight due to edema and increased blood pressure. Such untoward effects subside when the steroid is discontinued.)

3. The dose of the medication used (e.g., glucocorticoid) must be augmented during illness or stress.

CONGENITAL ADRENOGENITAL SYNDROME

1. If present at birth, the adrenal hyperplasia gives rise in the female to pseudohermaphroditism.

2. In female children, growth rate is accelerated.

3. Body hair growth may be excessive.

4. Masculine muscle development and torso with narrow hips are apparent.

5. Secondary female sexual characteristics are absent.

6. The clitoris is enlarged.

7. Laboratory Tests

a. *Plasma Sodium.* Normal or low, depending on severity of disorder

b. *Plasma Potassium.* Normal or high, depending on severity of disorder

c. *Urine 17-Ketosteroids.* Elevated

d. *Urine Pregnanetriol.* Elevated

e. *Urine 17-Hydroxysteroids.* Normal or low

f. *Plasma 17-Hydroxyprogesterone and Androstenedione.* Elevated in C21-hydroxylase deficiency (most common type)

g. *Metyrapone Test.* Marked increase in urine pregnanetriol and ketosteroid excretion

h. *Cosyntropin Stimulation Test.* Marked increase in plasma 17-hydroxyprogesterone and androstenedione (C21-hydroxylase deficiency)

POSTPUBERTAL ADRENOGENITAL SYNDROME

Basic Principles

1. The effects may vary from normal feminization to marked masculinization.

2. Body hair growth may be minimal or marked.

3. The clitoris may be normal or slightly enlarged.

4. Menstrual abnormalities are common—chiefly amenorrhea or anovulatory irregular menses.

5. Laboratory Tests

a. *Urine 17-Ketosteroids.* Elevated

b. *Urine Pregnanetriol.* Normal or elevated

c. *Urine 17-Hydroxysteroids.* Normal

d. *Metyrapone Test.* Marked increase in urine pregnanetriol and 17-ketosteroid excretion (only occasional increase in 17-hydroxysteroids)

e. *Plasma Sodium.* Normal

f. *Plasma Potassium.* Normal

Management

1. Therapy is the same for both the congenital and postpubertal syndromes. It includes the use of any one of the following preparations: Prednisone 5 to 7.5 mg. q.d., dexamethasone 0.5 to 0.75 mg. q.d., or hydrocortisone 20 to 30 mg. per day in divided doses.

2. A repeat 17-ketosteroid test is obtained 2 to 4 weeks later. If the levels are normal or low, the dose of corticoid is reduced to twice a day, and then further decreased depending upon 17-ketosteroid excretion.

3. Congenital adrenogenital syndrome must be treated for life.

4. Treatment for postpubertal adrenogenital syndrome may be discontinued in most patients after several months of treatment, with a permanent cure expected. (If therapy is discontinued in the congenital type, however, there is a marked increase in pregnanetriol.)

NEOPLASTIC ADRENOGENITAL SYNDROME

1. The clinical picture is the same as in congenital adrenogenital syndrome, except that the clinical changes appear so suddenly that defeminization is obvious and sudden in onset in the adult.

2. Increased hair growth, clitoral enlargement, decreased breast size, and oligomenorrhea terminating in amenorrhea are symptoms.

3. Laboratory Tests

a. *Urine 17-Ketosteroids.* Elevated (moderate to marked elevation)

b. *Urine Pregnanetriol.* Normal

c. *Urine 17-Hydroxysteroids.* Normal

d. *Glucose Tolerance.* Normal

e. *Plasma Sodium.* Normal

f. *Plamsa Potassium.* Normal

g. *Metyrapone Test.* No abnormal increase in steroid excretion

h. *Visualization by CT, MRI, and/or Arteriography.* To demonstrate presence of tumor

4. The adrenogenital syndrome in children is more likely to be caused by an adrenal tumor than by hyperplasia, and the tumor is commonly malignant. (In adults, such a tumor is more often benign.)

5. Sometimes the differential diagnosis between hyperplasia and tumor can be settled only by surgical exploration.

CUSHING'S SYNDROME

This is adrenocortical hypersecretion due to adrenal tumor, pituitary ACTH-secreting tumor, ectopic secretion of ACTH, or excess exogenous glucocorticoids.

Basic Principles

1. Clinical Features: Characteristic central obesity with dorsocervical fat pad ("buffalo hump"), thin arms and legs, muscle wasting, skin atrophy, presence of striae, and hypertension.

2. Laboratory Tests

a. *Urinary Free Cortisol.* Elevated

b. *Urinary 17-Hydroxysteroids.* Elevated

c. *Urinary 17-Ketosteroids.* Normal or elevated

d. *Plasma Cortisol.* Normal or elevated, with loss of diurnal rhythm; nonsuppressible with dexamethasone (see below)

e. *Glucose Tolerance.* May be abnormal (i.e., diabetes mellitus)

f. *Serum Potassium.* May be decreased

g. *Radiology.* CT and/or MRI may reveal adrenal tumor, pituitary tumor with bilateral adrenal hyperplasia, or occult carcinoma (producing ectopic ACTH) with bilateral adrenal hyperplasia. Osteoporosis is common, especially in the vertebrae. Delayed bone age is seen in children, with retarded growth; the sella turcica is rarely enlarged except with large pituitary tumors.

3. Provocative Tests

a. Dexamethasone Suppression Test. Plasma cortisol is normally suppressed below 5 μg. per 100 ml. at 8 A.M. after 1 mg. of dexamethasone given orally at 11 P.M. the night before. In patients with Cushing's syndrome, the plasma cortisol level after dexamethasone is above this level. A prolonged dexamethasone suppression test may be done, giving 0.5 mg. P.O. q.i.d. for 2 days, and collecting 24-hour urine on each day of the test; the urinary free cortisol and 17-hydroxysteroids should normally drop to not more than 50 per cent of baseline values.

4. Further Differential Diagnosis

a. In females, Cushing's syndrome must be differentiated from masculinizing syndromes such as occur with adrenogenitalism or arrhenoblastoma and other virilizing ovarian tumors.

b. Cushing's syndrome is characterized by muscle weakness, whereas adrenogenitalism is characterized by muscular strength.

c. Urinary 17-ketosteroids are markedly elevated in adrenal carcinoma, while they tend to be within the normal range with simple adenoma.

d. Urinary 17-hydroxysteroids usually are significantly elevated in all three types: adrenal carcinoma, adenoma, and hyperplasia.

Management

The prognosis may be poor unless the disease is arrested, with complications resulting from hypertensive cardiovascular disease. If any tumor is present, it should be removed surgically. For pituitary tumors, transsphenoidal microsurgical tumor excision is the preferred method of therapy. For adrenal adenomas, surgical excision should be performed. Adrenocortical replacement therapy is indicated for several months to 2 years postoperatively to allow for normalization of the hypothalamic-pituitary-adrenal axis.

PITUITARY DYSFUNCTION IN GYNECOLOGY

Basic Principles

1. The anterior pituitary gland secretes many important hormones:

a. Follicle-stimulating hormone (FSH)

b. Luteinizing hormone (LH)

c. Thyrotropin, or thyroid-stimulating hormone (TSH)

d. Prolactin (PRL)

e. Growth hormone (GH)

f. Adrenocorticotropin hormone (ACTH)

2. The concentration of circulating hormone from the target gland (e.g., ovary, thyroid, adrenal) exerts a negative feedback control on the secretion of its corresponding tropic hormone, the effect being at the level of the hypothalamus, the pituitary, or both.

3. Each pituitary hormone is regulated by hypothalamic hormones via the secretion of both stimulating and inhibiting factors.

4. A hypothalamic hormone with LH and FSH releasing activity (gonadotropin-releasing hormone, GnRH) has been isolated and synthesized. Normally, a midcyclic high estrogen peak triggers a midcyclic burst of GnRH, causing LH and FSH secretion.

HYPOPITUITARISM

Sheehan's Syndrome

1. Basic Principles

a. "Sheehan's syndrome" refers specifically to postpartum hemorrhage associated with pituitary necrosis.

b. The clinical features of Sheehan's syndrome are precisely the same as those seen when the pituitary gland has been destroyed by other processes (e.g., tumor, trauma, infection), except that the onset of symptoms is more often rapid. If severe and rapid onset of symptoms occurs, correct diagnosis and immediate replacement with glucocorticoids is lifesaving.

2. Clinical Features (chronic hypopituitarism)

a. Diminished or absent axillary or pubic hair

b. Premature aging of skin

c. The breasts are usually well formed and do not atrophy.

d. Cephalic hair is thick and coarse.

e. Pelvic examination shows atrophic vaginal mucosa and a markedly hypoplastic uterus and cervix, with the adnexa usually not palpable.

3. Laboratory Findings

a. Thyroid function tests (T_4, F T_4 I, T_3, TSH) are all low by RIA.

b. Adrenal function (plasma cortisol and ACTH, urinary free cortisol, 17-hydroxysteroids, and 17-ketosteroids) is low.

c. Adrenal response to exogenous ACTH or cosyntropin is delayed but elicitable.

d. On metyrapone test, decreased 11-deoxycortisol response

e. Gonadal function is suppressed, with low FSH and LH. Premenopausal patients generally have amenorrhea or menstrual irregularities. Ovarian function is elicitable if gonadotropin stimulation tests are performed, but there is no LH or FSH response to administration of GnRH.

4. X-ray Findings

a. CT or MRI is usually abnormal, with evidence of pituitary infarction.

b. The sella turcica is normal in Sheehan's syndrome, but may be markedly enlarged from a pituitary tumor or craniopharyngioma in patients with hypopituitarism not following pregnancy.

c. Osteoporosis of the skeletal system is generally noted in long-standing disease.

5. Management

a. Complete replacement therapy with glucocorticoid and thyroid hormone.

b. Ovarian replacement therapy: Oral Premarin 2.5 mg. q.d. (or Estinyl [estradiol] 0.1 mg. q.d.) administered continuously + Provera 10 mg. b.i.d. for 7 days per month.

c. Alternative treatments: Instead of oral gonadal steroids, one may give parenteral Depo-Estradiol 10 mg. at 3-week intervals, or Delestrogen 20 mg. at 3-week intervals. Progesterone 100 mg. in oil is then given I.M. at monthly intervals.

Amenorrhea With Persistent Lactation (Galactorrhea)

1. Basic Principles

a. This may occur postpartum (Chiari-Frommel syndrome) or may be unrelated to pregnancy.

b. Inappropriate lactation may also be caused by drugs, such as opiates, diazepines, tricyclic antidepressants, phenothiazines, and reserpine derivatives.

c. Excessive estrogen (e.g., birth control pills) can lead to galactorrhea via hypothalamic suppression.

d. Lactation is also associated with hypothyroidism, and less frequently results from stresses associated with surgery and anesthesia.

2. Laboratory and X-ray Findings

a. Almost all patients with galactorrhea have elevated serum prolactin levels (> 20 ng. per ml.).

b. CT and/or MRI of the sella turcica for pituitary tumor

c. Thyroid function tests for hypothyroidism. (Primary hypothyroidism is associated with hyperprolactinemia.)

d. Note: Even with no demonstrable pituitary tumor, a patient with a markedly elevated prolactin level may be harboring a small functional microadenoma that will eventually be radiologically detectable. Such patients should have periodic radiologic, endocrinologic (prolactin), and ophthalmologic (visual field) examinations with this diagnosis in mind.

3. Management

a. The treatment of choice for galactorrhea is bromocriptine. The usual dose is 2.5 mg b.i.d. or t.i.d. daily for 3 to 6 months, if needed. Spontaneous menses may occur within a few weeks.

b. Contraception (other than birth control pills) is advisable during this therapy.

c. For patients wishing to conceive, the drug is discontinued. Should amenorrhea (anovulation) with or without galactorrhea recur, clomiphene citrate may be used to induce ovulation, in doses of 50 mg. b.i.d. for 5 to 7 days. If this is ineffective, Pergonal may be tried.

d. Note: There are no dogmatic rules concerning the treatment of small pituitary tumors. Each case must be individualized as to whether to observe periodically to detect changes, to irradiate, or to remove surgically.

MISCELLANEOUS ENDOCRINE IMBALANCE

HIRSUTISM

Basic Principles

1. Hirsutism is an understandably distressing symptom for any woman and thus has both medical and emotional components.

2. Excessive hair growth in the female, with the exception of that which is genetically acquired, is caused by increased androgen secretion.

a. The source of increased androgen can be the ovary, the adrenal glands, or both.

b. So-called idiopathic hirsutism has been ascribed to end-organ response in the skin, i.e., an aberration of end-organ metabolism of androgen by peripheral conversion of plasma precursors.

3. Thorough history taking and physical examination are important.

a. The majority of patients with hirsutism report postpubertal onset (though it may be in the teens) and gradual, slow progression.

b. Later onset and/or rapid progression suggests organic disease.

c. Oligomenorrhea or secondary amenorrhea is common.

d. Other common complaints are acne, oily skin, and infertility.

e. Virilization suggests androgenic tumors, and the findings may include baldness (occipital or temporal), increased muscular size and strength, clitoral enlargement, and deepening voice. Androgenic tumor is also suggested by defeminization, such as decreased breast size and loss of female body contours.

4. Statistically, the vast majority of women with hirsutism, irregular menses, and acne, without other clinical evidence of androgen overproduction, do not have ovarian or adrenal tumors, nor do they have Cushing's syndrome.

5. Although tumors are rare, when they do occur most virilizing ovarian tumors are benign or of low-grade malignancy, while most virilizing adrenal tumors are malignant, especially in children.

Laboratory Tests

1. Basic Principles

a. The commonly employed substances tested for are urinary 17-ketosteroids and pregnanetriol, and plasma testosterone and 17-hydroxyprogesterone.

b. A urinary creatinine test is also helpful to exclude major collection errors.

c. The 17-ketosteroid excretion may be influenced exogenously. It is increased by cephalosporins, penicillin (large doses), erythromycin, and meprobamate; it is decreased by glucocorticoids, opiates, probenecid, Dilantin, and estrogens.

d. The metyrapone test is often used for "suppression." Metyrapone selectively inhibits β-hydroxylation, preventing the formation of hydrocortisone. This in turn increases ACTH secretion, with consequent adrenocortical stimulation and (normally) a rise in 17-ketosteroid excretion. The test consists of giving three tablets of metyrapone (each 250 mg.) q.i.d. for 6 doses, having previously obtained urinary 17-ketosteroid and pregnanetriol values. A second 24-hour urine collection is begun with the fifth dose—that is, on the second morning of metyrapone ingestion.

e. If mild C21-hydroxylase deficiency is suspected then a cosyntropin stimulation test, to reveal marked increase in 17-hydroxyprogesterone plasma level, should be done.

Identifying Tests

1. With this background, the following tests may be used to help identify the organ responsible for the excessive androgen secretion.

a. *Adrenal Glands.* 17-ketosteroid and pregnanetriol levels are obtained before and during administration of metyrapone, as describe above. If there is no inordinate increase in the excretion of both these steroids, then the likelihood of adrenal origin of the hirsutism is remote. If there is a significant increase in 17-ketosteroids and pregnanetriol, then the adrenogenital syndrome must be considered. On the other hand, if the metyrapone test fails to induce an elevation of 17-ketosteroids and pregnanetriol, the ovaries must then be considered as a possible source of androgens. The following method may be employed to demonstrate this.

b. *Ovaries.* Prednisone 5 mg. P.O. b.i.d. is given for 4 days prior to, and during, the administration of human chorionic gonadotropin (HCG). HCG is administered in doses of 4,000 I.U. during those days. A significant increase in 17-ketosteroid excretion points toward ovarian origin of the hirsutism. Failure of such an increase, however, does not rule out the ovaries as a source of androgens, and calls for additional testosterone determinations. A significant increase in testosterone levels from the blood and urine (as compared with levels before the prednisone-HCG test) suggests the ovary as a source of the hirsutism.

c. *Plasma Testosterone Levels.* These are normally 0.2 to 0.8 ng. per ml. and show some elevation in most women with hirsutism and anovulation, but there is much individual variation. The reason why serum testosterone is not often significantly elevated is decreased bound testosterone; it is the unbound fraction that produces the androgenic effect. Also, serum testosterone is elevated by estrogens, hyperthyroidism, and cirrhosis; it is lowered by progestins, hypothyroidism, and glucocorticoids.

d. Note: Ovarian and adrenal vein catheterization studies of women with hirsutism who had normal or slightly elevated urinary 17-ketosteroids have led to the observations that: (1) the ovary is a common source of androgen overproduction, (2) it is not uncommon to find that the source of androgen hypersecretion is from both the ovary and the adrenals, and (3) the various suppression tests do not really correlate well with the more direct catheterization findings in terms of pinpointing the exact source of androgen oversecretion.

Management

1. If the patient wishes to conceive, the infertility takes precedence over the idiopathic hirsutism. Clomiphene citrate (Clomid), or Pergonal if the clomiphene citrate fails completely, is the method commonly employed.

2. In patients who do not desire pregnancy, hirsutism is managed by suppressing ovarian steroidogenesis with progestin administration. Any low-dose combination oral contraceptive pill given in the usual cyclic fashion will suppress plasma testosterone levels after 6 to 9 months of treatment. This slow response to treatment should be explained to the patient beforehand.

3. If oral contraceptives are contraindicated, Depo-Provera may be used instead.

4. Although these suppressive treatments will suppress new hair growth after many months, they will not affect the hair already present. Thus the patient may wish to consider such additional methods as shaving, waxing, or depilatories, at appropriate intervals, once new hair growth has ceased. For permanent hair removal, electrolysis is used.

5. The above management applies to patients whose 17-ketosteroid suppression with dexamethasone is within the normal range of 5 to 11 mg. per day.

6. If the excretion of 17-ketosteroids is profoundly suppressed (e.g., $<$ 3 mg. per day), the suspected adrenal hyperplasia is treated with a glucocorticoid, such as prednisone 5 mg. orally daily, to maintain 17-

ketosteroid excretion within the normal range.

7. A complete lack of 17-ketosteroid suppression suggests an adrenal tumor (rare), which warrants further and separate investigation.

8. One must consider the possibility of an androgen-producing ovarian tumor, which also is relatively uncommon (but not as rare as adrenal tumor), if there is:

a. An enlarged ovary

b. No enlarged ovary, but abnormally high testosterone levels

c. No enlarged ovary, and normal testosterone levels, but no decrease in the original testosterone level after 6 months of treatment with progestational steroid suppression. One should not hesitate to do an endoscopy in any questionable case, to rule out a small ovarian tumor, or an exploratory laparotomy for virilizing tumor if there is definite enlargement.

EXCESSIVE LINEAR GROWTH IN FEMALES

Basic Principles

1. The patient is frequently a daughter of very tall parents.

2. If there is no family history of tallness, a history is taken and physical and routine laboratory examinations done. A hand-wrist radiograph for bone age is important. In the physical examination the degree of development of secondary sexual characteristics is most important, since the more advanced the patient's development the less likely it is that any treatment will influence her eventual height.

3. In general, a girl who is 5 feet 8 inches tall or more and in whom sexual maturation or menarche has not occurred is a possible candidate for preventive therapy. Ideally, treatment should begin as early as age 9 or 10, but in any case it should begin before menarche.

4. Once treatment has begun, it must be continued until the epiphyses are fused; otherwise further growth will take place.

Management

1. Treatment involves the use of high dosages of estrogens to close the epiphyses and inhibit growth hormone secretion from the pituitary.

2. The estrogen best tolerated for this purpose is conjugated estrogens (Premarin). It is given in high doses (10 mg. daily, in divided doses, if tolerated—otherwise at least 5 mg. daily) for the first 25 days of each calendar month.

3. During the last five days of estrogen therapy, medroxyprogesterone acetate (Provera) 10 mg. is added, to ensure withdrawal bleeding.

4. Both the patient and the parents should be told about possible side effects such as breast engorgement, menorrhagia, and water retention.

5. If the treatment is successful, epiphyseal closure occurs in 6 to 9 months. The overall growth achieved during this time is usually less than 2 inches, and frequently less than 1 inch.

OVARIAN DYSFUNCTION

Basic Principles

1. The two basic functions of the ovaries are to produce estrogen and to form ova.

2. Ovarian function is dependent upon pituitary stimulation.

a. Pituitary follicle-stimulating hormone (FSH) promotes follicular development.

b. Both FSH and LH (luteinizing hormone) from the pituitary are necessary for normal estrogen secretion and menstrual function.

c. Ovulation is triggered by a mid-cycle surge of LH which is also required for the formation and maintenance of the corpus luteum and the secretion of its hormones, including progesterone.

3. Pituitary function depends, in turn, upon hypothalamic stimulation.

a. Hypothalamic gonadotropin-releasing hormone (GnRH) has been synthesized; it acts to release pituitary LH and FSH.

b. The mid-cycle LH surge has been attributed to feedback of the chief ovarian estrogen (estradiol), perhaps mediated by GnRH release from the hypothalamus.

4. The goal in the evaluation of gonadal-pituitary function is to determine whether the ovarian dysfunction is due primarily to ovarian inadequacy or to selective pituitary insufficiency of gonadotropic hormones. Several diagnostic procedures may be undertaken to determine the functional state of the ovary.

Testing Ovarian Dysfunction

1. *Pregnancy Test.* This should be obtained for any patient with menstrual irregularities.

2. *Progesterone Test.* Oral medroxyprogesterone acetate (Provera) 10 mg. is given twice a day for 7 days, or progesterone in oil (100 mg.) is given I.M., in order to determine whether the patient with amenorrhea will menstruate.

a. Normally, menstruation should taken place within 2 weeks if the patient has adequate proliferative phase (estrogen) function, since progesterone cannot cause endometrial shedding unless there has been prior stimulation with estrogen.

b. Failure of menstruation to occur after the progesterone test indicates inadequate estrogen secretion, possible pregnancy, or persistent function of corpora lutea.

c. No other progesterone preparations should be used for this test, because of:

(1) Pain at the site of injection (aqueous suspension)

(2) Prolongation of effect (Delalutin or Depo-Provera)

(3) Inherent estrogenic activity of agents such as contraceptive pills

3. *Vaginal Smear.* An atrophic vaginal smear suggests complete ovarian insufficiency. A cornified or partially cornified vaginal smear indicates that there is at least some estrogen production, even if there is no ovulation (in cases of amenorrhea). A patient with an atrophic smear will not menstruate after the progesterone test; one with a cornified smear most probably will.

4. *Pituitary Gonadotropin Assay.* The FSH and LH levels may be obtained by blood (RIA) samples. A high gonadotropin level suggests primary ovarian inadequacy (premature menopause) and has a poor prognosis for fertility. Low gonadotropin secretion implies either pituitary insufficiency or hypothalamic disorder; with appropriate treatment the prognosis is good. A serum prolactin level should also be obtained, and, if it is high, pituitary CT or MRI performed.

5. *Estrogen Assay*

a. With ovarian hypogonadism, there is a low serum estradiol level by RIA.

b. With primary ovarian failure the FSH and LH are high.

c. With secondary ovarian insufficiency, both the serum estradiol and serum gonadotropins (FSH, LH) are low.

d. Although early follicular phase levels of estrogen may normally be low, estradiol levels that are repeatedly lower than normal follicular phase levels by RIA indicate ovarian insufficiency.

e. In contrast to measurements of estradiol, which is almost exclusively secreted by the ovaries, serum estrone measurements are of less value, since estrone may also be formed peripherally from adrenocortical androstenedione.

5. *Chromatin Pattern.* In cases of immature or poor secondary sexual development and primary amenorrhea, a chromatin-negative pattern points toward gonadal dysgenesis. A positive chromatin pattern combined with a high FSH points toward ovarian dysgenesis or agenesis. (Note: Whenever FSH values are inappropriately high [as in premature menopause or ovarian dysgenesis], it is also important to get a karyotype determination. If a Y chromosome is found, a testicular component within the gonad is suspected, and the patient should have a prophylactic gonadectomy before neoplastic changes occur. A blood assay for H-Y antigen may also be helpful in detecting testicular tissue, even in cases where the karyotype is apparently normal.)

Clinical Entities

1. Hypothalamic-Pituitary (Secondary) Amenorrhea of Short Duration. No specific clinical stigmata are apparent. Pregnancy should always be considered.

2. Hypothalamic Amenorrhea of Long Duration. This may be caused by:

a. Major weight gain or loss (including anorexia nervosa)

b. Cessation of oral contraception (post-Pill amenorrhea)

c. Psychological factors: severe emotional stress, occasionally pseudocyesis

d. Postpartum, including Sheehan's syndrome

e. Excessive prolactin secretion, with or without galactorrhea. (The serum prolactin level will clarify this.)

3. Primary Ovarian Failure

a. In the previously menstruating woman this occurs naturally as menopause or, if at a relatively early age, as premature menopause.

b. *Ovarian Dysgenesis (Turner's Syndrome).* The patient's secondary sexual characteristics are absent and she is of short stature, with a webbed neck; cubitus valgus; normal bone age, as a rule; normal thyroid function; high FSH; cardiovascular abnormalities; and abnormalities of the terminal or middle phalanges of the fourth or fifth fingers. There is a negative chromatin pattern—Barr bodies are absent on buccal smear.

c. *Prepubertal Ovarian Insufficiency (without Dysgenesis).* The patient has a eunuchoid build, and usually is excessively tall.

(a) Pubic and axillary hair may be diminished.

(b) Secondary sexual characteristics show poor development.

Management

1. General Principles

a. In the absence of local or systemic disease, tumor, congenital abnormality, or specific hormonal imbalance, amenorrhea per se requires no treatment unless the patient wishes to become pregnant. However, since absence of menstruation may cause emotional disturbance to some women by making them feel sexually inadequate or abnormal, and since absence of menstruation for a prolonged time may predispose to endometrial hyperplasia, it is generally prudent and helpful to induce artificial menstrual cycles.

b. Before hormonal therapy is begun, there should be an attempt to correct any dietary excesses or deficiencies and to relieve unfavorable emotional and environmental situations. Often such measures alone will result in the spontaneous resumption of menses.

c. The patient may be given conjugated estrogens (Premarin) 1.25 mg. q.d. for 21 days, or ethinyl estradiol (Estinyl) 0.05 mg. in the same manner. Medroxyprogesterone acetate (Provera) 10 mg. is given during the last 12 days of estrogen administration. Most patients will menstruate within 10 days of such therapy, which may then be repeated either monthly or every few months.

d. Failure to menstruate after such estrogen-progesterone administration is rare; it indicates endometrial failure, and generally has a poor prognosis. Before drawing that conclusion, however, one should try giving the progesterone parenterally instead of orally, since some patients do not absorb the oral medication well.

e. For those patients who wish to become pregnant, and in whom amenorrhea or faulty ovulation is the chief problem, the use of clomiphene citrate (Clomid) 50 mg. for 5 days starting on the fifth day of an induced menstrual cycle is often helpful in inducing ovulation and, thus, spontaneous menstruation. The dosage of Clomid may have to be increased according to the response, or lack of it, as determined by the basal temperature graph, endometrial biopsy, and pelvic examinations to detect any tendency toward cystic ovaries. In those infertility patients in whom pituitary insufficiency is the background cause of the ovarian problem, human menopausal gonadotropin (HMG, Pergonal) has been highly successful in inducing ovulation.

2. Turner's Syndrome

a. Conjugated estrogens (Premarin) 1.25 mg. b.i.d. may be given daily without interruption.

b. Provera 10 mg. b.i.d. is given for a week, beginning on the first day of each calendar month.

c. If the estrogen dose is not sufficient to adequately develop the patient, it may be doubled, and the Provera dose increased to 30 mg. per day. Ethinyl estradiol (Estinyl) may be substituted for the Premarin in doses of 0.05 mg. twice a day.

d. Estrogens should not be started unless the patient has reached her full growth potential, or unless she is so upset about her lack of secondary sexual characteristics as not to mind the prospect of not growing any more.

e. Since fertility is virtually absent in such cases, hormonal substitution therapy is all that can be offered.

f. However, it should be kept in mind that ovarian tumors (dysgerminomas, embryonal cell carcinomas) arise more often in dysgenetic ovaries. Tumor development is especially frequent when mosaicism is present, particularly in 45X/46XY individuals. For this reason, preventive oophorectomy should be done if the karyotype shows a Y chromosome.

3. Prepubertal Ovarian Insufficiency. This condition is treated only if the patient is excessively tall. High-dosage estrogen is given in an effort to close her epiphyses, thus preventing further growth. At the same time, progesterone is given to deciduate the endometrium monthly. Premarin may be given, 2.5 mg., two tablets twice daily. Provera 10 mg. t.i.d. may be given for one week of each month, during which time the patient does not take Premarin.

4. Uterine Agenesis

a. Basic Principles

(1) The patient is a normal-appearing female (normal feminization).

(2) Cyclic changes occur in the vaginal smear, but with no menstruation.

(3) The patient does not menstruate after treatment with progesterone, whether it is given alone or with estrogen.

(4) The vaginal introitus is shallow.

b. Management

(1) This is a congenital phenomenon caused by absent or rudimentary development of the uterus.

(2) Hormonal therapy is not indicated.

(3) If the vaginal introitus is too shallow for sexual intercourse, surgical correction of the vaginal defect is indicated.

5. Testicular Feminization Syndrome

a. Basic Principles

(1) The patient is a normally developed female, but with diminished or absent pubic or axillary hair and a short vaginal tract.

(2) The chromatin pattern is negative.

(3) The patient may have bilaterally palpable inguinal masses or hernias.

(4) The vaginal smear may show evidence of diminished estrogenic activity.

(5) The pituitary FSH may be high.

(6) The patient cannot be masculinized with androgens, nor does she

menstruate after progesterone given alone or in combination with estrogen.

(7) Vaginal dilatation may have to be performed in order to produce an adequate vaginal introitus.

(8) The patient may have a rudimentary uterus-like structure.

b. Management

(1) A patient with this syndrome must have her testes removed at about age 17 to 18 to avoid anaplastic changes.

(2) Replacement therapy with estrogen is necessary when such surgery is performed.

(3) It is unwise to tell the patient or family that "testicles" or other male features are present, since the mere knowledge of the presence of any features of the opposite sex may cause profound emotional distress.

MULTIGLANDULAR DYSFUNCTION STEIN-LEVENTHAL SYNDROME

Basic Principles

1. This syndrome, also referred to as polycystic or sclerocystic ovarian disease, is not a specific entity. It is associated with a thickened, fibrotic ovarian tunica and accompanied by an ovarian follicular cystic disorder. It is still unclear whether these abnormal ovarian changes constitute the etiological basis of the "syndrome," or whether they are simply one of the effects.

2. The following are frequent findings:

a. Failure to ovulate, or only occasional ovulation

b. Infertility, either primary or secondary

c. Hirsutism (in about half of cases)

d. Thickened ovarian tunica and multifollicle cysts (smooth white capsule)

e. The ovaries are usually, but not necessarily, enlarged.

f. Obesity may be present.

g. Menometrorrhagia, though uncommon, may occur between episodes of amenorrhea.

Laboratory and Other Findings

1. There are no "typical" laboratory findings in the so-called Stein-Leventhal syndrome.

2. Efforts to determine the source of increased androgens in women with polycystic ovarian disease are often difficult.

a. In the 25 per cent of patients in whom urinary 17-ketosteroids are significantly elevated, suppression by prednisone or dexamethasone (though inconsistent) appears to implicate the adrenal cortex. If suppression followed the administration of estrogen, an ovarian source of androgen would be implicated.

b. In about 50 per cent of patients with polycystic disease, there is elevation of the plasma testosterone and androstenedione. However, the testosterone level is usually well below 200 ng. per 100 ml. If levels are higher than this, one should suspect an androgen-secreting adrenal or ovarian tumor.

c. Ovarian and adrenal vein catheterization studies in women with excess androgens (but without distinct elevations of urinary 17-ketosteroids) have demonstrated that:

(1) The ovary is indeed a frequent source of androgen.

(2) Sometimes excessive androgen can arise from both an ovary and an adrenal gland.

(3) Suppression and stimulation tests appear to be of very little value in locating the source of excess androgen.

3. Characteristically, FSH levels are low or normal, while LH levels tend to be relatively high.

4. Estradiol levels are usually normal, while estrone levels are usually high.

5. Pelvic examination may reveal palpably enlarged ovaries.

6. The cervical mucus is typically profuse and clear, on account of unopposed estrogen production.

7. Endoscopy (either culdoscopy or laparoscopy) will confirm the presence of

polycystic ovaries. Sonograms are often helpful in suggesting this disorder.

Management

1. If fertility is not desired, one can consider the use of Provera 10 mg. b.i.d. for 7 days each month, for a limited time, to deciduate the endometrium.

2. A special problem exists for those women who plan to have no children: They are bothered mainly by hirsutism and functional uterine bleeding, and there is some evidence that untreated polycystic disease with amenorrhea may increase the potential for endometrial cancer. For these reasons it is desirable to suppress ovarian function by giving cyclic estrogen and progesterone. Oral contraceptives (such as those containing ethinyl estradiol and mestranol) help to replace endogenous estrogen and suppress ovarian androgen production. Continued use of oral contraceptives, by suppressing the pituitary, helps to arrest abnormal steroid secretion.

3. When pregnancy is desired, the drug of choice to induce ovulation is clomiphene citrate (Clomid). Starting with 50 mg. daily for 5 days from the fifth day of the cycle, the dose can be gradually increased up to 150 mg. The aim is to achieve ovulation, as demonstrated by the basal temperature graph, endometrial biopsy, serum progesterone, or sonograms. The patient must be monitored carefully by pelvic examination toward the end of the first cycle, to make sure there is no overstimulation (significant cystic ovarian enlargement). Such examination should be repeated if the dosage is increased.

4. If Clomid, or Clomid plus HCG, is unsuccessful in stimulating ovulation, human menopausal gonadotropin (Pergonal) may be tried, but with great care; women with polycystic ovarian disease are particularly prone to overstimulation. Monitoring should include frequent estrogen levels and pelvic sonograms. Clomid and Pergonal may also be used in combination.

5. In those rare instances where Clomid has failed and Pergonal is contraindicated or refused, wedge resection of the ovaries may be considered. The results are generally favorable as far as ovulation is concerned, and are further enhanced by the use of Clomid after the resection.

SEXUAL PRECOCITY

Basic Principles

1. The occurrence of menses prior to age 10 is considered precocious.

2. This may be the first symptom, though commonly there is also increased growth, followed by pubic hair and breast development.

3. Though most cases of sexual precocity in females are idiopathic, this diagnosis cannot be made except by exclusion, with careful follow-up in an effort to uncover a slow-growing lesion in the ovary, adrenal gland, or brain.

4. The history is important, since a familial occurrence makes the likelihood of tumors very small.

5. Premature development of the female secondary sex characteristics may be seen in patients with:

a. Idiopathic causes—i.e., constitutional sexual precocity (most common)

b. Space-occupying brain tumor, particularly in the region of the third ventricle

c. History of encephalitis or meningitis

d. Cranial injury

e. Hypothyroidism

6. Other neoplasms may induce sexual precocity, including tumors of the adrenal glands or of the ovaries—i.e., tumors primarily associated with increased estrogenic production, such as:

a. Feminizing tumor of the adrenals (very rare)

b. Theca cell tumors of the ovary

c. Granulosa cell tumors of the ovary
d. Brenner tumors of the ovary

Clinical Features

1. Precocious development of breasts and pubic and axillary hair

2. Height and weight much greater than in normal females of the same age

3. Premature menarche

Laboratory Findings

1. Increased estrogen level in 24-hour urine or in blood sample

2. Vaginal cornification

3. Low FSH in most patients; occasionally normal FSH

4. Both FSH and LH measurements are indicated to ascertain gonadotropic function. The urinary 17-ketosteroid should also be measured, and thyroid tests done. However, parameters of thyroid and adrenal function are usually normal.

Differentiation Between Neoplastic and Corticoidal Types

1. An initial vaginal smear is taken, and followed by the administration of 100 mg. medroxyprogesterone acetate (Depo-Provera) I.M. at weekly intervals for three injections. The smear is repeated each week.

2. A change in the vaginal smear from one with normal estrogenic activity to one with marked estrogenic deficiency is not a characteristic finding in patients with adrenal or ovarian tumors, and indicates premature release of pituitary gonadotropin. If the vaginal smear (after the injections) shows secretory activity without estrogenic deficiency, then the patient must be suspected of having an ovarian or adrenal tumor. In clinical practice, however, it is important to keep in mind that if a tumor is present, it is usually palpable; therefore, thorough physical examination is most important.

Management

1. Constitutional type (idiopathic): Treatment when no cause can be found is limited to the use of a potent progestational agent in order to inhibit gonadotropin production.

a. Administration of Depo-Provera in large doses, 400 mg. I.M. monthly for 3 months, then once every 3 months thereafter. The dosage and schedule may be modified according to the amount necessary to induce castration changes in the vaginal mucosa.

(1) This stops menstruation, and thus prevents the child from being psychologically upset by a physiological state which is greatly advanced beyond the norm for her age.

(2) Breast development decreases and stops. (Pubic hair will not disappear.)

(3) Premature closure of the epiphyses is delayed by this procedure. (Although the child is tall for her age, accelerated sexual development and secretion of estrogens, if unchecked by treatment, would cause premature closure of the epiphyses, with the result that she would eventually be much shorter than her agemates.)

(4) Because children lack the necessary self-possession, as well as the bodily strength, to resist improper advances, a sexually precocious girl may be preyed upon sexually and become impregnated at an early age. Depo-Provera prevents menses from occurring, and so makes impregnation impossible; in addition, it may curtail any libidinous drive the patient may have.

(5) Treatment should be continued until the chronological age matches the bone age, or until age 12 to 13. Hand-wrist films should be obtained every 6 months until epiphyseal closure has been demonstrated.

(6) If there is any breakthrough bleeding after the start of Depo-Provera therapy, it may be stopped by estrogen (e.g., Premarin 1.25 mg. daily for a week).

ANOVULATION

Basic Principles

1. Absence of ovulation is physiologically normal and expected during the first year or two after menarche, and again at the approach of menopause.

2. In the woman who is not interested in becoming pregnant, anovulation per se is unimportant if she has normal periods (anovulatory menses).

3. More frequently, anovulation is accompanied by abnormal bleeding (menorrhagia, metrorrhagia) or amenorrhea. These are often associated with the development of endometrial hyperplasia from unopposed estrogen stimulation.

4. The most frequent clinical manifestation of anovulation is amenorrhea of the hypothalamic type.

a. This may occur during any stressful experience—travel, overwork, etc.

b. Weight loss is another common cause—particularly "crash" diets. For reasons not clearly understood, weight loss may lead to a hypogonadotropic state.

c. Obesity may also be associated with anovulation, but here the amenorrhea is not usually associated with a hypogonadotropic state unless the patient has a concomitant emotional disorder.

Tests for Ovulation

1. Basal temperature chart which shows a biphasic curve

2. Change in vaginal smear from cornified to luteal type

3. Cervical mucus

a. Clear, thin, stretchable (*spinnbarkeit*) during and before ovulation

b. Thick, viscid, not stretchable postovulation

c. Ferning on microscopic examination of a dried smear from the cervix, which increases as ovulation approaches, then gradually disappears

4. Endometrial biopsy, showing postovulatory secretory phase.

5. Serum progesterone (by RIA) elevated after ovulation

All of the above criteria for ovulation are actually measures of increased progesterone production; on this basis ovulation is presumed.

Absolute Evidence of Ovulation

1. Direct observation of the ovaries by endoscopy or at laparotomy

2. Pregnancy

Induction of Ovulation

1. Before attempts to induce ovulation in a woman who wishes to conceive, the couple should be ascertained to be normal with regard to:

a. Tubal patency (Rubin test, hysterosalpingogram, endoscopy if needed)

b. Semen quality

c. Postcoital (Huhner) test

d. Thyroid, pituitary, and adrenal function, by tests previously outlined

2. There should be normal proliferative phase activity as evinced by:

a. Regular menses (even though anovulatory), or menses occurring at irregular intervals

b. Normal (cornified) vaginal smear

c. In the amenorrheic patient, menstrual response after administration of progesterone

d. Normal serum prolactin (and pituitary tomogram, if prolactin is elevated)

Management

1. Improvement of general constitutional state (environment, life-style stresses) and nutrition (obesity, underweight), as well as correction of any specific hormonal defect (e.g., thyroid) that may be found.

2. For women who do not wish to conceive, the use of cyclic estrogen and progesterone or one of the oral contraceptives will not induce ovulation but will deciduate the endometrium at regular intervals, thus preventing the development of hyperplasia or adenomatous hyperplasia.

3. For women who wish to conceive, and in whom estrogenic and pituitary function are normal, the following treatment is recommended:

a. Clomiphene citrate (Clomid) 50 mg. daily for 5 days starting on the fifth day of the cycle. If ovulation fails to occur, as determined by the basal temperature graph, endometrial biopsy, or progesterone levels, the dose of Clomid may be increased by 50 mg. daily up to 150 mg. per day. The Clomid is usually begun on the fifth day of a spontaneous or a progesterone-induced period, and the dosage is closely monitored by a pelvic examination, about 2 weeks after completion of medication, to determine if there is any evidence of ovarian cystic formation. If there is such overreaction, the drug may be stopped for the next month or two and then resumed more cautiously with smaller dose increments.

b. In some cases, induction of ovulation with Clomid is enhanced by the addition of HCG, 5,000 to 10,000 I.U. given about 3 to 5 days after the last Clomid medication.

c. The use of Pergonal (human menopausal gonadotropin—HMG) is indicated for a minority of cases of infertility where all factors are normal but the anovulation is due to a very low pituitary gonadotropin secretion (FSH). The dosages of Pergonal and HCG must be worked out individually, and the patient must be strictly monitored because of the tendency toward complications such as ovarian cysts, ascites, and multiple births.

d. Wedge resection of the ovaries (now rare) may be considered in women with polycystic ovaries, when Clomid has failed to induce ovulation and Pergonal is either contraindicated or refused.

MENORRHAGIA

Basic Principles

1. Excessive uterine bleeding may have either an organic or a functional origin; in this discussion we will assume that organic causes have been ruled out.

2. Functional uterine bleeding requires endocrine evaluation as well as hematologic examination to rule out bleeding tendency.

3. Such bleeding is most prevalent in adolescence and near menopause. In both of these situations, a common cause is anovulatory bleeding due to continued estrogen stimulation without progesterone formation.

4. The remaining causes of functional (or dysfunctional) uterine bleeding are probably endocrine imbalances involving the thyroid, pituitary, or adrenal glands. It can also follow estrogen (or progesterone) withdrawal.

Diagnostic Procedures

1. Laboratory blood studies

2. Endometrial biopsy

3. Rule out endocrine (thyroid, adrenal) dysfunction.

Management

1. Most patients with severe functional bleeding have proliferative endometrium, some to the point of hyperplasia. The first step, if menorrhagia is associated with anemia, is to stop the bleeding.

2. A potent progestational agent such as norethindrone acetate (Norlutate) 5 mg., three to four tablets at once, usually stops the bleeding promptly. The Norlutate can then be continued 5 mg. b.i.d. for the next 3 weeks. The drug changes the endometrium to a secretory phase, and its cessation promotes endometrial shedding.

3. The Norlutate can then be restarted on the fifth day of the next (induced) menstrual period (sooner if bleeding tends to be heavy again), and continued cyclically in doses of 10 mg. daily (or more, if needed), for 3 weeks at a time.

4. Anemia should be corrected by the simultaneous use of an oral iron preparation.

5. If there is specific thyroid or other endocrine dysfunction, therapy is directed toward that specific abnormality.

6. When the patient begins having normal "periods" from the cyclic progestational agent, it can be discontinued in favor of simply shedding the endometrium at monthly intervals with any progestational steroid, such as Provera in doses of 10 mg. b.i.d. for 7 days, for the next 2 to 3 consecutive months.

7. If parenteral preparations are preferred, progesterone in oil, 100 mg. I.M., is often effective in controlling bleeding.

8. Obviously, if severe bleeding is not reasonably controlled by any of these measures, the diagnosis of functional bleeding should be reassessed in favor of a previously missed organic cause, whether intrauterine pathology or adenomyosis, and appropriate measures taken (e.g., D&C, hysteroscopy).

9. Postmenopausal bleeding can also be functional (atrophic endometrium), but in such instances it is essential to rule out uterine pathology before coming to that conclusion.

MENOPAUSE

Basic Principles

1. The menopause, which means cessation of menses, is physiological and due to ovarian senescence and decline in estrogen production.

2. It is considered definitely established after 1 year of amenorrhea, at which time there is a concurrent loss of reproductive function.

3. The broader term *climacteric* refers to a general and gradual decline in ovarian function; it encompasses a span of years, during which time menopause occurs.

Symptomatology of the Climacteric and/or Menopause

1. Amenorrhea, usually preceded by irregular (progressively less frequent) menses

2. Anovulation

3. Vasomotor symptoms—flushes and sweating

4. Vaginal discomforts and/or dyspareunia due to atrophic vaginitis

5. Urinary discomforts due to atrophic urethritis and trigonitis

6. A host of other symptoms have often been attributed to "menopause" but, because of their emotional and psychosomatic components, might also be attributed to life-style factors and the multiple stresses of middle age. These include depression, insomnia, headache, fatigue, nervousness, backache, myalgias, etc. In any individual instance it is difficult to isolate the specific contribution that estrogen deficiency makes, for two reasons:

a. When estrogen replacement therapy puts an end to flushes, sweats, and atrophic vaginal discomforts, the patient will expectedly feel much better, and this may be reflected in an improvement in her vaguer emotional symptoms.

b. There may be a placebo effect when estrogen is given for "menopausal" symptoms.

Physical Findings

1. The physical changes most directly due to estrogen deprivation occur in the female genital tract. They include smaller uterus and ovaries, thin endometrium, and atrophic vaginal mucosa.

2. There may also be less muscle tone and fascial strength in pelvic structures, predisposing to pelvic relaxation and atrophy.

3. Additional atrophic changes are general loss of labial subcutaneous fat, sagging of the breasts, and markedly diminished cervical secretions.

4. Not all changes in muscle, skin, and bone (e.g., osteoporosis) are due to estrogen deficiency; other contributing factors are protein catabolism, degenerative changes of aging, and muscle disuse.

Laboratory Findings

1. Decreased estrogenic activity in the vaginal mucosa, as seen on wet or stained smear, showing gradually increasing numbers of intermediate and, finally, parabasal cells

2. Elevated FSH

Management

1. Management must be individualized.

2. A careful history taking and physical examination are essential. One cannot properly assess the multiple, often vague, symptomatology of "menopause" without knowing the patient's personal, marital, sexual, and socioeconomic history.

3. Vaginal discomforts and dyspareunia due to atrophic vaginitis are promptly relieved by the use of a local estrogenic cream, which can then be used preventively every 2 or 3 weeks.

4. Classic symptoms such as flushes and sweats can be dramatically eliminated by oral estrogen therapy.

a. The lowest dose that will make the patient comfortable is preferred. Therefore, one may start with conjugated estrogen (Premarin) 0.3 to 0.625 mg. daily. Higher doses may be necessary, according to clinical response.

b. A progestational agent such as medroxyprogesterone acetate (Provera) 10 mg. daily is given for 12 to 13 days each month to deciduate the endometrium.

c. Depending upon the response to treatment, medication may be gradually discontinued.

5. Even though estrogen is specifically helpful for the symptoms mentioned, the benefits of estrogen therapy must be reappraised in light of several reports that relate the prolonged use of estrogen with an increased risk of endometrial carcinoma.

a. The FDA requires that warnings of this possible effect be placed on all estrogen products, so it should be discussed with the patient.

b. It may be reassuring for the patient to know that there are additional measures that the physician can take to minimize this risk, whether real or potential:

(1) Careful history taking and physical examination have already been stressed.

(2) Preliminary screening of the endometrium by intrauterine Pap smears, endometrial biopsy, and/or office suction curettage is helpful in establishing a baseline.

(3) Thereafter, annual office suction curettage, or at least endometrial biopsy, would be a prudent follow-up for any patient on long-term therapy.

(4) Most important, the addition of a progestational compound, as outlined, minimizes concern about increased risk of endometrial cancer.

6. Estrogens are contraindicated in any woman with a history of, or in the presence of, cancer of the breast or endometrium, inasmuch as some of these tumors may be hormone-dependent and thus might be stimulated by estrogen therapy. In addition, estrogen should not be prescribed, or at least should be prescribed with great caution, to women with edema from cardiac decompensation, renal disease, or severe liver disease.

Estrogen Use in Prophylaxis

1. There is increasing evidence that coronary disease in postmenopausal women is diminished by *estrogen* replacement, probably by favorably altering lipoprotein levels. However, since the addition of progestins tends to reverse this beneficial effect, more epidemiological studies are needed to see of cardioprotection is still obtained. There are also ongoing studies in which the amount of progestin is greatly reduced but taken daily with the estrogen.

2. There are many studies favoring estrogen as a preventive measure against, and for treatment of, osteoporosis. The minimal effective dosage is thought to be 0.625 mg. of conjugated estrogens (Premarin) daily, which should be combined with Provera (10 mg.) for 12 to 13 days each month to minimize the risk of overstimulating the endometrium. Osteoporosis is a multifaceted disorder and is also influenced by other therapeutic measures, such as a high calcium intake, vitamin D supplementation, increased fluoride intake, and a systematic weight-bearing exercise program. It is prudent to have a preliminary bone density study to determine whether estrogen is needed and, if there is a demonstrable risk factor, to have comparative follow-up x-rays every year or two.

28 Family Planning

Hugh R. K. Barber

The purpose of family planning is to assist individuals in achieving their reproductive goals. Family planning is population control exercised at the individual rather than the national or global level.

There are three kinds of sexual intercourse (coitus): intercourse in order to procreate, intercourse to complement a relationship, and intercourse for pleasure. Contraception permits a couple to make a conscious decision about the purpose of an individual act of intercourse.

BASIC PRINCIPLES

1. Demographers report that the low reproduction rate and the inordinately high death rate of the human allowed for a stable population from the beginning of civilization until about 1850, when the population first reached 1 billion.

a. Since 1850, the world population has taken an incredibly sharp turn upward.

b. By 1930, in slightly less than 100 years, the population had doubled to 2 billion, largely due to the falling death rate and lowered infant mortality. Modern medicine and advances in nutrition have cut the death rate throughout the world, producing a fantastic population growth rate. Death rates for both children and adults have fallen sharply in recent years, due, in some part, to successful assistance in combating such ancient killers as malaria, cholera, typhus, typhoid, and smallpox.

c. By 1960, another billion had been added in less than half that time. The current rate of population growth is 2 per cent per year, or 76 million humans per year. In the developing countries, where population is increasing most dramatically, food production is rising at an average rate of 2.7 per cent annually. But the minimum food requirement considered sufficient to supply adequate diets is increasing at an even faster rate—4 per cent annually. If this gap is not closed through increased food production and decreased population growth, the great majority of people will be undernourished and unschooled, economically unproductive and living in hovels.

d. With the recent birth of a Yugoslavian baby, the world population reached 5 billion.

If world population growth continues at the annual rate of 2 per cent, as it has been since 1950, there will a doubling of the world population every 35 years. In the year 2022 there will be 10 billion people.

e. Among low-income, poorly educated parents surveyed, 56 per cent of their children were unplanned and 31 per cent were unwanted.

f. Over one-seventh (15 per cent) of all children in the United States under the age of 18 are reared in poverty. Over one-fifth (21 per cent) of the children in families with five or more children are being reared in poverty. Among whites, about one-ninth of all children (11 per cent) and over one-seventh of children in families with five or more children (15 per cent) are reared in poverty. Among blacks, over 40 per cent of all children and 44 per cent of children in families with 5 or more children are being reared in poverty.

g. It is estimated that by the year 2000, the world's population could reach 7 billion (highly theoretical) people (twice the world's population today).

h. Successful planned population control or some unforeseen catastrophe could change this trend.

2. Demographers agree that responsible parents today should plan a family of two, or not more than three, children, in an effort to replace but not increase the world population.

3. Acceptance of family planning must be voluntary. Motivation will determine who will participate.

4. It has been calculated that a single unprotected exposure, at any time in the menstrual cycle, regardless of cycle regularity, carries a pregnancy risk of 2 to 4 per cent, while one episode of intercourse every 5 days yields a 20-per-cent chance of conception in one cycle.

5. The patient's contraceptive method of choice should be prescribed unless there are medical contraindications.

6. Counseling allows the contraceptive user to make and implement an informed choice. It is the most important factor influencing correct usage of the chosen method, as well as assuring good continuation rates.

7. The moral and ethical values of the patient must be respected, and counseling must be carried out within the framework of those views.

8. Once an option has been selected, a complete physical examination, including a pelvic examination and appropriate laboratory testing, should be carried out.

9. Follow-up visits should be outlined.

METHODOLOGY

Abstinence

1. Despite the increase in pressure from society to participate in sexual activity, abstinence, or refraining from sexual intercourse, remains a commonly chosen contraceptive option in the United States and in other areas of the world. In fact, sexual abstinence has probably, historically, been the single most important factor in curtailing human fertility.

2. Couples should be queried about their moral and ethical views of sexual practices.

3. It is important to counsel them on methods of sexual fulfillment other than sexual intercourse. It is rare that this situation will arise, but it must be dealt with when it does.

4. If they elect to use contraception at a later date the couple should be made aware that it will be available to them.

Coitus Interruptus (Withdrawal)

1. In this method, the husband withdraws his penis just prior to ejaculation.

2. Coitus interruptus is used to a limited extent in the United States (by only about 2 per cent of couples using contraception); however, it is used extensively in some other nations. It is the approach used by 18 per cent of French couples, 29 per cent of Italian couples, and 30 per cent of couples in Poland.

3. For this method to be successful, the man must have good self-control and be highly motivated, with a strong sense of his responsibility to protect his sexual partner.

4. It is completely unsatisfactory for men with premature or early ejaculation. It is estimated that 50 per cent of all males are not able to use this method successfully due to an inability to control ejaculation.

5. Some pre-ejaculatory fluid (often said to be semen stored in the prostate or penile urethra or in Cowper's gland) can escape at any time prior to ejaculation. This fluid contains more sperm after recent ejaculation, though any drop may contain millions of sperm.

6. The failure rate of coitus interruptus is approximately 15 to 25 pregnancies per 100 woman-years in all users.

7. It has no medical side effects, no cost is involved, and it is always available.

8. Since withdrawal at the time of ejaculation is unnatural, it may diminish the sexual satisfaction of the couple.

Sex Without Intercourse

1. Intimate sex without intercourse is one of the contraceptive options a couple may choose. "Outercourse" (sexual alternatives to intercourse) has recently been hailed as a method of birth control which is 99-per cent effective, free from side effects, and simple to use and teach. It may lower the risk of acquiring sexually transmissible infections and may be helpful in dealing with common sexual problems.

2. Non-coital forms of sexual intimacy exist in many cultures. Sex without intercourse encompasses a continuum of activities from holding hands, hugging, kissing, massage, and dancing, to mutual masturbation, petting, oral-genital sex, and the use of stimulating devices such as vibrators.

Rhythm Method (Safe Period)

1. This method is based on three concepts:

a. that the fertilizable life span of an oocyte is no more than 24 hours after ovulation,

b. that sperm survival in the female genital tract is no greater than 4 days,

c. and that ovulation, which determines the rhythm of a cycle, occurs 14 days before the menstrual flow.

2. This means the avoidance of coitus around the time of ovulation. The woman must take her temperature every morning, watching for a drop followed by a sustained rise, which indicates ovulation.

3. Once the normal rhythm has been established, the woman may assume that ovulation occurs between days 12 and 14. Another day is added to allow for ovum survival, and, as sperm may live for at least 3 days, coitus must be avoided from the ninth to the eighteenth day (the seventh to twentieth day would be safer).

4. Even this semi-celibacy is unreliable because it depends too much on regularity of ovulation.

5. Failure rate is 38 pregnancies per 100 woman-years of use.

Natural Family Planning (NFP)

1. This has been referred to as the *mucus method.* In some women, changes in the character and appearance of cervical secretion and the cervix occur just before ovulation. In addition, women may experience ovulatory pain.

2. Observation of these physiological changes can help a woman determine at what point during her menstrual cycle she is fertile. When such observations are used for fertility control, this approach has been referred to as the *ovulation,* or Billings, method of natural family planning. Actually, all three fertility awareness methods—the calendar method, basal body temperature (BBT), and the mucus method—have historically been called natural family planning.

3. This is a summary of the mucus characteristics that should be used to train patients and staff:

a. *Amount* (volume) refers to the woman's subjective interpretation of what she feels with her fingers at the introitus and/or inside her vagina.

b. *Viscosity* means the consistency of mucus.

c. *Color* can vary quite a bit, and clear mucus may be tinged with blood at the time of ovulation.

d. *Spinnbarkeit* means (literally) *elasticity* (how far a mucus sample will stretch before it breaks).

4. The effectiveness of the mucus method, like the effectiveness of basal body temperature, is increased if intercourse is restricted to the post-ovulatory phase of the cycle.

Sheath (Condom, "French Letter")

1. A thin rubber sheath or a sheath made from a lamb's cecum is placed over the erect penis.

2. This is probably the most widely used mechanical contraceptive in the world.

3. The precautions that must be practiced with its use are:

a. To leave a "dead space" in the condom from which air has been expelled to receive the ejaculate (some have a built-in receptacle)

b. To use proper lubrication, if necessary (some are prelubricated)

c. To effect withdrawal before cessation of the erection

d. To grasp the ring of the sheath at the time of withdrawal to prevent it from slipping off

4. It protects against both pregnancy and venereal disease. It is most useful, therefore, in casual intercourse.

5. In men with premature ejaculation, the condom may blunt the sensation sufficiently to prolong the intercourse time.

6. It may also deleteriously interfere with sensation. In older men who have difficulty achieving full erection, it is impossible to use.

7. It may interrupt the mood, as application of the condom requires an erect penis.

8. Instruction of the partners in effective use can be aided by advising the female to apply the condom at the time of foreplay, which may offset the reduced sexual pleasure some couples say they experience.

9. It is not satisfactory in hot climates because of the deterioration of rubber.

10. The failure rate is 18 to 20 pregnancies per 100 woman-years of use. Failure in most instances is due to rupture of the condom, with the deposition of the entire ejaculate into the vagina.

The Vaginal Diaphragm ("Dutch Cap")

1. This is a rubber diaphragm which, when smeared with spermicidal cream, will prevent sperm from reaching the cervical canal.

2. It must fit snugly behind the pubic bone and over the cervix into the posterior fornix.

3. The diaphragm should not be removed until at least 8 hours after the last intercourse.

4. In the early days of marriage the most satisfactory method for using a diaphragm is to insert it each night with jelly or cream before retiring and to remove it, cleanse it, and reinsert it with jelly the following evening.

5. The failure rate is 15 pregnancies per 100 woman-years of use.

Chemical Methods (Aerosol, Foams, Jellies, Creams, and Suppositories)

1. The spermicidal ingredient used is usually p-triisoprophylphenolopolyetoxyethanol.

2. The aerosol and gels are effective immediately, whereas the tablets require from 5 to 10 minutes to dissolve before effectiveness.

3. The advantage of these methods is that they are inexpensive, easy to use, and require no instruction.

4. The disadvantage is that the woman or man may experience local irritation from them.

5. The failure rate is between 15 and 40 per 100 woman-years of use.

Vaginal Contraceptive Sponge

1. The vaginal contraceptive sponge is a soft, polyurethane foam sponge containing Nonoxynol-9 (a spermicide used by millions of women for more than 20 years), and other forms of intravaginal drug products.

2. It has a unique three-way action which provides safe and reliable protection without hormones and without the serious risk of dangerous side effects.

3. The vaginal contraceptive sponge

a. Continuously releases an extremely effective spermicide which quickly kills sperm on contact

b. Blocks the path of the sperm

c. Absorbs sperm

Intrauterine Devices (IUD)

1. A polyethylene spiral or coil is inserted into the uterine cavity and effectively prevents conception, although the mode of action is not known.

2. Ovulation is not prevented and no recognizable characteristic changes occur in the endometrium.

3. The great advantage of this method is the lack of necessity for high motivation. Once it is in place no further action is needed by the patient.

4. It should be placed in the uterus at the time of menstruation by an experienced gynecologist.

5. The disadvantages of this method are the menstrual complications which occur, i.e., excessive, profuse periods, irregular bleeding between periods, and abdominal cramps.

6. Major complications include pelvic infection, perforation, and pregnancy.

7. Medicated IUDs (those containing copper or progesterone) appear to have increased effectiveness when compared to inert plastic devices.

8. The copper IUD has two disadvantages: first, the introduction into the system of copper, a potentially toxic metal, and, second, the necessity for removal and reinsertion every 2 years.

9. If pregnancy occurs with an IUD in place, its removal will reduce spontaneous abortion from a rate of about 50 per cent to approximately 25 per cent.

10. Removal, if there is a pregnancy, reduces the likelihood of septic abortion.

11. If a pregnancy occurs, there is a relatively greater chance that it will be an ectopic pregnancy.

12. The failure rate is 2.3 per 100 woman-years of use.

13. Although the IUD has been removed from the market in the United States by most companies, it is still manufactured by at least two companies. It is therefore important for doctors to be familiar with its indications and contraindications.

Oral Contraception (OC)

1. These drugs are taken by mouth and permit the patient to indulge in normal coitus without the risk of conception.

2. The efficacy of the Pill in preventing pregnancy is the greatest of any form of contraception short of permanent sterilization.

3. The oral contraceptives are efficacious in preventing pregnancy primarily by inhibiting the midcycle release of luteinizing hormone (LH), thereby blocking ovulation.

4. Other changes contributing to preventing pregnancy are:

a. Changes in tubal transport

b. Changes to the nature of the endometrium and cervical mucus

5. The combination pill contains either mestranol or ethinyl estradiol and the progestin is usually norethynodrel or norethindrone.

6. The sequential types of oral contraceptive have been removed from the market.

7. The reported complications of OC use are:

a. Thrombophlebitis

b. Cancer of the endometrium

c. Hypertension

d. Postpill amenorrhea

e. Emotional lability and depression

f. Myocardial infarction

g. Cerebral infarction

h. Gallbladder disease and benign and malignant hepatomas

8. The failure rate is less than 1 pregnancy per 100 years of use in the combination method.

9. Contraceptive steroids may interfere with the treatment of hypertension because of their effect on blood pressure.

10. Conversely, some drugs effect the action of contraceptive steroids. These include the anticonvulsants. Breakthrough bleeding and failure of contraception may occur in patients taking diphenylhydantoin, rifampicin, griseofulvin, or phenobarbitone. This may result because these drugs increase the activity of hepatic enzymes which metabolize steroids. Antibiotics such as ampicillin, the tetracyclines, and neomycin prevent the absorption of estrogen and its reabsorption after excretion in the bile by killing the bacteria in the gut responsible for estrogen conjugation. As a result, the blood estrogen level falls, and the oral contraceptive pills may fail. A very high fiber diet may interfere with the recycling of estrogen.

Sterilization

1. Surgical Sterilization of the Female

a. This in practice means permanent interruption of the fallopian tubes.

b. Laparoscopy, laparotomy, and mini-laparotomy are used to produce sterilization in the female.

c. Most of the laparoscopic sterilizations use the standard electrocoagulation method. Although rare, bowel burn is one of the complications of this technique.

d. Nonelastic techniques include the clip or the band. The results are comparable to those experienced with electrocoagulation.

e. The mini-laparotomy has become popular and can be carried out under local anesthesia.

f. The techniques are:

(1) Pomeroy subtotal bilateral salpingectomy (most frequently used)

(2) Madlener—requires no cutting but is less reliable

(3) Irving—at the time of cesarean section the tubal stump is buried in the uterine musculature

(4) Cornual resection for interim, nonpregnant uteri

(5) Aldridge—reversible sterilization, buries the fimbriated ends between the leaves of the broad ligament

g. Hysterectomy is usually reserved for the patient with concurrent uterine or pelvic disease.

h. The only certain method of surgical sterilization is to remove the ovaries.

2. Surgical Sterilization of the Male

a. Vasectomy is the only popular method of male sterilization.

b. There are few immediate contraindications. These are local infection and bleeding disorders.

c. Sperm-agglutinating antibodies can be found in the serum of over half the men undergoing vasectomy, although the titer decreases with time.

d. More serious autoantibodies may form and in extremely rare cases have produced a clinical disorder with autoimmune characteristics.

e. There is a failure rate of about 0.4 per cent.

f. The advantages of vasectomy over surgical methods of sterilization in the female are simplicity, safety, low cost, and high effectiveness.

Estrogens and Postcoital Contraception

1. It has been estimated that approximately 60 per cent of first sexual exposures among young, unmarried women on university campuses are unprotected, while 40 per cent of subsequent intercourse is insufficiently protected.

2. The need for some form of postcoital contraception clearly exists; the only alternatives at present are endometrial aspiration, menstrual extraction, and abortion. They are costly, have side effects, and are inconvenient.

3. Postcoital contraception (PCC) has been defined as the pharmacological inhibition of implantation after unprotected intercourse. The term *interceptives* has been used to describe the use of estrogens as a method of preventing pregnancy after intercourse.

4. Diethylstilbestrol (DES), 50 mg., ethinyl estradiol, 5 mg., or conjugated estrogens, 30 mg., will be effective if given within 72 hours of the unprotected midcycle (ovulatory) exposure and continued for 5 days.

5. The preparations are potent and have side effects that contraindicate their use. Women suffering from thrombophlebitis, hypertension, cerebrovascular accident, epilepsy, migraine, or chronic liver or renal disease should not receive estrogen as a postcoital contraception.

6. If pregnancy occurs in a woman receiving estrogen as PCC, abortion should be recommended because of the teratogenic and carcinogenic effects reported in the offspring of mothers treated during pregnancy.

7. Since ectopic pregnancy has been reported following the use of PCC, great care must be taken when evaluating a patient complaining of abdominal pain who is known to have been exposed to high-dose estrogen therapy.

8. It is recommended that a signed and witnessed informed consent be obtained before instituting PCC. It should outline the known risks and limitations of high-dose estrogen therapy as well as the alternative treatments.

9. It must be emphasized that the use of high-dose estrogen is not a casual matter, that close observation is necessary, and that the patient's medical care is not complete until after the 6-week examination. Patients should be advised against having unprotected intercourse during or after treatment.

Methods Under Investigation

1. Chief among these is the male Pill, which is aimed at interruption of spermatogenesis or sperm maturation. A number of preparations are under trial, including androgens alone or in combination with progestogens or estrogens and the anti-androgenic compound cyproterone acetate.

2. Chinese researchers have developed a contraceptive for males, Gossypol, which shows some promise. This cottonseed derivative alters sperm structure and motility and decreases sperm production. It is being tested for use both as a male oral contraceptive and as a spermicide.

3. Synthetic analogs of gonadotropin-releasing hormone (GnRH) are possible contraceptives. If these are given continuously, rather than in pulses, they become fixed to pituitary receptors and block the action of GnRH, so that the output of gonadotropins falls and ovulation ceases.

4. Immunization against pregnancy has also reached the stage of clinical trial. This depends on immunization against the beta subunit of chorionic gonadotropin and might provide a simple and long-lasting method of contraception.

5. Medroxyprogesterone (Depo-Provera), a progestogen, acts on the hypothalamic-pituitary-ovarian axis to inhibit ovulation. As a consequence of this, it also has an effect on the endometrium and the cervical mucus.

a. There is some initial delay in the return of fertility following medroxyprogesterone use because of the time it takes to eliminate the drug completely and to resume ovulation.

29 Cytology

Hugh R. K. Barber

Cytology probably makes its greatest contribution as a screening method for the detection of cancer of the cervix in women. It is also used as a diagnostic method in detecting cancer in other organ systems. In addition, it has been employed as an index of hormonal levels.

Cytologic screening of women for cancer of the vagina, cervix, and endometrium may represent the most important advance in gynecology in this century. The technique was perfected by Dr. George N. Papanicolaou and is known as the Pap test, or Pap smear.

It is estimated that two or three (some studies report five to seven) unsuspected cases of cervical cancer per thousand women are usually found by this method.

NORMAL CYTOLOGY

1. In the normal menstrual cycle the majority of cells seen in Pap smears are squamous cells shed from the surface of the stratified squamous epithelium of the vagina and cervix. There are also varying numbers of polymorphs and histiocytes, endocervical columnar cells, and, during menstruation, endometrial cells.

2. The degree of quantification of the superficial cells of the squamous epithelium depends on the amount of circulating estrogens.

3. There is a great contrast between the histological appearance of the squamous epithelium seen at about the time of ovulation, when estrogenic activity is at its maximum, and that seen in an elderly, postmenopausal woman.

4. This is reflected in the type of squamous cell predominating in the vaginal smear. It is convenient to describe these cells as being of the superficial, intermediate, or parabasal type, according to which layer of cornified squamous epithelium they most resemble. However, these are merely descriptive terms.

5. The cells seen can only come from the surface layer, unless there is ulceration with exposure of the deeper layers; hence, if parabasal cells predominate, it means that the squamous epithelium has failed to develop to the mature cornified state.

BASIC PRINCIPLES

1. Due to the action of estrogen and progesterone, cyclical changes occur in the vaginal mucosa which can be identified by examining a stained smear. Such smears can to some extent be used as a rough guide to the hormonal status of the patient. The phases are:

a. *Postmenstrual.* The cells are mainly of precornified type; by Papanicolaou's stain the cytoplasm is stained blue-green.

b. *Proliferative.* The rising titer of estrogen increases cornification and causes glycogen to appear in the cells. Brown deposits of glycogen appear in the pink cytoplasm. The nuclei are small and pyknotic.

c. *Secretory.* The cornified cells diminish in number. Precornified cells with folded edges make their appearance and many polymorphs are seen.

d. *Premenstrual-menstrual.* The cells are clumped and degenerate. Debris and leukocytes are present, giving a "dirty" appearance to the smear.

2. Cells collected for hormonal evaluation should be taken from the anterior-lateral fornix.

3. Cytohormonal evaluation involves interpreting the intricate pattern resulting from epithelial maturation, secretory activity, cellular membrane status, inflammatory response, and many other features under endocrine influence.

4. The state of maturation that the cells of the vaginal epithelium have attained at the time of their exfoliation yields the most objective and reliable information.

5. The maturation index (MI) expresses the level of cellular maturation attained at the time of exfoliation. It is expressed as a ratio of the percentages present of parabasal, intermediate, and superficial cells, in that order. 0/55/45 represents the maturation index (MI) of a patient exfoliating no parabasal cells, 55 per cent intermediate cells, and 45 per cent superficial cells, which accurately reflects their ratio on the surface of the vaginal epithelium.

6. There were 12,800 new cases of invasive cancer of the cervix, with 6,800 deaths, anticipated in 1989. There has been a decrease in incidence of cervical cancer in the last 40 years. One of the main reasons for the relative decrease in the incidence of invasive carcinoma of the cervix is that so many lesions are now discovered by exfoliative cytology before invasion.

7. Exfoliative cytology (Pap test) is primarily a screening test. Obvious lesions must be biopsied.

Normal Cytohormonal Patterns of the Endocrine Periods:

Childhood—50/50/0
Perimenarchal—45/45/10
Reproductive period—ovulation, 0/40/60; menstruation, 0/70/33
Pregnancy—0/95/5
Postpartum—100/0/0
Postmenopausal—0/100/0 or 100/0/0
Atrophic pattern—100/0/0 (with estrogen therapy will approach 0/50/50)
Progestogens—0/100/0
Androgens—100/0/0
Cortisone—0/100/0
Presence of ovarian granulosa-cell tumors that produce estrogen produces a shift to the right—0/0/100
Vaginal inflammation—31/35/34
Turner's syndrome—0/100/0 (may shift, with age, to 100/0/0)
Symmond's disease—100/0/0

8. If the smears are properly taken and adequately interpreted, exfoliative cytology is accurate more than 95 per cent of the time in cases of carcinoma of the cervix.

9. On single smears there is a false-negative rate ranging up to 20 per cent. Therefore, it is important to have cytologic examinations at stated intervals.

10. The false-positive diagnosis, i.e., the presence of cells interpreted as malignant in the absence of histological confirmation, is more frequent than the false-negative. The consequences of a false-positive result, however, are not as grave as those of a false-negative.

11. The presence of endometrial cells on a routine Pap smear demands reevaluation and an endometrial aspiration.

12. The routine Pap smear is not adequate to screen the endometrium. Cervical scraping would give a low yield of positive cytology for endometrial cancer. The average return would be about 50 per cent, the posterior fornix would yield about 65 per cent, and endocervical aspiration about 75 per cent, but with the jet washer or a similar method or the Novak suction curettage the accuracy of diagnosis should exceed 90 per cent.

13. Collection of specimens for screening of the cervix may include swabbing, scraping, and aspiration of the cervical canal. A combination gives a higher yield.

14. Endocervical smears or aspiration should be routine. There is an increase in adenocarcinoma-in-situ as well adenocarcinoma of the endocervix.

COLLECTION OF A PAP TEST SPECIMEN

1. No lubricant should be used on the glove or speculum.

2. With the cervix visualized, a cotton-tipped applicator moistened with saline solution is introduced into the external cervical os and twisted. The cellular specimen is deposited on the slide by rolling, but not rubbing, the applicator tip against the glass surface. (Rubbing might streak or break the cells.)

3. The external os should be scraped with a wooden or plastic spatula. The end that is shaped to conform to the cervix is inserted in the external os. The spatula is rotated clockwise while moderate pressure is exerted on the edge in contact with the cervix. The sample is deposited on the slide by passing the tip of the spatula, and its slanted edges, slowly and firmly against the surface of the glass.

4. Some physicians prefer to aspirate the cervical canal. The tip of a glass or plastic cannula with an attached rubber bulb is introduced into the cervical canal and the contents of the canal are aspirated. The fluid from the syringe is emptied onto the slide. It serves the same purpose as cervical scraping or swabbing—i.e., detection of cervical carcinoma.

5. The superiority of aspiration over the other methods is debatable. A combination of aspiration and scraping enhances the sensitivity of the cytologic test for cancer detection.

6. Cytologic examination of the vaginal pool is the least reliable of the various methods used to detect cervical cancer. The vaginal pool usually contains a small amount of material, and there is poor preservation of the representative cells.

7. The laboratory request slip, in addition to the usual identifying data, should include the following information:

a. Last menstrual period

b. Pregnancy, if present

c. Use of oral contraceptives or intrauterine device (IUD)

d. History of hormonal imbalance or dysfunction

e. Current diagnosis

f. Previous surgery, particularly cervical surgery (conization, biopsy, etc.)

g. Radiation therapy and, if any, time of last treatment

h. History of previous cancer

REPORTING RESULTS

1. The cytologic diagnosis may be reported using a numerical classification system, a narrative description, or both.

2. The numerical classification introduces a great deal of subjective interpretation. Therefore, many laboratories report the results as positive, negative, or borderline.

3. A numerical classification based on Papanicolaou's original five-class system, or its modification, is most often used to report results. Papanicolaou's classification is:

a. *Class I—Negative.* Only normal cells are present.

b. *Class II—Negative.* There are no signs of malignancy; some atypical cells are present.

c. *Class III—Doubtful.* The smear contains cells with atypical features suggestive but not diagnostic of malignancy.

d. *Class IV—Positive.* Isolated atypical cells are present.

e. *Class V—Positive.* Numerous atypical cells or cell groups are present.

ENDOMETRIAL SCREENING

1. The routine cervical-vaginal smear is less effective for detection of endometrial cancer than for detection of cervical malignancy.

2. Screening methods employing cytology to detect endometrial abnormalities have been elusive.

3. Screening programs using cytology to identify early changes in cervical abnormalities have not yielded similarly useful results in picking up patients with early risk-associated changes in the endometrium. The pickup rate on routine screening for the asymptomatic patient is only about 3 per cent, or less, of all endometrial cancers.

4. Negative cytologic test results do not have the same accuracy in prognosticating that the development of cancer is highly unlikely, because on cytologic evaluation the preinvasive lesions are not diagnosed with the same accuracy as is obtained in cancer of the cervix.

5. It is unlikely that screening programs directed at detecting cancer of the endometrium will have a major impact on morbidity and mortality rates in the foreseeable future.

6. The cytologist can diagnose the benign or malignant endometrium with a high degree of accuracy, but has trouble detecting the "in-between" groups with adenomatous hyperplasia, dysplasia, or cancer in situ.

7. Endometrial hyperplasia develops into endometrial cancer in only 1.5 per cent of patients. Endometrial cancer patients do not have higher-than-normal estrogen titers; therefore, there must be factors other than simple prolonged estrogen stimulation at work.

8. The most optimistic estimate of the detection rate is 75 per cent.

9. A vaginal smear taken from the pool of secretion in the posterior fornix gives a relatively better chance of detection of endometrial cancer.

10. In screening for endometrial cancer, uterine aspiration or washing should be added to the routine Pap smear.

11. The rate of positive returns in asymptomatic women is low, and the discomfort is significant.

12. For women who have symptoms of endometrial cancer—even for those in whom there is only significant suspicion—fractional curettage is indicated.

30 Basic and Clinical Immunology

Hugh R. K. Barber

INTRODUCTION

1. Immunology is a relatively new discipline of medicine. Immunity has been recognized for centuries, and its study has been termed the study of resistance to infection. However, the concept of immunity has now expanded its scope and is now defined as the property whereby the lymphoreticular system makes a memorized response to an antigenic stimulus. This response may result in a state of *positive* reaction known as *sensitization* or a *negative* reaction known as *immunologic tolerance, enhancement,* or *immunosuppression.*

2. As a scientific discipline, *immunology* encompasses the study of *immunity,* which deals with the adaptive response to infective agents, *immunochemistry,* which concerns the chemical nature of antigens and antibodies, and *immunobiology,* which deals with the activity of the cells of the immune system and their relationship to each other and their environment. As a biological science, immunology includes developmental biology, genetics, biochemistry, microbiology, anatomy, and medicine. The basic concepts of immunology are fundamental to an understanding of the principles and practice of modern medicine.

3. Currently, immunology and immunotherapy have contributed little to the individual treatment of a patient. However, there is great promise for the future use of the principles of immunology in clinical medicine. Therefore, a summary of its basic principles is included here. On the other hand, immunology has played a key role in laboratory diagnoses. The following tests are listed—precipitation, immunodiffusion or gel diffusion test, immunoelectrophoresis, agglutination, mixed hemoadsorption, and the Coombs', Australian SH, complement fixation, fluorescent antibody, cytotoxic colony inhibition, migration inhibition, mixed lymphocyte culture, and radioimmunoassay tests—as those widely employed in clinical medicine.

BASIC PRINCIPLES

1. The cellular events in an immune response are fundamental to understanding the basic mechanisms of the development of both cell-mediated and humoral immunity.

2. The *macrophage* represents the keystone in the development of an immune response. The macrophage in blood is called a *monocyte;* in connective tissue a *histiocyte;* and in the spleen, lymph nodes, and thymus a *sinus-lining macrophage* or a *reticulum cell.* The macrophage has a wide distribution.

3. The *antigen,* or, more correctly, the immunogen (any substance foreign to the host), is processed by the macrophage if an immune response is to occur. The antigen is now a processed antigen.

4. Following contact of the antigen with the macrophage, the latter sends out a message in the form of an RNA or RNA-antigen complex. The uncommitted lymphocytes are transformed into *lymphoblasts.*

5. The transformed blasts (lymphoblasts) give rise to *sensitized lymphocytes* as well as to *plasma cells.*

6. The plasma cells (B cells) in turn produce a variety of *immunoglobulins;* five have been identified: IgM, IgG, IgE, IgA, and IgD.

7. The sensitized lymphocytes (T cells) are transformed into the so-called killer lymphocytes that have the ability to destroy cancer cells and produce lymphokines and delayed hypersensitivity.

8. The B cell must receive a stimulus from the antigen, plus one from the antigenically stimulated T cell, if it is to mature into a plasmocyte.

9. This helper function of the T cell appears to depend in a large measure on the T and B cells' sharing certain products of the major histocompatibility complex (MHC).

10. *T helper (Th) cells.* These T lymphocytes help B cell antibody. To make antibody to most antigens (T-dependent antigens), it is necessary that both T and B cells recognize different parts of the antigen.

a. T helper cells also cooperate with T cytotoxic cells and the recognition of allogenic cells and virally infected cells. They also release lymphokines which can activate macrophages and other cell types.

b. T helper cells recognize antigen in association with Class II molecules encoded by the MHC.

11. *T inducer cell* is a term used to describe the activity of T helper cells in activating other types of cells.

12. *T cytotoxic (Tc) cells* are capable of destroying allogenic cells and virally infected target cells, which they recognize by interaction with antigens and MHC Class I molecules on the target cell surface.

13. *T suppressor (Ts) cells* regulate the action of other T cells and B cells. They may be functionally divided according to whether their suppressive action is specific for cells with particular antigen receptors or nonspecific. Their actions are sometimes, but not always, MHC-restricted.

14. *Memory cells.* These are functionally defined lymphocytes which can be either B cells or T cells. They are responsible for the maintenance of the specific immunological memory following a primary immune response. Although the idea of memory cells is intellectually useful, there is not, as yet, any specific way of identifying them (although it has been suggested that memory B cells have completed a number of the differentiation steps and have little surface IgM).

15. *NK (natural killer) cells* are capable of killing a number of virally infected and transformed target cells to which they have not been previously sensitized. They have not been separated from K cells, although K cell activity and NK activity develop independently.

16. *K (killer) cells* are monocytes which can kill target cells sensitized with antibody, which they find via their Fc receptors; the majority are L cells [L cells/N cells, (non-T, non-B) cells/third population cells].

17. When the sensitized lymphocyte comes in contact with the antigen that sensitized it, the lymphocyte is stimulated to form an immunoblast which produces at least four mediators of cellular immunity, including transfer factor (TF), lymphocyte-transforming activity (LTA), migration inhibition factor (MIF), lymphotoxin (LT), and interferon (IFN).

DEVELOPMENT OF B AND T CELLS

1. Pluripotent stem cell gives rise to a variety of cells, only two of which will be described. They are distinct cell types clearly separable from one another in the process of differentiation. Pluripotent cells differentiate into the precursor stem cells of all of the major hematopoietic elements.

2. *Lymphoid stem cells* can function as prethymic cells and are processed in the thymus under the influence of thymosin (thymopoietin) to differentiate into T cells.

3. *Lymphoid precursor cells* are processed by an alternate pathway in a poorly defined organ in man, but have been extensively studied in birds (in the bursa of Fabricius) and in some mammals (in the fetal liver, probably under the influence of another hormone-like substance, "bursin"). They differentiate into B cells.

4. A subpopulation of thymus-independent lymphocytes (B cells) has been detected which mediates cytotoxic reactions on antibody-coated target cells in the absence of complement. These cells are called *K cells.* Sometimes they are referred to as null cells because they lack the markers characteristic of T or B cells.

5. In addition to the above three classes of lymphocytes, there is another population of circulating lymphocytes that have the characteristics of both T and B lymphocytes. These *double (D) cells* represent 2 to 3 per cent of the circulating lymphoid population. Their origin, function, and role in tumor immunology remain undetermined.

HUMORAL AND CELL-MEDIATED IMMUNE RESPONSES

The immune response takes two forms: A humoral response results from the transformed lymphoblast being converted to a plasma cell. It is a cell-free fluid containing antibodies which are circulating freely in the blood stream as well as in other body fluids. Also, a cell-mediated immunity is carried out by sensitized lymphocytes.

The Humoral Response

1. The humoral response (B cell) is mediated by immunoglobulins.

2. It is cell-free and is made up of the immunoglobulins IgG, IgM, IgA, IgD, and IgE.

3. For the cell-free antibody to have a killing or cytotoxic effect it must always have a third substance, complement, present.

4. Without complement, an antibody can bind to an antigen on a cell surface but cannot damage or kill the cell.

5. The humoral response offers a defense against most bacteria and some foreign proteins.

6. Bacterial vaccines inoculated into the organism result in the production of antibodies (immunoglobulins).

7. The humoral response includes B cells, K cells, and D cells.

The Cell-Mediated Response

1. The cell-mediated response (T cell) is mediated by sensitized lymphocytes.

2. In the cell-mediated immune (CMI) response, the antibody remains an integral part of the cells that produced it and is a cell-associated antibody.

3. Sensitized lymphocytes carrying such antibody are carried in the lymph to tumor cells, where their antibody combines with the antigen determinant on the surface of the tumor cell.

4. The cell-bound antibody then becomes capable of rupturing and killing tumor cells. It also produces potent mediators of cellular immunity, including TF, LTA, lymphocyte blastogenic factor, MIF, LT, and interferon.

5. The cell-mediated response is particularly important in graft rejection, eliminating viruses as well as intracellular bacteria and cancer cells.

IMMUNODEFICIENCY: NATURE'S EXPERIMENT TO DEMONSTRATE THE DIFFERENCE BETWEEN HUMORAL AND CELL-MEDIATED IMMUNITY

Immunodeficiency is often identified by the increased frequency of infection in patients. Impaired immunity is a consequence of any pathogenic infection, but immunodeficiency is primarily inherited and may affect any part of the immune system, including complement components, granulocytes, macrophages, and lymphocytes.

Any deviation in nature supplies valuable material for studying normal mechanisms. Nature has supplied such an experiment to study the role of the humoral and cell-mediated response.

Deficiency of Cell-Mediated Immunity (T Cell)

1. In the DiGeorge syndrome, there is dysplasia or hypoplasia of the thymus and often absence of the parathyroid glands.

a. The patient has no resistance to viruses or to other agents that are controlled by cell-mediated immunity, such as tuberculosis, brucellosis, leprosy, fungi, and parasitic diseases.

b. Patients do not have the immunologic capacity to develop a delayed hypersensitivity reaction or to reject grafts of foreign tissue.

c. They can produce circulating antibodies and have the ability to respond to bacterial vaccines by developing circulating antibodies (immunoglobulins).

d. Research programs have been structured to implant embryonic thymus glands with some success.

Deficiency of Humoral Immunity (B Cell)

1. In the Bruton type of agammaglobulinemia, there is a deficiency of immunoglobulin synthesis.

a. IgG is decreased tenfold and IgA and IgM about a hundredfold.

b. These patients do not have natural circulating immunoglobulins and are susceptible to bacterial infections.

c. They do not respond to bacterial vaccines by producing an increased antibody titer (immunoglobulins).

d. The cell-mediated immune mechanism functions normally, and they have the capacity to reject tissue or organ grafts and exhibit delayed hypersensitivity to the tuberculin skin tests.

e. Treatment with gamma globulin has served to help these patients resist bacterial infections.

Combined Deficiency of T and B Cells

1. In Swiss type agammaglobulinemia, which is an X-linked disease of male children, both cell-mediated and humoral mechanisms are deficient.

a. There is a block of the stem cell mechanism. These children cannot make humoral antibodies (immunoglobulins) or develop cell-mediated immune reactions.

b. They suffer from progressive bacterial and/or viral infections and die within the first two years of life.

c. Some highly selected patients have been treated with bone marrow that has been matched for major histocompatible antigens. The preliminary work has been promising and some success has been reported.

Other Immunodeficiencies

1. Currently, more than 30 phenotype patterns of immunodeficiency have been recognized in human beings.

2. In addition to T, B, and stem defects, other immunodeficiencies have been recorded.

3. The patient's phagocytic system may not function adequately to ingest and kill bacteria and fungi. Absence or malfunction of the complement system which normally aids in bacterial killing may give rise to serious illness.

4. Other significant immunodeficient states are hereditary ataxia telangiectasia, Wiskott-Aldrich syndrome, Chédiak-Higashi syndrome, selective IgA (immunoglobulin A) deficiency disorders, and chronic mucocutaneous candidiasis (moniliasis).

5. Acquired immunodeficiency syndrome (AIDS), which is contracted by children and adults, permits a variety of opportunistic infections and is associated with Kaposi's sarcoma. A human T lymphocyte cytotrophic virus (LAV or HTLV-III) is probably the cause.

AUTOIMMUNE DISORDERS

Introduction

1. *Autoimmunity* is the reaction of the immune system against the body's own tissue.

2. *Autoreactive cells* are lymphocytes with receptors for autoantigens. These cells can potentially produce an autoimmune response but do not necessarily do so.

3. *Forbidden clones.* Burnett proposed the theory to explain the way the body is normally tolerant to its own tissue. He suggested that autoreactive cells were effectively forbidden by being clonally deleted during embryological development. It is now known that autoreactive B cells are present, but they are not normally active.

4. Autoimmune disease occurs when autoimmune reactions result in pathological tissue damage. In general, the reactions are either organ-specific or organ-non-specific.

5. Clinical and experimental observations show that individuals can sometimes respond immunologically to certain of their own antigens (auto-antigens). These important exceptions to the principle of self-tolerance help to analyze the fundamental mechanisms of immunology, and they are frequently associated with disease. It is often not clear, however, whether these anomalous responses cause, or are the result of, disease; hence, it is necessary to emphasize the distinction between an autoimmune response, in which an individual makes antibodies or becomes allergic to self-antigen, and an autoimmune disease, which is a pathological condition arising from an autoimmune response. Autoimmune reactions can be both antibody- and cell-mediated. There is a great overlap between immunological deficiency diseases and autoimmunity.

Basic Mechanisms

1. Autoimmunity may arise whenever a state of immunologic imbalance exists in which B-cell activity is excessive and suppressor T-cell activity is diminished.

2. This imbalance occurs as a consequence of genetic, viral, and environmental mechanisms acting singly or in combination.

3. A central mechanism in this concept involves a disturbance of the delicate balance between the suppressor and helper activity of regulatory T cells.

4. Either an excess of helper-T activity or a deficiency of suppressor-T activity could lead to the development of autoimmunity.

5. The mechanisms by which such a balance may be upset are complex but may involve both viral factors and the abnormal production of thymic hormones.

6. The B cell has several different membrane receptors on its surface. There are immunoglobulin receptors for antigen and receptors for helper-T and suppressor-T cells.

7. The balance of the T-regulatory signals (helper T and suppressor T) arriving at the cell surface of the B cell determines whether the B lymphocyte remains inactive or goes into active synthesis and proliferation.

8. If the B lymphocyte represents a clone with the potential for producing an autoantibody, then this balance of signals determines whether autoimmunity appears.

9. Three general autoimmune diseases are: acquired (autoimmune) hemolytic anemia (AHA), systemic lupus erythematosus (SLE), and rheumatoid arthritis (RA).

HYPERSENSITIVITY

Definition

Hypersensitivity describes an immune response which occurs in an exaggerated or inappropriate form. These reactions have been classified into five major types (modified from Gell and Coombs) according to the speed of the reaction and the immune mechanism involved. Although they are classified separately, in practice they do not necessarily occur in isolation from each other. Furthermore, several different immune reactions may be subsumed under a single type.

1. Hypersensitivity is a state of the previously immunized (meaning a state of altered reactivity of a host to an antigen due to exposing the host to that antigen in such a way that it produces an immune response) host which results in tissue damage from an immune reaction to a further dose of antigen.

2. Hypersensitivity reactions may be antibody- or humoral-mediated, as in immediate hypersensitivity, or they may be a reaction of cell-mediated immunity, as in delayed hypersensitivity.

3. The term *hypersensitivity* implies a heightened reactivity to an antigen, but it is difficult to define all hypersensitivity reactions, particularly cell-mediated reactions, in such terms.

4. The hypersensitivity reactions have been classified into five types.

a. The first three develop as immediate reactions and are humorally mediated (type 1, anaphylactic reactions; type 2, cytolytic or cytotoxic reactions; and type 3, toxic-complex syndromes).

b. Although they are classified as immediate reactions, this may not be absolutely true.

c. Cytotoxic reactions may be delayed for hours, and, in the toxic-complex syndrome, serum sickness may develop after days or even weeks.

d. The humoral hypersensitivity reactions often dovetail in their responses and effects.

e. The fourth type of reaction is cell-mediated and is termed *delayed hypersensitivity.*

f. The fifth type has been added to the original Gell and Coombs classification. It is a stimulatory hypersensitivity which describes reactions where autoantibodies stimulate host tissue.

Basic Mechanisms

1. Type 1

a. Anaphylaxis occurs when the immunoglobulins of the IgE class interact with antigen, thereby causing the release of vasoactive substances which induce an immediate inflammatory response.

b. Examples: asthma, hay fever

2. Type 2

a. Cytotoxic hypersensitivity results when antibodies bind to self-antigens and destroy the host cells.

b. Examples: blood transfusion reactions, hemolytic disease of the newborn

3. Type 3

a. Immune complex, or toxic-complex, hypersensitivity occurs when antigen-antibody complexes are deposited at tissue sites and a subsequent destructive inflammatory response ensues.

b. A local version of immune complex hypersensitivity in which inflammation occurs 3 to 8 hours after cutaneous administration of antigen is termed an *Arthus reaction.*

c. A generalized inflammatory reaction characterized by inflammation of blood vessels, joints, and kidney, resulting from the formation of circulating antigen-antibody complexes, is termed *serum sickness.*

4. Type 4

a. Delayed hypersensitivity is an immunologic process. It is an acquired and transferable capacity which exhibits memory and specificity for the antigen. A sensitized lymphocyte reacts with specific antigens and releases lymphokines.

b. Thus, delayed hypersensitivity, a form of cell-mediated immunity, differs from immediate hypersensitivity, which is mediated by antibodies.

c. Examples: contact dermatitis, tuberculin reaction, skin and allograft rejection

5. A fifth type of hypersensitivity *(type 5, or stimulatory, hypersensitivity)* has recently been delineated which describes reactions where autoantibodies stimulate host tissue, such as the stimulation of thyroid by autoantibody binding to the TSH receptor which thus mimics thyroid-stimulating hormone.

THE IMMUNE DEFENSE SYSTEM

The logical question is: If tumor cells possess antigens on their surface capable of stimulating a specific immune response, why does cancer continue to grow in the presence of a mechanism designated to control its growth? The logical explanation is that the rate of growth exceeds the capacity of the immune response. However, from studies in animals, more specific reasons are now known for the failure of immune response to prevent the start and growth of cancer.

FAILURE OF THE IMMUNE RESPONSE

Immunosuppression

1. Many factors contribute to this. Among these factors are aging, the cancer itself, anticancer drug therapy, radiation therapy, genetic defects, and neonatal thymectomy. To a lesser extent, antibiotics, anesthetics, analgesics, and hypnotics contribute to immunosuppression.

2. In reality, it is often difficult to separate the contributions of drugs from those of disease in bringing about a state of immunosuppression.

3. Removal of a bulk of tumor reduces the immunosuppression of the host.

Immunological Tolerance

1. In a broad sense, this represents a form of immunosuppression.

2. It can occur with exposure to an antigen during embryonic or early neonatal life, before the immune system has matured. The latter then fails to recognize the antigen as nonself and is incapable of mounting an immune response.

3. Since cancer is considered to arise from a single cell clone, the tolerance theory for the progression of cancer is often suggested as an explanation. Choriocarcinoma has been advanced as a prototype for this theory.

4. The host is not immunologically tolerant in general, but only for that specific tumor antigen.

Acquired Tolerance

1. Was formerly called *immune paralysis.*

2. It is induced by injecting very small or very large doses of antigen into the body and persists as long as that antigen remains in the body.

3. In clinical practice, acquired tolerance or immune paralysis may suppress the immune response of the host in the presence of a large tumor.

4. Following removal of the tumor mass, the host exhibits resistance to the reimplantation of that tumor.

5. The conclusion is that there is no intrinsic failure of the immune response but that the response is overwhelmed by the volume of tumor.

6. Removal of the tumor or debulking the tumor may restore the integrity of the immune response.

Immunological Enhancement

1. This results in an increased growth of tumor in animals.

2. Animals transplanted with grafts of foreign cancer cells and then injected with antiserum against that cancer often experience a rapid growth of the cancer rather than the anticipated rejection of the tumor.

3. Obviously, the antibodies produced against the cancer and then injected into the host with the transplanted tumor were enhancing or blocking antibodies rather than cytotoxic antibodies.

4. These antibodies formed complexes with the antigens on the surface of the tumor and blocked the killer lymphocytes from attacking the tumor. The tumor was protected from destruction.

5. Immunological enhancement has indirectly been shown to play a role in the growth of choriocarcinoma.

6. Removal of a bulk of tumor, such as ovarian cancer, may suppress the enhancement phenomenon and permit the killer lymphocytes to successfully attack the tumor cells.

Immunoselection

1. Cancer develops from a clone of cells.

2. The cell has tumor antigens on the surface, and, as the tumor grows, the cancer cells have the same surface antigens.

3. During the course of many generations mutations occur. Some of the resulting cells have a greater number of antigens present and therefore stimulate a greater antibody production.

4. The cells with a greater number of antigens produce a significant number of antibodies which help to eliminate the cells with a strong antigenic component.

5. The cells that remain are those with few antigens present, and the result is a colony of cells with weak antigens followed initially by relatively slow growth of tumor.

6. It is conceivable that this leads to tolerance.

7. After a period of time the tumor cells develop autonomy and progressively greater invasive properties.

Antigen Modulation

1. This is a temporary change in antigenicity reflecting an adaptational alteration in an entire population of cells.

2. It can be stated that as soon as antibody is produced, cancer cells of certain leukemias in animals cease synthesizing antigens.

3. As a result, the immunological defense becomes ineffective.

4. In humans, this response has not been documented.

Unknown Factors

1. The tumor-bearing host may possess factors that depress the immunological reactivity in a nonspecific way, or the host may lack factors that are important for such reactivity.

2. This theory has been suggested by the poor response that the tumor-bearing host develops when tested for delayed hypersensitivity to a variety of antigens.

3. In vitro studies in this group have also shown a decreased ability to transform lymphocytes after stimulation with phytohemagglutinin (PHA).

BIOLOGICAL MARKERS AND MODIFIERS

1. The body's inherent biochemical capacity for killing cancer cells, joined with the new genetic technology, has given rise to biologic response modification—biomodulation for short. Biologic response modification is the new wave in cancer treatment.

2. The use of biologics and biologic response modifiers in the treatment of cancer is of recent origin. *Biologics* may be defined as any product of the mammalian organism, and *biologic response modifiers* are those agents and approaches that alter biologic responses in the host-tumor interaction.

3. The field encompasses not only traditional immunotherapy but also the use of molecular biology, recombinant genetics, and hybridoma technology, each of which produces highly purified biologic substances with anti-cancer activity.

4. The recognition of growth, differentiation, and maturation factors, as well as the possibility of making antagonist or competitive inhibitors to factors that support neoplastic growth, provides additional biologic approaches in this area.

5. Genetic engineering has brought about a revolution in the field of biology. It will continue to be at the front and center of research. In the future, genes will be implanted into bacteria, resulting in the production of any desired protein or enzyme in large quantities.

a. Medicine has already reaped many rewards from recombinant techniques that manufacture proteins in quantity by moving human genes into microorganisms. These genes can program the production of commercial quantities of human insulin, human growth factor, and interferon, as well as of genetically engineered vaccines.

b. It is possible that cancers of the reproductive tract will be controlled by the turn of the century. DNA probes and recombinant DNA experiments will change the face of obstetrics and gynecology as it is known today.

c. Gene therapy is medicine's next frontier. It is now possible to isolate a single gene from the DNA of an organism. It can be recombined with a carrier molecule of DNA.

d. It is now possible to introduce the recombinant DNA into a bacterial cell to produce an altered organism. Recombinant DNA technology, commonly referred to as genetic engineering, has provided science with the tools for the biosynthesis and subsequent mass production of a significant number of biologics. This should revolutionize the treatment of cancer over the next ten years.

e. The process involves the incorporation (recombination) of a segment of a DNA molecule containing a desired gene into a vector, usually a plasmid, which in turn is inserted into a host organism, usually *Escherichia coli,* although other bacteria, yeasts, insects, and mammalian cells have been used. *E. coli* are cloned and the organism producing the desired protein or polypeptide is selected.

f. This clone is mass-produced by fermentation techniques, and a protein molecule is harvested and purified. The resultant product is a highly purified protein solution, generally with greater than 95 per cent purity and with a highly specific activity, containing the greatest possible amount of biologic activity per mg. of protein.

g. By genetic engineering it is possible to produce, in fairly large quantities, alpha, beta, and gamma interferon. It is also possible to produce interleukin-2 (IL-2) produced by helper T cells. The presence of T-cell stimulants will stimulate and maintain in vitro the growth of normal activated T cells.

6. Tumor necrosis factor is being produced and is giving promising results. A whole field of diagnosis and therapy has been introduced with the use of monoclonal antibodies.

a. Monoclonal antibodies are homogeneous antibodies produced by a single clone. They are usually made by hybridomas, which are prepared by fusing immunized mouse or rat spleen cells with a non-secretor myeloma using polyethylene glycol (PEG). The fusion mixture is plated out in HAT medium.

b. HAT contains *h*ypoxanthine, *a*minopterine and *t*hymidine. Aminopterine blocks a metabolic pathway which can be bypassed if hypoxanthine and thymidine are present, but the myeloma cells lack this bypass and consequently die in HAT medium.

c. The spleen cells also die naturally in culture after 1 to 2 weeks, though a few cells survive since they have the immortality of the myeloma and the metabolic bypass of the spleen cells.

d. Some of the fused cells secrete antibody, and supernatants are tested in a specific assay. Cells which produce the desired antibody are then cloned.

CA-125

1. The work reported by Bast and colleagues on the use of monoclonal antibodies to monitor the course of epithelial ovarian cancer may some day be perfected so that it can be used for early diagnosis of ovarian cancer. Currently, the murine monoclonal antibody OC-125 reacts with the antigen CA-125, common to most non-mucinous epithelial ovarian cancers.

2. An assay has been developed to detect CA-125 in the serum. It has been reported that a rising or falling level of CA-125 correlates with progression or regression of disease in 93 per cent of patients.

3. One of the most exciting areas of gynecological oncology is the effort now being made to diagnose ovarian cancer with immunologic techniques. The progress is rapidly being made, and success at achieving diagnosis by a serologic method seems assured.

IN VITRO TESTING OF CANCER CELLS

1. Chemosensitivity testing is done to improve therapy by means of an individual (selective) cytotoxic chemotherapy; a bioassay technique facilitates drug selection.

2. The bioassay technique may be described as quantitation of differential sensitivity of human tumor stem cells to anticancer drugs. In using this technique, the evaluator should expect no better result than is achievable with studies of sensitivity to bacteria and antibiotics.

3. The current definition of sensitivity is an operational one. It has been shown, however, that there is a fairly high correlation between in vivo and in vitro sensitivity response.

FLOW CYTOMETRY

1. Flow cytometry has the potential to make a significant contribution to monitoring the response of the tumor to chemotherapy. By plotting a frequency of flourescence intensity, the relative DNA content of cells can be displayed.

2. The relative number of cells in each phase of the cell cycle can be determined. DNA analysis can help to determine the best time to administer chemotherapy.

3. By staining bone marrow cells with the DNA stain, the percent of abnormal cells in the S phase can be monitored. A schedule can be determined to administer an S-phase-specific drug, maximizing the kill of only abnormal S-phase cells.

4. It is possible to verify the long-term success of treatment. DNA analysis can monitor effects of chemotherapy by determining the relative number of cells in a tumor population at regular intervals.

5. Aneuploid cell populations in each phase of the cell cycle can be identified. These cells, containing an abnormal amount of DNA, can appear as separate populations on a DNA histogram.

6. In the future, the clonogenic assay and the flow cytometer may complement one another, or it may happen that the flow cytometer will render the clonogenic assay obsolete.

IMMUNOLOGIC TESTS

1. An *antigen* is a substance that binds to an antibody but does not always elicit an immune response. An *immunogen* is a molecule that has the ability to elicit an immune response. It should be noted that substances that are immunogenic are always antigenic, but that substances that are antigenic are not necessarily immunogenic. The expressions are currently used interchangeably, although this is not correct.

2. Antigens stimulate the production of immunoglobulins (antibodies). There are literally thousands of antigens, each capable of producing a specific antibody. The antigen may be potentially harmful, such as a virus or bacteria, or it may be an inert protein. The antibody produced can only combine with the antigen that is identical to it or nearly so. The antigen binding site links up with the Fab fragment on the immunoglobulin to form a complex. This reaction forms the basis for the detection of antigen-antibody by various laboratory tests.

COMMON CLINICAL LABORATORY TESTS

Immunoelectrophoresis

1. Electrophoresis. The combining of electrophoresis with precipitation in agar is a simple but exceedingly powerful method for identifying antigens in complex mixtures.

2. Technique. A glass slide is covered with an agar gel buffered at *p*H 8.8. Serum is placed into a well cut in the agar. A direct current is applied across the field for 1 to 2 hours.

3. Differential Migration of the Serum Components. The albumin migrates toward the anode, but, due to electroendosmosis, the IgG migrates toward the cathode in the agar support medium. The different serum components are not normally visible in agar but will show up if suitably stained.

After electrophoresis is carried out for 1 to 2 hours, a trough is cut longitudinally in the agar and an antiserum against the electrophoresed antigen is placed in the trough. The two components diffuse toward each other, and precipitin bands form where the antigen and antibody meet at equivalence.

4 Uses. This is a very powerful analytic technique and can reveal about 30 different components in human serum, as compared to the four or five revealed by electrophoresis alone.

Agglutination Test

1. Bacteria and other cells in suspension are usually clumped (agglutinated) when mixed with antisera prepared against them.

2. The antigen can be made part of some particulate material such as red cell, bacterium, or perhaps an inorganic particle such as polystyrene latex that has been coated with antigen. Antibody added to the suspension of such particles combines with surface antigens and links them together to form clearly visible aggregates or agglutinates.

3. This phenomenon is referred to as an *agglutination reaction.*

4. The steps of the agglutination test are outlined as follows:

a. The antigen is part of the surface of some particulate material (red cell, bacterium, or polystyrene latex).

b. Antibody is added to the suspension of such particles and links them together to form agglutinates.

c. The actual test is carried out by placing dilutions of the antiserum in round-bottom wells.

d. Doubling dilutions of antiserum are made up in tubes (1:2, 1:4, 1:8, 1:16, 1:32, etc.).

e. Particulate antigen is added.

f. After incubation at 37°C, agglutinate is seen in the bottom of the tubes.

g. The last tube showing clearly visible agglutination is the end point of the test.

h. The reciprocal dilution of the antiserum at the end point is known as the *titer* of the antiserum.

i. This measures the number of antibody units per unit volume of serum.

5. Uses are listed below:

a. The agglutination tests are employed routinely in the crossmatching of blood.

b. The Widal test is used for the demonstration of antibodies to salmonella in serum specimens in patients suspected of having enteric fever.

c. The agglutination test is used as a thyroid antibody test employing thyroglobulin-coated cells or latex particles.

d. Its principle is used in the hormone assay which employs an agglutination inhibition test as a reaction for pregnancy.

e. It is the basis for a virus infection.

f. *The immunological pregnancy test* is carried out as follows:

(1) *Control.* Red cells coated with hormone (HCG) are mixed with an antihormone antibody. Agglutination results.

(2) *Testing for the Unknown.* Antihormone antibody is added to known hormone molecules (HCG). An antigen-antibody complex is formed. The antigen-binding sites are thus blocked. The addition of hormone-coated red cells does not result in agglutination (because the antihormone antibody has already formed a complex with the hormone molecules in the urine or serum). There is agglutination inhibition. The test can be carried out quantitatively by comparing the activity of a known standard hormone preparation with the test sample. The test is not sensitive enough to measure below 3,000 or 4,000 I.U./liter.

The Coombs' Test—The Antiglobulin Test

1. The Coombs' test is a method for detecting incomplete or blocking antibodies.

2. The test exploits the ability of an antibody molecule to participate simultaneously in binding to an antigen on the red cell surface and in complexing with antibody to itself.

3. The direct Coombs' test is a test for incomplete antibodies attached to red cells.

4. The cells are washed several times and then mixed with Coombs' reagent (antihuman globulin). If incomplete antibodies are attached to the red cells, being human globulins, they will react with the Coombs' reagent, and the cells will agglutinate.

5. It has been demonstrated that the red cell antibody, probably because it is directed against an antigen situated deep in the cell wall, cannot link two red cells together for agglutination. Therefore, the addition of an antihuman globulin brings about agglutination by linking two attached immunoglobulins to one another.

6. This test is used extensively in testing the red cells of newborn babies and in investigating cases of hemolytic anemia.

7. In the indirect Coombs' test, cells of known antigenic content (Rh-positive cells) are mixed with serum suspected of containing the corresponding complete antibodies. After incubation, the cells are washed several times and Coombs' reagent is added, as in the direct Coombs' test. The cells are then examined for agglutination. If agglutination occurs, it proves that the corresponding antibodies are present in the suspected serum.

8. This test is used for checking the serum of pregnant women for incomplete antibodies and in crossmatching tests prior to blood transfusions.

9. The direct Coombs' test differs from the indirect test only in that Coombs' serum is added directly to a washed erythrocyte suspension in the direct test.

10. The indirect test requires the addition of serum from one individual (the prospective transfusion recipient) to a washed erythrocyte suspension from another individual (the prospective transfusion donor) before the addition of Coombs' serum to the system.

Complement Fixation (CF)

1. The ability of certain immune complexes to bind or fix the components of complement may be used as a test for antibodies if one has a known antigen or vice versa.

2. To detect the consumption of complement by the test system, indicator cells consisting of red cells coated with antibody are added. Complement is measured as an activity, as are other enzyme systems, and is expressed in terms of the degree of lysis of a standard suspension of optimally coated sheep red cells produced within a fixed time.

3. Sometimes an antigen-antibody reaction that is completely invisible occurs, in the course of which all available complement is used up or fixed. This is called *complement fixation.*

4. That complement is no longer available or that an antigen-antibody reaction has occurred is shown by adding red cells together with a hemolytic antibody.

5. If hemolysis now takes place, it must be assumed that complement was available. If hemolysis does not take place, it must be assumed that there was no complement available. Hence, an antigen-antibody reaction must have taken place with the original ingredient.

6. The test is performed as follows:

a. *Indicator System*

(1) Sheep red cells are coated with antibody to the sheep red cells.

(2) Complement (fresh guinea pig serum) is added.

(3) Complement reacts with anti–sheep red cell antibody.

(4) Lysis of cells occurs.

b. *Positive Test*

(1) An antigen is added to a specific antibody directed against that antigen.

(2) Complement is added.

(3) The antibody reacts with antigen, and complement combines with the antigen-antibody complex.

(4) Complement is used up and is no longer available.

(5) The addition of antibody-coated red cells does not then result in lysis.

7. The complement fixation test is used in identifying the Wasserman antibody in syphilis as well as in identifying an antigen such as a virus antigen.

Fluorescent Antibody Test (Coon's Test)

1. The fluorescent dye, fluorescein isothiocyanate, can be coupled onto antibody molecules by allowing the isothiocyanate group to react with free amino groups present on the antibody molecule.

2. The resulting antigen-antibody complex shows up as a brilliant yellow-green fluorescence when observed under the microscope using an ultraviolet light.

3. Rhodamine isothiocyanate is often used instead of fluorescein isothiocyanate. Rhodamine is more stable and gives a more brilliant fluorescence.

4. Because immunofluorescent staining reflects the serological specificity of the antibody employed, it is a highly specific histochemical tool.

5. The technique is more sensitive than precipitation or complement fixation techniques, and fluorescent protein tracers can be detected at a concentration on the order of 1μg. protein/ml. body fluid.

6. The Coon's fluorescent antibody test has been used for detection of antigens in bacteria, viruses, protozoa, and fungi as well as human tissue antigens.

7. There are two ways of applying the test in practice—the direct method and the indirect.

a. *Direct Method*

(1) The fluorescein-tagged antibody reacts with an antigen specific to it.

(2) The attached fluorescein-tagged antibody is visualized by use of the ultraviolet microscope.

(3) It is used as a diagnostic laboratory test to identify bacteria in tissue sections, blood, cerebrospinal fluid, urine, feces, or other clinical specimens.

b. *Indirect Method*

(1) Untagged antibody reacts with an antigen specific to it.

(2) The antibody attaches to the antigen determinant, forming an antigen-antibody complex.

(3) To the antigen-antibody complex is added a fluorescein-tagged antiglobulin serum (usually purchased from one of the commercial companies) specific for the globulin of the serum.

(4) The fluorescein-tagged antiglobulin reacts with the antigen-antibody complex.

(5) It is visualized by the ultraviolet microscope.

(6) The end point is much sharper and therefore easier to read than that seen in the direct method.

(7) This method is commonly used for detection of antibodies in serum.

Cytotoxic Tests

1. Cytotoxic tests are used in combination with red cell agglutinations for studying histocompatibility antigen system in tissue typing.

2. The purpose of these tests is to determine whether the permeability of the cell changes after incubation with an antibody and complement.

3. Cytotoxic antibodies have the ability to attach to a cell, activate complement components, and produce changes in the permeability of the cell membrane.

4. If the permeability of the cell membrane is changed, trypan blue will enter the cell and can be identified on microscopic examination.

5. The test has wide application but is usually chosen for work with blood leukocytes. It is less sensitive than the red cell hemagglutination test.

6. The test is performed as follows:

a. *Negative Test—No Antibody*

(1) Leukocytes react with trypan blue in the presence of complement.

(2) Dye is excluded from the cell.

(3) Antibody is not present—a negative test is reported.

b. *Positive Test—Antibody Present*

(1) Leukocytes react with trypan blue in the presence of complement.

(2) Antibody is present and forms an antibody-complement complex on the surface of the cell (antigen).

(3) The cell is rendered permeable to the dye.

(4) Dye enters the cell, proving that antibody is present—a positive test is reported.

7. A modification of this test, where eosin and trypan blue dyes are taken up by the damaged cell, employs radioactive chromium (^{51}Cr).

a. The ^{51}Cr is incorporated into the living cell after a period of incubation.

b. The addition of a specific antibody to the antigen on the surface of the cell in the presence of complement causes a change in the permeability of the cell membrane and results in ^{51}Cr leaking out of the cell.

c. This can be measured, and a judgment can be made on the titer of antibody present.

d. A cell incubated in the presence of a specific antibody directed against its surface antigen activates complement to produce an antigen-antibody complex which damages the cell.

e. The damaged cell is not able to utilize a radiolabeled precursor for the synthesis of nucleic acids and will not form colonies when plated in vitro.

f. Tritiated thymidine is used to label the precursor for this test.

Counter-Current Electrophoresis

Counter-current electrophoresis is a technique for detecting antigens and antibodies by forcing them to move together in an electric field. The technique is related to, but more sensitive than, immuno double diffusion.

Enzyme-linked Immunosorbent Assay (ELISA)

1. Enzyme-linked immunosorbent assay is used for detecting antibody. Antigen is adsorbed to a solid phase and test antibody is added, as in the radioimmune assay (RIA), but the ELISA ligand used to detect the antibody is an enzyme linked to a molecule specific for the bound antibody. Enzymes such as peroxidase and phosphatase are often used.

2. In the final stage a chromogenic substance is added which generates a colored end-product in the presence of the enzyme portion of the ligand. The optical density of this solution is measured after a defined period. This is proportional to the amount of enzyme, which in turn is related to the amount of test antibody. In comparison with RIA, this test has the advantage of stable reagents, but it is usually less sensitive.

3. Fluorescence-activated cell sorter (FACS) is a machine which can analyze the size and fluorescence intensity of single cells stained with specific fluorescent antibodies. The cells are then sorted according to their parameters under the conditions determined by the operator.

31 Diagnostic Radiology in Obstetrics and Gynecology

Hugh R. K. Barber

BASIC PRINCIPLES

The specialty of radiology will undoubtedly become known, in time, as "medical imaging."

1. The use of radiology in obstetrics has almost been phased out by the increased acceptance and use of ultrasonography. Radiologic studies in obstetrics are reserved for very rare cases where ultrasound has not provided positive diagnoses.

2. The use of radiology in obstetrics is limited because:

a. Fear of radiation injuries to the fetus, and to the ovaries of women of childbearing age, is widespread.

b. There is no known exposure threshold for gene mutation.

c. Estimates of the level of exposure at which the spontaneous mutation rate in man is doubled run from 10 to 140 roentgens (R).

3. The estimated threshold doses that may cause fetal damage in humans are:

First month of pregnancy	40 R
Second month of pregnancy	90 R
Third month of pregnancy	140 R
Fourth month of pregnancy	200 R
Fifth month of pregnancy	250 R
Sixth month of pregnancy	350 R
Eighth month of pregnancy	500 R
Tenth month of pregnancy	600 R

4. X-ray pelvimetry gives 1,200 mR to the skin and 1,300 mR to the female gonads.

5. A 14-by-7-inch chest film gives a skin dose of 100 mR, and 0.07 mR to the gonads.

6. Lymphocyte depression has been reported from doses of 50 R.

7. It is suggested, but not conclusively proved, that diagnostic radiation in the prenatal period may result in an increased incidence of leukemia in the children so exposed.

8. Long-term studies of the delayed effects of radiation on survivors of the atomic-bomb blasts in Japan have shown a significant lag in the growth and development of children whose mothers received a radiation dose of 50 rads or more.

9. Therapeutic levels of radiation for pelvic malignancy during pregnancy have resulted in approximately one-third of the babies being born with malformations. Microcephaly was the most frequently seen abnormality.

OBSTETRICAL RADIOLOGY

ANTENATAL FETAL STUDIES

Diagnosis of Pregnancy

1. Fetal skeletal parts such as the fetal skull, vertebral column, and ribs are visible by the fifteenth to eighteenth week.

2. Lower-limb ossification center appears in the femur at 9 weeks; epiphysis around the knee joint at 35 to 40 weeks.

Fetal Maturity

Although ultrasound is more commonly employed, occasionally a flat film of the pregnant abdomen is taken. It is interpreted according to these principles:

1. The epiphysis of the distal end of the femur ossifies at about the thirty-fifth week of gestation.

2. The epiphysis of the proximal end of the tibia ossifies between the thirty-sixth and fortieth weeks, usually indicating a full-term fetus.

3. If the biparietal measurement of the infant's head is more than 8.5 cm., the infant is estimated to be over $5\frac{1}{2}$ pounds.

Multiple Pregnancies

In multiple pregnancies, radiologic examination can reveal fetal presentation and position. In everyday practice it has been replaced by ultrasonography.

Fetal Death

Fetal death is detectable on radiograph by the overlapping of skull sutures (Spalding's sign) and by the presence of gas in the fetal circulatory system.

Abdominal Pregnancy

Radiologic studies can reveal malformations of the fetus. Hydrocephaly, anencephaly, lacunar skull (spina bifida), and long-bone deformities can be diagnosed.

Ultrasonography has almost entirely replaced antenatal radiologic fetal studies.

X-RAY PELVIMETRY

Basic Principles

1. Currently 5 to 7 per cent of all deliveries involve the use of x-ray pelvimetry.

2. The purpose of pelvimetry is to help the clinician decide whether to perform cesarean section.

3. Pelvimetry measures bony landmarks. It does not assess soft tissues, the moldability of the fetal head, the forces of labor, or the degree of relaxation of the pelvic ligaments.

4. Pelvimetry offers no information about uterine dysfunction.

5. Pelvimetry offers one set of parameters in a whole constellation of information from which the decision whether to do a cesarean section must be derived.

6. Pelvimetry is not always essential to this decision; the adroit obstetrician seldom uses x-ray pelvimetry.

Indications

1. There are no clear-cut, universally accepted indications for x-ray pelvimetry. At one end of the spectrum are those physicians who feel it has no place in the practice of obstetrics, while at the other end are those who have a record of heavy utilization.

2. There are three possible outcomes from x-ray pelvimetry:

a. The pelvic measurements are well within normal limits.

b. The measurements are clearly in the abnormal realm.

c. The measurements fall in the overlap at the lower limits of normal and the upper limits of the abnormal range.

3. If the obstetrician states that a particular patient's management will be influenced by the findings of pelvimetry, the study is then indicated. The usual indications are:

a. Clinical evidence of pelvic abnormalities:

(1) Biischial diameter less than 8.5 cm. in a primigravida

(2) Suspected clinical evidence of midplane contraction or other evidence of a contracted pelvis

(3) Diagonal conjugate less than 11.5 cm.

(4) Floating head at term in a primigravida

b. History of difficult forceps operation

c. History of pelvic trauma

d. Breech presentation in a primigravida

e. Obstetrical history suggestive of possible pelvic abnormality—e.g., stillbirth, hard or prolonged labor, unexplained neonatal death

f. Persistent fetal malposition

g. Lack of progress in labor with possible cephalopelvic disproportion (CPD)

h. Anticipated use of oxytocin in possible CPD

4. The views commonly taken are:

a. *Erect lateral view* (taken with the patient standing) showing:

(1) Obstetrical conjugate diameter, sacral angle, and the angle of inclination of the brim

(2) Anteroposterior diameter of the midpelvic cavity

(3) Anteroposterior diameter of the outlet

(4) Shape of the sacrosciatic notch, length and curvature of sacrum, and shape of ischial spines. The thickness and depth of the symphysis pubis can be estimated and the presenting part and its relationship to the brim assessed.

b. *Anteroposterior view* (taken with the patient lying down) showing:

(1) Transverse diameter of the outlet

(2) Interspinous diameter

(3) General shape and symmetry of the pelvic brim, and breadth and shape of the sacrum

c. *Outlet view* (taken with the patient sitting with legs spread and leaning as far forward as possible) showing:

(1) Shape of the subpubic arch. The angle may be measured by the lines joining the lower border of the symphysis pubis to the ischial tuberosities.

(2) Intertuberal diameter, measured 1 cm. above the tuberosities

(3) Subpubic capacity. A circle 9.3 cm. in diameter is applied to the subpubic area, and the distance between the symphysis and the circumference is measured. The measurement is the "waste space of Morris" and should not exceed 1 cm. The fetal head in labor, well flexed and molded, should approximate to 9.3 cm. (3 3/4 inches).

d. *Alternative View.* There is another view sometimes taken, with the patient reclining at an angle of 60° to bring the pelvic brim into the horizontal. This gives an excellent view of the brim shape but entails a high dosage of radiation for the fetal gonad in the vertex presentation (nearly twice as much as for the three other views). It is not commonly employed.

5. Because of these untoward effects and because of the difficulty of estimating the amount of radiation delivered to the maternal and fetal gonads, certain restrictions and precautions should be followed. These are:

a. Elimination of routine radiography of the abdomen for the purpose of diagnosing the presentation of the fetus or for pelvic measurements

b. Use of obstetric radiography only for significant clinical indications

c. Limitation of the number of exposures and use of the maximum tube distance when x-ray pelvimetry is employed

d. Use of such special devices as aluminum and brass filtration, high kilovoltage, fast screens, high-speed films, light localizers, adequate cones, and limiting diaphragms to reduce the area of exposure

e. Use of diagnostic techniques when applicable

X-RAY CLASSIFICATION OF THE PELVIS

Basic Principles

1. The Caldwell-Moloy system, introduced in 1933, classified pelves from the approach of the architectural structure.

2. X-ray films (anteroposterior, lateral, and stereoscopic) are necessary to identify the different types in this classification.

3. The portion of the pelvic cavity anterior to the longest transverse diameter was called the forepelvis, and the posterior portion the posterior or hindpelvis.

4. Caldwell and Moloy divided pelves into four main groups: gynecoid (true female), android (male type), platypelloid (flat), and anthropoid (apelike).

5. Not every pelvis falls definitely into one of these parent types.

6. The Caldwell-Moloy classification has now been altered to include 14 types based upon the shape of the anterior and posterior segments of the inlet.

7. With the addition of small, average and large sizes, the Caldwell-Moloy classification includes 42 different types.

Gynecoid Pelvis (True Female)

1. The gynecoid, or true female, pelvis is the most common type (normal) and is approximately round (or slightly oval).

2. The transverse diameter is a little longer than the anteroposterior diameter and is considerably anterior to the sacral promontory.

3. The hindpelvis is roomy, broad, and deep, leaving the foreplevis sufficiently roomy for vaginal delivery.

4. The sacrosciatic notch is broad, showing that there is ample room for normal birth in both the anterior and posterior pelvis.

5. The pelvic arch is wide.

6. Normal birth is the rule.

Android Pelvis (Male Type)

1. The inlet of the android, or male, type of pelvis is heart-shaped because the sacral promontory is pushed forward nearer the widest transverse diameter, making the posterior pelvis shallow.

2. The pubic arch is narrow.

3. The sacrosciatic notch is narrow, with the outlet diameter shortened.

4. This type of pelvis is a frequent cause of difficult labor.

5. The labor is difficult because of the masculine shape, angulated forepelvis, shallow hindpelvis, and narrow pubic arch.

6. Difficulties in labor arise from the pelvic brim to the outlet.

Platypelloid Pelvis (Flat)

1. The anteroposterior diameter is shortened.

2. The widest transverse diameter is relatively lengthened and lies approximately equidistant from the promontory and symphysis.

3. Both the forepelvis and hindpelvis are shortened.

4. The sacrosciatic notch appears narrowed, and the subpubic angle is usually relatively wide.

5. The fetal head enters the pelvic brim transversely in marked asynclitism.

Anthropoid Pelvis (Apelike)

1. The anteroposterior pelvic diameter is long and the transverse diameter is short, giving the inlet the shape of a sagittal eclipse.

2. Since the widest transverse diameter is so far from the promontory, the posterior pelvis is deep and the sacrosciatic notch is wide.

3. The head enters the pelvis obliquely (because of the relatively or actually short transverse diameter of the inlet).

4. The occiput frequently lies posteriorly, and not infrequently the infant may be born with the occiput persistently posterior.

PELVIC CONTRACTIONS

A contracted pelvis is one in which any important diameter is 1 cm. less than that of the normal gynecoid pelvis.

Inlet Contraction

1. The inlet is contracted if the anteroposterior diameter is 10 cm. or less, or if the greatest transverse diameter is 12 cm. or less.

2. When the diagonal conjugate diameter is less than 11.5 cm., it is assumed that the anteroposterior distance is under 10 cm.

3. The most common cause of pelvic inlet contraction is probably rickets in infancy.

Midpelvic Contraction

1. Average midpelvic measurements are:

a. Interspinous (transverse), 10.5 cm.

b. Anteroposterior (lower symphysis to junction of fourth and fifth sacral vertebrae), 11.5 cm.

c. Posterior sagittal (midpoint of interspinous line to same point on sacrum), 5 cm.

d. When the interspinous is below 9 cm. and the posterior sagittal measurement is below 4 cm., dystocia with a fetus of average term size can be anticipated.

2. Accurate midpelvic measurements are possible only by radiologic methods.

3. In Caucasian women, midpelvic contraction is more common than inlet contraction and leads to transverse arrest of the fetal head.

Contracted Outlet (Funnel Pelvis)

1. These are not as rare as was once supposed.

2. They may occur with all types of pelvis.

3. Complete perineal tears occur when funnel pelvis is not recognized.

4. When the transverse diameter of the outlet between the tuberosities of the ischium (normally 10 or 11 cm.) is 8 cm. or less, the outlet is contracted and the pubic arch (angle) is narrowed so that the baby's head cannot fit into it.

5. The head is forced back toward the tip of the sacrum.

6. If there is enough room in the hindpelvis, the head may pass the outlet.

7. When the outlet is adequate, spontaneous delivery will usually follow.

8. Forceps and a wide episiotomy may be indicated.

9. When the outlet is clearly inadequate, cesarean section should be elected before labor or at its start.

TRIAL OF LABOR

1. *Trial of labor* is the term used when the outcome of labor is uncertain.

2. Usually it means that the pelvic capacity for the baby is in doubt but that, given good uterine contractions and reasonable cranial molding, vaginal delivery is feasible.

3. A trial of labor is conducted in vertex presentations only and should never be used in breech presentation.

4. The term is sometimes used nowadays to mean the trial of induction of labor. If labor has not started or progressed well within some arbitrary time—e.g., 12 hours—then cesarean section is used for delivery.

5. The conduct of a trial of labor requires constant vigilance, frequent checking of descent of the head, cervical dilatation, and fetal heart rate, and monitoring of the labor.

6. In this group of patients cesarean section should be carried out at the earliest signs of fetal distress or lack of progress.

Indications for X-ray Pelvimetry

1. Because of the expense involved, as well as potential radiologic hazards, radiographic pelvic measurement is not necessary in the great majority of cases.

2. There are, however, certain clinical circumstances that point to the probability of pelvic contraction or potential dystocia and that may, at time, make x-ray pelvimetry a part of good obstetrical practice. These include previous injury or disease likely to affect the bony pelvis, and breech presentations in which vaginal delivery is anticipated.

3. Before obtaining x-ray pelvimetry, it is essential to ask: "Is the information to be obtained likely to affect the subsequent management of labor and delivery?" If cesarean section is almost certain to be performed irrespective of the x-ray findings, the use of x-ray pelvimetry is difficult to justify.

4. The slight risk from x-ray pelvimetry seems justifiable only if information critical to the welfare of the fetus or mother is likely to be obtained.

5. The American College of Obstetricians and Gynecologists, in cooperation with The American College of Radiology, has issued a statement of policy giving guidelines for diagnostic x-ray examination of fertile women. The recommended guidelines are as follows:

a. The use of x-ray examination should be considered on an individual basis. Concern about harmful effects should not prevent the proper use of radiation exposure when sufficient diagnostic information can be obtained. Pre-examination consultation with the radiologist may be useful in obtaining optimal information from the x-ray exposure.

b. There is no measurable advantage in scheduling diagnostic x-ray examination at any particular time during a normal menstrual cycle.

c. The degree of risk involved in an x-ray examination if the patient is pregnant, or may become pregnant, should be explained to her and the explanation documented in her record.

PLACENTAL LOCALIZATION

1. Soft tissue placentography, arterial placentography, intravenous placentography, and isotope placentography have been phased out with the wide acceptance of ultrasonography as an alternative.

2. Thermographic localization has a poor success rate (only 50 per cent) but is free of radiation danger.

3. Amniography has been reserved for certain suspected cases of hydatidiform mole in which ultrasound evaluation is not conclusive.

NONOBSTETRICAL RADIOLOGIC TECHNIQUES DURING PREGNANCY

Basic Principles

1. Routine chest radiographs should be avoided except in tuberculin-positive women or in those with signs of active chest disease. A 14-by-7-inch chest film gives 100 mR skin dose, and 0.07 mR to the female gonads. Chest photofluoroscopic film gives 1,000 mR skin dose, and 0.7 mR to the female gonads.

2. Unless absolutely necessary, radiographs should be deferred until the second trimester. The abdomen should be adequately shielded.

3. Gastrointestinal and gallbladder studies should be deferred until the pregnancy is terminated. However, in occasional cases it will be necessary to do such x-ray studies.

4. Intravenous pyelograms are difficult to interpret in pregnancy because of the gestational dilatation of the renal pelves and ureters. However, if they are indicated, the studies should be carried out. A pyelogram gives 1,200 mR to the skin and 1,300 mR to the female gonads.

5. Dental studies may be done with maximum shielding of the abdomen.

6. Bone studies associated with trauma should be done with maximum shielding of the abdomen. X-ray studies should not be ordered for the usual complaints of pubic symphysis or sacroiliac relaxations.

7. When a pregnant woman becomes ill, she deserves as complete an evaluation as if she were not pregnant.

a. If, in the considered judgment of her physician, radiologic examination may supply helpful information that could not be obtained more simply by other methods, then the study should be undertaken.

b. The patient should not be denied radiologic study if there is reasonable probability of its value.

c. Prior consultation between the referring physician and the radiologist will be of great benefit to the patient as well as to her baby.

DIAGNOSTIC ULTRASONOGRAPHY

1. Very-high-frequency sound, or ultrasound, is useful in diagnosis because it can be directed and penetrates the body, like x-rays, but does not cause ionization at the energy levels used.

2. Frequencies are in the range of 1 to 10 MHz, the most common being around 3 MHz—200 times the highest frequency that the average adult ear can hear.

3. Sound waves cause particles of the medium through which they are traveling to move over a minute distance, back and forth, along the direction of their path. Such waves are called *longitudinal* to indicate the direction of displacement of the particles supporting the wave.

4. The power to produce these waves is generated electrically; the device that transforms it into a sound power is called a *transducer.* A common form of transducer uses a thin slice of piezoelectric ceramic or quartz (T). These materials alter their thickness according to the voltage (V) applied between interfaces. The change in thickness is small—only a few microns in the highest-powered machines, producing wavelengths with displacement about 1 nm. which travel through tissue at about 1,540 m. per second.

5. *Intensity* is the amount of energy passing through a certain cross-sectional area, usually 1 square cm. It is usually expressed in watts per square cm.

6. The image is built up by the reflected energy of the beam emitted by the transducer. The reflections come from organ interfaces, vessel walls, and parenchymal tissue. The amount of energy reflected depends upon the orientations of the reflecting interfaces and the differences in acoustic impedance of the tissues at the interfaces.

7. If the beam passes through tissue, it is attenuated; the degree of attenuation determines the amount of energy reaching a given organ or interface. The ultrasonographic image is the result of the interplay of these two acoustic properties of tissue—reflection and attenuation.

8. A tissue may be reflecting or non-reflecting, attenuating or non-attenuating. The same transducer is used for both transmitting and receiving; several different methods are used for detecting and displaying reflected echoes.

A Mode or A Scan

In A mode, or scan, the echoes are displayed as vertical spikes along the baseline of a cathode ray tube, with the height of the spike related to the amplitude of the detected echo. One may use A mode in obstetrics to measure distance; for example, a biparietal diameter of the fetal skull.

B Mode or B Scan

1. B mode, or scan, represents a cross section of the body. A series of bright spots indicate the changing position of the echo as the probe moves across the surface of the abdomen. These spots "coalesce" to give an anatomic outline of the plane of scan.

2. The brightness of each spot corresponds to the intensity of the reflected echo.

3. B mode is used for two-dimensional scanning. B-scans can be produced in various ways. The original B-scanner was an articulated static scanner in which the image was obtained by movement of the transducer over the body's surface. Through the scanning of a number of overlapping areas, a compound picture was built up on the screen, each arc image being stored by the cathode ray tube (storage scope).

Real-Time Scanner

1. This is a machine that gives a moving picture of the fetus. The probe, a rectangular block, contains a large number of transducers (up to sixty-four) which are successively triggered at a rate of thirty impulses per second, so that the movement of the fetal limbs and trunk may be observed.

2. This form of B-scanning has almost completely replaced static B-scanning in routine obstetrical ultrasound practice. Real-time scanning does not require a storage scope.

3. The image is perceived as continuous if the frame rate exceeds "flicker fusion." "Flicker fusion" is the rate at which the viewer's persistence of vision smooths the transition from one frame to the next. The static scanner can cover a larger field of view, but the moving image of the real-time scanner allows the observer the best chance for making an intelligent assessment of three-dimensional anatomy, of noting moving structures, and of selecting the most clinically useful anatomic cross section.

4. Although the real-time scanner does not have a storage scope, the digital memory scan converter allows a high-quality freeze-frame to be held on the screen. Two categories of real-time scanners are in common use for obstetrical (and gynecological) scanning:

a. *Linear Ray.* In this machine the ultrasound beam is derived from a number of transducer elements arranged in a line and firing sequentially. The linear format is particularly suitable for fetal imaging and the machines have the advantage of being small and relatively portable.

b. *Mechanical Sector.* In this type of machine the transducer is oscillated around its own axis, thus giving a large field of view. The resolution obtained with these scanners is very good, which makes them particularly suitable for the detailed scanning required to detect fetal cardiac anomalies, for example; and, in gynecology, the growth and development of ovarian follicles.

5. In *gray-scale* ultrasonography the echoes are displayed in varying tones of gray that correspond to their respective intensities.

6. Ultrasonography is regarded as a noninvasive procedure that can be used at any time during pregnancy with a high degree of accuracy. The most common obstetrical indications include pregnancy dating; diagnosis of multiple pregnancy; monitoring of fetal growth, placental localization, presentation, and position and lie of the fetus; need for knowledge of positions of fetal parts when amniocentesis is anticipated; and detection of congenital anomalies.

The Safety of Ultrasound

1. Ultrasound has been widely used as a diagnostic tool in clinical medicine for more than 25 years. To date, no studies have shown any deleterious effects of ultrasound on the fetus or the mother. A good deal of research has been carried out on animals and tissues, but the adverse effects reported from some of these studies have occurred with ultrasound intensities, pulse durations, and exposure times far in excess of any that are currently used, or likely to be used, in obstetrical diagnostic ultrasonography.

2. The search for possible hazards continues; in the meantime, there is no reason to withhold the proven benefits of diagnostic ultrasonography.

3. Summary of Commonly Used Signal Processing and Ultrasound Systems

a. *A-mode (Amplitude Modulation).* Echo displayed as blip or deflection on oscilloscope. Size related to strength of echo.

b. *B-mode (Brightness Modulation).* Movement of transducer yields a series of dots which build a two-dimensional image

c. *Real-Time.* Transducer moved automatically (mechanically or electronically) to generate successive B-scans (typically 15 to 60 frames per second)

d. *M-Mode (Time-Position Mode).* B-scan displayed continuously with respect to time (i.e., demonstrates movements)

e. *Gray-Scale.* Selective amplification of low-level echoes from soft tissues

RADIOLOGY IN GYNECOLOGY

Basic Principles

1. Whenever possible, radiologic studies in females of childbearing age should be performed prior to ovulation (during the first half of the menstrual cycle).

2. Radiologic studies in gynecological patients have been generally related to:

a. The evaluation of problems of infertility

b. The evaluation of preoperative patients

c. Gastrointestinal studies and cholecystograms included in the gynecologist's area of interest as aids in differential diagnosis.

3. A metastatic workup of the patient with pelvic malignancy should include an intravenous pyelogram, upper and lower gastrointestinal series, and a bone survey.

HYSTEROSALPINGOGRAPHY

Basic Principles

1. This is an outpatient roentgenographic procedure requiring an aseptic technique, a radiolucent vaginal speculum, a cervical plug to prevent reflux, and contrast medium.

2. It is important to have taken a good history and to have done a thorough physical examination.

3. Excessive material exposes the patient to irritation from the medium and prevents proper interpretation.

4. Insufficient material results in an incomplete study.

5. Constant pressure, without excessive force, is maintained in the filled syringe.

6. Severe abdominal pain during the test demands termination of the test.

7. The optimal time for performing the procedure is one week after the menses.

8. Occasionally a sedative and/or an antispasmodic is indicated.

9. Indications are: evaluation of tubal patency, endocervical defects, myomas, polyps, congenital malformations of the uterus, and adenocarcinoma of the endometrium (questionable).

10. Image intensification and television fluoroscopy enable physicians to arrive at a proper conclusion promptly, safely, and with the greatest possible convenience to the patient.

Technique

1. A careful pelvic examination is carried out.

2. After cleansing of the vulva and perineum, a bivalve speculum is inserted into the vagina and the cervix is cleaned with antiseptic, followed by aspiration of cervical mucus.

3. A cannula, with a rubber acorn tip of proper size to occlude the external os, is inserted into the cervical canal. Before insertion of the cannula, the air in the cannula is replaced by a contrast medium.

4. A preliminary film is taken first.

5. For evaluation of the endocervix and uterine cavity, 1 ml. of contrast material is instilled under low pressure.

6. Small amounts of material are then instilled in increments of 1 to 2 ml., with films being taken after each increment.

7. For tubal evaluation it is necessary to instill approximately 6 to 10 ml. In a patient with an enlarged uterus and obstructed or distended fallopian tubes, an even larger amount may be necessary.

8. A 45-minute delayed film should be taken to evaluate peritoneal spill, and a 24-hour film in order to evaluate both spill and the presence of peritubal adhesions.

9. Water-soluble media, rather than oil media, are often chosen for evaluating the uterus. Films should be taken during, and within 5 to 10 minutes after, the instillation.

10. Image-intensified fluoroscopy and cineradiography add to the information provided by the test.

Potential Errors in Technique

1. Failure to take a preliminary film, especially if the patient has had a previous test with radiopaque material

2. Failure to test the equipment, especially the patency of the cannula, prior to the test

3. Too small an acorn on the cannula, which allows the contrast material to leak out

4. Failure to maintain even pressure during the instillation

5. Excessive or insufficient contrast medium

6. Failure to use an aqueous material when there is evidence of previous infection or tubal stenosis

7. Failure to take sufficient films, including laterals when necessary

Adverse Effects

Faulty technique and poor selection of patients usually are the causes of morbidity or are contributing factors in the untoward sequelae that occasionally follow hysterosalpingography.

The following complications can result from hysterosalpingography:

1. Mechanical Complications
- **a.** Pain
- **b.** Uterine perforation
- **c.** Tubal rupture
- **d.** Endometriosis
- **e.** Hemorrhage
- **f.** Shock

2. Chemical and Toxic Complications
- **a.** Granulomas
- **b.** Allergic reactions
- **c.** Iatrogenic thyroid dysfunction

3. Genetic Hazards

4. Intravasation
- **a.** Uterovenous intravasation
- **b.** Intravasation of lymphatic structures

Interpretation of Hysterosalpingogram

1. Intrauterine Adhesions. These are detected as lacunar shadows which are single or multiple, as well as large or small.

2. Infertility

a. This may be related to tubal lesions as well as to congenital anomalies.

b. Tubal obstruction is almost always secondary to salpingitis.

3. Tuberculosis

a. Multiple structures, dilatations, and sinus tracts may be present.

b. Tubes are obstructed, calcification is often present, and the tubes look like "pipe stems."

4. Malformations. Congenital defects or anomalies such as bicornuate uterus can be outlined.

5. Filling Defects

a. These are caused by polyps, hyperplasia, fibroids, synechiae, and adenomyosis.

b. Hydatidiform moles are easily detected.

c. Cervical-canal stenosis and atresia can be demonstrated.

PELVIC ARTERIOGRAPHY

Basic Principles

1. This method of demonstrating pelvic tumors directly is based upon observation of displacement of the normal arterial system, the presence of abnormal vessels, and the formation of communications to adjacent arterial systems, attesting to the invasiveness of such tumors.

2. It has very limited usefulness for assessing tumors of the pelvis exclusive of gestational trophoblastic disease.

3. Arteriography which is properly timed may help to diagnose a molar pregnancy. There is early bilateral filling of the uterine veins in the presence of mole or choriocarcinoma, presumably on the basis of arteriovenous shunts which may be present. The test cannot be applied except in rare cases, because it may expose a normal pregnancy to excessive radiation.

4. Arteriography may be useful in identifying a localized uterine disease that may be poorly responsive to systemic chemotherapy. If further reproduction is planned, arterial infusion chemotherapy may help such a patient. Otherwise, hysterectomy should be carried out.

5. Organs of interest to the urologist that are amenable to angiography include the kidney, adrenal gland, and bladder.

6. In the kidney, arterial patterns characteristic of tumors, cysts, arteriovenous fistulas, or other pathologic or normal processes, such as ectopic renal cortical tissue, are seen in detail.

7. Adrenal arteriography can accurately detect adrenal tumors, adenomas, and cysts.

8. Bladder arteriography has been used to detect invasion of bladder tumors into or through the bladder muscle. The bladder is partially filled with air to give better contrast. This procedure is only occasionally useful.

INTRAVENOUS PYELOGRAM

1. *Excretory urography* is a term used synonymously with *intravenous pyelography.*

2. This is a widely used test in which the calyces, renal pelvis, ureters, and bladder are delineated by renal excretion of intravenously given iodinated contrast medium.

3. This test should be preceded by an adequate plain film.

4. Cathartics and enemas are given to prepare the bowel.

5. Fluid intake is limited for at least 8 hours prior to the examination.

6. Before administration of the contrast medium, a careful history taking and physical examination should be carried out. Allergic reactions should be recorded. The patient's reactions to previous pyelographic studies should be determined.

7. Equipment and drugs necessary to treat an anaphylactic or allergic reaction should be readily available.

8. A pregnant patient should receive a pyelogram only if it is truly indicated.

9. Multiple myeloma has been considered to be a contraindication to intravenous pyelography because of the risk of subsequent acute renal failure. If the test is to be carried out, the patient should be thoroughly hydrated first.

10. Tomography is a roentgenographic technique that focuses on a desired level within the patient. This test should be ordered at the discretion of radiologist.

11. Pyelography gives a skin dose of 1,200 mR, and 1,300 mR to the female gonads.

INDICATIONS FOR ULTRASONOGRAPHIC DIAGNOSIS IN GYNECOLOGY

1. In contrast to the many valuable roles of ultrasound in obstetrics, its uses in gynecology are less distinct. When indicated, it can help to clarify diagnoses, but the results must be correlated with those from all other laboratory tests, the physical examination, and the patient's history.

2. There are three basic indications for ultrasonographic diagnosis in gynecology. These are:

a. Elimination of early pregnancy as a cause of gynecological symptoms.

b. Diagnosis of a hydatidiform mole. Ultrasonography is an extremely accurate method for this, provided that the mole is sufficiently developed. The scan must be carried out by an experienced operator. (The characteristic appearance of vesicle tissue can be mimicked by a septic abortion or a fibroid.)

c. Etopic pregnancy.

Evaluation of Pelvic Masses

Diagnosis of complications of intrauterine contraceptive devices (IUDs).

Pregnancy

Because many symptoms of early pregnancy can mimic those of pelvic disease, the ultrasonographic identification of an empty, nonpregnant uterus, or of the gestational sac of pregnancy, can greatly help in the evaluation of some patients.

Pelvic Masses

Ultrasonography can often give useful information about the nature of a pelvic mass. For instance, a cystic ovarian tumor can appear homogeneous on ultrasonography, whereas a malignant ovarian tumor can produce diffuse reflections that demonstrate its irregular internal pattern.

Loculations and a multicystic ovarian tumor can often be seen. It is rarely possible to differentiate between irregular types of gynecological tumors, such as tubal ovarian abscesses and cystadenomas of the ovary.

Ultrasonography can be useful in determining the size of a pelvic mass and then following its decrease or enlargement. However, there is no evidence that ultrasonographic evaluation of pelvic masses is any more reliable than clinical evaluation coupled with exploratory surgery when indicated. For example, in tubal pregnancies, if positive ultrasonographic diagnosis can sometimes be made, then only in a very few instances can it be relied on in preference to the doctor's suspicions and the results of other diagnostic procedures, such as the change in the beta subunit of human chorionic gonadotropin (HCG).

The localization and evaluation of intrauterine contraceptive devices (IUDs) have become important uses of diagnostic ultrasound in obstetrics and gynecology.

Ultrasonography can be most useful in managing patients who use IUDs.

32 Venereal Disease and Vulvovaginitis

Hugh R. K. Barber

SYPHILIS

Definition

Syphilis is an infectious disease caused by the human parasite *Treponema pallidum,* which ordinarily enters vulnerable mucous (anogenital, oral) or cutaneous surfaces during sexual contact.

The Centers for Disease Control (CDC) has reported an increase in the incidence of primary and secondary syphilis in the United States. The increase from 1986 to 1988 was greater for women than men, occurring most frequently in women between the ages of 15 and 40.

The highest incidence of syphilis occurs among individuals 20 to 24 years of age.

Basic Mechanisms

1. In women the primary chancre of syphilis frequently involves the vulva 3 to 4 weeks after exposure and is sometimes overlooked.

a. It presents as a small, rounded or ovoid ulcer, with raised indurated edges and a depressed center.

b. It is usually present on the labia, with associated edema and inguinal lymphadenitis. The initial lesion will regress in a month or so.

2. The incidence of syphilis has increased by 4 to 4.5 per cent in the past year. This may reflect the failure of the responsible physician to report cases of infectious syphilis to local health authorities so that all contacts can be adequately traced.

3. All contacts should be traced and treated, even if they are asymptomatic. They may be in the incubation period and lost to subsequent follow-up.

4. The incubation period is about 3 to 4 weeks.

5. It is accompanied by inguinal adenopathy. An afflicted gland is hard and enlarged but not tender. It is called an *inguinal bubo.*

6. Syphilis is a systemic disease which may be either acute or chronic and is capable of revealing itself through varied manifestations or of lying quiescent for months or years.

7. Primary syphilis is characterized by a lesion as described above.

a. It may occur on the inner surface of the labium (minus or major), on the clitoris or cervix, or as an extragenital lesion.

b. Diagnosis of primary syphilis is confirmed by examining the discharge from the lesion by dark field examination and by watching the movements of the treponemata.

8. Secondary syphilis appears a few months, usually 2 or 3, after the primary stage. It is a systemic infection with various skin rashes, usually symmetrical, of a copper-brown color like raw ham, and without irritation.

a. Snail-track ulcers and painless shiny gray patches appear in the mouth.

b. There may be sore throat, generalized lymph node enlargement, low fever, and malaise.

c. The gynecologist is usually consulted because of vulvar and perianal condylomata—multiple round and oval, and only slightly raised, warts.

9. The lesions are highly infective. Dark field is positive, and serological tests are positive.

10. Tertiary syphilis appears years (often many) after infection. The lesion is a localized swelling called a *gumma* and has the consistency of rubber.

a. The gumma does not contain treponemata and is not infective.

b. Gummata are irregular in distribution and may be found anywhere in the body.

c. A gumma may break down and result in a punched-out ulcer.

SYPHILIS IN PREGNANCY

Basic Principles

1. There is now a significant rise in the incidence of syphilis and a concomitant increase in the occurrence of congenital syphilis.

2. Effective prenatal screening of pregnant patients has resulted in treatment of those children whose congenital disease would otherwise be manifested at birth or in the immediate neonatal period.

3. Even before the advent of massive screening for *T. pallidum* in pregnancy, only about 10 per cent of cases of congenital syphilis were identified in the first year of life.

4. Recently there has been an increase in the maternal acquisition of syphilis in the period between the initial serological testing and parturition.

5. Organ pathology in congenital syphilis is not complete at the time of parturition but is a continuing organ-spirochete adverse effect well into the first two years of life.

6. By the early identification of a congenital infection and the institution of appropriate therapy, the disease process may be arrested and subsequent morbidity lessened.

7. Until the incidence of syphilis in the community is markedly reduced, the pregnant patient should be screened early and then again near parturition for evidence of infection with *T. pallidum,* especially if more than 90 days have elapsed between parturition and the initial serological test.

8. Adequate treatment of the mother during the first 18 weeks of gestation prevents infection of the baby (congenital syphilis), as the *T. pallidum* probably does not cross the placental barrier until the nineteenth week.

9. Treatment begun after the 18th week of gestation amounts to treatment of the baby in utero.

10. The fetus can be infected in utero. Abortion or stillbirth may result or the liveborn baby may be congenitally syphilitic.

11. The syphilitic placenta is a large, pale organ very like the placenta in hydrops fetalis, showing the microscopic changes of endarteritis and fibrosis.

Diagnosis

1. Dark field examination gives absolute diagnosis.

2. Serological tests used in the serological diagnosis of syphilis are of two main types, i.e., nontreponemal and treponemal tests.

3. *Nontreponemal Tests*

a. The Venereal Disease Research Laboratory (VDRL) test is well controlled, easily performed, and inexpensive. If VDRL is reactive, a quantitative test should be done.

b. Other nontreponemal tests such as the rapid plasma reagin (RPR) test and the automated reagin test (ART) are less specific and should only be used for screening when speed is essential.

4. If a screening test (such as RPR) is positive, the more specific VDRL test should be performed for verification and a quantitation for follow-up.

a. Conditions associated with false-positive VDRL reactions are narcotic addiction, aging, leprosy, and terminal malignancy.

b. Acute false-positive tests are seen in infectious mononucleosis, hepatitis, malaria, viral pneumonia, chickenpox, measles, and smallpox vaccination.

c. If a false-positive reaction is suspected, it should be validated by more specific treponemal tests.

5. Treponemal tests are those employed to detect specific antibodies to *Treponema pallidum.*

6. The fluorescent treponemal antibody test (FTA-ABS) is highly specific: it has only 1 per cent false-positive reactions.

a. False-positive FTA-ABS tests are limited to the group of diseases with abnormal and increased immunoglobulins, such as systemic lupus erythematosus and other autoimmune diseases.

b. Most FTA-ABS false-positive tests give an atypical beading fluorescent pattern which can be differentiated from the normal homogeneous treponemal fluorescence.

c. When there is a borderline FTA-ABS test, a *T. pallidum* immobilizing test (TPI) should be performed for verification.

7. Once the diagnosis of syphilis is made, the quantitative VDRL, not the FTA-ABS, test should be used for post-treatment follow-up.

Congenital Syphilis

1. The fetus can be infected in utero with resulting abortion or stillbirth, and the liveborn baby may be congenitally syphilitic.

2. If the cord blood is positive for VDRL in an asymptomatic infant, serial quantitative VDRL should be performed for a rise or fall of titer.

3. A falling titer indicates passive transfer of reagin from the blood of a mother who has been treated adequately before pregnancy.

4. A rising titer indicates active infection and the need for immediate treatment.

5. IgM antibodies represent fetal response to infection. A positive IgM-FTA-ABS test confirms active infection.

Management

1. In the adult, primary and secondary syphilis is treated with benzathine penicillin G, 2.4 million units I.M. divided into two equal doses given simultaneously.

2. Early and late latent syphilis should be treated according to whether the spinal fluid is positive or not.

3. If the spinal fluid is positive or if no spinal fluid examination is performed, aqueous procaine penicillin G (APPG), 2.4 million units, is given every 2 days for 10 treatments. Total dosage is 24 million units. Aqueous procaine penicillin results in higher penicillin levels in spinal fluid than does benzathine penicillin G.

4. If the spinal fluid is negative, 2.4 million units benzathine penicillin G, I.M., is divided into two equal doses and given simultaneously.

5. Late syphilis (excluding neurosyphilis) is treated with 6 to 9 million units of benzathine penicillin G, given according to the following schedule: 2.4 million units I.M. every 7 days on one or two separate occasions.

6. Syphilis in pregnancy under 16 weeks is treated according to the stage of disease as outlined above. If over 16 weeks, treatment with APPG, 2.4 million units every 2 days × 6 doses. The total dosage is 14.4 million units.

7. Treatment of infants is as follows: small infants are treated with APPG in equally divided I.M. doses every day for 10 days for a total dose of 100,000 to 200,000 units per kilogram body weight.

Alternate Treatment When Penicillin Is Contraindicated

1. Tetracycline 0.5 g. orally q.i.d. for 20 to 30 days (total dose in early syphilis is 40 g. and in late neurosyphilis is 60 g.).

2. Erythromycin base or stearate 0.5 g. orally q.i.d. for 20 to 30 days.

3. During pregnancy, under 16 weeks, erythromycin in the same regimen as for a nonpregnant patient. Over 16 weeks, cephaloridine, 1 g. I.M. daily for 10 days in early syphilis and for 20 days in late syphilis.

4. All treated patients should be followed with serology in the first, third, sixth, and twelfth months during the first year and every 6 months during the second year.

GONORRHEA

Definition

Gonorrhea is an infectious disease caused by the gram-negative diplococcus *Neisseria gonorrhoeae.*

Basic Principles

1. The incubation period for gonorrhea is 3 to 10 days from infection. It is a delicate organism that does not survive easily outside the body.

2. Gonorrhea is acquired by intercourse with an infected person, though it may be spread by clothing or towels, especially in young children.

3. It is an ascending infection of the female genital tract.

4. The clinical manifestations may present with the following stages:

a. *Stage I* (acute phase) is often of only a few days' duration. It may be accompanied by a history of urinary frequency and burning dysuria with a thick yellow discharge.

(1) At this time the patient may have a red urethra with a purulent urethral discharge, an inflamed cervix with a profuse mucopurulent discharge from the external os, swelling or abscess of either Bartholin gland, and acute skenitis.

(2) Many women have no acute phase, especially if the cervix is the primary source of infection.

b. *Stage II* (chronic phase) follows the acute phase. The ascending infection (occurring during menses) moves to the upper genital tract, with involvement of the tubes, ovaries, and pelvic peritoneum. Discharge may be the only complaint.

c. *Stage III* (carrier phase) follows Stage II, which lapses into a carrier state where symptoms are minimal but the ability to infect is present for many weeks.

5. Eighty-five per cent of all uncomplicated gonorrhea in the female is asymptomatic.

6. The most common site of infection is the endocervix.

7. Due to changes in sexual behavior, gonorrhea infections of the rectum and throat occur often enough that specific questions about anogenital and orogenital practices should be asked.

8. Pharyngeal infection occurred in 3 to 11.3 per cent of women examined in venereal disease clinics. Of these, 1 to 3 per cent had pharyngeal infection without demonstrable anogenital infection.

9. Nasopharyngeal culture for gonococcus should be obtained when pharyngeal symptoms are present in a patient suspected of having gonorrhea.

DISSEMINATED GONOCOCCAL INFECTION (DGI)

Basic Principles

1. DGI occurs in 1 to 3 per cent of patients harboring gonococci. Seventy-nine per cent of the patients who develop DGI are women.

2. Dissemination occurs during menstruation or pregnancy in 71 per cent.

3. It is more common in the second and third trimesters of pregnancy.

4. Arthritis is seen in 90 per cent of cases, dermatitis in 50 per cent, and endocarditis in 2 per cent of cases.

5. DGI is characterized by an initial "bacteremic stage" with polyarthritis, skin lesions, and positive blood cultures.

6. In 28 to 40 per cent of women with gonococcal arthritis, pregnancy is a precipitating factor.

Diagnosis

1. Diagnosis is confirmed by the presence of intracellular diplococci and by culture of the organism.

2. Cultures should always be taken from the cervix and anus. If there are any pharyngeal symptoms or if there is a history of orogenital sex, nasopharyngeal cultures should also be obtained.

3. The following technique should be followed for taking a cervical culture:

a. Remove cervical mucus plug with a cotton ball held in ring forceps.

b. Insert the cotton-tipped swab into the endocervical canal and move from side to side.

c. Allow 30 seconds for absorption of the organisms by the swab.

4. *Neisseria gonorrhoeae* grows best on chocolate-agar-based Thayer-Martin medium in a 5- to 10-per-cent CO_2 atmosphere. This agar has been modified recently by the addition of colistin, vancomycin, and nystatin to diminish the overgrowth of the commensal organisms.

Management

1. 4.8 million units of aqueous procaine penicillin G (APPG) I.M., divided into 2 doses. One gram of probenecid should be given orally one-half hour before the injection.

2. When parenteral administration is impossible, 3.5 g. of oral penicillin with 1 g. of probenecid is given orally.

3. If the patient is allergic to penicillin:

a. Spectinomycin 2 g. for males and 5 g. for females, given I.M.

b. Tetracycline 1.5 g. orally, followed by 0.5 g. q.i.d. for 4 days.

4. Penicillin is the only drug which is effective for simultaneously incubating syphilis. When regimens other than penicillin are used, follow-up serology for syphilis is mandatory.

Treatment of Complications

1. Pelvic inflammatory disease is treated with 10 to 15 million units of penicillin per day I.V., supplemented by other antibiotics effective against gram-negative organisms.

2. Patients with DGI should be hospitalized and given 6 to 12 million units penicillin I.V. followed by prolonged therapy for 10 to 14 days with ampicillin, 2 g. daily, once acute symptoms have subsided.

3. Neonatal conjunctival gonorrhea is treated with 150,000 to 600,000 units per day I.M. or I.V., supplemented with topical irrigations of the eye with aqueous solution of penicillin 10,000 U./ml.

CHANCROID (SOFT CHANCRE)

Definition

Chancroid is primarily a venereal infection and is caused by the gram-negative bacillus *Hemophilus ducreyi* (Ducrey's bacillus).

Basic Principles

1. The incubation period is 2 to 14 days.

2. The ulceration is irregular and ragged in outline. The edges are undermined, and the base is granulomatous and purulent. There is little or no surrounding induration, but there is erythema and edema, especially if the lesion is on the labia majora.

3. Pain is a common feature and differentiates chancroid from most of the other venereal diseases.

4. The inguinal lymph nodes enlarge and may suppurate.

Diagnosis

1. Diagnosis is made by the clinical picture of tender, necrotic ulceration and regional, tender, usually unilateral, lymphadenopathy.

2. Diagnosis is confirmed by the recovery of *H. ducreyi* from lesions or bubo aspirates.

3. Gram or Wright stain may be used to identify microscopically the short gram-negative rod in its characteristic parallel chains.

Management

1. Sulfisoxazole 4 g. initially, followed by 1 g. which may be given 4 times a day for 10 days or longer (up to 3 weeks).

2. Sulfamethoxazole (Gantanol) may be used in doses of 2 g. initially, followed by 1 g. twice a day for 10 days or longer (up to 3 weeks).

3. Tetracycline is also effective in a dose of 500 mg. 4 times a day for 2 weeks.

4. Resistant cases should be treated with kanamycin, 0.5 g., given I.M. twice a day for 2 weeks.

GRANULOMA INGUINALE

Definition

Granuloma inguinale is a chronic granulomatous and ulcerative lesion which is caused by *Klebsiella donovani* and is probably venereal in origin.

Basic Principles

1. It has a venereal spread, and the primary lesion is usually on the external genitalia but may be seen on the vagina, cervix, or groin.

2. It is found in tropical and subtropical regions and is more common among blacks.

3. Following a variable incubation period, one or more papular lesions occur, generally in the region of the labia minora.

4. The lesion is of the cutaneous and subcutaneous tissues. It is primarily a nodule which ulcerates and joins with other papules and ulcers to form a large raw area with rolled edges.

5. The disease progresses by fibrous healing. Scarring and ulceration are thus present together. Lymphatic blockage and vulvar elephantiasis can occur.

6. There is little tendency toward lymphadenopathy.

Diagnosis

1. Diagnosis is by recognition of Donovan bodies, small oval organisms contained in macrophages in the granulation tissue.

2. Biopsy should never be neglected.

3. Microscopically, there is an intense infiltration of leukocytes, plasmocytes, and mononuclear cells.

Management

1. Administer tetracycline, 500 mg. 4 times a day for 3 weeks.

2. For patients who do not respond to tetracycline therapy, intramuscular gentamicin in a dose of 40 mg. twice a day for 2 weeks should be given.

LYMPHOGRANULOMA VENEREUM

Definition

Lymphogranuloma venereum is a venereal disease acquired by direct sexual contact and caused by a virus that is related to the virus of psittacosis.

Basic Principles

1. It is caused by a large virus, *Chlamydia trachomatis,* which is also responsible for trachoma, inclusion conjunctivitis, some instances of nongonococcal salpingitis, urethritis, and cervicitis.

a. There are three immunotypes, L1, L2 and L3, of *Chlamydia* responsible for lymphogranuloma venereum (LGV). *Chlamydia* has evolved into a highly specialized bacterium, relinquishing many metabolic functions, and has thus become an intracellular parasite.

2. LGV is more common among blacks.

3. The incubation period is 5 to 21 days.

4. In women, there is initially a small vesicle or ulcer on the labia along with inguinal adenitis. This progresses to a large tumor-like mass which suppurates and discharges through many sinuses extending into the perineum and rectum (a condition known as *esthiomene*). This may cause elephantiasis of the vulva and stricture of the rectum.

5. The pathology involves primarily the inguinogenital and anorectal regions.

6. Signs and symptoms of systemic involvement may occur during lymphatic spread; these include malaise, anorexia, fever, chills, headache, abdominal and joint pain, toxic rashes or erythema, weight loss, pneumonitis, tachycardia, and, rarely, meningism and splenomegaly.

7. Proctitis may accompany the fever and weight loss. It is manifested by mucosanguineous discharge, tenesmus, constipation, diarrhea, and/or rectal pains.

Diagnosis

1. Diagnosis is by Frei's intradermal test. The test is negative until several weeks after infection and once positive remains so for life.

2. A person who has the disease is sensitive to an antigen prepared from the virus. Control material should be prepared as well. The reaction is positive in 48 to 72 hours.

3. Multiple biopsy in LGV and any other granulomatous disease should be performed to exclude an associated carcinoma, for several studies have indicated the frequency with which carcinoma may be associated with both granuloma inguinale and lymphogranuloma venereum.

Management

1. Tetracycline, 500 mg. 4 times a day for 3 weeks is given.

2. Sulfisoxazole, 4 g. initially, followed by 1 g. 4 times a day, is given for 10 days or longer (up to 3 weeks).

3. Sulfamethoxazole may be used in doses of 2 g. initially, followed by 1 g. twice a day for 10 days or longer (up to 3 weeks).

4. Surgery may have to be undertaken for correction of polypoid tumors or strictures that do not respond to dilatation.

TRICHOMONIASIS

Definition

1. Trichomoniasis may be expressed as an infection of the vagina, the vulva, and, less commonly, the urethra. It is rarely seen in the endocervix.

2. The causative organism is the protozoan *Trichomonas vaginalis;* it is globular or pear-shaped, is from 10 μm. to 30 μm. in length (somewhat larger than a polymorphonuclear leukocyte) and has four flagella at the anterior end. There is an eccentrically placed nucleus with attached axostyle.

Basic Principles

1. It is estimated that 2.5 million cases occur annually in the United States. The usual mode of transmission is by sexual contact.

2. Almost all of the female sex partners of infected men are infected.

3. In some patients there are no symptoms. Sometimes female patients may complain of a discharge which comes on during or immediately after menses and is relieved by douching.

4. Characteristically, infestation of the vagina results in symptoms of pruritus and leukorrhea. The discharge is often foul-smelling and may be accompanied by dysuria and dyspareunia.

5. Speculum examination reveals a frothy, bubbly, greenish-yellow vaginal discharge, slight-to-profuse in quantity.

6. There is an associated vaginal and cervical mucosal hyperemia. Not infrequently, hemorrhagic stippling of the posterior vaginal fornix and cervix occurs, resulting in the "strawberry cervix."

7. *p*H ranges from 5 to 7.

8. Vulvar edema, hyperemia, and vulvar excretions may occur.

9. The upper part of the vagina is most severely infected.

10. The infection appears to be chronic and relapses may occur.

Diagnosis

1. Diagnosis involves microscopic examination of a fresh, wet preparation of vaginal discharge in normal saline for evidence of actively motile flaggelate protozoa. Motility is necessary for identification on microscopic examination.

2. When the wet mount is negative, the trichomonads, if present, are easily distinguished from leukocytes after Giemsa staining.

3. Cultures of trichomonads are helpful in patients with small numbers of organisms which are not revealed by wet smear. Since the rate of multiplication of the organism is low, cultures must be observed for 10 to 12 days before they can be regarded as negative.

4. Studies indicate a sensitivity for the wet mount of 76 per cent and for the culture of 91 per cent.

Management

1. Metronidazole, 250-mg. tablet orally 3 times a day for 10 days.

a. When repeat courses are required, 4 to 6 weeks should elapse between courses, and total as well as differential leukocyte counts should be made before, during, and after treatment.

b. Because of metronidazole's reported toxicity in animals, every effort must be made to use it cautiously.

c. Alcohol should not be consumed during treatment because the patient may experience abdominal pain, flushing, and tremors.

d. The sex partner should be treated simultaneously in order to prevent exogenous reinfection.

2. Vagisec solution (1:100 strength) may be used locally.

3. Clotrimazole, 100 mg. vaginal suppository once daily for 7 days, has been found effective.

CANDIDIASIS (MONILIAL VAGINITIS)

Definition

Candidiasis is the name given to an infection, either acute or subacute, caused by the yeast-like fungus *Candida albicans* or by other species of *Candida.*

Basic Principles

1 Monilia is encountered in all parts of the world and may be seen in all age groups.

2. *C. albicans* is a normal inhabitant of the intestinal tract, and this is the source of autoinoculation.

3. Its overgrowth may be caused by pregnancy, use of oral contraceptives, antitrichomonal agents, antibiotics, or immunosuppressive drugs, and by diabetes mellitus.

4. Symptoms are pruritus vulvae and leukorrhea.

5. Speculum examination typically reveals a thick, white, patchy or cheesy vaginal discharge, with the vagina and vulva varying in appearance from normal to a state of acute inflammation.

6. *p*H ranges from 4 to 5.

Diagnosis

1. Diagnosis is by microscopic examination of a wet saline preparation of the vaginal discharge for evidence of pseudomycelia, the filamentous form of *C. albicans* to which potassium hydroxide has been added.

2. Culture techniques: Nickerson's medium, Monitube, Sabourand medium and speciated on cornmeal agar.

3. It is difficult to determine the significance of a positive culture because of the

frequency of candidal colonization in normal individuals.

Treatment

1. 100,000 units nystatin vaginal tablets deposited high up in the vagina by means of an applicator twice a day for 2 weeks.

2. In the gravid patient, a dose of one or two nystatin vaginal tablets daily for 3 to 6 weeks before term will probably prevent thrush in the newborn.

3. Miconazole cream should be applied to the vulva and perineum twice daily for 1 to 2 weeks.

4. Clotrimazole dispensed as 100-mg. vaginal suppositories may be used daily for 7 days.

5. Aqueous gentian violet 1-per-cent to 5-per-cent applied locally has been effective.

6. To prevent seeding of the perineum by fecal matter containing the organisms, nystatin, 500,000 units orally 3 times a day for 1 week to 10 days or longer, may be administered while continuing vaginal treatment.

7. The sex partner should be examined and treated, if symptomatic.

GARDNERELLA VAGINALIS

Definition

1. *Gardnerella vaginalis (Hemophilus vaginalis)* vaginitis is caused by *Hemophilus vaginalis,* now classified as *Corynebacterium vaginale.*

2. *Gardnerella vaginalis* is a gram-negative bacillus. The role of *Gardnerella vaginalis* as a pathogen causing vaginitis is controversial. The major problem concerning the significance of this organism as a pathogen is that it can frequently be isolated from asymptomatic women.

Basic Principles

1. Over 90 per cent of the vaginitides previously classified as nonspecific are caused by *G. vaginalis.*

2. It is probably transmitted sexually.

3. Females with normal ovarian function who have a gray, malodorous vaginal discharge that is relatively thin and has a *p*H of 5.0 to 5.5 are likely to have *G. vaginalis* vaginitis, provided that no trichomonads are demonstrable.

4. The usual complaint is a disagreeable odor.

5. The discharge is often gray and homogeneous.

6. It is not a tissue pathogen and does not cause irritation or soreness. It is simply a surface parasite that proliferates in the vagina to become the predominant organism.

Diagnosis

1. Microscopic examination after Gram staining reveals a predominance of vaginal epithelial cells with an almost complete absence of polymorphonuclear leukocytes.

2. The organism presents as a pleomorphic gram-negative body which adheres to cell surfaces (the so-called clue phenomenon). Sensitivity to Gram staining has been reported to be greater than 90 per cent.

3. Facilities for culturing *G. vaginalis* are not routinely available.

4. When *Gardnerella* vaginal infection is present, 10-per-cent KOH causes a burst of a fishy odor. This is an extremely reliable finding, and when one is new at recognizing "clue cells," the finding of this odor should prompt the search for clue cells because they will be present in nearly all cases.

5. Herman Gardner has said that if a patient has a malodorous discharge, a *p*H of 5.0 to 5.5, and no trichomonads on the wet smear, the patient invariably has *G. vaginalis* infection.

Treatment

1. Ampicillin, 500 mg. orally 4 times a day for 7 to 10 days.

2. Cephalexin monohydrate, 500 mg. every 6 hours for 6 days, or cephradine, 250 mg. every 6 hours for 6 days.

3. Triple sulfa vaginal tablets or cream are also effective.

4. Sex partners should be examined.

5. Appropriate tests for gonorrhea and syphilis should precede this treatment regimen so as not to mask concomitant infection.

MYCOPLASMAS

Definition

1. *Mycoplasma hominis* and *Ureaplasma urealyticum*, the latter formerly referred to as T-strain mycoplasma (T for "tiny"), are the smallest of free-living organisms capable of reproducing themselves without assistance from other forms of life.

2. They are extremely pleomorphic. They appear as granules, ring forms, filaments, coccoids, and other bizarre forms. They possess a limiting cellular membrane rather than a rigid cell wall.

Basic Principles

1. Mycoplasmas were formerly of most concern to veterinarians.

2. *Mycoplasma pneumoniae* has been implicated in human disease.

3. There are eight recognized species of mycoplasma found in humans.

4. *M. hominis* and *U. urealyticum* frequent genital sites from which they may be cultured by appropriate methods.

5. *M. hominis* and *U. urealyticum* are the principal mycoplasmas that have been isolated from the human genitourinary tract. They have been associated with nongonococcal urethritis, acute salpingitis, abortion, and postpartum fever.

Diagnosis

1. Techniques for identification have improved.

2. The samples are obtained from cervical and urethral swabs and from urine.

3. *M. hominis* forms colonies about 100 to 150 μm. in diameter which are just visible to the unaided eye.

4. A colony of *M. hominis* under the microscope has a dense granular center and a foamy peripheral zone ("fried egg" colony).

5. *U. urealyticum*, in contrast, forms tiny granular colonies with no peripheral growth and with an average diameter of 25 μm.

6. The possible role of mycoplasma in unexplained infertility and recurrent abortion remains to be clarified.

Management

All of the mycoplasma strains are sensitive to tetracycline and resistant to penicillin and other antimicrobial agents that act on the cell wall.

HERPES SIMPLEX VULVOVAGINITIS AND CERVICITIS

Definition

1. Herpesviruses are composed of a single molecule of double-strand DNA, one of the simpler forms.

2. Two major serotypes of herpesvirus have been identified and designated Type 1 and Type 2.

a. *Herpesvirus Type 1* (HSV-1), oral herpes, is most often involved in labial, upper respiratory, and central nervous system (CNS) infections.

b. *Herpesvirus Type 2* (HSV-2), herpes genitalis, affects the lower genital tract and causes prenatal infection of the newborn.

Basic Principles

1. Herpesviruses are probably the most widely disseminated human pathogens.

2. The incidence of herpes genitalis is far higher than is generally suspected. It may be the predominant cause of vesicoulcerative disease of the genitalia.

3. Patients observed with recurrent lesions outnumber those with primary lesions in the approximate ratio of 2 to 1.

4. The incidence of active recurrent or secondary disease has far exceeded the combined incidence of all major venereal diseases.

5. The majority of female patients with the primary disease are teenage girls and unmarried women.

6. The mean age of those with primary disease is 26½ years; of those with recurrent disease, 36½ years.

7. Once the infection is acquired, generally by sexual contact, the symptoms of the primary attack usually appear in 3 to 7 days.

8. The primary lesions are often extensive, and can involve all the vulvar tissues, the genitocrural folds, and the perianal skin, as well as the vaginal and ectocervical mucosa.

9. The primary lesions often appear as widespread indurated papules with vesiculations and ulcerations on the most dependent surfaces. A red areola is invariably present. The lesions often coalesce, forming bullae and large ulcerations, which may involve most of the vulvar and perianal skin.

10. Primary lesions last from 3 to 6 weeks. Complete healing without scarring will result unless there is a secondary infection.

11. The persistence of the herpetic stage of a lesion depends on the degree of moisture at the affected site and the degree of trauma to which the lesion is subjected.

12. Lesions within the labia minora (vestibule) will ulcerate within 24 to 48 hours, whereas those on dryer areas are less subject to maceration.

13. Inguinal lymphadenopathy is almost always present, and the majority of patients have a low-grade fever for several days.

Diagnosis

1. The culture is done on human fibroblasts. The material is collected by rubbing the lesions with a cotton-tipped applicator soaked in tissue culture medium. The material is then transferred immediately to tissue culture supplemented with protein. The cytopathic effect is evident after 24 to 48 hours in tissue culture.

2. The material should be stained by the Papanicolaou technique. A saline-soaked cotton-tipped swab is wiped on the lesion and smeared on a dry slide, which is immediately fixed in a standard fixative. Staining will demonstrate characteristic nuclear changes with or without intranuclear inclusions. These techniques have given a low yield of positive isolations.

3. Serologic testing may be employed to establish the diagnosis of primary herpetic infection. Germs should be obtained during the acute episode and during the convalescent phase. It is preferable to obtain acute serum shortly after the vesicles appear and a sample of convalescent serum in ten days.

4. The convalescent serum should have a higher titer of herpetic antigen than the serum obtained during the acute phase. The rise in antibody titer can be taken to mean that the patient has experienced primary herpetic infection.

5. In the face of recurrent infection, the antibody titers of acute and convalescent sera will be similar. This is due to the fact that recurrent disease is a local phenomenon, and no systemic manifestation occurs.

Management

1. The management of genital herpes is directed mainly at relieving symptoms. Many agents have been recommended, but when proper double-blind studies were performed, these agents proved either ineffective or potentially toxic.

2. The only agent thus far approved by the FDA for the treatment of herpesvirus 1 or 2 infection is acyclovir (chemical name: 9-[(2-hydroxyethoxy)methyl] guanine sodium). Activation of acyclovir requires that the compound first be phosphorylated, which occurs preferentially in the infected cells via HSV-thymidinekinase.

3. The concentration of phosphorylated acyclovir in virally infected cells is approximately 40 to 100 times greater than in uninfected host cells.

4. Phosphorylated acyclovir actively inhibits viral DNA polymerase.

5. The concentration of phosphorylated acyclovir required to inhibit host cell growth is 3,000 times the concentration required to inhibit viral DNA polymerase. This propensity for viral thymine kinase and viral DNA polymerase makes acyclovir a promising agent, not only for the treatment of herpes simplex in the nonpregnant patient but also in the pregnant patient. Acyclovir can be administered as a topical ointment, by intravenous infusion, or by mouth.

6. Symptomatic relief is with wet dressings and sitz baths (1 part Burrow's solution to 20 parts water).

7. An ice bag applied to the lesion over a towel may give relief from pain.

8. Antibiotic ointment (bacitracin) should be used to prevent secondary infection.

9. Urinary antiseptics and analgesics, such as phenazopyridine hydrochloride (Pyridium) 200 mg. 3 times a day, may give relief from dysuria.

10. Percodan may be required for pain.

11. Hospitalization may be required for patients with extensive vulvovaginal lesions, pelvic lymphadenopathy, and fever.

12. Idoxuridine (Stoxil) applied locally may give relief from the acute symptoms.

13. Inoculation with smallpox vaccine has been used for the prevention of recurrent herpes but is not recommended.

14. Photodynamic inactivation gives symptomatic relief rapidly in 75 per cent of recurrent infections and in almost all primary infections.

a. The technique is to apply neutral red dye 1-per-cent or proflurine 0.1-per-cent directly to the lesion.

b. The physician then exposes the area to light (using a 100- to 150-watt incandescent bulb) for 10 to 15 minutes.

c. The bulb is held about 6 inches from the lesion.

d. Exposure to the light is repeated in 6 to 8 hours and again in 24 hours.

15. The potential effect of producing defective oncogenic viruses in laboratory animals has been demonstrated. There is little evidence to indicate this side effect in humans. Use of acyclovir has practically phased out this method of management.

16. The suspected association of cervical cancer and untreated genital herpesvirus 2 must be considered.

CONDYLOMATA ACUMINATA (VENEREAL WARTS)

1. Genital warts, condylomata acuminata, is an ancient disease; mention is made of it as early as the Greek and Roman civilizations. The disease is caused by the human papillomavirus, which is a member of the papovavirus group.

2. The papillomavirus has been demonstrated in genital warts. These are small DNA viruses. After gaining entrance to a host cell, they attach to the nucleus. Although the papillomavirus is the etiologic agent of verruca vulgaris (the common skin wart), the two strains are antigenically different.

Definition

1. They are the visible manifestations of a viral venereal disease (they are also known as *venereal warts*). Condylomata acuminata are the common form of vulvar papilloma but are granulomatous rather than true neoplasms.

2. The infecting agent of genital warts has been identified with the electron microscope as a papillomavirus.

3. Condylomata acuminata result from infection with the human papillomavirus. There are many subdivisions of the human papillomavirus at present.

Basic Principles

1. The lesion is usually pedunculated, and there is no induration around the base of the lesion.

2. No ulceration is seen as a rule, but when secondary infection is present, all the patterns of infection, with polymorphs, plasma cells, and vascular proliferation, may be seen below the epithelial layer.

3. The patient frequently gives a history of a sexual partner having a similar growth, but not always.

4. In most areas the growth becomes luxuriant. Discharge, secondary infection, and bleeding are common.

5. Genital warts seldom grow outside the anogenital areas. They may spread into the rectum.

6. Monilia infection is seen more often with genital warts than without.

7. Poor personal hygiene seems to play some role in the female.

9. Pregnancy appears to act as a marked stimulus. Some grow so large that a cesarean section is necessary.

9. Genital warts occasionally disappear spontaneously.

Diagnosis

1. Biopsy should be carried out. Concomitant vulvar cancer may be present.

2. The diagnosis can occasionally be made by cytology.

Tests to Detect Human Papillomavirus (HPV)

Pap smear
Indirect immunofluorescence
ELISA
Western blot analysis
Southern blot test
Competition radioimmunoprecipitation with purified HIV and specific antibody
Vira Pap test
Vira type test (as yet does not have FDA approval)
In situ hybridization

Polymerase chain reaction (PCR) will be used in the near future.

Management

1. Podophyllin 25-per-cent is effective when applied to the condylomata acuminata.

a. The surrounding skin must be carefully protected.

b. Podophyllin should not be used in pregnancy.

2. Halogenated acetic acid (Nevitol) is effective when applied locally.

3. Triple sulfa cream locally has been reported to be effective.

4. Cryosurgery and hot cautery have been quite successful in eradicating condylomata acuminata.

5. Large condylomata may require surgery and in some instances even vulvectomy.

6. Laser surgery has been employed with excellent therapeutic and cosmetic results. In the large condyloma, it is the treatment that is most often and most effectively chosen.

7. Cancer chemotherapy drugs (thiotepa, methotrexate, 5-fluorouracil cream, and bleomycin) have not given a predictably good response.

8. Autogenous vaccines have been reported to be effective.

MOLLUSCUM CONTAGIOSUM

Etiology

1. Molluscum contagiosum is probably due to a DNA virus belonging to the poxvirus group.

2. The typical lesion appears after an incubation period of 3 to 6 weeks and characteristically is asymptomatic. The mode of transmission is thought to be physical contact, frequently sexual intercourse.

Clinical Manifestations

1. The lesion appears as raised papules which are smooth, hemispheric in shape, and centrally umbilicated. The lesions are frequently found on the vulva, lower abdomen, thighs, and perineum. They are usually asymptomatic but may become pruritic, especially when irritated by friction of clothing. They can become inflamed and secondarily infected. Infected lesions of molluscum contagiosum are often associated with a local lymphadenopathy, and the lesions tend to resemble furuncles.

2. Secondary bacterial infection is not a common sequela to initial infection with molluscum contagiosum.

Diagnosis

1. The diagnosis can be determined first by the typical appearance of the lesion, the umbilicated papule. The content of the papule is curd-like or cheese-like material which consists of nonviable epithelial cells and keratin.

2. Cytologic examination of these cells will reveal the presence of large cytoplasmic inclusion bodies. The lesions may persist for anywhere from months to as long as 2 years and tend to resolve spontaneously.

Treatment

1. Treatment can consist of observation until the disease resolves spontaneously. The lesion can also be sprayed with ethyl chloride and then opened, and the base of the lesion curetted. An application of silver nitrate or ferric subsulphate (Monsel's) solution, or electrodesiccation, should follow to prevent bleeding.

2. Pregnancy has not been known to exacerbate the disease.

33 Acute and Chronic Pelvic Inflammatory Disease and Pelvic Tuberculosis

Hugh R. K. Barber

DEFINITION

1. *Pelvic inflammatory disease* is a generalized term describing acute, subacute, recurrent, or chronic infections in the cervix, uterus, fallopian tubes, and ovaries, with or without involvement of adjacent supportive tissues or of the peritoneum or intestines.

2. These infections may be bacterial, fungal, parasitic, or viral in origin.

3. Though commonly used as a diagnosis for any pelvic complaint, the term "pelvic inflammatory disease" should be replaced by specific descriptive terms as to the type of involvement and causative agent of the infection, if known.

NATURE AND MODE OF INFECTION

There are five causes and types of salpingitis:

1. **Gonorrhea.** This is an ascending infection which progresses up along the endometrial surface from the cervix to the fallopian tubes and peritoneum. Acute attack usually happens at the end of menstruation.

2. **Puerperal and Postabortal Infection**

a. This is nearly always hemolytic streptococcus, either alone or associated with staphylococcus or *E. Coli.*

b. It occurs during the early stage of the uterine infection, during the second or third week after labor.

c. The path of infection differs from that in gonorrhea insofar as it spreads by the lymphatics of the broad ligament and mesosalpinx to those of the tubal wall. It is truly a parametritis.

3. ***Chlamydia trachomatis.*** This has been investigated as a possible etiologic agent in pelvic inflammatory disease (PID). It seems likely, at least in Scandinavia, where the most detailed studies have been carried out, that the majority of cases of PID are caused by chlamydia. It is thus important that antibiotic regimes for the treatment of PID should incorporate a drug that eradicates chlamydia.

4. **Direct Extension from Acute Pelvic Appendicitis.** This infects the serous coat of the tube—not the lumen.

5. **Tuberculosis.** The majority of cases of salpingitis are secondary to tuberculotic infection of other organs.

BASIC MECHANISMS

1. PID is usually a problem of young women and women of low-parity.

2. Pelvic infection has always been a formidable problem in obstetrics and gynecology. With the present rapid rate of increase of venereal disease, this problem has become more formidable and widespread de-

spite current advances in antibiotic therapy.

3. The most frequent cause of acute salpingitis is the gonococcus (*Neisseria gonorrhoeae*), the gram-negative intracellular diplococcus, which invades the pelvic adnexa by direct extension from the lower generative tract.

4. It is difficult to assess the true role of the gonococcus in the disease process, because the patient may be asymptomatic initially.

5. With repeated contacts and reinfection or exacerbation, the disease process spreads throughout the reproductive system, crippling it in most cases.

6. In the adult, the method of transmission of the disease is usually sexual contact. In female children, direct nonsexual contamination may occur.

7. The incubation period is from 3 to 8 days. The organism primarily infects the urethra, Skene's ducts, Bartholin glands, and cervical glands. Recently there has been an increased incidence of pharyngitis and anal contamination.

8. The fallopian tubes and peritoneum may become involved later by direct extension, especially following the menstrual period.

9. Extension of the disease may take place through the blood stream and involve joints, the heart, meninges, and skin.

10. When acute salpingitis is diagnosed and treated in its early stages, the prognosis is excellent.

11. The patient and her sexual partner(s) should be reported to the local Department of Health.

12. The organisms most commonly involved in pelvic infections are:

a. *Bacteria. N. gonorrhoeae, Streptococcus* sp., staphylococcus, *Escherichia* sp., *Proteus* sp., bacteroides, *Aerobacter aerogenes, Pseudomonas aeruginosa, Mycobacterium tuberculosis,* and, more recently, an epidemic of chlamydia.

b. *Virus.* Myxovirus (mumps).

c. *Parasite. Schistosoma haematobium, S. mansoni.*

d. *Fungus. Actinomyces bovis, Blastomyces dermatitidis.*

13. Most infections of the pelvis are polymicrobial (aerobic-anaerobic) infections.

ACUTE SALPINGITIS

Basic Principles

1. Pain. Sudden, severe, in the hypogastrium.

2. Temperature. Raised to 102 to 103°F at onset. Irregular and intermittent. The patient may have chills.

3. Tachycardia is present.

4. Vomiting is not usual.

5. The patient may occasionally have vaginal bleeding.

6. There is a foul-smelling discharge. The patient may pass tissue via the vagina.

7. In milder cases, the disease process usually subsides with 4 to 7 days of bed rest.

8. Relapses on getting up too soon are likely.

9. At first there is extensive endosalpingitis with marked edema, hyperemia, and a heavy purulent discharge.

10. As the process extends, all layers of the fallopian tube are involved. Pus escaping from the fimbriated end of the tube may result in frank pelvic peritonitis. If the tube is closed at its fimbriated end it may become grossly distended with pus and form a pyosalpinx.

11. Tubo-ovarian abscess is a frequent complication.

12. Drainage of pus out of the tube may become loculated by loops of bowel or mesentery, producing a pelvic abscess.

Orders

1. Bed rest
2. CBC
3. SMA-12

4. Urinalysis
5. Sedimentation rate
6. Measure fluid intake and output
7. Chest radiograph
8. Flat plate of abdomen
9. Intravenous pyelogram and sonogram—optional
10. Smears from urethra, cervix, and anus for aerobic and anaerobic incubation and sensitivity studies
11. Blood cultures
12. Regular diet
13. Infusions as needed. The I.V. may facilitate the antibiotic regimen.
14. Percodan q.3h. p.r.n. for pain
15. Mineral oil } 15 ml. of each per os at bedtime
16. Milk of magnesia }
17. Dulcolax rectal suppositories as needed
18. To each 1,000 ml. I.V. fluid add 10 to 20 million units of penicillin.
19. If the patient is sensitive to penicillin, administer cephalothin sodium, 2 to 4 g. as stat I.V. push, then 2 g. every 4 to 6 hours, totaling 12 to 24 g. per 24 hours.
20. Kanamycin sulfate, 1 g. daily, added to penicillin or cephalothin sodium therapy
21. Chloramphenicol has been a valuable drug in doses of 4 to 6 g. per 24 hours. It can be used only as a last-resort drug, because of its reported complications.
22. Change antibiotic therapy as indicated after cultures are reported.
23. Nasogastric tube, if indicated
24. Nasal oxygen, if indicated
25. Central venous pressure monitoring as indicated

Management

1. As outlined under "Orders," above
2. Cultures of cervix, urethra, and anus
3. Cul-de-sac aspirates
4. Fluids and antibiotics as outlined above
5. Semi-fowler's position
6. Reevaluate every 12 hours

CHRONIC SALPINGITIS WITH PELVIC INFLAMMATION

Basic Mechanisms

1. The acute inflammation process will subside into subacute or chronic stages either spontaneously or after treatment, although there is marked tendency to repeated re-exacerbations.

2. Chronic salpingitis is often the result of pelvic inflammation which has been inadequately treated and then complicated by the superimposed secondary invasion of other strains of bacteria. When this occurs the patient may be acutely ill.

3. The patient may have remarkably few symptoms.

   a. The chief disability is fatigue or pain following exertion. While the patient is resting there may be no symptoms.

   b. The symptoms usually associated with chronic salpingitis are: pain, menorrhagia, leukorrhea, dyspareunia, and sterility.

4. Abscess formation and pelvic peritonitis may complicate chronic salpingitis; then the clinical picture is similar to that seen in acute PID.

Orders

As for acute salpingitis (above)

Pelvic Abscess

1. If a pelvic abscess is present in the posterior fornix, carry out wide colpotomy drainage.

2. Perform gentle digital exploration of the cul-de-sac area to break down pockets of exudate.

3. Keep the patient in the semi-Fowler's position.

4. Place adequate and large drains in the lateral pelvis and flanks, if possible.

5. Continue this regimen as long as the response is satisfactory.

6. In obstetrics and gynecology, pelvic abscesses are always polymicrobial (aerobic-anaerobic) infections.

7. If the condition deteriorates it may be necessary to do an exploratory laparotomy. The technique is described below.

8. The rate of mortality from ruptured tubo-ovarian abscess prior to 1950 was reported to be between 80 and 100 per cent. It has now been reduced to 6 per cent.

Ruptured Pelvic Abscess

1. Orders, fluids, and antibiotic therapy as outlined for acute salpingitis (above)

2. Aspirate pus by culdocentesis to serve as a guide to laparotomy.

3. Do cultures for anaerobic and aerobic organisms.

4. Remove only infected organs, unless the infection is so widespread that more extensive surgery is necessary.

5. Explore above and below the liver and spleen to rule out pockets of exudate.

6. Run the small and large bowels to break up sacculations of pus.

7. Aspirate all obvious exudate.

8. Thoroughly wash the pelvis and abdomen with saline.

9. Secure hemostasis.

10. Use drains through the vaginal cuff as well as through the right and left lower quadrants. The drains should be large.

11. Close the abdomen with retention sutures.

12. Drain above and below the fascia.

13. Sepsis and septic shock are discussed in Chap. 20.

14. Since pelvic abscesses are usually polymicrobial infections, it is important that the antibiotic regimen cover both aerobic and anaerobic organisms. The patient should be given gentamicin and, particularly, metronidazole, because of its ability to penetrate tissue. Cefoxitin or ampicillin should be included in the regimen as well.

PELVIC TUBERCULOSIS (GRANULOMATOUS SALPINGITIS)

Basic Principles

1. The causative organism is the acid-fast tubercle bacillus.

2. The majority of cases are secondary to tuberculotic infection of other organs.

3. Pelvic tuberculosis may be transmitted through the bloodstream from a primary lesion in the lungs, kidney, or peritoneum. Rarely, it is transmitted by a male sexual partner who has tuberculosis of the genitourinary tract.

4. About 8 per cent of women who die of pulmonary tuberculosis are found postmortem to have tuberculosis of the genital tract.

5. The diagnosis is often made during investigation of infertility problems.

a. The physician may inadvertently discover tubercular lesions in the endometrium by biopsy or curettage.

b. Genital tuberculosis is the cause of infertility in about 5 per cent, or more, of women seeking help in infertility clinics.

c. When tubercular lesions are found in the endometrium, it can be assumed that the patient has tuberculosis of the fallopian tubes.

6. The frequencies of tuberculotic involvement of the various organs in genital tuberculosis are: fallopian tubes, 90 to 100 per cent; uterus, 50 to 60 per cent; ovaries, 20 to 30 per cent; cervix, 5 to 15 per cent; and vagina, 1 per cent.

7. The frequencies of presenting manifestations in female genital tuberculosis are: sterility, 45 to 55 per cent; pelvic pain, 50 per cent; poor general condition, 26 per cent; menstrual disturbances, 20 per cent; and vaginal discharge, 4 per cent.

8. Most patients are young women. The most common complaints are primary infertility and abdominal pain with menstrual disturbances.

9. Genital tuberculosis has a reputation for appearing unexpectedly; but any complaint suggestive of pelvic inflammation, especially in a patient who is infertile, should be regarded with suspicion.

Physical Examination

1. On palpation, the abdomen may feel doughy.

2. Ascites, either general or sacculated, may produce distension of the abdomen.

3. Irregular masses may be felt, caused by the matting together of intestines, omentum, and pelvic organs.

4. On pelvic examination the tubes may not be palpable. One may palpate a unilateral mass, with the uterus displaced and tender. The mass is usually completely fixed and tender. The consistency of the mass is not uniform; both firm and fluctuant areas can be palpated.

Diagnosis

1. Symptoms as outlined above.

2. Histological evidence from endometrial curettings is the most easily obtained evidence.

a. When signs of tuberculosis are seen in the endomentrium, it is assumed that the tubes are also infected.

b. A negative report may indicate that the infected area was missed, the biopsy was not taken at or during menstruation, and that the infection may not yet have spread from the tubes.

3. Bacteriological evidence should always be looked for, and curettings sent for Ziehl-Neelsen staining, cultures, and guinea pig inoculation. Growth is slow; at least 6 weeks must be allowed.

4. Biopsy should be made of any ulcerated area in the cervix, vagina, or vulva.

5. If all findings are negative but clinical suspicion remains, a laparotomy or laparoscopy and biopsy of any infected area should be carried out.

6. Once evidence of genital infection is obtained, a search should be made for signs of active tuberculosis elsewhere, particularly in the respiratory and urinary tracts.

Aids in Diagnosis

1. X-Ray. Chest radiograph

2. Tuberculin Test. Intracutaneous injection of first-strength purified protein derivative (PPD) on the flexor surface of the forearm. If after 48 hours the transverse diameter of edema and redness measures 10 mm. or more, the result is considered positive.

3. Hysterosalpingography. (Always use a water-soluble contrast medium, never Lipiodol or any other oily liquid.)

a. The tubal lumen appearances are: rigid "pipe-stem," straight shadow, and "fluffy" outline due to thickened mucosa. A tube may be closed, but often tuberculous tubes are open; this is a sign of adhesions.

b. This test may be dangerous in the presence of active or secondary infection.

Management

1. One must first rule out extragenital tuberculosis.

2. Minimal genital tuberculosis is treated with isoniazid, 300 mg. daily, and ethambutol, 20 mg. per Kg. of body weight, or approximately 1,200 mg. daily.

3. At 6 and 12 months, endometrial curettages or biopsies are examined bacteriologically. If negative, a hysterosalpingogram is done.

4. If curettings become positive or tubo-ovarian masses appear during treatment, rifampin, 600 mg. daily, is added for 3 months, and the patient is subjected to laparotomy.

5. If no complications arise, isoniazid and ethambutol are continued for at least 2 years.

Management of Advanced Genital Tuberculosis

1. The regimen includes isoniazid, 300 mg. daily, and ethambutol, 20 mg. per Kg. of body weight, or approximately 1,200 mg. daily.

2. The patient is reexamined every 4 weeks.

3. For the first 2 months most adnexal masses get smaller.

4. If tubo-ovarian masses are still present after 3 to 4 months of isoniazid and ethambutol therapy, laparotomy is indicated.

5. One week before laparotomy, streptomycin, 1 g. per day I.M. is given and continued until 2 weeks after surgery.

6. Depending on whether or not residual tuberculosis foci are left in the abdomen, streptomycin administration may be continued twice weekly for a total of three months.

7. Isoniazid and ethambutol are given postoperatively as they were before the operation.

8. Rifampin, 600 mg. daily, may be used in place of streptomycin. (Hearing loss has been associated with long-term use of streptomycin.)

Indications for Surgery

1. Antituberculotic drugs should be started immediately and administered for 3 to 4 months, after which removal of the tuberculous lesions is made easier.

2. Persistence, or increase in size, of adnexal masses after a course of antituberculotic drugs as outlined above

3. Recurrence of endometrial tuberculosis after 1 year of antimicrobial therapy

4. Persistence of pelvic symptoms after long antituberculotic drug therapy

5. Age of 40 years or more in a patient who will not continue long-term therapy or return for follow-up

6. Fistulas that fail to heal

Important Points in Management

1. A preoperative course of antituberculotic drugs is indicated.

2. Antituberculotic drugs should be given postoperatively for 18 months or longer.

3. Preoperative use of antituberculotic therapy makes the surgical procedure technically easier and reduces the risk of operative and postoperative complications.

4. Genital tuberculosis is more quickly cured with surgery than with antituberculotic drugs alone.

ACUTE PELVIC PARAMETRITIS OF NONVENEREAL ORIGIN

Basic Principles

1. Parametritis is an inflammation of the parametrial tissue with cellular infiltration of the broad, cardinal, and uterosacral ligaments. The inflammation is described as being of ligneous consistency.

2. The infection travels directly, by lymphatic vessels and veins, to the loose areolar tissue in the pelvis at the bases of the broad ligament and the sides of the uterus.

3. Factors predisposing to the development of parametritis are: surgical, including conization, cauterization, cervical biopsies, tubal insufflation, hysterosalpingography, dilatation, uterine sounding, and abortion.

4. Traumatic factors include coital trauma, postabortal or post-delivery laceration of the cervix, douche under high pressure, foreign body, and intrauterine device (IUD).

5. The patient becomes acutely ill and develops sustained fever (103°F) and rapid pulse. If there is associated thrombophlebitis, chills and a spiking temperature will also be noted.

6. Rectovaginal examination reveals thickening and tenderness in both fornices, and eventually a hard cellular infiltration of the uterosacral ligaments and parametria.

7. The WBC and sedimentation rate are elevated.

Management

1. Bed rest.

2. Antibiotic therapy. Type will depend on the organism cultured. Preliminary broad-spectrum antibiotic therapy should be started.

3. Activity and intercourse are contraindicated for at least one month.

4. Antibiotics should be continued for 2 to 4 weeks.

5. Surgery is indicated to manage abscess formation.

CHLAMYDIAL INFECTIONS

Basic Principles

1. Chlamydial infections are epidemic in the United States.

2. There has been an alarming nationwide increase in the number of cases of ectopic pregnancy and salpingitis, a large proportion of which may result from chlamydial infections. Since each of these ectopic pregnancies represents one fetal death, they contribute to the epidemic of fetal deaths.

3. Chlamydial infections during pregnancy should receive much more attention than they do. They may lead to postpartum endometritis in the mother and may be transmitted to the infant, causing pneumonia or eye infection. Chlamydial infections in pregnancies raise rates of premature birth, stillbirth, and neonatal death.

4. Current failure rates, against chlamydia, of conventional ambulatory therapy for non-gonococcal PID are unacceptably high.

5. Greater awareness, better diagnosis, and better treatment of chlamydial infections, as well as treatment of the sexual partners of patients with chlamydial infections, might have a major impact on the epidemic.

6. The respective prevalences of gonorrheal and chlamydial infections have been compared in populations cultured for both agents. In some sexually transmitted disease (STD) clinics, chlamydial infection is found to be about 50 per cent more common than gonorrhea.

Differences Between Chlamydial PID and Gonococcal PID

1. Women with chlamydial PID have a less acute presentation than women with gonococcal PID. Their symptoms are of longer duration and they have higher sedimentation rates. They also tend to have more-prominent adenexal masses.

2. Reports indicate that the risk of infertility is higher after an episode of non-gonococcal PID than after an episode of gonococcal PID; it follows that infertility from tubal scarring might be more often related to chlamydial infection than to gonococcal infection.

3. Chlamydial infection causes scarring in the submucosal area of the fallopian tube, which makes the tube narrower and interferes with peristalsis. This may account for the relatively large numbers of ectopic pregnancies seen with chlamydial infection.

4. In women who have chlamydial infection the organism lives in the columnar epithelium of the endocervix. Women taking oral contraceptives appear to be at about twice the normal risk of having a positive cervical culture for chlamydia. This may be the result of the oral contraceptives' causing ectopia of the cervix, which may make it more susceptible to infection because the columnar epithelium becomes exposed on the exocervix.

5. After infection, mucopurulent cervicitis—characterized by edema and friability of the ectopic epithelium and the presence of inflammatory cells in the cervical mucus—develops in some women. Without treatment, complications will develop in an unknown proportion of women. The organism can extend upward into the endometrium and produce endometritis. It may also extend into the fallopian tubes and cause salpingitis.

6. Direct culture of the organism is difficult and used to require cumbersome techniques. There is an immunofluorescent antibody test available, and also a monoclonal antibody test that is reliable and easy to carry out.

Treatment

1. Tetracycline is the drug of choice for chlamydia. However, it is only moderately active against anaerobes and facultatives.

2. Since many of the pelvic infections are polymicrobial, other broad-spectrum antibiotics should be added.

Conclusion

1. *Chlamydia trachomatis* is a pathogen commonly found in the genital tracts of men and women. Although infected patients may be asymptomatic, there is accumulating evidence that the microorganism is responsible for a wide range of diseases almost certainly including cervicitis and salpingitis, and probably acute bartholinitis, perihepatitis, and urethral syndrome.

2. Infected patients should be treated with tetracyclines or erythromycin. Their sexual partners should be investigated.

3. In the absence of culture evidence of infection, the management of patients with suspected chlamydial infection depends upon a mixture of epidemiological evidence and clinical acumen.

ACQUIRED IMMUNODEFICIENCY SYNDROME (AIDS)

1. AIDS is a virus-induced disease in which the virus attacks and destroys selected cells in the immune system. The destruction of these cells leaves the body vulnerable to a number of microorganisms which, under normal circumstances, do not produce disease in immunologically intact persons. These are called opportunistic pathogens, and have the potential to kill their hosts.

2. There are 1 million to 1.5 million Americans currently infected with human immunodeficiency virus (HIV, the causative agent of AIDS). Of these, 20 to 30 per cent are expected to develop the disease by 1990.

3. In the next few years the number of cases among heterosexuals and pediatric patients will increase considerably.

4. The AIDS virus has been variously termed:

a. Human T-lymphotrophic virus Type III (HTLV-III)

b. Lymphadenopathy-associated virus (LAV)

c. AIDS-associated retrovirus (ARV)

d. Human immunodeficiency virus (HIV)

5. There is no definitive test for AIDS. What we have are tests for HIV infection, which may progress to AIDS.

6. The diagnosis of AIDS is made on clinical grounds. The initial Centers for Disease Control (CDC) definition was the presence of brown-proven Kaposi's sarcoma in a person younger than 60 years of age and/or *Pneumocystis carinii* pneumonia, or other opportunistic infection, in a person who has no obvious underlying cause for immunosuppression.

Symptoms

1. In its early stages, AIDS may not cause any symptoms. The symptoms that AIDS victims eventually develop are primarily related to the diseases or infections that attack them because of the body's inability to fight off infection.

2. These symptoms are persistent and may include:

a. Extreme tiredness, sometimes combined with headaches, dizziness, or lightheadedness

b. Continued fever and night sweats

c. Weight loss of more than 20 pounds not due to dieting or increased physical activity

d. Swollen glands in the neck, armpits, or groin

e. Purple or discolored growths on the skin or the mucous membranes (inside the mouth, anus, or nasal passages)

f. Heavy, continual dry cough that is not due to smoking, or that has lasted too long to be due to an upper respiratory infection or influenza

g. Continuing bouts of diarrhea

h. Thrush—a thick whitish coating on the tongue that may be accompanied by sore throat

i. Unexplained bleeding from any body opening or from growths on the skin or mucous membranes

j. Tendency to bruise more easily than normal

k. Progressive shortness of breath

3. Most people infected with HIV develop specific antibodies within two or three months of infection. The interval to onset of symptoms after infection with HIV virus is thought to range from 6 months to 6 or 7 years. Most people exposed to the virus have not developed AIDS.

Dissemination of AIDS Through Blood Supply

1. All blood collected in the United States for transfusions is now being tested for antibodies to HIV. Blood that tests positive is removed from the transfusion pool.

2. The process involves use of an ELISA (enzyme-linked immunosorbent assay) screening test, with confirmation of positive results through a more specific antibody test known as the Western Blot. Blood that is positive on the initial ELISA is retested by the same ELISA method. If it is reactive on a repeat ELISA test, a Western Blot test is conducted to confirm the result. Blood that is positive for antibodies to HIV on any of these tests is removed from the transfusion pool.

3. All studies indicate that the HIV antibody test is highly effective in eliminating from the donor pool blood that may be infected with HIV.

AIDS-Related Complex (ARC)

1. *AIDS-related complex* is the term that has been adopted to describe clinical signs and/or symptoms that seem related to AIDS syndrome but do not specifically meet the CDC's criteria for the disease.

2. AIDS-related complex manifests itself as fatigue, weight loss, chills, fever, night sweats, and swollen glands in the neck, armpits, or groin. These symptoms last longer than they would with most illnesses with which they might normally be associated.

3. Symptoms of disease must persist for at least 3 months, in conjunction with antibodies to HIV, in order to meet the criteria established for ARC. Some patients with ARC may never develop AIDS.

Vaccine

1. At present there is no vaccine to protect a person from the HIV virus or from AIDS. The development of a successful vaccine will require a great expansion of our base of knowledge.

2. The properties of the retrovirus suggest that the development of a vaccine will be difficult. Because the virus can alter its form in the human body, researchers in the United States and other countries are working diligently to develop an AIDS vaccine.

Chemotherapy

1. Within the next few years, dramatic advances will be made in the fight against the AIDS virus and the infections it causes.

2. Improved understanding of how the HIV reproduces itself in the T-4 helper lymphocyte and brain cells has opened up several potential avenues for successful therapy.

3. Tests of the compound azidothymidine (AZT) have demonstrated that by chemical modification of the building blocks of DNA it can stop the replication of the virus. However, the prevention of further replication of the virus cannot undo damage already done to an immunosuppressed patient.

34 Fluid and Electrolyte Problems

Hugh R. K. Barber

FLUIDS AND ELECTROLYTES

DEFINITIONS

1. Basic Type Body Fluids. The plasma and the interstitial and intracellular fluids consist of water, electrolytes, and protein.

2. Electrolyte. A substance that is capable of conducting an electric current when it is placed in a solution.

3. Ions. Electrolytes dissociated into electrically charged substances.

4. Ionized Solution

a. The ions that migrate to the negative electrode (*cathode*) of the cell have a positive charge and are called cations, e.g., Na^+, K^+, Ca^{++}, Mg^{++}.

b. The ions that migrate to the positive electrode (*anode*) of the cell have a negative charge and are called anions, e.g., Cl^-, HPO_4^{--}, SO_4^-, HCO_3^- (without equivalent base).

ACIDOSIS AND ALKALOSIS

1. The hydrogen ion concentration determines whether a solution is acid or alkaline.

2. An increase in hydrogen ion concentration leads to an acid solution, whereas a decrease leads to an alkaline solution.

3. There must always be an equal number of positively charged ions (*cations*) and negatively charged ions (*anions*) in a solution.

4. The hydrogen ion (H^+) concentration, the ion that determines acidity, will bear a direct relationship to the total number of anions present and a reciprocal relationship to the other cations present.

5. It is common usage (but not chemically correct) to associate base in terms of cations other than hydrogen.

6. Sodium (Na^+), potassium (K^+), magnesium (Mg^{++}), and calcium (Ca^{++}) are called bases.

a. They are called bases inasmuch as they replace, and are equivalent in electrical charge to, hydrogen ions in maintaining an equal balance of positive and negative ions.

b. Their presence in the body reduces the hydrogen ion concentration.

7. Chloride (Cl^-), phosphates (PO_4^{--}), sulfates (SO_4^{--}), and much of protein (proteinates) increase the hydrogen ion concentration and act as acids.

8. Although the hydrogen ion concentration per se in a liter of plasma is small, and the balance between cations and anions greatly influences the hydrogen ion concentration, in the final analysis it is the hydrogen ion concentration that determines acidity or alkalinity.

pH (POTENTIAL OF HYDROGEN)

The term *p*H (potential of hydrogen) is a simple way of representing hydrogen ion concentration.

1. $pH = -\log (H^+)$ or $pH = \log \frac{1}{H^+}$.

2. *p*H represents the negative logarithm of the hydrogen ion concentration.

3. As the hydrogen ion concentration increases, the *p*H decreases, and the solution contains more acid.

4. Conversely, as the hydrogen ion concentration falls, the *p*H rises, and the solution contains more alkaline.

5. Normal plasma *p*H is 7.40, with a range of 7.38 to 7.42.

6. In strict chemical terms, the plasma, with a *p*H of 7.4, is on the alkaline side.

Henderson-Hasselbalch Equation

1. $pH = pK + \log \frac{\text{salt}}{\text{acid}}$

2. It is possible to calculate any of the three unknown variables (*p*H, $NaHCO_3$, or H_2CO_3) if two are known by direct measurement.

3. At the normal *p*H of plasma (*p*H = 7.4), the relation of sodium bicarbonate (salt) to carbonic acid (acid) is $\frac{20}{1}$.

4. In metabolic imbalances of acidosis or alkalosis, it is the numerator, or salt value, that is altered.

5. In respiratory imbalances of acidosis or alkalosis, it is the denominator, or acid value, that is altered.

6. Diagrammatically:

a. Metabolic Acidosis

$$pH\downarrow = pK + \log \frac{\text{salt}\downarrow}{\text{acid}} \; (pH\downarrow CO_2\downarrow)$$

b. Metabolic Alkalosis

$$pH\uparrow = pK + \log \frac{\text{salt}\uparrow}{\text{acid}} \; (pH\uparrow CO_2\uparrow)$$

c. Respiratory Acidosis

$$pH\downarrow = pK + \log \frac{\text{salt}}{\text{acid}\uparrow} \; (pH\downarrow CO_2\uparrow)$$

d. Respiratory Alkalosis

$$pH\uparrow = pK + \log \frac{\text{salt}}{\text{acid}\downarrow} \; (pH\uparrow CO_2\downarrow)$$

7. If the $\frac{\text{salt}}{\text{acid}}$ ratio stays at $\frac{20}{1}$, the *p*H will remain at 7.4.

8. The *p*H does not depend on the total sodium bicarbonate or the total carbonic acid but rather on the relative ratio of salt to acid.

9. Elevation of the sodium bicarbonate fraction without an increase in carbonic acid, $\frac{NaHCO_3\uparrow}{HHCO_3}$, will result in an elevated *p*H and a metabolic alkalosis.

10. If the carbonic acid is elevated at the same time, $\frac{(NaHCO_3\uparrow)}{HHCO_3\uparrow}$, as the sodium bicarbonate, and the ratio of $\frac{20}{1}$ is maintained, no change in *p*H will occur, and a compensated state will exist.

11. By the same token, a decrease in the sodium bicarbonate fraction without a decrease in carbonic acid $\frac{NaHCO_3\downarrow}{HHCO_3}$ will result in a decrease of *p*H.

12. If carbonic acid content is decreased at the same time as the sodium bicarbonate fraction $\frac{NaHCO_3\downarrow}{HHCO_3\downarrow}$ so that the $\frac{20}{1}$ is maintained, no change in *p*H will occur.

a. *Illustrated by Use of Formula for Metabolic Alkalosis*

$$pH = 6.1 + \log \frac{27}{1.3} = 7.4 \text{ Normal}$$

$$pH = 6.1 + \log \frac{36}{1.3} = 7.6 \text{ Uncompensated}$$

$$pH = 6.1 + \log \frac{36}{1.8} = 7.4 \text{ Compensated}$$

Equivalent and Milliequivalent

1. It is an ion's power to combine, and not its weight, that is important in body fluids.

2. The terms *equivalent,* and, more specifically, *milliequivalent* (mEq.), have been designated to represent the "horsepower" of a given electrolyte.

3. An equivalent, as the name implies, means equal to something. The hydrogen ion (H^+), with a valence* of one, has been used as the basis for comparison.

---

* Valence of an atom depends on how many atoms of hydrogen (H^+) it can combine with or displace. The monovalent atoms (Na^+, Cl^-) displace one atom of hydrogen, while the divalent atoms (Ca^{++}) displace two atoms of hydrogen.

4. An *equivalent* is that weight of an element which has a combining or reacting value equal to one gram atom of hydrogen ion in change.

a. A *milliequivalent* is 1/1,000 of an equivalent.

5. Equivalent $= \frac{\text{atomic weight}}{\text{valence}}$

Equivalent (sodium) $= \frac{23}{1} = 23$ g.

Milliequivalent (sodium) = 1/1,000 of an equivalent = 0.023 g. = 23 mg.

6. For divalent ions, such as calcium, with a valence of two:

Equivalent (calcium) $= \frac{40}{2} = 20$ g.

Milliequivalent (calcium) = 1/1,000 of an equivalent = 0.020 g. = 20 mg.

MOL

1. A *mol* is equal to the molecular weight of a substance.

2. It is independent of valence.

3. A *millimol* (mM.) is 1/1,000 of a mol.

4. Univalent ions (Na^+, Cl^-) have equal values for milliequivalent and millimol.

5. For divalent ions, millimol is twice the milliequivalent weight.

6. Examples

a. 1 milliequivalent of potassium (K^+) = 39 mg.

b. 1 millimol of potassium (K^+) = 39 mg.

c. 1 milliequivalent of calcium (Ca^{++}) = 20 mg.

d. 1 millimol of calcium (Ca^{++}) = 40 mg.

OSMOL AND MILLIOSMOL

1. The unit of osmotic pressure is termed the *osmol.*

2. Like the milliequivalent, the milliosmol (mOsm.) is the smallest unit of measure.

3. Each substance exerts an osmotic effect.

4. Substances that dissociate give rise to dissociated ions, each producing an independent osmotic effect.

5. Valence is *not* considered in calculating milliosmols.

6. An equivalent of a univalent substance exerts a pressure of one osmol.

7. Divalent substances such as calcium (Ca^{++}) require two equivalents to produce a pressure of one osmol.

1 mOsm. calcium/liter $= \frac{10 \times 10}{40} = \frac{100}{40} =$ 2.5 mOsm.

1 mEq. calcium/liter $= \frac{10 \times 10 \times 2}{40} = \frac{200}{40} = 5$ mEq.

8. A gram of sodium chloride produces a much greater osmotic pressure than a gram of glucose because of the larger number of particles in an ionized solution of the former.

9. One millimol of NaCl (58.5 mg.) in solution in one liter of water has a milliosmolar (mOsm.) effect of two milliosmols, one each for sodium (Na^+) and chloride (Cl^-). The following is an example:

a. 23 mg. Na per liter = 1 milliosmol per liter

35.5 mg. Cl per liter = 1 milliosmol per liter

58.5 mg. NaCl per liter = 2 milliosmols per liter

b. 39 mg. K per liter = 1 milliosmol per liter

35.5 mg. Cl per liter = 1 milliosmol per liter

74.5 mg. KCl per liter = 2 milliosmols per liter

c. 180 mg. of glucose per liter = 1 milliosmol per liter

d. 60 mg. of urea per liter = 1 milliosmol per liter

e. The milliosmolar concentration of 0.9-per-cent NaCl is

9 gm. NaCl per liter $= \frac{9{,}000}{58.5}$

$= 154$ mEq. Na^+
154 mEq. Cl^-
308 milliosmols

f. Milliosmolar concentration 5-per-cent glucose in water.

$$50 \text{ g. glucose per liter} = \frac{50{,}000}{180} = 278$$

milliosmols

10. Sugar and urea do not dissociate and only produce an osmotic effect equal to their molecular weight and concentration.

11. Therefore, in disease states, greatly increased concentrations of glucose and urea can raise the osmolarity of the extracellular water with resulting physiologic consequences.

12. One milliosmol/liter =

$$\frac{\text{mg. of substance or ion per liter}}{\text{atomic weight of substance or ion}}$$

$$\text{One mOsm./L.} = \frac{\text{mg. per 100 ml.} \times 10}{\text{atomic weight}}$$

DAILY BASELINE REQUIREMENT, EXTRARENAL LOSSES, DEFICITS, OR EXCESSES

Basic Principles

1. Fluid and Electrolyte Replacement. The problem of fluid and electrolyte replacement resolves itself into three parts:

a. What are the normal daily baseline requirements?

b. What are the extrarenal losses?

c. What are the deficits or excesses that are present at the beginning of treatment?

2. Fluid Replacement. Daily baseline requirements represent the fluid and electrolyte needs for the day of an average patient who is being maintained on parenteral therapy, has no abnormal losses, and does not have an excess or deficit present at the start of therapy.

Water Requirements

1. Insensible loss of 700 to 1,000 ml.

2. Urinary output of 800 to 1,500 ml.

3. Total water requirement of 1,500 ml. to 2,500 ml. This is replaced as 5-per-cent glucose and water.

4. The above is based on findings that the average adult requires 35 ml. of water per Kg. of body weight and that the obese elderly female requires only 25 ml. per Kg. of body weight.

Electrolyte Requirements

1. Maximal need for sodium chloride is 77 mEq. Na^+ and 77 mEq. of Cl^-. It is supplied by administering 500 ml. of 0.9-per-cent sodium chloride.

2. Approximately 30 to 40 mEq. KCl (2 to 3 g. of KCl) supplies the daily baseline requirement. A urinary output of at least 1,000 ml. in 24 hours must be present before potassium can be added safely.

Calories

1. It is difficult to supply an adequate number of calories with intravenous fluids. In short-term replacement therapy it is not necessary.

2. By giving 100 g. of glucose (2,000 ml. 5-per-cent glucose and water) a day, the nitrogen loss of proteins is cut by 50 per cent. 100 g. of glucose can supply only about 400 calories per day.

3. The body can only utilize about 0.5 to 0.7 g. of glucose per Kg. of body weight per hour. An infusion of 5-per-cent glucose and water should not be run faster than 600 ml. per hour, if dehydration is to be prevented.

Vitamins

1. The average postoperative Ob-Gyn patient does not need intravenous vitamin supplements.

2. Vitamins B and C are water soluble and, when given by the intravenous route, are excreted in the urine in high concentrations.

Amino Acids

1. There are practically no indications for the use of amino acids in the average postoperative Ob-Gyn patient. In the immediate postoperative period, the enzyme systems are not working at maximum efficiency, and, as a result, amino acid preparations are excreted at a rapid rate.

2. The reactions associated with protein hydrolysates make their use undesirable unless they are absolutely necessary.

Extrarenal Losses

Extrarenal losses are those losses that are going on under observation. They are replaced in kind, in amount, and at a rate equal to that at which they are lost; and they are divided into external and internal losses.

1. External Losses

a. Vomitus

b. Tube suction

c. Stomach—has a high concentration of chlorides

d. Small bowel—has a high concentration of bicarbonate

2. Surface Losses From Wounds

a. Groin dissection wounds, burns, exenterations, and abdominal perineal resections

b. The losses may be of sufficient magnitude to produce a severe electrolyte problem, especially in the elderly patient.

c. Excessive sweating

d. Hemorrhage—must be replaced at the rate it is lost

3. Internal Losses

a. Ileus

b. Peritonitis—resembles a third-degree burn

c. Raw pelvic surface—as seen after radical hysterectomy, pelvic exenteration, or an abdominal perineal resection

Excesses and Deficits

1. Excess

a. Expanded extracellular space—may be seen in cirrhotics, cardiacs, and nephrotics

2. Deficit—Dehydration

a. *Rapid*—less than 48 hours in duration, as seen in acute obstruction or ileus. It involves mainly the extracellular space.

b. *Slow*—over a longer period than 48 hours; as seen in pregnancy, ileus, or large bowel obstruction. It involves the intracellular, as well as the extracellular, space.

Management

Replacement of Fluids and Electrolytes After Rapid Dehydration

1. Apply the empiric formula of H. T. Randall to determine fluid-replacement requirement:

$$\left(1 - \frac{\text{Normal hematocrit}}{\text{Found hematocrit}}\right) \times \begin{array}{c}\text{20\% body}\\ \text{weight in}\\ \text{Kilograms.}\end{array}$$

2. Hematocrit is obtained and is designated as the *found hematocrit.*

3. The normal hematocrit for women is usually 40.

4. The weight in Kg. is obtained by dividing the weight in pounds by 2.2.

5. The weight in Kg. is multiplied by 20% and equals the liters in the extracellular space, i.e., 20% × 60 Kg. = 12 liters.

6. Assume that a 60-Kg. female is admitted with a diagnosis of acute obstruction and a history of vomiting for 12 hours.

a. Hematocrit on admission is 60 (found hematocrit).

7. By application of the formula:

$$\textbf{a.}\ 1 - \frac{\text{Normal hematocrit}}{\text{Found hematocrit}} \times \begin{array}{c}\text{20\% body}\\ \text{weight in}\\ \text{Kg.}\end{array}$$

$1 - 40/60 \times 20\%$ of 60

$1 \times 2/3 \times 12$ L. $\quad (3/3 - 2/3 = 1/3)$

$1/3$ of $12 = 4$ L. deficit

b. Inasmuch as the deficit is 4 L. and the patient normally has a 12-L. extracellular space, there are only 8 L. present.

c. 4 liters must be replaced.

8. The electrolyte content of the replaced fluid is determined as follows:

a. A serum chloride is obtained.

b. Assume that it is returned as 90

mEq./L. and that the laboratory normal is 100 mEq./L.

c. The amount of electrolytes to be replaced is worked out as follows:

(1) The value should be:
12 L. × 100 mEq. Cl = 1,200 mEq. Cl^-

(2) The actual value is:
8 L. × 90 mEq. Cl = 720 mEq. Cl^-

(3) Therefore the deficit is:
480 mEq. of Cl^-

d. In each 1,000-ml. bottle of 0.9-per-cent saline there are 154 mEq. Na^+ and 154 mEq. Cl^-.

e. To find the amount of saline to give, divide: 480/154 = 3.1 L.

f. Of the 4-liter deficit in the extracellular space, 3.1 L. must be replaced as saline or saline and glucose.

g. This leaves 900 ml. that must be replaced as glucose and water.

h. The daily requirement consists of:

(1) Daily baseline requirement:
1,000 ml. 5-per-cent g/w
500 ml. 5-per-cent g/s
1,000 ml. 5-per-cent g/w
40 mEq. KCl—if urinary output is over 1,000.

(2) Extrarenal losses.

(3) Deficit.

HELPFUL HINTS IN MANAGEMENT OF FLUID AND ELECTROLYTE PROBLEMS

Fluid and Electrolyte Imbalance

1. A high sodium level is almost invariably associated with dehydration.

2. Normal adults maintained exclusively on intravenous fluids lose 200 to 300 g. of body weight a day.

3. The maximum amount of water that the kidney can excrete is about 15 ml. per minute, or 900 ml. per hour.

4. 500 ml. of citrated whole blood transfused to an adult will raise the hemoglobin about one g., or 7 per cent.

5. Ten per cent of the total body weight can be lost before clinical signs of dehydration start to become obvious.

6. At first, salicylate poisoning gives rise to a state of respiratory alkalosis; if untreated, it leads to a metabolic acidosis.

7. The patient who complains of restlessness, fatigue, dizziness, chest pain, numbness, tingling, and syncope, particularly when under stress, may be suffering from a hyperventilation syndrome.

8. The administration of excessive amounts of intravenous sodium may give rise to hoarseness.

9. The normal urinary flow is 50 to 100 ml. per hour. In treating dehydration, a urinary output of about 40 ml. per hour indicates that the dehydration is being corrected.

10. A low serum potassium level means a low cellular, as well as low extracellular, level, whereas a high serum level does not necessarily mean that a high cellular level is present.

11. To each 1,000 ml. of replacement fluid for gastric or small-bowel losses, add 20 mEq. of potassium chloride.

12. Every seriously ill surgical patient who is being maintained on intravenous fluids should be weighed daily, and an accurate intake and output record should be kept.

13. An intravenous solution of 5-per-cent glucose and saline is hypertonic and should be given at a rate no greater than 300 ml. per hour if dehydration resulting from excess diuresis is to be prevented.

14. Inasmuch as the body is only able to metabolize about half a gram of glucose per Kg. of body weight per hour (0.5 g. × Kg. per hour), it is important to administer an intravenous 5-per-cent glucose and water solution at a rate no greater than 600 ml. per hour, if dehydration is to be prevented.

15. It is important to administer plasma in cases of peritonitis and also to guard against calcium deficiency, which may occur in these cases.

16. There are cases in which the electrolyte imbalance is not appreciated and incorrect therapy is given.

Examples:

a. The use of antibiotics for dehydration fever.

b. The use of the Miller-Abbott for intestinal distension that is secondary to a low serum potassium.

c. Cardiovascular disease or heart failure is often diagnosed when a salt depletion syndrome is actually present.

17. Never give sodium lactate* in the presence of:

a. Liver disease
b. Shock
c. Anoxia
d. Cardiac decompensation
e. Respiratory alkalosis

18. All electrolyte problems are caused by:

a. Disturbance of volume
b. Disturbance of osmotic pressure
c. Disturbance of *p*H

19. The average adult intake of sodium is about 100 mEq. per day and almost all of it is excreted in 1,000 ml. to 1,500 ml. of urine.

20. An early ileus may be detected by noting a decrease in the output with an increase in urine specific gravity.

21. Early in septic shock, arterial blood gases frequently reveal a mild respiratory alkalosis.

22. Central venous pressure (CVP) monitoring measures only the function of the right side of the heart.

23. Studies have shown the superiority of pulmonary artery pressure (PAP) and pulmonary wedge pressure (PWP) monitoring by means of a Swan-Ganz catheter over CVP as an index of left ventricular competence.

24. Any rise in either pulmonary artery pressure (PAP) or left atrial wedge pressure is a sign of early pulmonary insufficiency.

* Ringer's injection, rather than lactated Ringer's injection, has been widely employed in these situations.

25. Following the successful control of septic shock, the patient may develop acute respiratory distress syndrome (ARDS, or shock lung or wet lung of World War II).

26. Therapy for ARDS should include volume-cycled ventilation with PEEP (positive end-expiratory pressure) as well as frequent higher-dose albumin and lasix than is usually given. Careful digitalization, if not already accomplished, should be considered to improve inotropic status.

27. Patients in labor who receive general anaesthesia should be given antacids preoperatively.

28. A low pO_2 and pCO_2 are nearly constant findings in acute pulmonary embolism, and if there is a normal pO_2 it is possible to rule out pulmonary embolism shock.

29. Patients with massive pulmonary embolism shock will benefit from immediate and total heparinization.

30. The lifesaving capabilities of intravenous hyperalimentation have been confirmed in many clinical studies involving intestinal fistulas, renal and hepatic disease, severe burns and trauma, cancer, congenital malformations, and prematurity.

ILEUS

Definition

Obstruction of the intestines.

Types of Ileus

1. Adynamic—inhibition of bowel motility, which may be produced by many causes, e.g., peritonitis.

2. Dynamic—related to mechanical obstruction.

3. Ileus versus Mechanical Obstruction. Ileus is probably one of the most frequent complications seen in the period following gynecological surgery or cesarean section. It may vary in severity from mild distension to a full-blown picture of paralytic ileus, with its accompanying electrolyte, water, and acid-base imbalances. It is extremely important to make certain that the problem is one of paralytic ileus and *not* one of mechanical small-bowel obstruction. Although the fluid and electrolyte replacement may be the same, the definitive approach to the underlying problem is different.

Basic Principles

Ileus is most often preceded by a diminution in urine volume. Fluids and electrolytes collect in the intestines. The extracellular fluid is therefore decreased, and this in turn leads to a decrease in glomerular filtration, with a drop in the urinary output.

1. Vomiting and distension occur on the second or third day after an operation or following a traumatic delivery.

2. Vomitus first consists of mucus, then bile, and, later, altered blood.

3. Constipation is the rule.

4. Abdomen rapidly distends with gas.

5. Peristalsis is absent.

6. Bowel sounds are absent.

7. Pain is usually absent but, if present, is never colicky.

8. Patient becomes dehydrated.

9. Pulse becomes rapid.

10. Respiratory rate, temperature, and leukocyte count rise.

11. Urinary output drops.

12. Patient becomes toxic.

13. Flat plate of abdomen shows:

a. Gas-distended loop and multiple fluid levels in the small bowel.

b. A little gas may be present in cecum and pelvic colon.

14. Ileus must be differentiated from a mechanical obstruction. The four cardinal symptoms of mechanical intestinal obstruction are:

a. Colicky abdominal pain—intermittent, comes on suddenly, reaches a peak, and subsides. Auscultation at time of pain reveals loud, metallic, high-pitched peristaltic rushes. This is a most important difference from ileus.

b. Vomiting—frequent and copious

c. Distension

d. Obstipation

Changes Caused by Ileus

A full-blown ileus gives rise to changes in bowel, kidney, and lung function (see Fig. 34-1). This is demonstrated as follows:

1. Intestines

a. Fluids and electrolytes pour into the intestines.

b. The extracellular fluid is decreased in direct proportion to that lost to the intestines.

c. Hematocrit, hemoglobin, and plasma protein concentration reflect this shift by showing an increase in concentration in the intravascular compartment of the extracellular space. (Hct. increases, Hgb. increases, protein increases.)

d. The loss of fluids to the intestine leads to dehydration, which decreases glomerular filtration and may be followed by vasomotor instability.

2. Kidneys

a. Glomerular filtration rate (GFR) is decreased secondary to the diminished extracellular fluid and to the abdominal distension.

b. Urinary output is decreased. It may occur before the problem of ileus is appreciated. This indicates the importance of following the daily urine output as well as its specific gravity.

c. Specific gravity of the urine is increased.

d. The decreased glomerular filtration leads to an elevation of the urea nitrogen, sulfates, and phosphates. This will increase and aggravate the metabolic acidosis that is present.

3. Lungs

a. The diaphragm is elevated secondary to the abdominal distension.

b. Carbon dioxide retention occurs secondary to the elevated diaphragm and causes a respiratory acidosis.

c. Atelectasis may occur.

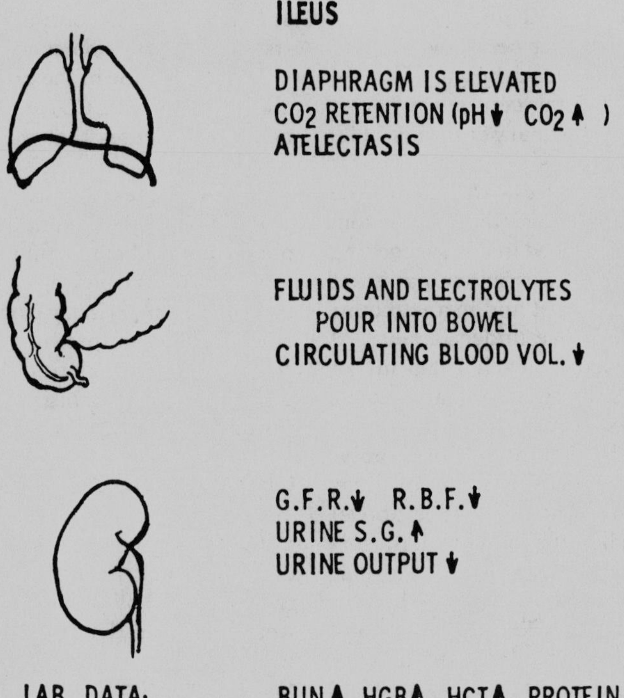

Figure 34-1. Changes caused by ileus.

Management

1. The replacement of fluids and electrolytes that have been lost by vomiting or that collect in the intestines during the development of an ileus is usually an easy matter. The use of the empiric formula

$$\left(1 - \frac{\text{Normal hematocrit}}{\text{Found hematocrit}}\right) \times \begin{array}{l}\text{20\% body}\\ \text{weight in}\\ \text{kilograms}\end{array}$$

suggested by Randall provides a useful guide in evaluating the deficit that must be replaced. In addition, the daily baseline requirements and extrarenal losses must also be supplied. Although a decreased red cell mass, such as follows cesarean section, causes the formula to lose some of its value, it still serves a useful purpose if the daily weight, urine volume, and specific gravity and laboratory findings are evaluated in setting up an intelligent fluid and electrolyte regimen. Because the daily baseline losses are recorded, only the deficit remains to be corrected. The deficit can be estimated as follows:

a. By the time the obstruction or ileus is identifiable on a scout film the deficit is at least 1,000 to 1,500 ml.

b. In well-established obstruction or ileus, the deficit is at least 3,000 ml.

c. In an ileus or obstruction in which the pulse rate is elevated and there is a drop in the blood pressure, the deficit may be 4,000 to 6,000 ml.

2. Outline for fluid and electrolyte replacement (following plan set up on p. 334 under "Daily Baseline Requirement, Extrarenal Losses, Deficits, or Excesses").

a. Daily Baseline Requirements
1,000 ml. 5-per-cent g/w
500 ml. 5-per-cent g/s
1,000 ml. 5-per-cent g/w
plus 40 mEq. KCl, if urinary output is 1,000 ml. or over in 24 hours.

b. *Extrarenal Losses*—represent the losses from vomiting or tube aspiration. These losses are replaced in kind according to the level in the gastrointestinal tract from which they are lost and in an amount equal to that lost. (See under *Deficit.*) 20 mEq. KCl is added for each 1,000 ml. of replacement, but only if the urinary output is 1,000 ml. in 24 hours.

c. *Deficit.* This is replaced by supplying fluid and electrolytes similar to those found in the small intestine. (See above) The amount can be calculated from the formula

$$\left(1 - \frac{\text{Normal hematocrit}}{\text{Found hematocrit}}\right) \times \begin{array}{l}\text{20\% body}\\ \text{weight in}\\ \text{kilograms}\end{array}$$

or can be judged from the response of the patient to replacement as well as the urinary output, its reaction, and specific gravity.

d. Total fluids replaced in 24 hours should *not* exceed 10 per cent of the body weight.

e. The average early case of ileus occurring in obstetrics and gynecology can be handled by giving the daily baseline requirements and replacing vomitus or intestinal aspirate as described.

f. In treating these cases, it is important to follow carefully the urinary output, its specific gravity, and the reaction of the urine.

g. A metabolic acidosis with accompanying hypotension that cannot be explained points to an intra-abdominal catastrophe.

h. A fixed specific gravity near 1.010 and a low urinary output points to impending renal failure.

i. A specific gravity of 1.028 to 1.030 and a low urinary output indicates that a state of dehydration exists.

j. Acid urine in the presence of plasma alkalosis (elevated CO_2 and chlorides below normal) indicates that more potassium is needed.

k. Alkaline urine with normal plasma potassium and adequate potassium replacement indicates that more saline is needed. This is based on the assumption that there is no urinary tract infection present and that the specimen tested is a fresh specimen. A urinary tract infection caused by a urea-splitting organism gives rise to alkaline urine.*

CHRONIC SHOCK

Definition

Chronic shock is a metabolic imbalance characterized by reduced blood volume as well as protein deficiency.

Basic Principles

1. Hemoglobin and hematocrit may be normal despite the markedly decreased blood volume. There are two important reasons for this:

a. Blood volume may vary independently from the concentration of substances within a given volume. The decrease in volume may also parallel the decrease in the concentration of the substances.

b. There may be a compensatory vasoconstriction working, which reduces the area containing the volume as well as the concentration of substances in that volume.

---

* The presence of a urinary tract infection can be determined by culture or by an analysis of the ammonia content of alkaline urine. Ammonia is not normally excreted by the kidney when there is alkaline urine. Ammonia present in alkaline urine indicates the presence of a urea-splitting organism.

2. Clinical states in which chronic shock is seen:

a. Bleeding submucous fibroids

b. Intermittent and prolonged bleeding in placenta previa

c. Poor nutrition

d. Carcinoma

3. Review of normal values of total blood volume, red cell mass, and plasma volume:

a. *Normal Blood Volume*—represents 7 to 8.5 per cent of body weight in Kg.

60 Kg. × 7% = 4.2 L. or 4,200 ml.

b. *Normal Red Cell Mass*—represents 3 to 4 per cent of body weight in Kg.

60 Kg. × 3% = 1.8 L. or 1,800 ml.

c. *Plasma Volume*—roughly 4.5 per cent of body weight in Kg.

60 Kg. × 4.5% = 2.7 L. or 2,700 ml.

Application to Clinical Problems

The ideal blood volume, red cell mass, and plasma volume are calculated from these figures after corrections are made for obesity, age, sex, and weight loss. The values obtained are compared with the actual values reported by the laboratory. By this approach an abnormality in the blood volume can be found and corrected.

Examples

1. Age and Sex

a. The average female under 50 years of age has a red cell mass of 32.6 ml. ± 4 ml. per Kg. of body weight. Beyond the age of 50 the red cell mass is 28.6 ± 3 ml. per Kg. of body weight.

2. Weight

a. *Obesity.* The obese patient has a lower blood volume than would be expected for her weight. The amount of obese weight over ideal weight increases the blood volume by one-fourth of that expected on a weight basis. This is shown as follows:

(1) If the ideal weight is 120 and the patient weighs 140, the obese weight is 20 pounds.

(2) 1/4 × 20 (obese weight) = 5 pounds.

(3) The ideal weight in calculating the blood volume is 120 pounds plus 5 pounds = 125 pounds. It is this weight that is used to calculate the blood volume.

3. Weight Loss

a. If the weight loss has occurred over a period of less than 2 months, the original weight is used.

b. If the weight loss has occurred over a period of 2 to 6 months, the present weight plus one-half of the weight loss is used.

c. If the weight loss has occurred over a period of 6 months to a year, the present weight plus one-fourth of the weight loss is used.

d. If the weight loss has occurred over a 1-year period, the present weight is used.

e. *Application*

(1) A female who has lost weight over a 6-month period.

(2) The original weight was 160 pounds, and her present weight is 140 pounds. The weight loss is 20 pounds.

(3) 20 pounds (weight loss) × 1/2 = 10 pounds.

(4) 140 pounds plus 10 pounds = 150 pounds.

(5) This is the weight that should be used in calculating the blood volume.

4. Explanation

Blood volume contracts continually to keep pace with the weight that is being lost. The weight loss is not obese weight but is loss from the ideal weight.

5. Application

a. The ideal blood volume, plasma volume, and red cell mass for a 53-year-old female who has not lost weight nor is obese for her height can be determined as follows:

(1) 60 Kg. × 28.6 ml./Kg. = 1,716 ml. red cell mass

(2) 60 Kg. × 4.5% body weight = 2,700 ml. plasma volume

(3) Total blood volume 4,416 ml.

(4) If the actual calculations are reported from the laboratory as:

(a) 1,200 ml. red cell mass

(b) 2,300 ml. plasma volume

Then:

	Red Cell Mass	*Plasma Volume*	*Total Blood Volume*
Ideal value	1,716 ml.	2,700 ml.	4,416 ml.
Actual value	1,200 ml.	2,300 ml.	3,500 ml.
Deficit	516 ml.	400 ml.	916 ml.

6. Conclusions

Inasmuch as each 500 ml. of whole blood contains about 225 ml. of red cell mass, it would require about two and one-half transfusions of 500 ml. each to restore the red cell mass to normal values as determined by the above calculations. It is important to restore the values to normal before major surgery is undertaken.

Alternate Approach

1. The hospital may not have the facilities for carrying out blood volume determinations. In a patient suspected of having a contracted blood volume, it is possible to evaluate her response to transfusions by the use of serial hematocrits.

2. If the clinical history and physical examination suggest that the blood volume is decreased, a transfusion can be given and the result evaluated in 24 hours by the hematocrit. A hematocrit change in the range of 0.5 to 2 per cent indicates that more blood is needed, whereas a hematocrit change of 3 to 6 per cent indicates that the blood volume has been restored to normal. It is important to make certain that the patient is in a state of normal hydration.

3. Graphically, this is shown as follows:

Total Blood Volume	*Red Cell Mass*	*Hematocrit*	*Per Cent of Change*
4,000 ml.	2,000 ml.	35	—
500 ml.*	225 ml.		
4,500 ml.	2,225 ml.	36.2	1.2%
500 ml.*	225 ml.		
5,000 ml.	2,450 ml.	39.8	3.6%
500 ml.*	225 ml.		
5,000 ml.	2,675 ml.	44.0	4.2%

* Transfusion

Explanation

It has been shown that the vascular compartment contracts and adjusts to a smaller blood volume. However, the vascular compartment resists overexpansion after transfusions have restored the blood volume to normal. Further transfusions will cause the red cell mass to expand, and at the same time the plasma portion will be dispersed from the vascular compartment. This supplies an explanation for the hematocrit changes found after giving a transfusion. In the above illustration the blood volume was restored to normal after the second transfusion, and the next transfusion did not change the total blood volume. The red cell mass expanded at the expense of the plasma portion, which is dispersed from the vascular compartment. The hematocrit takes about 18 to 24 hours to stabilize after a transfusion has been given.

Protein Replacement

Transfusions are not a good way to replace protein deficiency. Because each 100 ml. of blood contains only 7 g. of protein, a transfusion of 500 ml. supplies only 35 g. of protein. A patient whose blood protein determination is found to be 5 g. per 100 ml. is deficient 2 g. per 100 ml. of extracellular fluid. The extracellular fluid in a patient who weighs 70 Kg. is 14 L. (20% × 70 Kg. body weight = 14 L. or 14,000 ml. extracellular fluid). In such a patient the extracellular protein deficit would be 14,000/100 = 140 × 2 or 280 g. of protein. Since each transfusion of 500 ml. of blood supplies only

35 g. of protein, in order to replace the protein deficit in the extracellular fluid alone it would be necessary to give 8 transfusions.

PERITONITIS

Definition

An inflammation of the peritoneum; a condition marked by exudation of serum, fibrin, cells, and pus in the peritoneum.

Basic Principles

1. Peritonitis may result from many causes, such as a ruptured tubo-ovarian abscess, ruptured viscus, ruptured ovarian cyst, or bacterial contamination.

2. The electrolyte, water, and acid-base problems that arise during the development of peritonitis parallel closely the problems encountered in the treatment of burn cases. The patient with peritonitis usually pours plasma, proteins, water, and electrolytes into the affected area. This gives rise to a depletion of the blood volume, with its unstable vasomotor response, shock, and diminution of glomerular filtration.

3. Although antibiotics may control or alter the signs and symptoms and check the septicemia that so often accompanies peritonitis, an alteration in fluid and electrolyte imbalance still occurs.

Diagnosis

1. Initial stages depend on the mode of infection.

2. Temperature is elevated.

3. A most important sign of pelvic peritonitis following operation is a pulse that is more rapid than would be expected from the amount of temperature elevation.

4. Once peritonitis is established, the picture is characteristic.

5. Pain spreads with the spread of infection.

6. Vomiting is usual.

7. Constipation is more common than diarrhea.

8. The patient lies motionless and supine, most often with legs drawn up.

9. The patient's expression is anxious, and face drawn.

10. Abdominal muscles over the inflamed site are tightly contracted.

11. In diffuse peritonitis, the whole abdomen is rigid, wooden, and motionless; there is no movement of the abdomen with respiration.

12. Paralytic ileus.

a. Result of direct paralysis of Auerbach's plexus.

Management

1. Because peritonitis resembles a 15- to 30-per-cent third-degree body burn, the basic principles suggested by Evans for fluid and plasma protein replacement in burn cases can be adapted to the patient who has peritonitis. Evans administered 1 ml. of colloid (plasma) and 1 ml. of crystalloid (isotonic saline) per kilogram per cent of body burn, or, more specifically in these cases, as per per cent peritonitis. In applying this concept to replacement therapy in a 60-kilogram female with pelvic peritonitis, we have:

a. 60 Kg. × 15% (pelvic peritonitis) = 900 ml. colloid. 60 Kg. × 15% (pelvic peritonitis) = 900 ml. isotonic saline.

This represents extrarenal loss, and if peritonitis has been present for a few days prior to therapy, it may also represent deficit.

2. Fluid Regimen

a. *Daily Baseline Requirements*

1,000 ml. 5-per-cent g/w
500 ml. 5-per-cent g/s
1,000 ml. 5-per-cent g/w

Need for potassium will be based on serum findings as well as on the urinary findings.

b. *Extrarenal Losses.* Represent the abnormal losses that are going on under observation. Kilogram body weight × per cent of peritonitis = amount of colloid. Kilogram body weight × per cent of peritonitis = amount of crystalloid.

c. *Excesses and Deficit.* Calculated as indicated if the process has been going on for more than 24 hours.

d. Calcium gluconate as needed.

e. Continue regimen until peritonitis is controlled.

f. As the peritonitis resolves, fluids and electrolytes will be absorbed back into the extracellular space.

g. The clinician must be prepared to supply an extracellular space during the time that fluid and plasma proteins are lost to the site of peritonitis and be prepared to withhold fluids during the time that the third space is resolving.

h. In addition to fluids and electrolyte replacement, the patient should be given the benefit of antibiotics, oxygen, surgery, or any supportive therapy deemed necessary at the time.

Treatment (Four Essentials of Therapy)

1. Nothing by mouth.

2. Levin, Cantor, or Miller-Abbott tube connected to continuous suction.

a. Measure intake and output and record.

3. Maintain fluid and electrolyte balance.

4. Antibiotic regimen (early and in adequate dosage): gentamicin up to 1.6 mg./Kg. I.M./I.V. 3 times a day; ampicillin 2 g. I.M./I.V. 4 times a day.

a. If anaerobes are present, add clindamycin 300 mg. I.M. 3 times a day.

b. In the critically ill patient there is justification for administering ampicillin and Chloromycetin 1 g. in the volutrol every 6 hours for 2 days and then dropping the dose to 500 mg. q.6h.

35 Acidosis and Alkalosis

Hugh R. K. Barber

BASIC PRINCIPLES

1. Acidosis and alkalosis are not diseases in themselves, but chemical states that are seen in a wide variety of diseases.

2. Clinically, the terms *acidosis* and *alkalosis* represent shifts from normal of the hydrogen ion concentration of the plasma, and therefore of the cells.

3. Acidosis and alkalosis may be further subdivided into metabolic and respiratory types. Both may originate from either internal errors in metabolism or externally introduced substances or physical circumstances, such as medications, anesthesia, or pneumothorax.

4. There are four basic types of *p*H changes: metabolic acidosis, metabolic alkalosis, respiratory acidosis, and respiratory alkalosis.

5. The diagnosis of an acute change is dependent on the patient's history and on clinical observation. Its type may be revealed by chemical analysis of the plasma, particularly by plasma *p*H.

6. As compensations take place, changes in the major electrolytes of the plasma, in the *p*H and sometimes in the electrolytes of the urine, and in the electrocardiogram, as well as the presence of abnormal substances in the urine, assist substantially in making the diagnosis.

7. The *p*H of the blood or plasma represents one of the most important laboratory determinations since it measures directly the hydrogen ion concentration and the direction, as well as the degree, of change from normal.

8. CO_2 content, chloride determination, sodium, potassium, and other anions contribute further information to assist in diagnosis.

9. There are buffers in the plasma. In addition, the hemoglobin of the red cells buffers the change in *p*H of the plasma. It does so by the chloride shift, as follows:

a. The HCO_3 of the plasma and red blood cells decreases.

b. The chloride content of the red blood cells increases.

c. The chloride content of the plasma decreases.

d. The total fixed cation content of the red blood cells does not change.

e. The water content and volume of the red blood cells decrease.

f. These changes occur in the reverse direction in the capillaries of the tissues.

10. The extravascular buffering that is associated with the movement of K^+ into and out of the extracellular fluid (ECF) with changes in *p*H is probably of the greatest importance clinically.

METABOLIC ALKALOSIS (*p*H ↑ CO_2 ↑) (TABLE 35–1)

Etiology

1. The plasma bicarbonate must be primarily elevated. This may be brought about by:

a. Ingestion or infusion of $NaHCO_3$

b. Inappropriate retention of bicarbonate by the kidney, which often occurs in potassium deficit

c. Vomiting in a person who produces HCl in stomach secretions and therefore loses HCl and chlorides

Table 35-1. Metabolic Alkalosis (pH ↑ CO_2 ↑)

Mechanism	State	Major Plasma and Urinary Changes
Total base in excess of total anion (except HCO_3^-)	Excess of alkali	Na± ↑ K± ↓ HCO_3 ↑ Cl ↓
	Iatrogenic heartburn	Urine is alkaline.
	Excessive I.V. $NaHCO_3$	
Chlorides are lost in excess of base	Vomiting	Na± ↓ K ↓ HCO_3 ↑ Cl ↓
	Tube aspiration	Urine is alkaline.
Potassium deficiency	Inadequate intake	Na± ↓ K± ↓ HCO_3 ↑ Cl ↓
	Stress	Urine is acid.
	Diarrhea	
	Diuretics	
	Adrenal hormone therapy	Na± ↓ K ↓ HCO_3 ↑ Cl^- ↓
Mixed state	Combination of above	Urine is acid.

Basic Principles

1. Metabolic alkalosis is a state of decreased hydrogen ion concentration (pH ↑ $NaHCO_3$ ↑) owing to causes other than hyperventilation.

2. It occurs when there is either an increase in base from exogenous sources, a loss of anion (other than HCO_3) in excess of base, or a loss of potassium ion.

3. Addition of excess alkali usually results from the ingestion of large amounts of sodium bicarbonate by patients suffering from peptic ulcer or gastric neuroses. It may be iatrogenic from excessive administration of sodium bicarbonate or lactate.

4. In surgery the most common cause of metabolic alkalosis is the loss of chloride by vomiting or gastric suction.

a. In the stomach the chloride ion exceeds sodium by a ratio of 3 : 2 in the normal resting state; the ratio may rise as high as 4 : 1, with chloride concentrations of up to 150 mEq. per liter.

b. As much as 2,500 ml. gastric juice may be lost in 24 hours, although the average gastric suction in unobstructed cases is usually around 1,000 ml.

c. Even larger volumes may be lost when contents of the small bowel are regurgitated into the stomach.

5. With the excess intake of bicarbonate, 67 per cent of the bicarbonate remains in the ECF. Most of the remainder is buffered by H^+ moving out of cells in exchange for Na^+.

a. A small amount of bicarbonate is converted to H_2CO_3 by the production of lactic acid. The H_2CO_3 is then dissociated to CO_2 and H_2O, and the CO_2 blown off by the lung.

b. K^+ probably moves into cells in metabolic alkalosis.

6. Potassium deficiency is now widely recognized as a complication of surgical illness and its management.

a. Potassium cannot be completely conserved by the kidneys; normal dietary intake of 60 to 90 mEq. must be supplied to surgical patients who are unable to ingest potassium-containing food.

b. Potassium losses increase with the alarm response. Often, large amounts are lost extrarenally from the gastrointestinal tract and through wounds.

c. Alkalosis from other causes results in a shift of potassium intracellularly and also in an increased renal loss, so that plasma levels fall. The plasma level, however, is not a reliable index of the total potassium loss.

d. As potassium is lost, there develops an alkalosis which is characterized by an elevated CO_2, a moderately decreased chloride, a low-normal to low serum potassium level, and a relatively normal sodium. The urine in this condition is acid. The alkalosis does not respond to the administration of NaCl or NH_4Cl, but only to potassium administration.

7. Mixed hypochloremic and hypokalemic alkalosis eventuates in many patients, particularly those who are on parenteral fluids without potassium for more than 3 or 4 days, and especially if they are subjected to upper gastrointestinal tract drainage.

a. Often a patient on gastric drainage starts off with chloride loss, mild alkalosis, and, with sodium chloride replacement, alkaline urine.

b. After 2 to 4 days of this the alkalosis increases despite adequate sodium chloride replacement, and the urine becomes acid.

c. Only the additional administration of potassium will correct the alkalosis.

8. The alkalotic hypokalemic patient is hypersensitive to digitalis. Great caution must be exercised in its use.

MAJOR PLASMA ELECTROLYTE IMBALANCES AND URINARY CHANGES OCCURRING IN METABOLIC ALKALOSIS

Basic Principles

1. Metabolic alkalosis is a state of decreased hydrogen ion concentration (pH ↑ $NaHCO_3$ ↑) owing to causes other than hyperventilation.

2. It occurs when there is an increase in base (i.e., Na^+) from exogenous sources; when there is loss of anion (i.e., Cl^-) in excess of base; or in potassium-deficient state.

Compensation

1. Dilution. Extracellular fluid space is increased due to the alkali load.

2. All alkali above 27 mEq. per liter of $NaHCO_3$ is excreted by the kidneys.

3. Potassium leaves extracellular fluid and goes into the cells or is excreted by the kidney.

4. If potassium is not replaced, an increased amount of alkali is reabsorbed by the tubules. A metabolic alkalosis with acid urine results.

5. Acid urine is secondary to the alteration in the $\frac{KHCO_3}{HHCO_3}$ buffer system in the cell. The numerator ($KHCO_3$) is decreased, but the denominator ($HHCO_3$) is not changed. The hydrogen ion concentration in the cell increases and the kidney is stimulated to absorb bicarbonate in larger amounts. $\frac{KHCO_3 \downarrow}{HHCO_3}$ = more acid intracellular environment.

6. Respiratory compensations do not occur. If they did, the $HHCO_3$ fraction of the equation would increase, and bicarbonate reabsorption would be elevated. The renal compensation would be ineffectual.

Management

1. Correct the underlying disease state causing the imbalance.

2. Rehydrate.

3. Replace gastric losses in equal volume to that vomited or aspirated as:

a. Two-thirds in the form of 5-per-cent glucose and saline

b. One-third in the form of 5-per-cent glucose and water

4. Add 20 mEq. KCl for each 1,000 ml. of aspirated gastric contents replaced.

5. Only the addition of KCl will correct a persistent plasma metabolic alkalosis in the presence of acid urine.

6. Add daily baseline requirements.

7. Add only potassium after an output of at least 1,000 ml. in 24 hours (40 ml. per hour) is assured.

8. With the mixed type of alkalosis, both sodium and potassium chloride are re-

Table 35-2. **Metabolic Acidosis (*p*H ↓ CO_2 ↓)**

Mechanism	*State*	*Major Plasma and Urinary Changes*
Total anion is increased in relation to total base	SO_4^{--} HPO_4^{--} elevated Shock, renal insufficiency Septic abortion Incompatible blood transfusion Premature separation of placenta	Na ↓ K± ↑ Ca± ↓ HCO_3^+ ↓ Cl ↓ HPO_4 ↑ Urine is acid.
	Keto acids elevated Diabetic acidosis Starvation	Na ↓ K± ↑ HCO_3^- ↓ Keto acid ↑ Urine is acid.
	Lactic and pyruvic acids elevated Adrenal insufficiency Postpartum vasomotor collapse, hypoxia	Na ↓ K± ↑ HCO_3^- ↓ Cl± ↓ Lactic acid ↑ Pyruvic acid ↑ Urine is acid.
	Chlorides elevated NH_4Cl, Diamox, ureterosigmoid, transplant	HCO_3^- ↓ Cl ↑ Urine is acid.
Excess loss of base over anion, especially chlorides	Excess loss of base over chlorides Small-bowel losses Diarrhea Small bowel fistula Long-tube suction	HCO_3^- ↓ Cl ↑ Urine is acid.

quired. The urine will again become alkaline when sufficient potassium is being administered if chloride loss continues.

METABOLIC ACIDOSIS (*p*H ↓ CO_2 ↓) (TABLE 35–2)

Etiology

1. Loss of bicarbonate may occur through buffering of strong acids, i.e., diabetic acidosis. Lactic acid may be produced in excess, or strong acids may not be excreted if kidney disease is present. Ketosis and the production of strong acids may occur in starvation.

2. Loss of bicarbonate may occur directly as the result of any body fluid's containing HCO_3^- in a concentration that is higher than that in plasma, e.g., diarrhea, vomiting of duodenal contents, small-bowel fistulas, long-tube suction, pancreatic and biliary fistulas, etc.

3. In certain renal diseases there may be excessive and inappropriate loss of bicarbonate. Retention of fixed acids occurs in chronic renal disease.

Basic Principles

1. Metabolic acidosis (*p*H ↓ CO_2 ↓) is a state of increased hydrogen ion concentration of plasma and cells due to causes other than the retention of CO_2.

2. Metabolic acidosis occurs when there is either an increase in total anion (except

HCO_3^-) without equivalent base or a loss of total base (for example, Na^+) in excess of anion (e.g., Cl^-).

3. Metabolic acidosis may occur as a result of one or more of the following clinical circumstances:

a. Increase of normal inorganic sulfate and phosphate, as the result of failure of renal excretion of these ions in acute or chronic renal failure

b. The appearance of large amounts of organic acid radicals normally present in small or trace amounts—e.g., keto acids in diabetic acidosis or lactic and pyruvic acids in shock and hypoxia

c. Administration of certain drugs, such as NH_4Cl and/or Diamox.

d. Sodium may be lost in excess of chloride in diarrhea, small-bowel fistulas, long-tube suction, and pancreatic or biliary fistulas.

4. In severe acidosis, a little over half of acid is buffered in some other manner than by red cells and plasma.

a. Hydrogen ions leave the ECF in exchange for both Na^+ and K^+.

b. The exchange for K^+ represents about 15 percent of the total buffering, and the exchange for Na^+ about 36 per cent. This exchange is mainly across cell membranes.

5. The patient is often lethargic and may be comatose. Respirations are increased in depth and rate.

MAJOR PLASMA ELECTROLYTE IMBALANCES AND URINARY CHANGES OCCURRING IN METABOLIC ACIDOSIS

Basic Principles in Summary

1. Metabolic acidosis occurs when the hydrogen ion concentration $\frac{HCO_3^-}{HHCO_3}$ is elevated from causes other than retention of CO_2 (pH ↓ CO_2 ↓).

2. It occurs when there is a loss of total base in excess of anion or an increase of total anion (except HCO_3^-) without equivalent increase of base.

Compensations for Metabolic Acidosis

1. Dilution. There is a shift of water, sodium, and potassium to the extracellular compartment.

2. Relation Between Intracellular and Extracellular Space. Chlorides to intracellular space; Na^+, K^+ to extracellular space

3. Buffer System. Handles about 50 per cent of acid base; $BHCO_3 + (H)(Acid) \rightarrow$ B Acid + $HHCO_3$

4. Kidney Compensations

a. Titratable acid (substitute H^+ for Na^+).

$$H_2CO_3 + B_2HPO_4 \rightarrow \underset{\text{(to urine)}}{BH_2PO_4} + \underset{\text{(to plasma)}}{BHCO_3}$$

b. Substitute NH_4^+ for Na^+.

$$NH_4HCO_3 + BCl \rightarrow \underset{\text{(to urine)}}{NH_4Cl} + \underset{\text{(to plasma)}}{BHCO_3}$$

Management

1. Correct the underlying disease state.
2. Rehydrate.
3. Restore electrolyte balance.
4. Keep CO_2 above 15 mEq. per liter.
5. Give potassium as needed after urinary output is at least 1,000 ml. in 24 hours.
6. Add daily baseline requirements.
7. Calculate and give infusions over 24-hour period.

RESPIRATORY ALKALOSIS (TABLE 35–3)

Etiology

1. Something must happen to cause the individual to excrete CO_2 at a rate greater than it is produced. This lowers pCO_2.

***Table 35-3.* Respiratory Alkalosis (*p*H ↑ CO_2 ↓)**

Mechanism	*State*	*Major Plasma and Urinary Changes*
CO_2 is blown off in excess quantities by hyperventilation.	Hysteria Fever Early salicylate poisoning Ammonium toxicity Respirators High altitude Eclampsia Panting in labor Early septic shock	Na ↓ K ↓ HCO_3 ↓ Cl± ↑ HPO_4 ↓ Lactic acid ↑ Ketones ↑ Early, urine is alkaline; later, after compensations occur, urine is acid.

2. The respiratory center may be stimulated abnormally and directly as:

a. In encephalitis or meningitis

b. In hypoxia

c. Secondary to anxiety or hysteria

d. Following ingestion of drugs such as aspirin

e. In high fever

f. From ammonium toxicity in patients with liver disease

Basic Principles

1. Respiratory alkalosis is a state in which pCO_2 is reduced by hyperventilation, with a rise in *p*H as the result of a reduction of the $HHCO_3$ fraction of the bicarbonate buffer system.

2. Tetany may be present transiently.

3. In the presence of a high *p*H with low pCO_2, the dissociation of oxygen from oxyhemoglobin is impaired, and relative tissue anoxia results. The venous blood tends to be redder than normal.

4. In respiratory alkalosis, the plasma bicarbonate is lowered by other mechanisms besides renal compensation. In the early phase of the imbalance they are more effective than renal compensation. The bicarbonate can be lowered by the chloride shift. It can also be lowered further, by about the same amount, by increased production of lactic acid. Another means of medication is by exchange of Na^+ and K^+ in ECF for intracellular H^+. The exchange for Na^+ is about four times the exchange for K^+. The two combined represent one-fifth of the total buffering in an animal without kidneys.

MAJOR PLASMA ELECTROLYTE IMBALANCES AND URINARY CHANGES OCCURRING IN RESPIRATORY ALKALOSIS

Basic Principles in Summary

This is a state of decreased hydrogen ion (H^+) concentration $\frac{BHCO_3}{HHCO_3 \downarrow}$ secondary to hyperventilation.

Compensation

1. Acute respiratory alkalosis is compensated for by a renal mechanism.

2. Excess respiratory loss of CO_2 $\frac{(NAHCO_3)}{(HHCO_3 \downarrow)}$ results in a decrease in the hydrogen ion concentration.

3. The kidney attempts to restore the ratio by excreting bicarbonate.

4. It excretes bicarbonate with water, resulting in dehydration.

5. Chlorides shift from the cells to the extracellular space.

Table 35-4. Respiratory Acidosis (pH ↓ CO_2 ↑)

Mechanism	*State*	*Major Plasma and Urinary Changes*
Secondary to inability to blow off CO_2	Narcotic Barbiturate Pneumonia Atelectasis Emphysema Anesthesia Large abdomen in pregnancy Postoperative abdominal distension	HCO_3 ↑ Cl ↓ Urine is acid.

6. There is also a derangement in the deposition of glycogen, as well as in the utilization of glucose, with an accumulation of lactic acid and ketones in the ECF.

a. Lactic acid and ketones are buffered, with the result that the bicarbonate value is decreased ($BHCO_3$ + H Acid → B Acid + $HHCO_3$).

b. $HHCO_3$ is converted to H_2O and CO_2.

c. CO_2 is released from the lungs.

7. Low potassium values, which may occur in respiratory alkalosis, result in increased absorption of bicarbonate by the kidney tubules, with the formation of acid urine.

8. The late phase of respiratory alkalosis closely resembles metabolic acidosis.

Management

1. Correct the underlying disease state.

2. Give 10-per-cent CO_2, ideally by nasal catheter.

3. Prevent and/or correct dehydration.

4. Do not give bicarbonate in the acute phase. The kidney is excreting it in an attempt to return the ratio of $\frac{NaHCO_3}{HHCO_3}$ back to $\frac{20}{1}$.

5. Sodium lactate should not be given, because the lactic acid value is already elevated and any interference with the metabolism of the lactate ion will merely increase the amount already present.

6. If metabolic acidosis and dehydration result, sodium bicarbonate and water must be given.

RESPIRATORY ACIDOSIS (TABLE 35–4)

Etiology

The concentration of H_2CO_3 increases because of the retention of CO_2, which is caused by some impairment in pulmonary function. This may be caused by:

1. Poor exchange of CO_2 across an alveolar membrane when it is thickened

2. Inadequate ventilation

3. Increased CO_2 concentration in the inspired air

Basic Principles

1. Respiratory acidosis develops when there is interference with the respiratory exchange of CO_2 and thus an increase in the $HHCO_3$ fraction of $\frac{BHCO_3}{HHCO_3}$ of the bicarbonate buffer system. As $HHCO_3$ rises, H rises and *p*H falls.

2. Respiratory acidosis in the acute form is often seen in surgical patients, particularly under anesthesia during surgery and in the immediate postanesthetic period.

3. Pneumothorax, atelectasis, and pneumonia are fairly common as acute postoperative complications, and may produce acute respiratory acidosis.

4. If the respiratory acidosis persists, compensations take place as in chronic respiratory acidosis.

5. The increase in pCO_2 in respiratory acidosis is buffered by a rise in bicarbonate due to factors other than renal compensation.

a. About 33 per cent of the rise of these mechanisms is accounted for by the chloride shift.

b. Approximately 15 per cent is brought about by the exchange of ECF $[H^+]$ for intracellular K^+. This tends to raise the ECF $[K^+]$, but if the renal function is normal the K^+ will be excreted.

c. A small amount of increase in $[HCO_3^-]_p$ is brought about by a reduction in the organic acid content of plasma.

d. There is a further rise in $[HCO_3^-]_p$ that is thought to be caused by cellular mechanisms, but the exact nature of the mechanism is not known.

MAJOR PLASMA ELECTROLYTE IMBALANCES AND URINARY CHANGES OCCURRING IN RESPIRATORY ACIDOSIS

Basic Principles

This is a state of increased hydrogen ion concentration $(H^+)\ \frac{(NaHCO_3)}{(HHCO_3\uparrow)}$ secondary to some interference in the ability to blow off CO_2.

Compensation

1. CO_2 retention is in the form of carbonic acid ($HHCO_3$), which changes the ratio of

$$\frac{NHCO_3}{HHCO_3} = \frac{20}{1}$$

$$\text{to}\ \frac{NaHCO_3}{HHCO_3\uparrow} = \frac{20}{1\uparrow}$$

2. Electrolyte shifts occur. Sodium shifts to the extracellular space.

3. The main compensation is renal.

a. There is increased renal tubular reabsorption of bicarbonate and base.

b. This restores the ratio of $\frac{20}{1}$, a compensated state.

Management

1. Correct the underlying disease state.

2. Give oxygen. If the problem has been long-standing, oxygen may cause cessation of breathing, because the respiratory center now depends on anoxia for its stimulation.

3. Bronchodilators

4. Cold steam

5. Expectorants

6. Antibiotics

7. Tracheostomy

36 Cystocele, Urethrocele, Rectocele, and Enterocele

Hugh R. K. Barber

Urethrocele and cystocele should be discussed together. Although they may occur independently of each other, they are commonly present together.

URETHROCELE

Definition

Urethrocele is a protusion downward of the urethra from its attachment just beneath the symphysis pubis.

Basic Principles

1. Results from the inability of the musculofibrous structure to give the urethra normal support.

2. There is a descent of the urethra from its position under the pubic arch.

3. It may be a cause of stress incontinence and may exist by itself or in company with a cystocele.

4. Childbirth injuries to the urogenital trigone and the pubovesicocervical fascia are chiefly responsible for this condition.

5. When it occurs in a nulliparous woman, metabolic and/or neurologic disease should be ruled out.

6. Aside from the bulging there may be no inconvenience except for the stress incontinence previously described.

7. A urethrocele must be differentiated from a urethral diverticulum.

Management

1. The urethrocele may be repaired at the time of cystocele repair. The procedure will be discussed later.

2. The stress incontinence should be corrected by a suitable operation after careful urological evaluation. This is described in Chap. 37, "Urinary Incontinence."

CYSTOCELE

Definition

Cystocele is a herniation of the bladder, causing the anterior vaginal wall to bulge downward.

Basic Principles

1. It is usually the result of childbirth. The baby's head may stretch the pubococcygeal fibers of the levator ani muscles, permitting gradual sagging of the vaginal walls.

2. Probably the most important factor in the development of a cystocele is incompetency of the pubovesicocervical fascia.

3. Obesity and asthma and other upper respiratory conditions are often associated causes of cystocele. Cystocele alone with uterine descent rarely produces appreciable symptoms and usually does not necessitate surgical repair.

4. One of the most common descriptions of the complaint is the feeling that there is a ball bulging between the patient's legs.

5. With a large cystocele, frequent cystitis may occur as well as retention of urine. Some women report that they must shove the mass back to void.

6. A large cystocele may stretch the trigone and cause urgency and frequency without evidence of any infection.

7. A cystocele seldom causes stress incontinence.

8. An asymptomatic cystocele and/or urethrocele does not require correction.

Indications for Surgery

1. A large cystocele that causes discomfort on sitting or walking.

2. Inability to void without pushing up the anterior vaginal wall manually.

3. Marked stretching of the trigone resulting in urinary frequency and urgency.

4. Overflow incontinence and/or, rarely, stress incontinence.

5. Difficulty with intercourse.

6. Bleeding and ulceration secondary to trauma from the mass.

7. Repeated bladder infections secondary to retention of urine.

Management

1. A pessary may be used to support the bladder while treating infections in the bladder, thus reducing the amount of residual urine and increasing the probability of successful eradication of the infection.

2. A pessary supporting the bladder often results in incontinence.

3. The pessary is rarely successful in controlling the overall clinical problems related to the cystocele but may be helpful in the treatment of urinary infections preoperatively.

4. The definitive treatment of cystocele and urethrocele is surgical.

5. Since both cystocele and rectocele occur so frequently together, the operations for both conditions are often combined.

6. The most important and essential step in the cure of these two conditions is restoring support to the urethra and/or bladder by proper use of the pubovesicocervical fascia.

7. Care must be exercised not to advance the bladder excessively or the urethrovesical angle may be increased with resulting stress incontinence.

8. If there is stress incontinence, which is rare, restoration of the urethrovesical angle must be carried out with meticulous care. A slight tug on a Foley catheter placed in the bladder helps identify the urethrovesical angle, permitting precise placement of sutures.

9. A careful urologic and medical workup is indicated, and then the following preoperative orders are routinely carried out:

a. Sulfa vaginal cream twice a day for 2 days.

b. Estrogen vaginal cream for 2 days if the mucosa is very atrophic.

c. Soap suds enema until clear.

d. Crossmatch 1,000 ml. blood.

e. N.P.O. for 8 hours before the operation.

f. Nembutal 100 mg. or Seconal 100 mg. for sleep.

g. Demerol 50 mg. or Seconal 100 mg. plus atropine 0.4 mg. on call to O.R.

h. Infusion of 1,000 ml. 5-per-cent glucose with heparin 1,000 ml. to be started the evening before surgery, to run during the operation and for 2 or 3 days postoperatively.

Postoperative Orders

See "Stress Incontinence," Chap. 37.

RECTOCELE AND ENTEROCELE

Definition

1. Rectocele. Protrusion of the rectum into the vagina. It is usually accompanied by some deficiency of the perineal body.

2. Enterocele. High, posterior vaginal herniation of the small bowel, peritoneum, and fascia, bulging forward at the apex of the vagina. It usually dissects down between the rectum and the vagina. Unlike a rectocele it is a true hernia. Enterocele may occasionally occur after the uterus has been removed by abdominal or vaginal hysterectomy and is usually combined with some degree of prolapse of the vaginal wall.

3. Cystocele or rectocele, or both, may occur without uterine descent, but uterine prolapse is accompanied by descent of the bladder because of the close attachment of the bladder to the anterior aspect of the supravaginal cervix.

a. Descent of the rectum does not necessarily accompany uterine prolapse because the prolapsing vaginal wall easily becomes separated from the rectum.

Basic Principles

1. If the prolapse is at the level of the middle third of the vagina, the rectovaginal septum is often involved and the rectum prolapses with the vaginal wall. This is a true rectocele.

2. If the lowest part of the vagina prolapses, the perineal body is involved rather than the rectum, resulting in a relaxed vaginal outlet.

3. If the upper part of the posterior vaginal wall prolapses, the pouch of Douglas is elongated and small bowel or omentum may descend, pushing peritoneum in front of it. This is called an *enterocele.* Enterocele is usually associated with uterine prolapse and is sometimes called *vault prolapse* or *hernia of the pouch of Douglas.*

4. The causes are generally the same as those listed for uterine prolapse and cystocele.

5. Anterior and posterior herniations usually occur concomitantly.

6. Hemorrhoids are frequently associated with the relaxed condition and may contribute to the general perineal discomfort.

7. The rectocele may give rise to very definitive symptoms that require relief.

Indications for Surgery

1. The protruding mass may be annoying, particularly when the patient is walking.

2. The patient may be troubled by a collection of feces in the rectocele pouch, and pressure may be required on the mass through the vagina in order to effect an evacuation of the bowels.

3. Interference with sexual intercourse. The complaint may be legitimate but may really represent sexual incompatibility.

Management

1. A pessary is rarely helpful.

2. Perineal exercises are of little value.

3. Surgery is the treatment of choice.

4. Repair of a relaxed vaginal outlet and repair of a rectocele are two distinct operative procedures.

5. They are frequently done together, but perineal repair is often done when a rectocele is not present.

6. Rarely, a rectocele may be present and require repair in a women whose outlet is not relaxed.

Vaginal Approach

The aim is to reduce herniation and build a supportive floor from the adjoining muscles and fascia. The cure rate is about 95 per cent.

1. Rectocele

a. A high dissection of the rectum is done from the posterior vaginal mucosa.

b. Imbricate the rectum using the prerectal tissue.

c. Build a firm support utilizing the levator muscles and fascia.

d. The muscles are ensheathed in fascia, and it is not wise to dissect the fascia from the muscles because the firmest union is obtained by the healing of fascia to fascia.

e. The excess vaginal mucosa is trimmed and then closed with continuous or interrupted sutures. It is wise to include some of the prerectal tissue. This closes dead spaces and adds to the support.

2. Enterocele

a. In addition to the symptoms listed for rectocele, the enterocele may give symptoms of pulling in the upper abdomen. This results from a pull on the mesentery of the bowel as the small bowel protrudes into the vagina.

b. The dissection must free the vagina from the rectum and must be carried as high as needed to identify the peritoneal sac.

c. The peritoneal sac should be opened and the contents pushed back into the pelvis.

d. The repair is the same as for any hernia and should include high ligation of the sac with excision of the excess peritoneum, approximation of the fascia, and also approximation of the uterosacral ligaments.

e. Then continue as for the repair of a rectocele.

Abdominal Approach

1. Enterocele

a. Indications are:

(1) Failed previous vaginal repair.

(2) Dense vaginal scarring.

(3) Anatomically short vaginal canal and desire to preserve the existing depth.

(4) When the abdominal cavity has already been opened for exploration and an enterocele is known to exist.

b. Obliterate the cul-de-sac. It is important to obliterate the space below the level of the uterosacral ligaments (Moschcowitz operation).

c. The uterosacral ligaments must be approximated. Care should be taken to avoid including the uterers in the sutures.

PROLAPSE OF THE UTERUS

Definition

Uterine prolapse is a herniation through the pelvic diaphragm with resultant protrusion into the vagina and, sometimes, beyond the introitus.

Basic Principles

1. The uterus and vagina are held in the pelvis by the cardinal and uterosacral ligaments and by the pelvic floor musculature, mainly the levator ani muscles. When these ligaments and muscles become ineffective, the uterus and vagina descend (prolapse) through the gap between the muscles. Descent of the uterus is only possible if the fascial structures which support it are injured or atrophic.

2. The causes of prolapse are:

a. The stretching of muscle and fibrous tissue which occurs with repeated childbirth.

b. Increased intra-abdominal pressure, as seen in obese women with chronic coughs and in women who undertake heavy industrial work.

c. A constitutional predisposition to stretching of the ligaments presumably as a response to years in the erect position.

d. When a nulliparous woman develops a prolapse, she should have a careful metabolic and neurologic workup.

e. Obstetrical trauma with injury to the fascia, muscles, and ligaments that maintain the uterus in its normal position.

Clinical Features

1. Sensation of something hanging out when the patient stands or walks.

2. Backache. It may be related to other causes than the prolapse.

3. A bearing-down sensation.

4. Frequency of urination.

5. Difficulty in voiding or moving the bowels.

6. Rarely, stress incontinence.

7. The uterus gradually descends in the axis of the vagina, taking the vaginal wall with it. It may present at any level but is usually classified as one of three degrees.

8. The degree of descent of the uterus is sometimes difficult to evaluate because in most cases the cervix usually becomes hypertrophied and elongated.

a. *First Degree, or Slight.* The uterus has descended only a slight distance into the vagina.

b. *Second Degree, or Moderate.* The cervix appears outside the vulva. The cervical lips become congested and ulcerated.

c. *Third Degree, or Severe.* Complete prolapse. This is called a *procidentia* (meaning "a falling forward"). The uterus protrudes through the introitus.

Morbid Anatomy

Most of the anatomic changes in prolapse have been listed above, but other, secondary, changes should be mentioned.

1. The vaginal epithelium becomes stretched and increased in area, and if it is exposed it soon becomes thickened and sometimes ulcerated. Ulceration may also arise from a neglected ring pessary.

2. In cases of gross prolapse of the vaginal walls, the drag of these structures on the cervix may lead to elongation of the supravaginal cervix and to edema and enlargement of the vaginal portion.

3. If the cervix is exposed, it may become ulcerated, and secondary infection gives rise to mucopurulent or blood-stained discharge.

4. If there is a large cystocele, the bladder often empties incompletely, and cystitis from bacterial infection is a common sequela. In cases with uterine descent, the ureters are carried downward with cardinal ligaments but are not usually obstructed.

Symptoms

Symptoms connected with prolapse of the uterus include local discomfort, backache, urinary symptoms, bowel symptoms, ulceration, and bleeding.

Management

1. Pessary

a. When surgery is contraindicated or refused by the patient, the pessary may provide partial or complete relief of symptoms.

b. The patient must have careful follow-up to detect any ulcerations or pathology that may develop.

c. Sulfa vaginal and estrogenic hormone creams should be prescribed once a week.

2. Surgery

a. The treatment must be individualized and the surgery tailored to fit the patient and the extent of her prolapse.

b. Factors to be considered are:

(1) The age and general physical condition of the patient

(2) The desirability of preserving menstruation

(3) The desirability of preserving the childbearing function

(4) The degree of descensus

(5) The condition of the cervix and the corpus uteri

(6) The presence and degree of cystocele

(7) The presence and degree of rectocele and enterocele

3. Manchester (Donald or Fothergill) Operation

a. Curettage should be done in conjunction with an anterior and posterior repair. The anterior parametrial pillars are cut and plicated in front of the cervix. The cervix is amputated. Scar tissue forms at the level of plication of the cardinal ligaments and gives firm support. Sturmdorf sutures are used to close the mucosa over the amputated cervix.

b. The success rate is high and there are few complications.

c. The procedure is possible with almost any degree of prolapse if there is no disease in the uterus.

d. The best results are obtained with first and second degree descensus, particularly if the uterus is not in retroposition.

e. Approximating the uterosacral ligaments prevents the development of an enterocele.

4. Vaginal Hysterectomy

a. Many consider this the procedure of choice for uterine prolapse, particularly if any uterine pathology is present.

b. After the uterus is removed the surrounding supportive ligaments must be shortened and approximated. Any enterocele must be corrected, and, if none is present, the uterosacral ligaments must be approximated to prevent one from occurring postoperatively. An anterior and posterior repair are usually indicated and should be carried out.

c. The cure rate is not as good as those reported for the Manchester operation, but this may be because of the selection of patients with the most severe prolapse for vaginal hysterectomy.

d. The complications most frequently encountered are bleeding during and after surgery, urinary tract injuries, urine retention in the postoperative period, and vaginal vault infections.

e. Complications can be kept to a minimum by adequate exposure, careful dissection, and good hemostasis.

5. Abdominal Suspension Operations

a. A variety of operations have been described in the literature. There are few indications for this approach. The operation is mainly used to hold the uterus from the cul-de-sac after endometriosis and endometriomas have been resected.

b. In young women in whom future pregnancies are expected, a modified Gilliam operation is considered the operation of choice.

c. The uterosacrals should always be approximated to prevent the development of an enterocele.

6. LeFort Operation

a. This is a short and simple procedure, designed for frail old women who would not be fit for a more extensive operation.

b. It is not, however, as reliable as the Manchester repair and has been made almost obsolete by modern advances in anesthesia and postoperative care.

c. The patient's symptoms must be due to the prolapse. This is confirmed if the symptoms are relieved by a pessary.

d. The patient must complain about the prolapse.

e. The operation is carried out by removing a triangular strip of tissue from each vaginal wall. The edges are sutured together, anterior wall to posterior wall. The vagina is now formed into two parallel small vaginas.

f. The disadvantages are that there is no vagina and some patients develop stress incontinence.

7. Choice of Operation

a. A vaginal hysterectomy is the procedure of choice for a uterus with pathology.

b. For a young woman who wishes to maintain menstruation and preserve childbearing, a vaginoplasty and abdominal suspension may be indicated. If a vaginal repair is undertaken in this patient, the cervix should not be amputated and the cardinal ligaments should not be plicated.

c. In women who work in industrial jobs and do heavy lifting, the Manchester operation is the best.

Other Operations

In addition to the operations listed above, others include the Spalding-Richardson procedure, the Watkins transposition operation, the modified Coffey procedure, the modified Gilliam suspension, Olshausen's procedure, and a variety of fascial slings that are attached to the lower part of the uterus and/or cervix and then secured against the sacrum.

Preoperative Orders

1. Routine orders for gynecological surgery

2. A careful genitourinary workup with cystoscopy and pyelography is indicated.

Postoperative Orders

Routine for vaginal procedures (see "Stress Incontinence," Chap. 37).

37 Urinary Incontinence

Hugh R. K. Barber

STRESS INCONTINENCE

DEFINITION

1. *Stress incontinence* is the involuntary loss of urine at the time of any sudden increase in intra-abdominal pressure, as in sneezing, coughing, laughing, or lifting with the patient in the upright position.

2. To qualify for this diagnosis a patient must have an intact functioning neurogenic system, and the bladder and urethra must be free of disease.

Classification of Urinary Incontinence

1. Genuine stress incontinence (urethral sphincter incontinence)

2. Unstable bladder (neurogenic bladder), detrusor dyssynergia, bladder hyperreflexia

3. Retention of urine with overflow incontinence

4. Congenital causes

5. Urinary fistulas and diverticula

6. Functional disorders

BASIC PRINCIPLES

1. This is a common disorder. The patient complains that a small quantity of urine escapes involuntarily whenever the intraabdominal pressure is suddenly raised by an exertion, such as coughing, sneezing, laughing, or even walking.

2. Stress incontinence is most commonly seen in parous women and is usually the result of damage to the pelvic floor during delivery, but it is sometimes noticed for the first time during pregnancy.

3. It may occur in a nulliparous patient, and it may occur for the first time, or get worse, after menopause.

4. About half of the patients who have mild cystoceles have stress incontinence, but it can occur without evident prolapse.

5. The essential problem is loss of muscular support at the junction of the bladder and urethra, combined with descent of base of the bladder. In many cases of stress incontinence, cystography shows that the normal angle between the posterior aspect of the urethra and the bladder base is lost; but sometimes the angle is lost in patients who have no incontinence.

6. There may be more than one defense against urinary leak.

7. Even if the attachment of the pubococcygeal muscle to the urethra—which accounts for the possible vesicle-urethra angle—is damaged, the patient may still have control if other mechanisms remain effective. It is for this reason that in mild stress incontinence the patient should first be tried on perineal exercises.

8. Only some of the possible causes of urinary incontinence can be treated by surgery. Accurate diagnosis of the cause of stress incontinence requires some consideration of the problems of bladder physiology.

9. The physiology of micturition is as follows:

a. The bladder stores urine at a low pressure. As the volume of urine increases, the bladder wall relaxes its tone. Pressure rises very little until over 400 ml. of urine is contained. The pressure does not exceed 20 cm. of water until the bladder is full (600 ml.).

b. The urethra can normally resist pressures between 20 and 50 cm. of water, which is much higher than the bladder exerts until it is full. The pressure in the urethra is maintained by the urethral wall as well as by the sphincter muscle function, which is served by the entire urethra.

c. Urine is contained in the bladder as long as the intra-urethral pressure is greater than the intravesical pressure.

10. The nervous control of micturition is not completely understood.

a. Micturition may be described as an autonomic reflex that can be consciously inhibited or facilitated in trained individuals.

b. A desire to void reaches consciousness when about 300 ml. of urine is in the bladder.

c. The stimulus passes via the parasympathetic system. Reflex detrusor contractions can be inhibited until about 700 ml. is secreted.

d. The urethra is strongly contracted.

11. Relaxation of the urethra (which is smooth muscle extending from the detrusor to the end of the urethra) is usually a conscious act at the onset of micturition. It may be psychologically inhibited, as in a patient who is not used to using a bed pan or to micturating when someone else is present.

12. At the end of micturition the urethra contracts and forces the last drops of urine back into the bladder (the urethra is normally empty).

13. Disturbed bladder function may be due to urgency incontinence, fistula, overflow incontinence, neurologic disease, frequency, nocturnal frequency, dysuria, or hematuria.

14. Most physicians agree that the basic problem in the etiology of stress incontinence is inadequate support of the bladder base, vesical neck, and proximal urethra. If the urethra is properly supported, the proximal two-thirds is intra-abdominal.

15. Some physicians believe that stress incontinence results from dilatation of the urethra and the urethrovesical junction with funnelling. About 30 per cent of patients with stress incontinence do not have funnelling.

16. Reports indicate that the posterior urethrovesical junction and the urethral axis are crucial factors in the etiology of stress incontinence and its successful correction. The posterior urethrovesical angle in the continent female is usually about 90° to 100°. The vertical urethral axis is equally important. A vertical line drawn posterior to the urethrovesical junction is used as the base of an angle drawn to the urethra. Normally, the angle should be 15° to 30°. Management varies for abnormal anterior and posterior angle or combinations.

17. There is not total agreement on the role that the posterior urethrovesical angle and the loss of the normal urethral inclination play in producing stress incontinence.

18. Ninety-five per cent of significant stress incontinence occurs in multiparas.

19. It is found more frequently in Caucasian women who have delivered vaginally, and is aggravated by the erect position with Valsalva stress.

20. One study showed that fifty per cent of nulliparous college women experienced stress incontinence at some time or other.

21. Only about 25 to 30 per cent of women with symptomatic cystoceles have concomitant stress incontinence. There is no correlation between the degree of cystocele and the frequency of stress incontinence.

22. In the presence of a cystocele, if the herniation occurs anterior to the interureteric ridge the patient usually shows evidence of stress incontinence. If the herniation is posterior, in most cases the patient does not have stress incontinence. Of course, there may be a combination of these conditions.

23. The hypothesis that a short urethra is a primary cause of urinary stress incontinence has not been confirmed.

24. Marked peri-urethral adhesions with distortion of the normal urethra may interfere with urinary continence. The urethra may be a stiff tube through which urine flows. When this occurs it is necessary to release all adhesions before normal function can be restored.

25. Most gynecologists agree that if vesical funnelling, bladder neck descent, and the like are present, it is because of inadequate support of the bladder neck by components of the levator ani in the erect position, as well as loss of adequacy of the attachments of the urethra to the symphysis pubis. This permits the bladder neck to be the target point in the transmission of force from the dome to the base of the bladder. The chief cause is trauma that may not show up until after menopause.

26. With the patient in the upright position, straining and coughing should not result in urine loss. Another evaluation test that may be helpful is asking the patient to void and voluntarily stop urine flow.

27. Detrusor instability is defined as a detrusor contraction exceeding the urethral pressure producing incontinence, occurring during filling of the bladder or when the patient is standing erect or coughing and straining. This may also cause involuntary incontinence, but the mechanism is altogether different from that of genuine stress incontinence.

DIAGNOSIS

History

1. One must differentiate stress incontinence from urgency incontinence, irritable bladder secondary to infection, and neurologic disorder.

2. The psychological stability of the patient must be evaluated.

3. Failure of bladder sensation is a result of diseases that interrupt the posterior columns of the cord, such as tabes, syringomyelia, and, occasionally, multiple sclerosis. Chronic overdistension leads to an atonic bladder; overflow incontinence and infection are common complications.

Physical Examination

1. This should include a general physical evaluation.

2. It is important to evaluate the tone of the levators, the tone of the vagina, and the sensation of the perineal area.

Tests to Perform During the Examination

1. Cotton-Swab Test. This may show an abnormal urethrovesical junction. A lubricated cotton swab is placed into the urethra to the bladder neck with the patient in lithotomy position.

a. In the normal patient the swab will be angled 13° to 16° above the horizontal and will remain at this angle when the patient strains.

b. In patients with stress incontinence, straining will increase the upward angulation by 20 degrees or more, with the majority producing an angle of 50 to 70 degrees. This demonstrates the detachment of the urethra from the symphysis pubis.

2. Marshall-Marchetti Test

a. 250 ml. of sterile saline is instilled into the bladder.

b. The vagina is infiltrated with a local anesthetic in the area of the bladder neck.

c. Two Allis clamps are placed so that the bladder neck can be elevated without obstructing the urethra.

d. The patient is asked to cough, and the results are noted.

3. Bonney Test. This is similar to the Marshall-Marchetti test. The neck of the bladder is elevated by placing two fingers at the bladder neck; after the bladder is elevated toward the symphysis, the patient is asked to cough and the results are observed.

4. Hodgkinson Test. The largest contraceptive diaphragm fitting ring that the patient can comfortably accommodate is inserted. The patient is then asked to cough and the results are recorded.

5. Cystometry

a. Cystometry recording demonstrates the timing of events:

(1) Intra-abdominal pressure increases (measured per rectum).

(2) The detrusor contracts (intravesical pressure increased).

(3) The sphincter relaxes (electromyogram of anal sphincter).

(4) Urine flow begins.

b. The intravesical pressure is recorded continuously as the bladder is filled.

c. Twin-channel cystometry measures the rectal pressure, which represents intra-abdominal pressure. This is simultaneously recorded by a transducer in the rectum. Electronic circuitry subtracts one channel from the other, thus recording the true intravesical pressure.

d. Modern urodynamic apparatuses also measure detrusor pressure and urethral activity.

e. Cystometry determines the bladder's tone and its response to gradual distension with normal saline at body temperature.

f. This provides a measurement of capacity (the normal bladder can hold about 400 to 700 ml.) and of residual urine after voiding (as with cystocele).

g. About 50 ml. is instilled at a time, and the bladder wall given time to accommodate.

h. The manometer indicates detrusor contractions. If these are frequent, and occur early on, an "irritable bladder" is diagnosed. Cystometry cannot determine the cause.

i. The patient should be questioned as to her sensitivity to cold and warmth.

j. The ability to start and stop the urinary flow at will is important.

k. Bladder hypertonicity is characterized by a contracted, spastic bladder with limited capacity and increased tone.

l. Bladder hypotonicity, which is characterized by low pressures and an increase above the usual capacity of the bladder, may be caused by neurogenic dysfunction.

m. The majority of patients with stress incontinence have hypotonic bladders, with a low resting pressures of 5 to 10 cm. of water.

(1) A sudden increase in the intravesical pressure of an additional 25 to 35 cm. of water is enough to cause urinary loss.

(2) With a low resting pressure, the spill pressure is correspondingly low.

(3) Although in the continent patient an increase in intravesical pressure of 40 to 60 cm. of water is necessary for voiding, the incontinent patient sometimes spills with a rise to only 15 to 20 cm. of water.

6. Urethrocystography

a. The bladder is filled with a contrast medium, and lateral x-ray pictures are taken at rest, straining, and micturating.

b. In the normal resting radiograph there is a well-formed urethrovesical angle.

c. In the normal micturating radiograph, there is urethral dilatation, downward displacement of the urethrovesical junction, and flattening of the urethrovesical angle.

d. If micturition occurs on straining, stress incontinence is diagnosed.

e. Urethrocystography is a difficult and specialized technique, uncomfortable for the patient, and not infallible; but it is the best way of demonstrating urethral mobility in cases where there is neither obvious prolapse nor much peri-urethral scarring.

7. Urethroscopy

a. It is very important to rule out pathology. Diverticula, local disease, tone and length of the urethra, inflammatory changes, neurogenic disease, tumors, fistulas, ectopic ureters, and other pathology of the bladder and/or urethra can be diagnosed.

b. To undertake the repair of stress incontinence without preliminary cystourethroscopy will reduce the likelihood of cure.

8. Chain Cystograms

a. The use of chain cystograms was once considered an essential part of the workup for stress incontinence. Recently there has been controversy over its value.

b. Green* has been most consistent in reporting its value. He describes two basic types of anatomic configuration encountered in patients with stress incontinence, as revealed by the lateral standing-straining view of the urethrocystogram. In both Type I and Type II, the posterior urethrovesical (PUV) angle is lost; in Type II there is, in addition, an increase in the angle of inclination of the urethral axis, varying from 45° to 120°, depending on the amount of rotational descent of the urethra.

c. Green's major contribution is that with Type I cystograms, vaginal repair is usually successful (90 per cent). On the other hand, with Type II, only 50 per cent were corrected by vaginal operations, while if a Marshall-Marchetti-Krantz procedure was undertaken as the primary therapy, the success rate was 93 per cent.

d. The exact diagnosis is indispensable in treating both hypotonic and hypertonic bladder. One must remember that in addition to neurological examination, cystometry, cystoscopy, and urethroscopy are mandatory.

e. Older women may have urinary incontinence due to impaired central nervous system control. This is secondary to advanced arteriosclerosis. Little can be done to help this group.

9. Laboratory Tests

a. Routine urinalysis

b. Midstream culture of the urine should be carried out.

c. Clearance tests should be ordered as indicated.

d. Intravenous pyelograms should be done routinely before surgery.

10. Videocystourethrography (VCU). This elaborate technique demonstrates bladder neck activity by means of cineradiography and at the same time measures changes in intravesical pressure. It gives the most reliable evidence of the presence or absence of detrusor instability, but its cost is against its use for a routine screening. It is carried out as follows:

a. The bladder is filled with contrast medium and is seen on the screen. Bladder neck incontinence is diagnosed by the presence of an open bladder neck at rest or on coughing.

b. Electrodes in the bladder and rectum record the required pressure.

c. The flow meter records the rate at which urine is voided.

11. Indications for Urodynamic Assessment. These investigations are invasive (carrying a 2-per-cent risk of infection) and also costly, but their application is justified in the presence of the following indications:

a. Continuing difficulty in distinguishing genuine stress incontinence from detrusor instability

b. Failure of surgery to relieve a complaint of incontinence

c. Other complicating factors, such as neurologic disease

d. Difficulty in voiding urine, whether complained of or suspected. (Such a condition may be encountered after pelvic surgery and leads to incomplete emptying and, perhaps, retention overflow.)

---

* Green TH: Urinary Stress Incontinence: Differential Diagnosis, Pathophysiology, and Management. *Am J Obstet Gynecol* 122:368, 1978

MANAGEMENT

Nonsurgical—Medical

1. Tincture of hyoscyamus, 10 drops t.i.d.

2. Propantheline bromide (Pro-Banthine), 15 mg. t.i.d., and 30 mg. at bedtime.

3. This management may be helpful if there is an additional complication of urgency incontinence.

4. Estrogens may help to alleviate the symptoms of stress incontinence associated with postmenopausal atrophy. Excessive use of estrogens, on the other hand, may produce or aggravate stress incontinence.

Exercises

1. Perineal exercises (Kegel) increase pubococcygeal muscular control as well as urogenital diaphragm control.

2. A good voluntary sphincter mechanism alleviates the distress of stress incontinence by permitting a quick forceful contraction of these muscles, thus reducing the involuntary loss of urine under stress.

3. Voluntary contractions of these muscles should be done for 3 or 4 minutes, four times a day.

Pessaries

1. Elevation of the neck of the bladder with a pessary may provide control of the stress incontinence. This is used only when the patient is not a good candidate for surgery.

2. In some instances, use of a pessary may produce or aggravate the problem.

Urethral Dilation

This may relieve a few cases of stress incontinence. Dilation of the urethra up to a No. 28 French dilator is adequate treatment. The results are unpredictable, and the technique often unsuccessful.

Surgery

1. Basic Principles

a. The only type of incontinence that is helped by surgery is stress incontinence.

b. Urgency incontinence must be ruled out before surgery for stress incontinence.

c. Cystocele is rarely associated with stress incontinence. Over-vigorous correction of a cystocele may lead to stress incontinence.

d. All infections of the urinary tract must be controlled before surgery.

e. The operation should be tailored to the pathologic findings and to the physiological and anatomic imbalance.

f. The initial result is often good. However, over 5 to 10 years only about 50 to 60 per cent of operations prove to be successful.

g. The failure rate for repeat operations is high.

Types of Operation

1. Vaginal Urethroplasty (Kelly's Operation)

a. This is the most common operation and is usually the first choice.

b. It is sometimes called a buttressing, or Kelly, operation.

c. It is an attempt to prevent urethral dilatation on straining by tightening the para-urethral tissues; and to raise and support the urethra by suturing the fascia beneath it.

d. The injection of phenylephrine hydrochloride (Neo-Synephrine) (1 ml. in 60 ml. of saline) reduces the amount of oozing and permits a better dissection of the planes.

e. The anterior wall is carefully dissected from the urethrovesical area.

f. At the level of the urethrovesical junction, a silk suture picks up the periurethral fascia on either side of the urethra. This suture is repeated above and below.

g. After the silk sutures are tied, the bladder fascia (sometimes called pubocervical fascia) is pulled together with catgut to give added support.

h. The cystocele, if present, is now repaired in the usual way.

2. Marshall-Marchetti-Krantz Operation

a. If the bladder neck is elevated and fixed in the presence of stress incontinence, the primary approach should be suprapubic or a combination of the suprapubic and vaginal operations.

b. The basic functions of the Marshall-Marchetti operation are the elevation of the urethrovesical junction and posterior rotation of the bladder.

c. Marked vaginal and urethral scarring is a contraindication to the Marshall-Marchetti-Krantz operation, unless it is combined with release of scars from below.

d. The urethrovesical junction is made to adhere firmly to the anterior vaginal wall by the suturing of the vaginal tissue to the back of the symphysis pubis in the Marshall-Marchetti-Krantz operation. The main steps of the operation are outlined below.

e. The urethrovesical junction is exposed in the Retzius space. Adhesions are divided and all bleeding points picked up. The urethra must be dissected to within 1 cm. of the external meatus.

f. A Foley catheter in the bladder helps to identify the urethrovesical junction. Silk sutures pick up vaginal tissue on either side and suture it to the pubic periosteum.

g. Additional sutures may be added between the bladder muscle and rectus muscles.

h. Hematuria is common; continuous catheterization is required for 7 days.

i. Periostitis occurs in about 3 per cent of patients.

j. If too acute an angle is produced, the patient may have difficulty in emptying her bladder.

k. The object of this operation is to provide elevation and support for the urethrovesical junction and the proximal urethra.

l. A 90-per-cent immediate success rate and an 85-per-cent long-term success rate are reported.

3. Modifications of the Marshall-Marchetti-Krantz Operation

a. *Lapides' Operation.* The urethra itself is sutured to the symphysis and periosteum. The object is to correct the accordion-like shortening of the urethra on straining, which is thought to be a factor in the causation of stress incontinence. This operation is more traumatic to the urethra than the standard Marshall-Marchetti-Krantz operation.

b. *Burch Operation*

(1) This is an additional suprapubic approach for urinary stress incontinence. Basically, this operation anchors the vagina, lateral to the urethra, to the Cooper's ligament on each side. The main advantages are a low surgical morbidity, diminished chance of fistula, decreased postoperative pain, virtual absence of hematuria, and a minimal chance of osteitis pubis.

(2) The disadvantages are that voiding in the postoperative period is slow and incomplete. However, as time passes, the patient begins to void normally.

c. *Ball's Operation*

(1) This operation involves combined repairs from below and above. It has been promoted on the grounds that freeing the urethra and repairing it from below prevents failure of the suprapubic suspension. It also involves suspending the neck of the bladder to the rectus muscle rather than the periosteum of the symphysis pubis, on the grounds that this eliminates periostitis, chronic suprapubic pain, and osteomyelitis.

(2) The operation consists of an anterior plication of the urethrovesical junction with the posterior urethroplasty, so as to create good anterior and posterior urethrovesical angles. To do this, the urethra must be well mobilized and all bleeding controlled.

(3) The theoretical basis of Ball's operation is the ability of the intact urethra to contract by itself, if free to do so, and the equal distribution to urethra and bladder of raised intra-abdominal pressure.

4. The Pereyra and Inco procedures to correct stress incontinence have given disappointing results. The initial results were good, but long-term follow-up has been reported to show a 50-per-cent failure rate with a high complication rate.

URINARY INCONTINENCE NOT CURABLE BY SPHINCTER PLICATION

Sling Operations

1. These have been popular for many years, but the number of patients treated by sling operations has decreased since the introduction of the Marshall-Marchetti-Krantz operation.

2. The Goebell-Frangenheim-Stoeckel operation has been cited as the first sling operation described. It has been modified several times.

a. It involves a combined vaginal and abdominal approach.

b. One or two teams attach strips of rectus fascia through the Retzius space on each side of urethra, thus encircling it. This permits elevation of the urethral base.

c. The tension should be adjusted so that the bladder neck lies behind the upper half of the symphysis pubis.

3. Aldridge's operation and Moir's operation are modifications of the original sling operation.

Millin's Operation

1. This is a sling operation done entirely through an abdominal incision.

2. The abdomen is opened through a lower transverse incision down to the fascia. Fascial strips are cut and are left attached laterally.

3. The urethra is freed from the vaginal wall by the same approach used in the Marshall-Marchetti-Krantz operation.

4. The slings are led through the recti and under the urethra and sutured in front of the urethra.

5. If the sling is too tight, voiding is difficult and a urethrovesical fistula may develop. If it is too loose the operation will be ineffective.

Indications

The indications for these operations are a failed Marshall-Marchetti-Krantz operation and a short anterior vagina which cannot be elevated behind the symphysis pubis.

URGENCY INCONTINENCE

It is important to rule out urgency incontinence in evaluating patients with stress incontinence. Two out of three patients with stress incontinence have at least minimal urgency incontinence.

Basic Principles

1. The patient with urgency incontinence is unable to inhibit detrusor contraction and must void urine immediately. She has the sensation of wanting to void, but loses her urine before reaching the bathroom.

2. The most common cause is irritability due to cystitis, but all forms of bladder pathology must be considered, including tuberculosis, calculus, and carcinoma. Urethritis and even vaginal discharge from cervicitis are also causes. Remember that urgency and stress incontinence may occur simultaneously.

3. Urgency incontinence may be neurogenic (seen in conjunction with spina bifida, multiple sclerosis, or diabetes) or may be due to local disease of the bladder, such as interstitial cystitis, cystitis, or trigonitis.

4. If the patient has a cystocele, this may stretch the trigone and produce postural frequency.

5. A difficult problem is presented by the patient with urgency or urgency incontinence, usually combined with frequency, in whom no organic lesion is discovered.

6. Such patients are strictly the responsibility of the urologist, but in practice many of them present to the gynecologist.

7. The cause may also be psychological or environmental. Precipitating factors may include marital problems, widowhood, or accidents or illnesses to close relatives, together with postoperative retention and cystitis.

Management

When there is a diagnosis of urgency incontinence and no organic reason has been discovered:

1. The underlying dysfunction may be poor cortical processing of the stimuli resulting from bladder distension. This may be helped by a regimen of "bladder drill."

2. The bladder drill starts with filling the bladder to capacity at the time of cystoscopy. Instead of draining it at the completion, fluid is left in, and on recovering consciousness the patient voids what is usually a very much larger volume of fluid than she has done for a long time.

3. The psychological influence of the anticipated improvement following the bladder drill may have a good effect on the patient.

4. The patient is kept in the hospital and a regimen of voiding "by the clock," regardless of whether or not she desires to micturate, is initiated.

5. Starting half-hourly, the interval between voidings is increased by one-half hour daily, up to 3 or 4 hours. Even if 2 hours is the longest that can be achieved, this is usually a great improvement over the previous situation.

6. The success of this regimen is often helped by prescription of a mild tranquilizer or sedative, especially at bedtime.

7. Pro-Banthine 15 mg. t.i.d., plus 30 mg. at bedtime, or atropine, belladonna, or flavoxate hydrochloride (Urispas), may diminish the desire to void too frequently. (Rule out glaucoma before using these drugs.)

8. Dilation of the urethra until it admits a No. 28 French catheter may be helpful. The rational is unclear, unless it be that some factor causing irritation in the proximal urethra is relieved by stretching.

9. Bladder infection is one of the main causes of urgency incontinence, and a basic part of therapy is to eliminate it if it exists.

10. It cannot be too strongly emphasized that full genitourinary tract investigation must be performed before one embarks on the type of regimen outlined above.

11. If this is not done, from time to time a patient with serious and treatable pathology of the urinary tract, such as tuberculosis, may be denied specific therapy.

THE URETHRAL SYNDROME

1. The urethral syndrome includes complaints of frequency, dysuria, urgency, and a sensation of incomplete emptying in a patient in whose urine no evidence of infection can be found. The cause is not known; there are several hypotheses about it.

2. Urinary infection is strictly defined as being present only when ten or more typical urinary pathogens are grown per ml. of freshly voided midstream urine. It may be that the urethral syndrome is simply a condition caused by fewer than the usual number of organisms, or by organisms that cannot be cultured in the media used for conventional organisms.

3. Clinically, a patient with this syndrome must be regarded as suffering from a urinary tract infection, and one must persevere in the investigation. Even if no evidence of infection is found, some empirical treatment must be given.

4. Some pharmacies will make up urethral suppositories of nitrofurantoin (Furadantin) and estrogen. These, placed just inside the urethra and rubbed carefully after they melt, will get into the various little crevices and sinuses and provide relief. It is also important in these patients to apply a vaginal hormone cream, taking care to rub it in under the urethra and around the external part of the meatus.

38 Benign Tumors of the Ovary

Hugh R. K. Barber

BASIC PRINCIPLES

Eighty-five per cent of ovarian tumors are benign. The incidence of benign tumors approximates 7 per cent for all females.

Classification

1. **Cystic**
   a. Non-neoplastic
      (1) Surface müllerian epithelial cysts
      (2) Follicular
      (3) Corpus luteum
      (4) Theca lutein cysts
      (5) Stein-Leventhal (polycystic ovary)
   b. Neoplastic
      (1) Germ cell
         (a) Benign cystic teratoma (dermoid)
      (2) Epithelial
         (a) Serous
         (b) Mucinous
         (c) Endometrioid
2. **Solid**
   a. Fibroma
   b. Brenner
   c. Other associated rare lesions (e.g., pregnancy luteoma)

DIAGNOSTIC SYMPTOMS AND SIGNS

1. Often no symptoms or signs are present.

2. In many instances, the first symptoms noted is a palpable mass or abdominal enlargement.

3. Vague heaviness, pressure, and dull aching may occur.

4. As a rule, there is no destructive influence exerted on menstrual function.

5. Often, because of the lack of any specific symptom, an uncomplicated tumor has grown large by the time the doctor is consulted.

6. Symptoms are usually related to whatever complications occur.

PHYSICAL SIGNS

1. Small tumors remain in the pelvis and are detected only on bimanual examination.

2. Larger tumors fill the pelvis and usually lie between the uterus and the sacrum. If the patient is not too fat, the uterus can be distinguished on palpation as separate from the tumor.

3. A tumor occupying the abdomen causes a midline swelling and is usually tense.

4. Little can be done at this stage to classify the tumor or exclude malignancy. A very large tumor is likely to be benign; a primary malignant tumor would probably have killed the patient before reaching such a size.

5. If the patient is very thin, irregularities may be palpated, and sometimes two tumors may be suspected.

6. A tumor of moderate size may have a long pedicle composed of the attenuated broad ligament and fallopian tube, which allows the tumor to be displaced from side to side or to occupy a high abdominal position.

7. Adhesions, inflammation, and displacement of pelvic organs may all exist along with a tumor, and may confuse the examiner.

DIFFERENTIAL DIAGNOSIS

1. Full bladder
2. Ascites
3. Pregnancy
4. Myomata
5. Pelvic inflammatory disease
6. Diverticulitis
7. Appendiceal abscess
8. Distended cecum
9. Pancreatic cyst
10. Mesenteric cyst
11. Broad ligament cyst
12. Pelvic kidney
13. Retroperitoneal tumors

COMPLICATIONS

1. Torsion of pedicle
2. Rupture of cyst
3. Suppuration of cyst
4. Hemorrhage
5. Malignant change

NON-NEOPLASTIC (PHYSIOLOGICAL) CYSTS

Non-neoplastic cysts of the ovary are quite common and almost all ovaries examined at intra-abdominal surgical procedure or during autopsy show one or more small cystic structures, including generations of developing or regressing follicles. Cysts and related disorders may be due to changes in the surface of the müllerian epithelium or in the ovarian follicles in the surrounding ovarian stroma.

SURFACE (MÜLLERIAN) EPITHELIAL CYSTS

1. These cysts, which are also known as germinal inclusion cysts, occur frequently near and after menopause. They are usually small and close to the surface of the ovaries. These cysts are thought to be derived from invaginations of the surface epithelium following rupture of graafian follicles, or to result from scarring of the ovary; or they may be due to implantation of tubal epithelium or to tubo-ovarian adhesions.

2. The cysts are lined by one layer of cuboidal or partially ciliated columnar epithelium. The epithelium may show tubal or endometrial metaplasia and calcification of luminal contents. Although these cysts are asymptomatic, they are considered to be the site of origin of some true neoplasms of the ovary.

FOLLICULAR CYSTS

Basic Principles

1. Persistence of an enlarged follicle may lead to temporary enlargement of the ovary.

2. A follicular cyst may result when a follicle does not rupture at the time of ovulation.

3. These cysts are usually small but may attain a size of 6 cm.

4. They are unilateral.

5. Most follicular cysts disappear after one or two menstrual cycles.

6. Most patients are asymptomatic, but some complain of fullness or pain in one adnexal area.

Management

1. Observation and re-examination after two menstrual periods.

2. Surgical intervention is indicated only if a complication arises.

CORPUS LUTEUM CYSTS

These cysts develop from excessive secretion and accumulation of fluid associated with the involution process.

Basic Principles

1. Most corpus luteum cysts are larger than follicular cysts; they may increase to 8 cm. in size.

2. Most of these cysts are due to vascular or lymphatic disturbance.

3. The symptoms are similar to those seen with follicular cysts.

4. A corpus luteum cyst may be asymptomatic or may mimic a tubal pregnancy. It may be associated with amenorrhea, pain, and a mass.

5. A ruptured hemorrhagic cyst may produce typical signs of intraperitoneal bleeding.

6. Halban's syndrome is characterized by a persistent corpus luteum cyst, amenorrhea followed be irregular uterine bleeding, unilateral pelvic pain, and a small, tender, movable adnexal mass. It is obvious that in most cases the syndrome is diagnosed after ectopic pregnancy has been ruled out.

Management

1. Laparoscopy, culdoscopy, colpotomy, or, occasionally, exploratory laparotomy is needed for diagnosis and therapy, if there is no accident in the cyst or the diagnosis is unclear.

2. In this age group it is possible to follow the patient through one or two periods to see if there is regression of the mass.

THECA-LUTEIN CYSTS

Basic Principles

1. The development of a corpus luteum cyst is preceded by ovulation; in the instance of theca-lutein cyst or cysts, the abnormality occurs in the absence of ovulation.

2. These cysts may be unilateral and solitary, but more often are multiple and bilateral.

3. They result from disturbances in the hypothalamic-pituitary-gonadal axis in which an elevated gonadotropin level is observed.

4. Theca-lutein cysts may be iatrogenic.

5. They usually regress without treatment.

6. Theca-lutein cysts may be found in the newborn, with hydatidiform mole, choriocarcinoma, twin pregnancy, or erythroblastosis fetalis, or with the use of clomiphene citrate (Clomid) or Pergonal.

Management

1. Management is conservative.

2. Surgery is not necessary except in the management of complications.

Stein-Leventhal Syndrome (S-L)

1. This may be referred to as the polycystic ovary syndrome (PCO). It is characterized by amenorrhea or oligomenorrhea, infertility, and, usually, clinical evidence of excess androgenicity.

2. The ovaries are often bilaterally enlarged, but may be of normal size; or only one ovary may be affected.

3. The ovaries usually are enlarged and have thick gray capsules and numerous subcapsular cysts (oyster or potato ovary). There are varying degrees of theca-cell hyperplasia.

Diagnosis

1. The diagnosis is usually made on clinical grounds.

2. Confirmatory laboratory findings include moderately elevated serum testosterone (usually not over 200 ng. per 100 ml.), normal urinary 17-hydroxycorticosteroids, normal or slightly elevated urinary 17-ketosteroids (rarely over 25 mg. per 24 hours), elevated serum luteininzing hormone (LH), and normal serum follicle-stimulating hormone (FSH).

3. Occasionally, if the diagnosis is in doubt, visualization of the ovaries by laparoscopy, culdoscopy, or laparotomy may be necessary.

Differential Diagnosis

1. Adrenal hyperplasia
2. Adrenal tumor
3. Pituitary tumors

Management

1. If pregnancy is not desired, menstruation should be induced by medroxyprogesterone acetate (Provera) or one of the oral contraceptive agents.

2. If there is evidence of adrenal hyperplasia, cortisone should be given and the hyperplasia monitored by following the 17-ketosteroid levels.

3. If pregnancy is desired, the patient will probably ovulate in response to clomiphene. If there is no response to clomiphene and if other factors contributing to infertility have been ruled out, Pergonal and human chorionic gonadotropin (HCG) may be used.

4. Surgery offers an opportunity to explore the patient. In some patients who do not respond to medical therapy, a wedge resection of the ovary is indicated. This requires excision of about half of the ovarian tissue. The resection must be carried to the hilus of the ovary.

NEOPLASTIC OVARIAN CYSTS

BENIGN CYSTIC TERATOMA (DERMOID)

Basic Principles

1. Dermoids are rarely large, but are often bilateral (25 per cent).

2. They are usually found in women of childbearing age, but may be present at any age.

3. Grossly, there is a rather thick, opaque, whitish wall, and on opening the cyst one frequently finds hair, bone, and cartilage as well as a large amount of greasy fluid, which rapidly becomes sebaceous on cooling.

4. There are no pathognomic signs. In pregnancy the cyst frequently lies anterior to the uterus, overlying the bladder.

5. The malignancy rate is low; it has been reported as from 1 to 3 per cent.

6. The possible complications are torsion, hemorrhage, rupture, and infection.

Management

1. Resection of the cyst. If this is not possible, excision of the ovary.

2. The other ovary should be bisected, inspected, and biopsied.

3. In the over-age-35 patient, the treatment of choice is total hysterectomy and bilateral salpingo-oophorectomy.

NEOPLASTIC EPITHELIAL CYSTS

SIMPLE SEROUS CYSTS

Basic Principles

1. These make up 15 per cent of all benign ovarian tumors.

2. They may vary in size from a few centimeters to a huge cyst occupying the entire abdominal cavity. They usually measure about 5 to 6 cm.

3. They are usually unilateral.

4. Usually there are no symptoms unless torsion, rupture, or hemorrhage occurs.

Management

1. Resection of the cyst in the younger age group

2. In the over-35-years age group, hysterectomy and bilateral salpingo-oophorectomy is indicated.

SEROUS CYSTADENOMA

Basic Principles

1. This is a unilocular or multilocular cyst lined by epithelium similar to the fallopian tube.

2. It is common and accounts for 20 per cent of all ovarian neoplasms.

3. It is smaller than its mucinous counterpart (below) and grows to a maximum of 10 cm. in diameter.

4. About one-third of cases are bilateral.

Management

Management depends upon the age of the patient. In a young woman a unilateral salpingo-oophorectomy is sufficient therapy. However, in peri- or postmenopausal patients and patients over age 35, total hysterectomy and bilateral salpingo-oophorectomy is the treatment of choice.

PAPILLARY SEROUS CYSTADENOMA

Basic Principles

1. This tumor accounts for 10 per cent of all benign ovarian tumors.

2. It is most common in women in their reproductive years.

3. In 50 per cent of cases, this type of tumor appears bilaterally.

4. Grossly, papillary serous cystadenomas are globular and multiloculated.

5. They reveal intracystic and extracystic papillary growths.

6. They may show clinically malignant tendencies.

Management

1. After age 35 years, a total hysterectomy and bilateral salpingo-oophorectomy is indicated.

2. A more conservative operation may be carried out during the childbearing years, if the patient is willing to accept a concomitant risk of developing a more serious future problem, such as recurrence of the cyst with possible malignant potential.

MUCINOUS CYSTADENOMA

Basic Problems

1. This is a unilocular or multilocular cyst of the ovary, lined by tall columnar epithelium resembling that of the cervix or large intestine.

2. It may reach a very large size, occupying the whole abdomen.

3. It is the second most common type of ovarian tumor. It accounts for 15 per cent of all ovarian tumors and 25 per cent of all benign ovarian tumors.

4. It is usually unilateral.

5. Malignant changes occur in about 5 per cent of cases.

6. Torsion is common because of the well-defined pedicles that are often present.

Management

As for serous cystadenoma

FIBROMA

Basic Principles

1. This tumor is composed of fibrous tissue and resembles fibromata found elsewhere.

2. It is common in the elderly.

3. It accounts for about 5 per cent of all ovarian tumors.

4. It may represent a thecoma that has undergone fibrous transformation.

5. It may be associated with Meigs' syndrome. When hydrothorax is present, the right side is involved in 75 per cent of cases, the left side in 10 per cent; and both sides are involved in only 15 per cent of cases.

Differential Diagnosis

1. Malignancy with pulmonary metastases

2. Cardiac or renal disease with fluid retention
3. Hepatic cirrhosis
4. Tuberculous peritonitis

Management

1. In the peri- or postmenopausal patient, hysterectomy and bilateral salpingo-oophorectomy is indicated.
2. In a younger patient a conservative operation is acceptable.

BRENNER TUMOR

Basic Principles

1. This is a rather uncommon type of ovarian neoplasm; grossly it is identical to a fibroma.
2. It accounts for 1 to 2 per cent of all ovarian tumors.
3. It is most common in the sixth decade.
4. It is rarely malignant.
5. Microscopically, the epithelial cells show a "coffee bean" pattern due to the longitudinal grooving of the nuclei.

Management

As for fibroma

PREGNANCY LUTEOMA

Basic Principles

1. This is not a true neoplasm, even though it may attain a diameter of 15 cm. and have numerous mitoses.
2. It is best interpreted as a focus of reversible, nodular, lutein-cell hyperplasia, since it depends on HCG stimulation for its structural and functional integrity.

Management

1. Management is conservative, since pregnancy luteoma is reversible in most instances.
2. Surgery is reserved for the complications that may arise, such as torsion or hemorrhage.

39 Benign Uterine Tumors

Hugh R. K. Barber

ENDOMETRIAL POLYPS

Definition

1. The term *polyp* is a clinical rather than a pathologic one, referring to a growth that is attached by a pedicle or stem, and not indicating in any way its histological character.

2. The polyp has a structure like that of the endometrium itself, consisting simply of a localized heaping-up of the latter. Most polyps reveal only estrogen response—i.e., proliferation or hyperplasia.

3. Most polyps are benign growths that occur after the age of 35 years. They may be single or multiple.

4. Polyps form sessile or pedunculated masses of endometrial tissue. They are usually single, grayish-pink, soft-to-firm lesions. The tumors frequently arise from the fundus and may be pedunculated to the extent of protruding from the external os.

5. If large in size, they may distend and distort the endometrial cavity. In a curettage specimen, endometrial polyps stand out as firm fibrotic structures, compared to the fragile, soft-or-rubbery normal endometrial tissue.

Basic Principles

1. Endometrial polyps may be small, or may be large enough to fill the uterine cavity.

2. It is impossible to assess their frequency.

3. Most endometrial polyps are asymptomatic.

4. Some may be associated with menorrhagia, postmenstrual staining, and postmenopausal bleeding.

5. There is cramping pain, usually mild, as the uterus tries to expel the polyp.

6. The polyp may be present at the external os.

7. The histological types of endometrial polyps are:

a. Those made up of functional endometrium

b. Those made up of immature endometrium

c. Adenomatous polyps

8. Endometrial polyps undergo malignant degeneration, particularly in the postmenopausal period.

9. They may cause chronic vaginal discharge.

Diagnosis

1. The diagnosis may be suspected on the basis of the patient's history.

2. Pap smear

3. Hysterogram (fractional—should be carried out with a water-soluble dye)

Management

1. Remove the polyp with a tonsil snare or twist it off with polyp forceps.

2. A fractional curettage and cervical biopsies should be carried out.

3. The base of the polyp must be carefully curetted.

ENDOMETRIAL HYPERPLASIA

Definition

1. This is a uterine condition in which the endometrium remains in the proliferative phase for many weeks or years, which results in hyperactivity and growth of both glandular and stromal elements of the endometrium.

2. Endometrial hyperplasia is a common condition and is seen in 5 to 10 per cent of all diagnostic curettages.

3. Possible causes include anovulatory cycles, Stein-Leventhal syndrome, and estrogen-secreting ovarian tumors, such as granulosa or theca cell tumors.

Basic Principles

1. The majority of patients are between the age of 35 and menopause, but this condition may affect young women and even postpubertal adolescents.

2. Functional (dysfunctional) uterine bleeding presents without a causative uterine lesion (such as tumor, infection, or complication of pregnancy), although frequently there may be associated follicular cysts of the ovary.

3. *Functional bleeding* is a clinical term, while *hyperplasia* is a histological diagnosis.

4. The underlying cause is excessive or unopposed endometrial stimulation by estrogen in the absence of progesterone.

5. Functional bleeding is usually associated with anovulation or extended periods of amenorrhea. It may be secondary to ovarian unresponsiveness, disturbed pituitary gonadotropin secretion, Stein-Leventhal syndrome, adrenocortical hyperplasia, functioning ovarian tumors, and administration of estrogens.

Symptoms

1. Hemorrhage is common, irregular, often continuous for weeks, and liable to be profuse.

2. Amenorrhea intervenes for 1 or 2 months between spells of hemorrhage.

3. Anemia may be marked.

Diagnosis

1. History indicating anovulation or prolonged periods of amenorrhea

2. Endometrial biopsy

3. Fractional curettage

Management

1. Puberty to Age 30

a. Improve diet and recommend more rest. Anemia, obesity, and underweight for height should be corrected.

b. Rule out endocrine, metabolic, and other pathologic states.

c. Progesterone in oil, 100 mg. I.M.

d. Provera, 10 mg. q.4h. until improved.

e. Combined estrogen-progesterone pill for three cycles.

f. Premarin 20 mg. I.V. in emergency cases; response is seen usually in one hour; if not, repeat the dose q.3 to q.4h. times three doses.

g. Give cyclic progestin therapy after the immediate bleeding problem is over.

2. Age 30+ to Menopause

a. Rule out pathologic conditions, i.e., fibroids, chronic pelvic inflammatory disease, etc.

b. Correct anemia if it is present.

c. Fractional curettage is indicated.

d. Rarely is hysterectomy required to control the bleeding.

3. Postmenopausal Patient

a. Rule out pathologic condition, i.e., carcinoma of the endometrium, ovarian tumors, etc.

b. Fractional curettage with cervical biopsies

c. If bleeding occurs, do a repeat fractional curettage.

d. Hysterectomy may become necessary for recurrent bleeding.

e. If the patient is not a good candidate for surgery, she may be treated with large doses of Depo-Provera or Delalutin, which produces hemostasis through the production of endometrial atrophy.

ADENOMATOUS HYPERPLASIA

Definition

Adenomatous hyperplasia, a typical precancerous lesion, may be a focal or general change. Its greatest prevalence is in women of perimenopausal age with dysfunctional bleeding.

Basic Principles

1. Histological examination of curettings shows the glands to be back-to-back; there is pseudostratification of the glandular epithelium and, in the most intense form, a characteristic pallor or eosinophilic stain reaction of these glands with intense proliferation of the glandular epithelium, forming buds and islands within the gland lumen.

2. In contrast to carcinoma in situ of the cervical squamous epithelium, adenocarcinoma in situ of the endometrium is less well-defined. The term "adenocarcinoma in situ" is seldom used, because of the lack of precision in the literature as to the exact definition and clinical significance of this lesion. For these reasons an increasing number of authors prefer the term "atypical endometrial hyperplasia."

3. Adenomatous hyperplasia is a precursor lesion. Patients who have it are at high risk for later invasive carcinoma of the endometrium.

4. A young woman may have a syndrome of the cystic ovary and oligomenorrhea and may present with adenomatous hyperplasia in her reproductive years.

5. Classifications of endometrial hyperplasia are almost as numerous as authors who have written on the subject, although there is widespread agreement that some classification system is necessary to distinguish these hyperplasias, with minimal associated risks of progression to cancer, from those that are more likely to progress if left untreated.

6. A simple system is to designate hyperplasias as adenomatous (architectural atypia without cytological atypia) or atypical (both architectural and cytological); it has been reported that the latter have a substantial risk of progression to carcinoma.

Management

1. Young Women

a. Fractional curettage is indicated if there is any lawless bleeding.

b. Induction of ovulation and the subsequent progestational effect on the endometrium can reverse the pattern of adenomatous hyperplasia and restore normal cycling of the endometrium.

c. This may be achieved by giving progesterones, Clomid, or cortisone, and, in some instances, by wedge resection of the ovary.

2. Peri- and Postmenopausal Years

a. Fractional curettage and hysterectomy will confer upon the patient a lasting prophylaxis without the requirement for further follow-up.

b. If hysterectomy is not indicated at that moment, a repeat curettage should be done 4 months after the initial diagnosis.

c. If adenomatous hyperplasia is not present, the patient may be followed with endometrial biopsies at 6-month intervals.

d. If adenomatous hyperplasia is present at the time of the second curettage, a hysterectomy is indicated. In this age group the ovaries should also be removed.

e. Treatment with progesterones is not indicated in this age group.

ENDOMETRIAL METAPLASIAS

1. The differential diagnosis of endometrial carcinoma includes not only the well-known hyperplasia, but also a group of epithelial metaplasias, some appearing from known etiological stimuli and others occurring without known antecedents.

2. The endometrial metaplasias have been classified into seven categories:

- **a.** Morules and squamous metaplasia
- **b.** Papillary metaplasia
- **c.** Ciliated-cell or tubal metaplasia
- **d.** Eosinophilic metaplasia
- **e.** Mucinous metaplasia
- **f.** Hobnail metaplasia
- **g.** Clear-cell metaplasia

3. Their importance is that they may be mistaken for carcinomas.

4. Squamous metaplasia and morules are likely to be confused with adenoacanthoma.

5. The clinician must appreciate that adenoacanthoma, like any other carcinoma of the endometrium, is diagnosed primarily from the glandular component; thus, if the glands are benign in appearance and do not invade their own stroma it is safe to assume that the overall lesion is benign.

6. Papillary metaplasia has also been called *syncytial surface metaplasia* because it tends to occur at or near the endometrial surface and is characterized by cells that form papillary projections and syncytia. The appearance is often reminiscent of microglandular hyperplasia of the endocervix, but this endometrial lesion is usually seen in patients receiving exogenous estrogens rather than progestins.

7. In tubal, ciliated-cell, or eosinophilic metaplasia, glands are sometimes aligned by cells with bland nuclei and brightly eosinophilic cytoplasm. The cilia are usually easily identified. When they are not, the term *eosinophilic metaplasia* may be used. The lesion resembles metaplasia toward a type of epithelium identical to that seen in the fallopian tubes, and is most likely to be confused with atypical hyperplasia or adenocarcinoma in situ.

8. The distinction is made largely on this basis: ciliated cells are present in tubal metaplasia, and nuclear stratification and atypia are absent.

LEIOMYOMAS (FIBROIDS)

Definition

1. A *leiomyoma* is a benign, well-circumscribed tumor of nonstriated muscle with supporting fibrous tissue. Though not encapsulated, it can be shelled out from the uterine muscle.

2. It may arise from immature or undifferentiated cells in the myometrium, or possibly from cells in blood vessel walls. It has been definitely shown that the tumor arises from a muscle cell, probably from an undifferentiated myoblast.

3. Rarely, leiomyomas are found in the ovary or the round ligament.

Basic Principles

1. The fibroid is the most common tumor found in women (present in 15 to 20 per cent), especially after 35 years of age.

2. The locations of fibroids describe their types. They may be conglomerate or multiple and vary in size from tiny (millet seeds) to several centimeters in diameter.

3. Some fibroids develop long pedicles and present as polyps.

4. They are seemingly hormone-dependent and will continue to grow with varying degrees of rapidity during the menstrual era, with postmenopausal regression and shrinkage.

5. As leiomyomas contain either A or B type G-6-PD, but not both, they are considered to arise from single cells and are therefore neoplasms.

6. Fibroids bind approximately 24 per cent more estradiol per mg. of cytoplasmic protein than does the normal myometrium.

7. Erythrocytosis associated with uterine fibroma is mediated through direct production of erythroprotein by the tumor.

8. Abnormally large venous spaces in the endometrium overlying fibroids may be an objective source of associated menorrhagia. The finding is usually associated with glandular atrophy and stromal hyperplasia, not an uncommon finding in anovulation associated with fibroids.

9. Varieties According to Position

a. *Interstitial* or *Intramural.* Probably all fibroids begin to grow in the substance of the uterine wall. As they grow they continue to be surrounded by a layer of muscle of varying thickness. Most fibroids, as they increase in size, pass into one of the following positions: subserous (subperitoneal), submucous, or cervical.

b. *Subserous* develops on the outer surface of the uterus. It may become very large and cause only minimal symptomatology. It may be sessile or pedunculated and may become intraligamentous, retroperitoneal, or parasitic, depending upon growth.

c. *Submucous* migrates toward the uterine cavity and projects therein. It is probably the most important myoma, since it involves the endometrial cavity and leads to increased bleeding and cramps.

10. Cervical fibroids make up about 5 per cent of all fibroids. They are always solitary tumors and may attain large sizes.

11. Secondary changes with myomas include hyaline degeneration (most common), cystic degeneration, infection, calcification, necrosis, fatty degeneration, and sarcomatous degeneration (in 0.5 per cent or less, usually postmenopausal). Carneous degeneration is a particularly interesting degenerative process, which most often is a curious phenomenon of pregnancy and is probably related to impaired circulation in the myoma.

Special Types of Leiomyoma

Some leiomyomas have unusual histological features. These include:

1. *Epithelioid,* or *bizarre,* leiomyomas. These are smooth-muscle tumors composed of epithelial-like cords or nests of cells rather than the usual elongated spindle cells. The cells in these tumors may be bizarre or atypical.

2. The *leiomyoblastoma* variant is composed of round or polygonal cells with clear cytoplasm, especially around the periphery, resembling a fried egg. These cells are arranged in sheets or cords.

3. *Plexiform tumorlet* is considered by some authors to be a subtype of epithelial leiomyoma. It is usually located in a superficial part of the myometrium. Its histogenesis is controversial; some authors prefer to use the term "glomus tumor," or "angioma," for this type of neoplasm, while others feel it may originate from endometrial stroma or perivascular mesenchyma.

4. The *symblastic* or *pseudosarcomatous* leiomyoma is another type of benign leiomyoma. The neoplastic cells are giant, bizarre, and multinucleated. Similar cells may occur as a manifestation of focal degeneration. (This is common in pregnancy and with the use of birth control pills.) This type differs from leiomyosarcoma in being focal rather than diffuse. The cells are separated by pale bands of collagen that may be hyalinized, in contrast to the hypercellularity of sarcomas. Hyperchromasia of the nuclei is associated with karyorrhexis and lack of mitotic figures, features not seen in the actively growing sarcoma.

5. Other extremely rare types include benign leiomyomas with dissemination inside the uterine veins, which constitute a condition known as *intravenous leiomyomatosis.* Occasionally they spread to the lungs; then they are known as *benign metastasizing leiomyomas.* Sometimes they spread within the peritoneum; this condition is called *leiomyomatosis peritonealis disseminata.* The latter may be a form of subserosal mesenchymal metaplasia to smooth muscle, and is not related to uterine leiomyomas.

Symptoms and Diagnosis

1. In many instances the patient is totally asymptomatic.

2. There is a history of heavy menstrual periods.

3. Pain is not a symptom of myoma unless there is torsion of a pedunculated lesion.

4. There may be a palpable abdominal tumor.

5. Vaginal examination reveals an irregularly enlarged uterus and bulky ovaries.

6. As the tumor grows there may be pressure symptoms, according to the location.

7. If bleeding is sufficient there may be associated anemia.

8. Fractional curettage is indicated in the presence of lawless bleeding.

Management

Management depends upon:

1. Associated symptoms
2. Size and location of tumors
3. Patient's age
4. Patient's childbearing status

Conservative Treatment

1. Asymptomatic Tumors. Most fibroids are small and free of symptoms. They are found on routine examination and require no treatment other than periodic follow-up examinations in the absence of any developing symptoms.

2. Symptomatic Tumors

a. Treat conservatively if fibroids are small.

b. Give analgesics for dysmenorrhea and minimal pressure symptoms.

c. Perform a fractional curettage for any abnormal bleeding so as to rule out endometrial polyps, hyperplasia, submucous fibroids, and carcinoma of the endometrium.

Surgery

1. Indications for Surgery

a. Excessive size (generally 16 weeks or more)

b. Exclusive of pregnancy, excessive or rapid growth may be associated with sarcomatous changes.

c. Submucous fibroid associated with heavy and recurrent bleeding

d. A pedunculated fibroid may be susceptible to torsion and possible necrosis.

e. Pronounced pressure symptoms on the bladder or rectum; obstruction to ureter

f. Cases in which myomas, by size or location, are believed to contribute to infertility, habitual abortion, or premature labor

2. Type of Surgery

a. Myomectomy is usually reserved for patients in whom the preservation of reproduction is important.

b. Patients so treated have a high incidence (5 to 40 per cent) of subsequent myomas necessitating further surgery. If in the interim the patient has one or two full-term deliveries, this is a small price to pay.

c. Morbidity is slightly higher than with hysterectomy.

d. Hysterectomy is the usual and preferable procedure, particularly in older women and when the myomas are large. Ideally, a fractional curettage should be carried out prior to hysterectomy.

e. If at the time of curettage (for heavy and repeated bleeding in women over age 40 years) a diagnosis of submucous fibroid is made, hysterectomy is probably indicated.

Radiotherapy

1. Today there is scant indication for an irradiation menopause. Most gynecologists prefer surgical treatment.

2. Rarely in the occasional bad-risk patient, radiotherapy is effective. A fractional curettage or endometrial biopsy should be done prior to the radiotherapy.

3. It is contraindicated in the presence of submucous fibroid, pedunculated subserous myoma, degenerated myoma, pelvic infection, or a myoma exceeding 12 weeks' size.

Adenomyosis

See Chapter 40.

Plexiform Tumorlets

Plexiform tumorlets found in the endometrium are benign. They are incidental lesions of stromal-cell origin, are noted microscopically, and are associated with a high incidence of uterine fibroids.

Hemangiopericytoma

1. This is a cellular tumor, rarely malignant, found in the uterus and in other parts of the body as well.

2. It is a vascular lesion, like the glomus tumor, and may be distinguished by a tendency toward concentric arrangements of pericytes around capillaries.

3. The malignancy rate is reported as 20 to 25 per cent.

4. Differential diagnosis includes endometrial stromatosis and sarcoma.

Müllerian Adenofibroma (Papillary Cystadenofibroma)

1. This tumor is considered to be a benign counterpart of the malignant mixed müllerian tumor. Adenofibroma is a common tumor in the ovary that can also occur in the uterus, cervix, and fallopian tubes.

2. The broad-based polypoid mass protrudes from the endometrial cavity and has a papillary surface.

3. Microscopically, the cyst and glands are lined by one or more types of müllerian epithelium, such as the endometrial endocervical and tubal types. The stroma is fibrous, forms papillary structures covered by the epithelium, and may protrude into the cystic area.

4. Occasionally the stroma is of the endometrial stromal type; or it may be formed of nondescript spindle cells that condense around the cyst, giving an appearance like that seen in adenosarcoma. However, the stromal cells lack the mitotic activity that is seen in stromal sarcoma and adenosarcoma.

OTHER BENIGN NEOPLASMS

Angiomas, lipomas, lipomyomas, and adenomatoid tumors may occur in the uterus. The adenomatoid tumor is derived from the mesothelial cells on the surface. It occurs with equal frequency in the fallopian tubes and uterus. Although this neoplasm is often circumscribed, it lacks a capsule. The cells tend to form solid cords and eventually cleft-like spaces develop within these nests; cellular atypia and mitotic activity are not seen.

40 Adenomyosis

Hugh R. K. Barber

DEFINITION

1. *Adenomyosis* is characterized by benign invasion of the myometrium by the endometrium, which normally lines the uterine cavity superficially.

2. It continues to be an elusive disease of the perimenopausal years.

3. Adenomyosis is also known as *endometriosis interna.*

4. Careful examination of hysterectomy specimens demonstrates such foci of ectopic endometrial tissue in 8 to 27 per cent of cases in different series.

5. The condition may be associated with leiomyomas in about 50 per cent of cases and with endometriosis of other organs in approximately 10 to 15 per cent of cases.

BASIC PRINCIPLES

1. Adenomyosis results from direct extension of the basal endometrium down into and, rarely, through the myometrium. Serial sections will reveal this direct continuity.

2. Previous pregnancy seems to play a role in etiology; fewer than 6 per cent of patients are nulliparous.

3. Although no firm relationship between adenomyosis and a precancerous or malignant condition of the uterus has been established, on a few occasions adenocarcinoma has been reported as arising from adenomyosis in conjunction with a normal-surface endometrium.

4. On occasion the adenomyosis may penetrate through the uterus and involve the rectosigmoid or uterosacral ligaments and other adjacent organs.

5. Close examination of the cut surface shows a trabeculated appearance with numerous small dark areas, these being cystic spaces containing thick, tarry menstrual blood.

6. Histological examination shows interlacing muscle bundles and fibrous tissue, together with numerous islets of endometrial tissue.

7. Stromal cells are found surrounding the typical endometrial glands; occasionally, the glands are few or completely absent.

8. The cervix is rarely involved.

9. The presence of concomitant pelvic endometriosis is frequent.

DIAGNOSIS

1. The clinical diagnosis is presumptive. It is based on the following three findings:

   a. Progressive severe dysmenorrhea, with or without menometrorrhagia

   b. Normal to slightly-enlarged, globular uterus

   c. Patient age of 35 to 45 years

2. The diagnosis is only made definitively if the uterus has been removed and the diagnosis is confirmed on histological examination.

MANAGEMENT

1. The progress of adenomyosis depends on continued ovarian function.

2. If the patient is immediately premenopausal and the symptoms are mild, conservative therapy is indicated.

3. Menopause will completely correct the condition.

4. When the symptoms are severe and getting progressively worse, hysterectomy is indicated. In this age group oophorectomy should also be carried out.

41 Endometriosis

Hugh R. K. Barber

DEFINITION

1. Endometriosis is a disorder characterized by the presence of functioning endometrial tissue outside the uterine cavity.

2. Aberrant tissue may be found in many locations, including the ovaries, uterosacral and other pelvic ligaments, rectovaginal septum, pelvic peritoneum, umbilicus, laparotomy scars, hernia sac, bowel or bladder, lower genital tract, tubal stumps, and lymph nodes.

3. Endometriosis is a rather ubiquitous, potentially disabling disease that seems to be increasing in incidence. It is a frequent cause of infertility and has been reported to account for 25 to 30 per cent of fertility problems in human females.

4. If male factors were excluded, endometriosis would probably be the most common cause of infertility in women over age 25.

BASIC PRINCIPLES

1. The development and extension of endometrial tissue into the myometrium is termed *adenomyosis*. This disease entity seems histogenetically unrelated to endometriosis and is characterized by an entirely different clinical situation. Furthermore, findings on pelvic examination show none of the characteristics of endometriosis.

2. Endometriosis implies proliferating growth and function (usually bleeding) in an extrauterine site.

3. An *endometrioma* may be defined as an area of endometriosis, usually in the ovary, that has enlarged sufficiently to be classified as a tumor.

4. When the endometrioma is filled with old blood (resembling tarry or chocolate-colored, syrupy fluid) it is commonly known as a "chocolate cyst."

5. While the complaint of infertility should be sufficient to alert the physician to the possibility of endometriosis, the index of suspicion is elevated if the woman has progressively severe dysmenorrhea, dyspareunia, or pain on defecation.

6. Endometriosis is found in about 15 per cent of pelvic operations.

7. It is a disproportionately common problem among women of the higher socioeconomic groups. As such, it has been correlated with delayed or deferred motherhood.

8. Endometriosis has been called "the disease of civilization."

9. The median age of patients at the time of diagnosis is approximately 37 years, but approximately 15 per cent of patients are under age 30 years.

10. Several possible routes of histogenesis of endometriosis have been proposed: transplantation, or tubal regurgitation; coelomic metaplasia; lymphatic spread; the hematogenous route; and a composite, or unified, histogenic process.

11. More recently, two other explanations of the etiology of endometriosis have been proposed: genetic and familial origin, and autoimmune pathogenesis.

12. Certain racial influences may also be present, as suggested by the higher-than-average incidence found in Japanese women.

13. The development of an antibody complement system that triggers immune responses by action of surface-cell antigens called *HLA antigens* is an interesting part of animal and human evolution. Many diseases are associated with particular HLA antigens. These surface-cell antigens play an ever-growing role in the field of organ transplantation, and may come to play a significant part in the investigation of the etiology of endometriosis.

14. Recent work has supported prostaglandin studies that have shown significant elevations of prostraglandin levels ($PGF_{2\alpha}$) in the peritoneal fluid of endometriosis patients compared to levels found in controls. Normally, physiological levels of prostaglandin are necessary for ovum release, normal tubal motility, uterine relaxation, and steroidogenesis.

15. An increased concentration of prostaglandins in peritoneal fluid may result in altered tubal motility, ovum release, and steroidogenesis.

The significance of this finding, of course, is that prostaglandins, which are the end products of arachidonic metabolism, are produced in the presence of hypersensitive autoimmune response.

MANEUVERS TO AVOID

1. Pelvic examination during the menstrual period or after diagnostic dilatation and curettage.

2. At the time of menstruation or just premenstrually, uterotubal insufflation should not be done.

3. Pelvic examination after endometrial biopsy is contraindicated because of the possibility of endometrial spillage inside the peritoneal cavity.

4. Cryosurgery should be avoided in young females because of the high incidence of subsequent cervical stenosis.

DIAGNOSIS

Diagnostic Triad

1. A period-linked symptom that gets progressively worse.

2. An interval of 5 years since the last delivery, regardless of the number of previous deliveries.

3. Tender nodules in the cul-de-sac, uterosacral ligaments, and ovaries, particularly noticeable during menstruation. A fixed retroversion of the uterus may be present.

Diagnostic Aids

1. Ultrasonography
2. Laparoscopy
3. Barium enema
4. Intravenous pyelogram
5. Cystoscopy
6. Examination under anesthesia
7. CA125 (Low level)

Differential Diagnosis

1. Chronic pelvic inflammatory disease
2. Ovarian tumor or cancer
3. Rupture of an ovarian endometrial cyst may simulate an attack of pelvic peritonitis or appendicitis, an ectopic pregnancy, an ovarian cyst with twisted pedicle, a ruptured dysfunctional ovarian cyst, or carcinoma of the rectosigmoid.

MANAGEMENT

1. Asymptomatic endometriosis may be safely dealt with by close observation. Mild pain can be controlled by analgesics.

2. For more pronounced symptoms, surgery and hormone treatment are still the only available therapeutic options.

Surgery

1. Endometriosis is probably best treated primarily by surgery. This is mandatory if there is an adnexal mass.

Table 41–1 **AMERICAN FERTILITY SOCIETY CLASSIFICATION OF ENDOMETRIOSIS**

Stage		Score
Stage I	(Mild)	1–5
Stage II	(Moderate)	6–15
Stage III	(Severe)	16–30
Stage IV	(Extensive)	31–54

PERITONEUM	Endometriosis		1cm	1–3 cm	3 cm
			1	2	3
	Adhesions		filmy	dense w/partial cul-de-sac obliteration	dense w/comlete cul-de-sac obliteration
			1	2	3
OVARY	Endometriosis		1cm	1–3 cm	3 cm or ruptured endometrioma
		R	2	4	6
		L	2	4	6
	Adhesions		filmy	dense w/partial ovarian enclosure	dense w/complete ovarian enclosure
		R	2	4	6
		L	2	4	6
TUBE	Endometriosis		1 cm	1 cm	tubal occlusion
		R	2	4	6
		L	2	4	6
	Adhesions		filmy	dense w/tubal distortion	dense w/tubal enclosure
		R	2	4	6
		L	2	4	6

*This classification is based on the work of V. C. Buttram, Jr., R. W. Kistner, A. M. Siegler, and S. J. Behrman.

2. Hormone therapy over a long period of time is expensive and often unsatisfactory, and the result is not predictable.

3. Where the disease is very extensive with adnexal masses, particularly in older women, hysterectomy and bilateral salpingo-oophorectomy is indicated.

4. In young women with less extensive disease than described above, it is possible to preserve an ovary, since hysterectomy alone will relieve most, if not all, symptoms. (With the various forms of pregnancy that can be carried out—e.g., in vitro, GIFT, and surrogate motherhood—it is important to save ovarian tissue whenever possible, especially in young women.)

5. In young women desiring pregnancy, conservative surgery should be carried out if possible. It should include resection of endometrial cysts, unilateral adnexectomy

CLASSIFICATION OF ENDOMETRIOSIS

STAGE I (Mild)

Broad ligaments:
No implants more than 5 mm.

Tubes:
Avascular adhesions, fimbria free

Ovaries:
Avascular adhesions no fixation

Cul-de-sac: No implants more than 5 mm.
Bowel: Normal Appendix: Normal

STAGE IIA (Moderate)

Broad ligaments:
No implants more than 5 mm.

Tubes:
Avascular adhesions, fimbria free

Ovaries:
Endometrial cyst 5 cm. or less — A1 stage; over 5 cm.— A2; ruptured — A3

Cul-de-sac: No implants more than 5 mm.
Bowel: Normal Appendix: Normal

STAGE IIB (Moderate)

Broad ligaments:
Covered by adherent ovary

Tubes:
Adhesions not removable by endoscopy; fimbria free

Ovaries:
Fixed to the broad ligament; implants over 5 mm.

Cul-de-sac: Multiple implants, no adherent bowel or fixed uterus
Bowel: Normal Appendix: Normal

STAGE III (Severe)

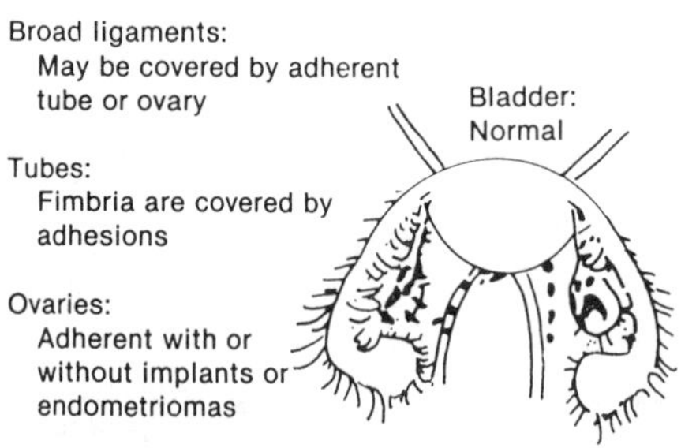

Broad ligaments:
May be covered by adherent tube or ovary

Bladder: Normal

Tubes:
Fimbria are covered by adhesions

Ovaries:
Adherent with or without implants or endometriomas

Cul-de-sac: Multiple implants, no adherent bowel or fixed uterus
Bowel: Normal Appendix: Normal

STAGE IV (Extensive)

(Usually combined with stages I, II, III)

Bladder: Implants

Uterus:
May be fixed and adherent posteriorly

Cul-de-sac:
Covered by adherent bowel or fixed retrodisplaced uterus

Bowel: Adherent to the cul-de-sac, uterosacral ligaments, or corpus
Appendix: May be involved

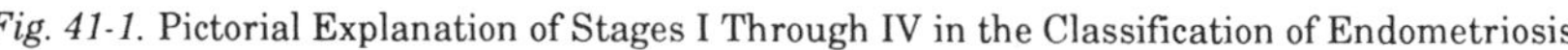

Fig. 41-1. Pictorial Explanation of Stages I Through IV in the Classification of Endometriosis

if required, fulguration of implants, suspension of the uterus, and presacral neurectomy.

6. If there is a recurrence of the endometriosis following conservative surgery that requires a second operation, it should probably include castration. After castration surgery, hormonal replacement therapy in the premenopausal woman is an accepted practice.

7. Laser surgery has been used to eradicate all macroscopic evidence of endometriosis. It will take time to evaluate the overall results.

8. Pregnancy rates following conservative surgical procedures depend upon the stage of disease. The literature reports a pregnancy rate of 76 per cent in Stages I and II, and a rate of 38 per cent in Stages III and IV.

Hormonal Therapy

1. The aims of treatment are to secure relief of pain, to permit adequate coitus, to prevent abnormal bleeding, and, of course, to preserve or increase the possibility of pregnancy.

2. Hormonal therapy is indicated in patients with Stage I or Stage IIA disease. A variety of methods have been devised for the medical management of this illness. The hormonal pseudopregnancy approach yields pregnancy rates of 45 to 55 per cent in Stages I and IIA.

3. Pregnancy has often been suggested as the optimum prophylactic and therapeutic treatment for endometriosis.

4. Regression of endometriosis following suppressive hormone therapy is probably due to a combination of anovulation and amenorrhea brought about by adenohypophyseal suppression.

5. Hormones that have given subjective or objective relief of signs or symptoms are: estrogens, androgens, progestins, combined estrogen-progesterone pill, hydroxyprogesterone caproate, and medroxyprogesterone.

6. A new testosterone derivative, 2,3 isoxazol ethisterone (danazol), with weak androgenic and no estrogenic or progestational activities, is also reported effective in suppressing endometriosis. It acts by inhibiting gonadotropins or gonadotropin-releasing factors. More clinical trials are necessary to evaluate its overall value in the management of endometriosis.

7. Hormonal therapy consists of: pseudopregnancy and progestins, androgen, danazol, and, more recently, gonadotropin-releasing hormone (GnRH) agonist.

8. GnRH agonist brings about a medical oophorectomy, which allows temporary suppression of ovarian function without the transient stimulation of estrogenic substances or the inconveniences of androgenic ones.

9. A 28-day pilot study of five women with proven endometriosis, who were treated daily with subcutaneous doses of a potent GnRH agonist, showed suppression of ovarian estrogens and androgen levels similar to that reported in oophorectomized women. This has popularized the potential use of medical oophorectomy for endometriosis.

10. Contraindications to Hormone Therapy

a. Unproved endometriosis, especially in the presence of adnexal masses

b. Large myomas that might be stimulated to grow by hormone therapy

c. Excessive side effects, whether physical or psychological

d. Hepatic disease

e. Previous thrombophlebitis or embolic phenomenon

f. Previous mammary cancer

g. Age greater than 35 years

h. Excessive use of cigarettes

11. Prolonged therapy is appropriate in:

a. Patients with maximal symptoms and minimal palpable findings in whom a biopsy diagnosis has been established

b. Patients with persistent or recurrent disease after previous conservative surgery

12. Short-term hormonal therapy is indicated:

a. Prior to conservative surgery

b. Subsequent to conservative therapy, in order to inhibit ovulation and prevent reactivation of the disease

Results

1. Only a 25-per-cent rate of successful pregnancy is reported after hormone therapy that results in pseudopregnancy.

2. A 50- to 60-per-cent rate of successful pregnancy is reported after surgery.

3. Surgery not only eliminates endometriosis but also can correct tubal distortion and uterine fixation.

COMPLICATIONS

1. Endometriosis, untreated, is rarely a fatal disease. The complications arising from it are few.

2. Occasionally there is some obstruction of the rectosigmoid at the level of the cul-de-sac.

3. Obstruction of the small bowel is infrequent but may occur. It is usually in the low ileum or at the ileocolic junction. It is most likely due to adhesions between loops of the intestine, which may produce kinking and obstruction.

4. An ovarian endometrial cyst may rupture and become infected. Occasionally this is associated with malignant changes.

5. The ureters may be invaded, although this is very rare.

CONCLUSION

The enigmatic disease of endometriosis continues to baffle both scientists and clinicians. An encompassing theory of pathogenesis has failed to emerge from contemporary understanding of the immunological manifestations, the hormonal aberrations, and the evasive infertility associated with endometriosis.

Similarly unsettling is the failure of medical and conservative surgical maneuvers to eradicate endometriosis in a manner commensurate with the past situation. We must hope that further research in these areas will resolve both of these dilemmas, and, more specifically, that the technique of laser ablation of all remaining macroscopic evidence of endometriosis may allow a significant improvement in the fertility rate.

42 Gynecological Cancer

Hugh R. K. Barber

Exclusive of the ovary and the fallopian tube, carcinoma in the female reproductive system can be readily detected early by presently available diagnostic techniques. The question is raised, and rightfully so, if indeed this is the situation, then why are cancers of the vulva, vagina, cervix, and corpus not diagnosed at an early stage? Why have screening programs failed to accomplish this? The blame must be shared by the patient as well as the doctor. Only a well-informed public and profession can work cooperatively together to search for cancer in its early, most curable stage. Each doctor's office should serve as a screening clinic for detection of gynecological cancer.

BASIC PRINCIPLES

1. Exclusive of choriocarcinoma, there are only two definitive types of therapy that result in cure in a significant number of gynecological cancers, i.e., surgery and radiation.

2. The essential question in the philosophy of treatment has changed from what is the best form of treatment for a given cancer, to what is the best form of treatment for a given patient. Individualization has replaced standardization.

3. Chemotherapy—the treatment of cancer with drugs and with hormones—can be used effectively for disseminated as well as localized cancer. It has not only added to the longevity of the patient with gynecological cancer but has also improved the quality of life.

4. Therapy is no longer rigidly instituted for a state of disease but rather to eradicate a volume of cancer in a patient.

GENERAL MANAGEMENT

1. Although there are individual variations in the management of patients with different forms of gynecological cancer, there is an overall plan for all of these patients.

2. The patient admitted to the hospital for treatment of cancer is subject to a general evaluation of her physical status. A complete history is taken, and specific answers to the following questions are included: duration of present symptoms, history of weight change, previous neoplastic disease at any site, family history of neoplastic disease, whether she is a twin, menstrual history, abortions, histories of pregnancies, and previous operations of any kind.

3. In the routine physical examination, a careful pelvic and rectal examination should be carried out on admission and recorded. The speculum examination should not only visualize the cervix but should be manipulated to expose the entire vagina.

4. A patient who has cancer generally suspects the nature of her illness; or, as often happens, she has been told the diagnosis or that such a diagnosis is to be ruled out. When entering the hospital she is apprehensive, regardless of appearance. A well-organized admission routine can be most reassuring.

5. The admitting doctor or house officer should refrain from general discussion of neoplastic disease, methods of treatment, specific diagnoses of her case, and prognosis. The terms *tumor* and *growth* should be used in relation to her condition and not the word *cancer.*

6. On admission, the patient should be put at ease and medication should be prescribed to attain two objectives: tranquilizing drugs that allay apprehension should be given as necessary; to ensure sleep, medication should be given at a stated time so that the patient does not have a restless night.

7. If pain is present, the patient is asked what she has been taking and with what effects; the medication is ordered immediately and, if necessary, in increased doses to insure maximal relief.

LABORATORY DATA

1. Papanicolaou smears of the vagina, cervix, and endometrium should be obtained.

2. Complete blood count.

3. Urinalysis, including cultures and sensitivity.

4. SMA-12 (total protein, albumin, calcium, cholesterol, glucose, blood urea nitrogen, uric acid, creatinine, total bilirubin, alkaline phosphatase, LDH, SGOT).

5. SMA-6/60 (chloride, CO_2, potassium, sodium, BUN, glucose) as indicated.

6. CEA and AFP as indicated.

7. Clotting mechanism is assessed by thrombin time, prothrombin time, and partial thromboplastin time. Bleeding time, platelet count, and clot retraction are optional.

8. *Roentgenologic Studies.* Chest radiograph, intravenous pyelogram, and, in indicated cases, a bone survey.

9. Electrocardiogram.

10. Proctoscopy and cystoscopy as indicated.

11. Sonogram (ultrasonography).

12. Barium enema and GI series are optional.

13. Lymphangiography is optional and is not recommended in the elderly.

14. Computed tomography as indicated.

15. Liver scan if deemed necessary.

16. Magnetic resonance imaging (MRI) can eliminate many of the x-ray examinations that were previously included under the metastatic work-up.

PREOPERATIVE REGIMEN FOR RADICAL ABDOMINAL SURGERY

1. The general principles in preparation for laparotomy and major pelvic surgery are followed, with the addition of the list below for radical pelvic surgery.

2. The preparation for intracavitary radiation does not need to be as extensive but should include certain of the following orders as deemed appropriate for the patient.

3. Upon return of laboratory reports, any abnormal values are rectified by appropriate measures—i.e., blood transfusions for anemia, plasma for hypoproteinemia, indicated parenteral fluids for chloride, potassium or sodium deficiencies, vitamin K for prolonged bleeding and clotting time, and so on.

4. In debilitated patients, preoperative blood volume studies may be carried out and blood replacement ordered as needed and indicated. Ordinarily such studies are not necessary.

a. If the blood volume is thought to be depleted and facilities for blood volume determination are not available, it is possible for a blood volume determination to be made by watching the response of the patient's hematocrit to transfusions.

b. If there is a rise of 2 to 3 per cent after the transfusion of 500 ml. of whole blood, it can be assumed that the blood volume deficit has been overcome.

5. In certain debilitated patients in whom it is felt that there is a chance for cure or significant palliation, hyperalimentation (TPN—total parenteral nutrition) should be administered.

6. Counseling of the patient should be intensive, and the husband or another relative should be involved. The type of procedure, the complications, and the period of hospitalization must be presented.

7. The team of social workers, oncology nurse, and inhalation therapist, as well as others, should be involved preoperatively.

Preoperative Bowel Preparation

1. Ideally, the intestinal tract should contain the minimal amount of material, but stringent measures are not necessary. Regular diet may be permitted up to and including the evening meal prior to the day of operation. Nothing by mouth is permitted after midnight.

2. Enemas are ordered daily and until clear the evening before surgery. It is to be emphasized that mechanical cleansing is the most important factor in a bowel prep.

3. 60 ml. of 50-per-cent magnesium sulfate is given twice a day for 2 days prior to surgery.

4. 45 ml. of castor oil is given in the afternoon before surgery. It serves to flatten the small intestine.

5. Neomycin, 1 g. q.1h. × 6 doses, is given in the afternoon and evening before surgery. Erythromycin is often added to the regimen of neomycin. It has proven a worthwhile combination.

6. Sulfathalidine, 2 g. 4 times a day for 1 week, provides an excellent bowel prep.

7. If the patient has had any barium studies, it is important to take a flat plate of the abdomen the evening before surgery to make sure that there is no residual barium.

Additional Preoperative Measures

1. The patient is given a pHisohex shower the night before surgery.

2. A sulfa cream or antibiotic suppositories are inserted into the vagina the day before surgery.

3. No pelvic laparotomy for cancer should be undertaken without adequate blood readily available for transfusion. Thus, typing and crossmatching of several units of blood is a routine order, the number depending on the anticipated magnitude of the procedure.

4. The vagina is prepared with Betadine in the operating room.

5. If the patient has a carcinoma in situ, it is better not to prepare the vagina because the superficial layer of cells may be denuded.

Management in the Operating Room

1. After induction of anesthesia, the patient is placed in lithotomy position and pelvic examination is performed. With complete relaxation, palpation often permits different impressions than can be obtained with the patient awake, uncomfortable, and exhibiting varying degrees of muscle rigidity.

2. A Foley catheter is inserted into the bladder. Care must be taken to ensure that it is not in the vagina or the urethra but is well placed in the bladder.

3. In undertaking radical surgery, a Swan-Ganz catheter is often inserted prior to the start of surgery.

a. The relative fluid balance of the patient in shock can be assessed via a flexible catheter introduced into the great intrathoracic vessels by way of the antecubital, external or internal jugular, or subclavian veins. In patients with no cardiopulmonary disease, monitoring of central venous pressure with monitoring of the vital signs as well as the input and output and other clinical signs may provide sufficient guidance for fluid resuscitation.

b. Central venous pressure monitoring may be accomplished with a simple manometer, which avoids several of the complications of the pulmonary artery (Swan-Ganz) catheter.

c. The Swan-Ganz catheter is being employed with greater frequency.

d. The Swan-Ganz catheter provides an accurate picture of the left ventricle and also pulmonary artery wedge pressures.

4. The indicated operation is then carried out.

POSTOPERATIVE MANAGEMENT AFTER RADICAL SURGERY

1. Immediately following surgery, the vital signs, i.e., blood pressure, pulse, and respirations, are noted at 15-minute intervals until sensoria are fully recovered.

2. Special attention is directed to the pulmonary response and ventilation.

3. Urine output per catheter is recorded at hourly intervals. Forty ml. per hour is considered satisfactory.

a. In the immediate postoperative period urinary output may be minimal, but after 12 hours the normal rate of excretion generally increases if fluid intake is adequate. An excess secretion of antidiuretic hormone (ADH) may decrease the urinary output.

b. A good urinary output indicates good tissue perfusion. An output of 1,000 ml. a day is considered adequate.

c. Absence of urine indicates a mechanical block. Caution must be exercised in administering fluids.

d. The urine excretion from ileal or colon conduits should be especially noted. In case of ileal conduits, prompt urine flow is anticipated, but not infrequently the first 24-hour output may be less than normal.

e. In the case of colon conduits, urine excretion may be delayed for several hours or even 1 or 2 days. This is because of the usual excessive edema that may occur at the uretero-colon implantation sites as compared with the uretero-small bowel implantation sites.

f. In the case of wet colostomy there may be little or no urine excretion for 1 or 2 days. These patients must be carefully observed and controlled.

4. The insertion of a nasogastric tube is carried out at the discretion of the operator.

5. Oral ingestion of fluids is not permitted until the bowel sounds are completely normal.

a. When oral feedings are started, it is best to give 60 ml. of water each hour as desired by the patient. If the patient is reluctant to take fluids or has any nausea, fluids should be withheld.

b. Generally, fruit juices and milk produce an increased amount of gas accompanied by gas pains that may be severe. They should not be given.

6. The use of prophylactic antibiotics in the postoperative period should be individualized.

7. Fluid and electrolyte intake is discussed in Chap. 34.

8. The treatment of ileus, intestinal obstruction, and peritonitis is discussed in Chap. 34, as well.

9. When large denuded areas have been created, such as result from radical Wertheim hysterectomies with pelvic node dissection, pelvic exenterations, and radical vulvectomies, excessive exudation from these sites may result in significant fluid, electrolyte, and protein loss. This should be corrected by the addition of 250 to 500 ml. of plasma added to the daily baseline fluid and electrolyte replacement.

10. Blood chemistry studies should be obtained at least every other day.

11. The protein level should be maintained at a minimum of 6 g. per 100 ml. and the hemoglobin at at least 11 g.

12. The extended radical procedure that includes excision of the hypogastric arteries and veins results in removal of the branches of the autonomic nervous system and interferes with bladder and bowel function.

a. In this instance, the catheter should be kept in place for at least 6 weeks. This keeps the bladder from overdistending, reduces residual urine with its accompanying infection, and maintains the ureters in a position where there is no pull on their blood supply.

b. If a lesser procedure is carried out, the catheter can be removed in 2 weeks. The patient should be catheterized for residual urine until the residual is below 150 ml.

43 Cancer of the Lower Genital Tract

Hugh R. K. Barber

CANCER OF THE VULVA

Basic Principles

1. Cancer of the vulva accounts for 0.7 per cent of all female cancers, at a rate of 1.8 per 100,000 females. It is the fourth most common malignant tumor of the female genital tract, accounting for 3 or 4 per cent of all gynecological malignancies.

2. It occurs most frequently after the age of 65 years; it makes up 30 per cent of the malignant gynecological tumors arising in the seventh decade. It is rare under age 45 years and is very rare in pregnancy.

3. There are about 500 deaths annually in the United States from vulvar carcinoma.

4. Cancer of the vulva is usually diagnosed in the localized stage—i.e., in about 60 per cent of all cases.

5. Surgery is the usual treatment in over 80 percent of all cases. The 5-year survival rate is 64 per cent.

6. Almost all lesions are squamous-cell in origin, although adenocarcinomas of Bartholin's glands, basal cell carcinoma, malignant melanomas, and malignant sweat-gland tumors also occur.

7. The most common symptom of vulvar carcinoma is long-standing pruritus.

a. Chronic inflammatory changes are always present for varying periods, sometimes for several years, before cancer appears as an ulcerating lesion, with raised rolled borders and surrounded by induration of the uninvolved skin and subcutaneous tissues.

b. Rarely, one or more other cancerous lesions are present simultaneously in different portions of the vulva. They may appear as "kissing" lesions, one ulcer on each side, directly opposite one another.

8. Approximately 50 per cent of patients with cancer of the vulva have positive lymph node involvement. About 30 per cent have superficial involvement, and about 15 per cent have superficial and deep involvement; only about 3 per cent have deep involvement as the only metastases.

9. The most frequent site of the initial lesions is the labia majora, in the mid or anterior portion.

a. The clitoris is also a common site.

b. Encroachment upon the urethra, or actual involvement of it, occurs in larger lesions.

c. Less frequent primary sites are the region of the fourchette and posterior labial areas.

10. In the differential diagnosis other common conditions to be considered are: lymphogranuloma inguinale, chancre, chancroid, and condylomata acuminata.

11. All white lesions of the vulva must be biopsied if short-term medical treatment is unsuccessful.

12. Any suspicious lesion should be biopsied immediately.

PRECANCEROUS LESIONS

Vulvar Carcinoma In Situ (VIN)

There are two kinds of vulvar intraepithelial neoplasia (VIN):

1. Squamous cell carcinoma in situ

2. The rare adenocarcinoma (Paget's disease)

Basic Principles

1. The condition is being seen with increased frequency, especially in younger age groups (third and fourth decades).

2. Many lesions are asymptomatic and suspected on routine examination of the vulva. Itching is common.

3. The clinical appearances are highly variable. The skin may be white or pigmented—that is, darker than normally pigmented skin—and the lesions may resemble vulvar warts.

4. Twenty-five per cent of patients have a history of pre-malignant or malignant change in another organ. Half of these are carcinoma in situ of the cervix and/or vagina.

5. Condylomata acuminata are increasingly associated with VIN, and occur in 7 to 31 per cent of cases. The human papilloma virus (HPV) has become the prime suspect in vulvar neoplasms.

6. In the past, vulvectomy was most often indicated. Today newer and more conservative modalities are generally recommended.

7. Whatever the initial treatment, recurrences and new intraepithelial occurrences are common.

8. Diagnosis is usually made after the application of toluidine blue, which is allowed to dry and is then rinsed with 1-per-cent aqueous acetic acid or 4-per-cent acetic acid; examination under the colposcope helps in identifying the lesion. Multiple punch biopsies are required for accurate diagnosis.

9. Treatment should be individualized. Several options are available:

- **a.** Wide local excision
- **b.** Simple vulvectomy
- **c.** Skinning vulvectomy
- **d.** CO_2 laser
- **e.** Cryosurgery
- **f.** Nonsurgical methods (e.g., topical 5-FU)

10. CO_2 laser ablation is currently preferred to the other methods, especially in young patients with large lesions. The major advantage is the excellent cosmetic result.

Paget's Disease of the Vulva

1. The mean age of patients at diagnosis is 63 years.

2. The lesions characteristically present clinically as white islands of hyperkeratosis over a bright red base.

3. The disease is usually confined to the apocrine gland (sweat gland) region of the vulva.

4. Histologically, it is characterized by the presence of Paget's cells. One-third of patients have underlying sweat-gland carcinoma, which can be diagnosed only after excision.

5. Twenty-five per cent of cases are associated with a prior malignancy elsewhere, most frequently in the breast.

6. Wide excision (down through the fat to the fascia) should extend at least 2.5 cm. beyond visible margins. (Lines of incision must be checked histologically for Paget's cells.)

7. If there is no evidence of invasion, this constitutes the treatment.

Microinvasive Vulvar Carcinoma

1. When squamous cell carcinoma is 2 cm. or less in diameter, with 5 mm. or less of stromal invasion, it is termed *microinvasive.* The presence of vascular confluency, vascular channel permeation, and cellular anaplasia does not exclude a case from this category.

2. Microinvasive cancer constitutes up to 17 per cent of all vulvar cancers. The mean age of patients at diagnosis is in the late 50s. The disease is being reported with increasing frequency in younger women, and is now commonly reported in women in their 20s.

3. The most common site is the labia majora, but any part of the vulva, perineum, or anal or perianal epithelium may be affected. The lesions are frequently multifocal.

4. Antecedent or coexisting vulvar dystrophy is a feature in 80 per cent of cases; the associated lesion may be atrophic or hypertrophic, with or without a typical epithelial hypertrophy or intraepithelial neoplasia.

5. Vulvar condylomata precede, or coexist with, over 10 per cent of microinvasive vulvar lesions. The lesion may be present as a condyloma.

6. The true incidence of involvement of lymph nodes remains to be determined. Data from several series indicate that 8 per cent of patients have superficial (femoral and inguinal), and 2 per cent deep (pelvic), node metastases. The incidence depends on the grading of tumors as well as on their size and depth of penetration.

7. The treatment options vary from wide local excision to radical vulvectomy, with or without superficial (inguinal or femoral), and with or without deep (pelvic), lymphadenectomy. Sexual function should be conserved whenever possible.

8. In some minimal microinvasive lesions where invasion has been ruled out, CO_2 laser ablation can provide adequate treatment.

9. The extent of surgery is individualized. Surgical options include:

a. Wide excision biopsy

b. If penetration extends beyond 1 mm., wide excision is combined with ipsilateral superficial node dissection.

c. Vulvectomy is used as a diagnostic and therapeutic measure, and may be indicated in the presence of widespread dystrophy. Clitoral conservation is almost always possible and is desirable unless the lesion involves the clitoris or adjacent area.

d. Radical vulvectomy with lymphadenectomy is indicated for tumors measuring between 1 and 2 cm. with clinically suspicious nodes or involving the clitoris, urethra, or adjacent tissues, or showing the following histological features: cellular anaplasia, lymphatic or vascular permeation, or stromal invasion exceeding 2 mm.

INVASIVE TUMORS OF THE VULVA

Basic Principles

1. Vulvar malignant tumors make up 3.5 per cent of all gynecological malignancies. Over 80 per cent are squamous carcinomas. Other types include malignant melanoma, adenocarcinoma (usually in Bartholin's gland), sarcoma, and basal cell carcinoma.

2. These lesions may be unilateral or bilateral. Vulvar lesions may be divided into central (clitoral) and lateral (labia, including fourchette and perineum) in view of different routes of lymph drainage.

3. Twenty per cent of patients have inguinal node metastases, and one-quarter of these have pelvic node metastases. The incidence of metastases bypassing inguinal glands to involve pelvic glands directly is 3 per cent.

4. The standard operation is extended vulvectomy with bilateral inguinal and pelvic lymphadenectomy. More recently, individualization of surgical therapy has been recommended.

5. Pelvic lymphadenectomy is omitted on occasion (unless cytology shows metastases in inguinal glands). A more conservative surgical approach has been advocated for Stage I lesions. It has been recommended that hemi-vulvectomy and ipsilateral lymphadenectomy be carried out in selected cases of Stage I tumors.

6. The vulvar region tolerates radiation poorly, because of constant moisture and friction. Hence radiation therapy as a primary treatment is not desirable.

7. An acute painful reaction to radiation therapy may occur. Possible late complications include edema and radionecrotic ulcers. The principle use of radiation in vulvar cancer is as an adjuvant to surgery in patients in whom surgery has a high risk of failure.

8. The overall survival rate with current methods of management should approach 75 per cent in the presence of node involvement and 90 per cent in its absence.

Staging of Carcinoma of the Vulva

A case should be classified as carcinoma of the vulva if the primary site of growth is in the vulva. Tumors that are present in the vulva as secondary growth from either genital or extragenital sites should be excluded from registration, as should cases of malignant melanoma.

Stage O	Carcinoma in situ, e.g., Bowen's disease, noninvasive disease, noninvasive Paget's disease.
Stage I	Tumor confined to the vulva, 2 cm. or less in largest diameter. Nodes are not palpable or are palpable in either groin, not enlarged, and mobile (not clinically suspicious of neoplasm).
Stage II	Tumor confined to the vulva, more than 2 cm. in diameter. Nodes are not palpable or are palpable in either groin, not enlarged, and mobile (not clinically suspicious of neoplasm).
Stage III	Tumor of any size with adjacent spread to the urethra and any or all of the vagina, the perineum, and the anus, and/or nodes palpable in either or both groins (enlarged, firm, and mobile, not fixed but clinically suspicious of neoplasm).
Stage IV	Tumor of any size infiltrating the bladder mucosa, the rectal mucosa, or both, including the upper part of the urethral mucosa, and/or fixed to the bone or other distant metastases.

International Federation of Gynecology and Obstetrics (FIGO) Method of Staging: TNM Classification

1. T—Primary Tumor

a. T1—Tumor confined to vulva—2 cm. or less in larger diameter

b. T2—Tumor confined to vulva—more than 2 cm. in diameter

c. T3—Tumor of any size with adjacent spread to the urethra and/or vagina and/or perineum and/or anus

d. T4—Tumor of any size infiltrating the bladder mucosa and/or the rectal mucosa or both, including the upper part of the urethral mucosa and/or fixed to the bone

2. N—Regional Lymph Nodes

a. N0—No nodes palpable

b. N1—Nodes palpable in either groin, not enlarged, mobile (not clinically suspicious of neoplasm)

c. N2—Nodes palpable in either one or both groins, enlarged, firm, and mobile (clinically suspicious of neoplasm)

d. N3—Fixed or ulcerated nodes

3. M—Distant Metastases

a. M0—No clinical metastases

b. M1a—Palpable deep pelvic lymph nodes

c. M1b—Other distant metastases

Treatment

1. Radiation therapy is not suitable for established invasive malignant disease of the vulva.

a. The blood vessels in the vulva are end-type vessels with poor collateral circulation. As a result, endarteritis with necrosis may follow radiation therapy.

b. Many vulvar lesions are very big and therefore not suitable for implantation with radium or newer radioactive substances.

2. Invasive cancer must be treated by radical vulvectomy. This means removal of the entire vulva, including the labia majora, labia minora, hymenal remnants, and clitoris.

a. The lateral incision is made at the labiocrural fold; superiorly, the mons pubis is removed; inferiorly, the perineum is incised near the anus; and the medial incisions usually lie just outside the level of the urethral meatus.

b. The procedure must encompass the disease even if the distal half of the urethra has to be removed.

c. The superficial nodes bilaterally are excised. A decision must be made about the removal of the deep nodes.

d. Recently there has been a move toward more conservative surgery. Options include:

(1) Radical vulvectomy with superficial lymphadenectomy only

(2) Radical vulvectomy with clitoral conservation where there is no clitoral involvement

(3) Wide local excision with ipsilateral or bilateral superficial lymphadenectomy

Radiotherapy

Radiotherapy has a limited place in management. It may be appropriate:

1. Preoperatively, in advanced primary lesions and in lesions close to the urethra and anus, to lessen the risk of local occurrence

2. Postoperatively, when there is concern over the adequacy of excision and/or there are lymph node metastases

3. In patients unsuitable for surgery

Chemotherapy

Bleomycin or a combination chemotherapy—(cisplatin, vinblastine, bleomycin), or (methotrexate, fluorouracil)—is used in advanced and recurrent carcinoma.

Postoperative Management

1. Hemovacs are used to facilitate the apposition of flaps and prevent the accumulation of serum. The hemovacs are removed when the daily drainage is less than 50 ml.

2. Postoperative ambulation is begun the day after surgery and progresses rapidly each day.

3. Postoperative antibiotic therapy is ordered as indicated.

4. Oral feedings are usually started the day after surgery.

5. The catheter is removed on the tenth postoperative day.

6. Sitz baths are started within the first week.

7. Wound breakdown at the margin of the skin flaps continues to be a problem.

a. The wound should be denuded and an enzyme ointment applied to, and in, the debridement.

b. Most close without requiring a skin graft.

8. Certain cases of recurrence can be managed by pelvic exenteration.

Results

1. The cure rate ranges around 60 per cent in most cases.

2. Patients with positive superficial nodes have a 40-per-cent cure rate. In patients with negative nodes the cure rate approaches 80 per cent. Approximately 60 per cent of patients have negative nodes.

CANCER OF THE VAGINA

Basic Principles

1. Cancer of the vagina is extremely rare. It accounts for less than 1 per cent of all genital malignancies.

2. Cancer of the vagina usually occurs after the age of 70 years.

3. There are about 300 deaths from cancer of the vagina each year in the United States.

4. Cancer of the vagina is usually diagnosed in the localized (43 per cent) or regional (36 per cent) stage.

5. The ratio of incidence of cancer of the cervix to vaginal cancer is roughly 50:1. It is often difficult to tell whether the tumor arises primarily in the vaginal epithelium or extends to it from a primary locus in the cervix. When both are involved together, the cervix is considered the primary locus.

6. The usual treatment is radiation—it is used in 60 per cent of all cases.

7. The 5-year survival rate is 45 per cent.

8. Persistent bloody vaginal discharge, at first relatively painless, is the initial sign of primary vaginal cancer.

9. Because of its relative infrequency, primary vaginal cancer is not often considered; if an ordinary solid-blade speculum is used for examination, the instrument may cover the anterior midportion of the vaginal tube, at which point the lesion frequently originates.

10. The most common form of primary vaginal cancer is the squamous cell type. Macroscopically, it presents as a rounded or elongated ulcer with raised rolled edges and central excavated ulcer.

11. Vaginal cancer generally arises in the upper third of the posterior wall of the vagina and involves the rectovaginal septum early.

12. As the cancer invades and spreads, usually it destroys the cervix and then invades the parametria. Involvement of the vulva is rare, and spread to the lymph nodes is usually late.

13. Occasionally, adenocarcinoma is seen. In the face of this diagnosis it is important to determine whether the lesion is primary or is actually a metastasis from an unsuspected primary cancer elsewhere.

14. Cancer of the endometrium is prone to metastasize to the vagina, and when it does so is almost always found on the anterior wall.

15. Less often, secondary vaginal lesions may have their origins in the ovary, paraurethral glands, or gastrointestinal tract (especially the colon), or may originate from hypernephroma or uterine choriocarcinoma.

16. Since many alleged primary vaginal cancers are really metastases from unsuspected primary cancers elsewhere, it is important to have a careful workup including biopsies and fractional uterine curettage.

17. Clear-cell adenocarcinoma (müllerian type) is discussed elsewhere.

VAGINAL INTRAEPITHELIAL NEOPLASIA (VAIN)

1. The concept of cervical intraepithelial neoplasia (CIN) has been extended to a similar disturbance in the vaginal canal: vaginal intraepithelial neoplasia (VAIN).

2. The condition, like its counterpart in the cervix, usually presents through an abnormal smear. Routine colposcopy during cervical examination assists detection.

3. The incidence of VAIN is increasing. This may be coupled with the increased incidence of wart virus in the genital field. All condylomata and wart-like lesions of the lower genital tract warrant thorough vaginal survey.

4. The lesion most often occurs in the 4 per cent of transformation zones that extend from the cervix onto the vaginal wall. This site may be missed at hysterectomy so that the lesion persists and is erroneously diagnosed, later, as a recurrence. The transformation zone in a female who has been exposed to diethylstilbestrol (DES) extends to the vaginal wall in 85 percent of cases.

Diagnosis

1. Four-per-cent acetic acid is used to saturate the vagina. The lesions are usually aceto-white with clearly demarcated borders.

2. Schiller's iodine (the solution used in Schiller's test) is also used to identify the lesion.

3. The diagnosis is made by biopsy.

Treatment

1. The following methods are available and permit an individual approach:

a. Biopsy excision

b. CO_2 laser, cryosurgery, electrocoagulation diathermy under anesthesia

c. Local chemotherapy

d. Surgical excision

e. Radiation therapy

2. The laser is preferred and allows for more controlled destruction. The technique is similar to that for the cervix, but one vaporizes only to a depth of 3 mm.

INVASIVE TUMORS OF THE VAGINA

1. Squamous carcinoma is the predominant histological type of invasive tumor of the vagina.

2. The majority of malignant vaginal tumors result from metastasis or extension from nearby organs.

3. This disease is often regarded as having a poor prognosis; in recent series, though, overall 5-year survival rates have approached 40 to 50 per cent. Localized disease is as curable as cervical carcinoma, whereas there are few recorded 5-year survivals for invasive vaginal tumors diagnosed in Stages III and IV.

4. In general terms, lesions of the upper third of the vagina have a better prognosis than those of the lower third; annular and full-length lesions have a very poor prognosis.

Staging of Carcinoma of the Vagina

Excluded from this classification are secondary cancers in the vagina, cervical cancers involving the vagina, and malignant lesions extending into the vagina from the urethra or vulva.

Stage O	Carcinoma in situ; intraepithelial carcinoma
Stage I	The carcionma is limited to the vaginal wall.
Stage II	The carcinoma has involved the subvaginal tissue but has not extended to the pelvic wall.
Stage III	The carcinoma has extended to the pelvic wall.
Stage IV	The carcinoma has extended beyond the true pelvis or has involved the mucosa of the bladder or rectum. Bullous edema as such does not permit a case to be allotted to Stage IV.
Stage IVA	Spread of the growth to adjacent organs.
Stage IVB	Spread to distant organs

Treatment

Since the 5-year survival rate in primary epithelial cancer of the vagina is approximately 45 per cent with primary radical surgery with or without supplemental radiation, it is important to concentrate on making an early diagnosis.

1. Upper Two-Thirds of the Vagina

a. *Stage O (Carcinoma In Situ).* Simple excision or, in select cases, total hysterectomy and total vaginectomy.

b. *Stage I.* Radical hysterectomy, bilateral pelvic node dissection, and total vaginectomy. Radiation therapy is an alternate that is chosen for certain patients.

c. *Stage II.* Radical surgery as listed above. If it is not possible to encompass the cancer, radiation therapy, both external and intravaginal, should be carried out. Exenteration is reserved for recurrent cases of cancer of the vagina.

d. *Stage III.* Primary radiation therapy

e. *Stage IV.* Primary radiation therapy. It may be necessary to divert the fecal and/or urinary stream before therapy.

2. Lower Third of Vagina

a. Stage O. As listed above

b. *Stage I.* Total hysterectomy and total vaginectomy plus radical vulvectomy and bilateral groin node dissection. Radiation therapy may be chosen and be followed by a groin dissection.

c. *Stage II.* As for Stage I

d. *Stage III.* Primary radiation therapy

e. *Stage IV.* Radiation therapy with or without diversion of the urinary and fecal streams, depending on the condition of the patient

CLEAR-CELL ADENOCARCINOMA (MÜLLERIAN TYPE)

It was reported that a study at Massachusetts General Hospital revealed a highly significant association between the treatment of mothers with DES during pregnancy and the later development of adenocarcinoma in their daughters.

Basic Principles

1. The natural estrogens have apparently not been associated with this problem.

2. Nonsteroidal estrogens—i.e., DES, dienestrol, hexestrol, and benzestrol—have also been associated with this type of vaginal and cervical cancer.

3. The incidence rate for the development of clear-cell carcinoma of the vagina or cervix is approximately 0.1 per cent in females whose mothers took DES during pregnancy.

4. About 80 to 90 per cent of these patients develop adenosis of the vagina or have a congenital anomaly of the cervix and/or vagina. From these observations it was suggested that DES acts as a teratogen rather than a carcinogen.

5. Any teenage girl with irregular periods should receive a thorough pelvic examination, including palpation and direct visual inspection of the cervix and vagina, plus cytologic studies.

6. DES-exposed females should start to have regular pelvic examinations after their first periods—and at any age if they have symptoms.

7. Although the cytology studies are often negative because the tumors have a low grade of malignancy and are often covered with either intact mucosa or slough, the studies should still be carried out. It is suggested that the lesions or fornices be scraped with a spatula.

8. In all cases of clear-cell adenocarcinoma with a history of DES ingestion by the mother, adenosis has been found.

a. Adenosis is defined as the persistence of glandular elements in and under squamous epithelium of the vagina.

b. There is no current evidence that adenosis is a precursor of clear-cell adenocarcinoma.

9. In studies carried out with the microspectrophotometer, all clear-cell adenocarcinomas had aneuploid DNA distribution; all areas of adenosis had diploid or tetraploid distribution patterns, which are usually seen in proliferating epithelium.

Diagnostic Signs

1. Often the anterior fornix appears shortened and is less elastic than usual.

2. A cervical hood may be present. This gives the appearance of a cockscomb.

3. The cervix appears red.

4. There is often a red granular mucosa, small cysts, or a papillary lesion that may be multicentric in appearance.

5. On palpation there is a sandy irregularity.

6. The involved area takes Schiller's or Lugol's stain poorly, if at all.

7. The same findings may exist in patients with adenocarcinoma. Usually the findings are more marked; polypoid, nodular, or papillary lesions often are present.

Treatment

1. After representative biopsies, the general program for managing adenosis is close observation and repeated examinations. Adenosis is benign, and there is no evidence that it will turn directly to cancer.

2. Although some authors recommend partial or total vaginectomy for vaginal adenosis, treatment is conservative in most institutions. Laser therapy is being tried in a few centers.

3. Clear-cell adenocarcinoma of the cervix and fornices is best treated with radical surgery. Early lesions (Stage I vaginal or cervical carcinomas) can, and do, metastasize to regional pelvic lymph nodes.

4. The procedure consists of radical hysterectomy, pelvic lymph node dissection, and placement of split-thickness graft from the buttock into the area from which the vagina was excised.

a. The ovaries are preserved unless they are diseased.

b. Pelvic exenteration has been employed to encompass disease too extensive to be cured by a less radical surgical procedure.

5. Clear-cell adenocarcinoma can also be treated and cured by radiation.

a. Many radiotherapists are reluctant to deliver large doses of cancericidal radiation to a young woman.

b. However, radiation therapy is considered by some physicians to be preferable to pelvic exenteration as therapy for the more advanced lesion.

6. The criteria for prognosis are the degree of mitotic activity (one or more mitoses per high-power field carries a bad prognosis), the degree of involvement of regional lymph nodes, and the stage of disease.

7. The recent observation of pulmonary and/or supraclavicular lymph node metastases indicates that prolonged follow-up of treated individuals is essential.

EMBRYONAL RHABDOMYOSARCOMA (BOTRYOID TYPE) OF THE VAGINA

Basic Principles

1. This is an uncommon, highly malignant neoplasm, which is encountered in infants and young children and has a very poor prognosis. It may be seen in adults.

2. When seen in the vagina it usually starts as a small, broad-based, polypoid mass. As it grows it takes on the typical appearance of lobulated masses of vesicular or hemorrhagic polyps, which soon fill the vagina and project through the vaginal introitus.

3. Widespread metastases are the rule rather than the exception.

4. The most common metastatic sites are the lungs and the regional lymph nodes.

5. Bloody discharge and vaginal bleeding and/or mass are the most common signs.

6. Formerly, pelvic exenteration with pelvic node dissection was the treatment. Now, however, the favored approach is to perform a less radical procedure and treat the patient with combination anticancer chemotherapy.

CANCER OF THE CERVIX

Cancer of the cervix is a disease of the inner city. About 1.6 per cent of today's newborn girls, or 1 out of 63, will develop invasive cancer of the cervix uteri sometime during their lives. In 1989 the estimated number of new cases of cancer of the cervix will be 13,000, with 6,000 deaths.

Basic Principles

1. The high-risk group includes those starting intercourse in their teens, having multiple sex partners, or having many children, and women from the low socioeconomic groups.

2. The age of peak incidence for carcinoma in situ of the cervix is between 30 and 40 years, whereas for invasive cancer it is between 40 and 50 years.

3. In understanding the natural history of cancer of the cervix, it is important to know the causes of death from the disease. Uremia leading to infection and hemorrhage is the leading cause of death from invasive cancer of the cervix, but some women die from distant metastases.

CERVICAL CARCINOMA IN SITU AND DYSPLASIA (CIN)

Basic Principles

1. The term *cervical intraepithelial neoplasia* (CIN) denotes all precursors of squamous cervical cancer and embraces a continuum ranging from CIN I (minor dysplasia) through CIN II (moderate dysplasia) to CIN III (major dysplasia and in situ carcinoma).

2. Adenocarcinoma in situ is uncommon.

3. The condition usually presents as an abnormal smear.

4. Intraepithelial lesions, in most cases, occur within the transformation zone, which is usually visible in its entirety with the colposcope.

5. Failure to diagnose CIN on colposcopy may be due to:

a. A lesion high in the canal. This is more likely to occur in post-menopausal women.

b. Intercurrent acute cervicitis, often with contact bleeding

c. Warty atypia due to subclinical human papilloma virus infection, which can complicate the colposcopic interpretation

6. Invasive cancer can usually be excluded by colposcopically directed punch biopsies without need to resort to conization. Rates for cone biopsy have been reduced to about 5 per cent of those cases requiring further evaluation of an abnormal smear.

7. The management of CIN follows the exclusion of invasive cancer. It involves evaluation by colposcopy, diagnosis by biopsy, and individualized treatment by the most appropriate method. Endocervical curettage should always accompany the colposcopically directed biopsies.

CERVICAL ADENOCARCINOMA IN SITU AND ADENOSQUAMOUS CARCINOMA IN SITU

1. Adenocarcinoma in situ is an uncommon entity. It tends to be recognized via distinctive changes in the Pap smear.

2. Adenocarcinoma in situ is frequently associated with squamous lesions (CIN). In such cases the lesions are called *adenosquamous carcinoma in situ.*

3. On colposcopy the lesions, when visible, closely mimic the villous outgrowth of normal columnar epithelium. The distinguishing feature of the villi after application of acetic acid is their striking white color, which has been described as pearly-white.

4. Often the lesions are multifocal.

5. Invasive cancer may coexist deep in the cervical clefts or glands.

6. Cone biopsy is necessary to exclude invasive cancer. In younger patients this procedure can serve as definitive therapy.

7. Careful follow-up is necessary.

Preclinical Cervical Carcinoma (Microinvasive and Occult Invasive Carcinoma)

1. The term *preclinical invasive cervical squamous carcinoma* denotes all cases not recognizable by traditional methods of clinical examination.

2. The new classification established by the International Federation of Gynecology and Obstetrics (FIGO) has taken Stage IA preclinical carcinomas of the cervix, that is, those diagnosed only by microscopy, and subdivided them into Stage IA1, minimal microscopically evident stromal invasion, and Stage IA2, lesions detected microscopically that can be measured. The upper limit of the measurement should not show a depth of invasion of more than 5 mm. taken from the base of the epithelium, either surface or glandular, from which it originates; and the second dimension, the horizontal spread, must not exceed 7 mm. Larger lesions should be staged as IB.

3. The lesions should be evaluated colposcopically and adequate biopsies, with endocervical curettage, should be taken.

4. The therapy should be individualized.

5. The addition of colposcopy to traditional histology allows much more rational management than prevailed in the past. The colposcope can frequently discern lesions of high significance requiring radical management, leaving the remainder to be treated by appropriate conservative methods.

6. Preclinical invasive adenocarcinoma is usually diagnosed after cone biopsy for suspected cervical squamous or adenosquamous carcinoma, or adenocarcinoma, in situ.

7. Treatment is individualized and depends on the extent of the lesion. Conization, hysterectomy, hysterectomy with pelvic lymphadenectomy, and radical hysterectomy with pelvic lymphadenectomy are the options.

Diagnosis

1. There are no symptoms characteristic of cancer of the cervix. A high index of suspicion is necessary.

2. Bleeding is probably the most common symptom associated with cancer of the cervix and is usually bright red and "lawless." It may result from contact ("contact bleeding").

3. The cervix should be examined carefully, with rotation of the speculum in order to see all fornices as well as the entire cervix.

4. A cervix involved with a malignant process may show nothing if the disease is localized in the canal or if the lesion is smaller than an ulcerated mass.

5. The spectrum of findings may include red areas, erosions, ulcers, nodularity, an exophytic or endophytic lesion, or nodularity with ulceration.

6. An accurate histological diagnosis is essential before definitive treatment is instituted.

7. The differential diagnosis should rule out chancres, tuberculosis, granuloma inguinale, lymphogranuloma venereum, condyloma acuminatum, and radium eschars.

8. A point to emphasize is that each of these lesions can be present concurrently with cancer. This argues strongly for biopsy proof of disease.

9. The Pap smear is merely a screening method, and has its greatest application in the asymptomatic woman.

a. Any lesion visible on the cervix should be biopsied, since an obvious lesion may result in a negative Pap smear despite the invasive nature of the lesion.

b. The combination of Pap smear and biopsy gives a high yield of positive results in those patients in whom "early" cancer is present.

10. Pregnant patients represent a captive group and afford the physician the opportunity not only to do Pap smears but also to train patients in the need for routine physical examination, cytology, and biopsy screening.

11. When positive or suspicious cells are reported on Pap smear examination, it is important to take a systematic approach to diagnosis.

a. Repeat smears are submitted to another laboratory.

b. A colposcope can be used to outline the lesion and obtain colposcopically directed biopsies.

c. On an outpatient basis, punch biopsies of the Schiller's- or toluidine-blue-treated cervix and vagina are taken. Endocervical curettage with a small curette may be performed.

d. The patient may be admitted to the hospital or to ambulatory surgery for fractional D & C, further biopsies, or conization of the cervix, if necessary.

e. Biopsy revealing invasive cancer obviates conization.

f. Vaginal bleeding is evaluated systematically.

g. The D & C is preceded by a careful pelvic examination under anesthesia.

h. The endocervix is carefully curetted with a small curette, and the tissue sent as a separate specimen.

i. Next, the depth of the uterine cavity is determined with a sound.

j. The cervix is then dilated, and the uterine cavity explored with a polyp forceps.

k. The endometrial cavity is systematically curetted, including the top of the fundus and both cornua. An attempt should be made to identify the site of the tumor.

l. Multiple punch biopsies are then taken of the cervix.

Definitions of the Clinical Stages in Carcinoma of the Cervix Uteri

(Correlation between the FIGO, UICO, and AJCC nomenclatures.)

Stage O Carcinoma in situ, intraepithelial carcinoma. Cases of Stage O should not be included in any therapeutic statistics for invasive carcinoma.

Stage I The carcinoma is strictly confined to the cervix (extension to the corpus should be disregarded).

Stage IA Preclinical carcinomas of the cervix—that is, those diagnosed only by microscopy.

Stage IA1 Minimal microscopically evident stromal invasion.

Stage IA2 Lesions detected microscopically that can be measured. The upper limit of the measurement should not show a depth of invasion of more than 5 mm. taken from the base of the epithelium, either surface or glandular, from which it originates, and a second dimension, the horizontal spread, must not exceed 7 mm. Larger lesions should be staged as IB.

Stage IB Lesions of greater dimensions than Stage IA2 whether seen clinically or not. Preformed space involvement should not alter the staging but should be specifically recorded so as to determine whether it should affect treatment decisions in the future.

Stage II The carcinoma extends beyond the cervix, but has not extended on to the pelvic wall. The carcinoma involves the vagina, but not as far as the lower third.

Stage IIa No obvious parametrial involvement.

Stage IIb Obvious parametrial involvement.

Stage III The carcinoma has extended onto the pelvic wall. On rectal examination there is no cancer-free space between the tumor and the pelvic wall.
The tumor involves the lower third of the vagina.
All cases with a hydronephrosis or non-functioning kidney should be included, unless they are known to be due to other cause.

Stage IIIa No extension onto the pelvic wall, but involvement of the lower third of the vagina.

Stage IIIb Extension onto the pelvic wall or hydronephrosis or non-functioning kidney.

Stage IV The carcinoma has extended beyond the true pelvis or has clinically involved the mucosa of the bladder or rectum.

Stage IVa Spread of the growth to adjacent organs.

Stage IVb Spread to distant organs.

Notes on staging. Stage IA carcinoma should include minimal microscopically evident stromal invasion as well as small cancerous tumors of measurable size. Stage

---

Published with the permission of FIGO.

IA should be subdivided into those lesions with minute foci or invasion visible only microscopically as Stage IA1 and the macroscopically measurable microcarcinomas as Stage IA2 in order to gain further knowledge of the clinical behavior of these lesions. The term "IB occult" should be omitted.

The diagnosis of both Stage IA1 and IA2 should be based on microscopic examination of removed tissue, preferably a cone, which must include the entire lesion. As noted above, the lower limit of Stage IA2 should be that it can be measured macroscopically (even if dots need to be placed on the slide before measurement) and the upper limit of IA2 is given by measurement of the two largest dimensions in any given section. The depth of invasion should not be more than 5 mm. taken from the base of the epithelium, either surface or glandular, from which it originates. The second dimension, the horizontal spread, must not exceed 7 mm. Vascular space involvement, either venous or lymphatic, should not alter the staging but should be specifically recorded as it may affect treatment decisions in the future.

Lesions of greater size should be staged as IB.

As a rule, it is impossible to estimate clinically whether a cancer of the cervix has extended to the corpus. Extension to the corpus should therefore be disregarded.

Treatment

1. Dysplasia, when moderate (CIN2) or marked (CIN3) is usually adequately treated by conization or multiple biopsies plus endocervical curettage. This is followed by Pap smears. Cautery and cryotherapy should only be used after a firm histological diagnosis has been established.

2. Carcinoma in situ should be treated only after accurate clinical and histological findings are determined.

a. Colposcopically directed biopsies, with an endocervical curettage, should be performed.

b. In most cases, with the exclusion of invasive cancer by combined colposcopic-histological study, the management of CIN becomes an academic matter. Methods employed are electrocoagulation, cryosurgery, and laser therapy.

c. In young women desiring children, cone biopsy should be avoided if at all possible.

d. Older women should be given the option of hysterectomy after an invasive lesion has been ruled out. This is a controversial decision; only the physician taking main responsibility for the patient's care should make the judgment.

e. Cautery, cryotherapy, and laser ablation are recommended only if the lesion is visible, does not go beyond the squamocolumnar junction, and does not cover too large an area.

3. Stage IA1 can be treated as an in situ lesion in most instances. However, IA2 requires treatment that is individualized according to the age of the patient, the extent of the disease, and the histological features of the lesion.

4. Stage IB is usually treated by radical hysterectomy and bilateral pelvic lymphadenectomy. Radiation therapy is chosen for patients in whom surgical therapy is not to be performed because of age or general health.

5. Stage IIA receives the same treatment as Stage IB.

6. Stages IIB, IIIA, and IIIB are treated by primary radiation. External therapy is started first, followed by intracavitary radiation.

7. Stage IV is generally treated by primary radiation therapy. This therapy may require preradiation diversion of the fecal and/or urinary stream. Primary pelvic exenteration may be selected for those patients with central disease that extends into the bladder (usually with a vesicovaginal fistula) in whom it is possible to completely encompass the disease.

Cancer of the Cervix Complicating Pregnancy

1. Approximately 1 pregnancy in 3,000 is complicated by cervical cancer.

2. The disease is not different from that found in the nonpregnant state.

3. A comparison of cure rates in comparable stages of disease between pregnant and nonpregnant patients shows no difference.

4. Prognosis depends on the extent of the disease.

5. The primary treatment usually chosen is surgery. Radiation therapy gives equally good results, but produces more late side effects in these relatively young patients.

PREOPERATIVE CHEMOTHERAPY OR RADIOTHERAPY

1. These modalities are recommended for all large, fungating tumors. The purpose is to reduce the bulk of the tumor and thus facilitate surgical excision.

2. Recently, in selected patients, three courses of chemotherapy (cisplatin, vinblastine, and bleomycin) have been used preoperatively instead of the more traditional radiation therapy.

3. The latter approach is designed to complement any subsequent irradiation, should this be indicated postoperatively.

POSTOPERATIVE ADJUVANT THERAPY (CHEMOTHERAPY AND RADIOTHERAPY)

Indications

1. All nodal metastases, even if microscopic

2. Incomplete excision as determined by histological examination of the operation specimen

3. Incomplete lymphadenectomy

4. Aggressive histological types—i.e., adenosquamous, anaplastic, or glassy cell tumors (not an absolute indication)

Surgical Exclusions

1. Patient's age greater than 65. (This is not an absolute contraindication.)

2. Intercurrent illness—e.g., severe cardiac disease, severely impaired renal function

3. Obesity (node dissection is less effective and surgical morbidity is higher)

4. These patients are treated by radiotherapy and chemotherapy.

Radiotherapy as Primary Therapy

1. External Radiation

a. The treatment volume includes the central disease and its direct extensions in continuity with the internal, external, and common lymphatics.

b. The average dose is about 5,000 rad in 5 weeks.

2. Intracavitary Irradiation

a. This is required to boost the dose to the central disease area and is used as soon as is practical immediately before, during, or after the course of external therapy.

b. The total rectal dose should not exceed 6,000 rad.

Follow-up

1. Follow-up is best undertaken by the same observer who was responsible for the initial management.

2. Since 75 per cent of deaths of patients who have had primary radiotherapy occur during the first two years after treatment, special attention must be given to this time interval.

3. Careful documentation of the following is necessary: pain, discharge, cough, body weight, leg edema, supraclavicular nodes, abdomen including girth and liver, vaginal examination, rectal examination, and rectovaginal examination

4. Carcinoembryonic antigen (CEA) is a valuable marker; a rising level is frequently an early sign of recurrent disease, particularly in adenocarcinoma.

5. Blood chemistries and IVP where indicated

6. Ultrasound, CT scan, MRI, and/or chest x-rays as indicated

7. Estrogen replacement therapy if indicated

8. The patient should be followed every 3 to 4 months for the first 18 months, then at 6-month intervals for the next 3 years, and annually thereafter.

Recurrent Cervical Cancer

Only patients with central cancer should be considered for pelvic exenteration. If metastases are found in nonpelvic locations either preoperatively or at laparotomy, or in the para-aortic area on frozen section, the operation should be carried out only if the case is unusual.

Persistent or Recurrent Disease

1. Chemotherapy is the treatment of choice.

2. Exenteration has a place in cases where the disease is central. Total pelvic exenteration should be used in previously irradiated patients, because of complications associated with subtotal exenteration.

3. Radiotherapy should be used on any patient not previously irradiated.

4. Urinary-stream diversion is rarely indicated for palliation. It should be reserved for cases where there is some prospect of cure.

5. Palliation includes surgery for fistulas and bowel obstruction.

44 Cancer of the Upper Genital Tract

Hugh R. K. Barber

Carcinoma of the upper genital tract includes cancers of the endometrium, ovary, and breast. These cancers share similar epidemiologic findings and hormonal relationships.

CANCER OF THE ENDOMETRIUM

Basic Principles

1. Cancer of the endometrium is a disease of suburbia.

2. About 2.2 per cent of newborn girls, or 1 in 45, will develop cancer of the corpus uteri sometime during their lives.

3. Malignant neoplasms of the corpus uteri generally occur in patients a decade older (of peri- and postmenopausal age) than those who develop cancer of the cervix.

a. Five per cent of cases occur in women less than 40 years of age. It has been found as early as age 17 years.

b. More than 70 per cent of the cases occur after age 50, while 20 per cent occur between the ages of 40 and 50.

c. There is an increasing number of patients in the older age group presenting with adenosquamous cancer of the endometrium.

4. Early diagnosis is the key to successful treatment in cancer of the endometrium.

5. The physical habitus of these patients is well known to the gynecologist.

6. They are patients with an abnormal pituitary function and a long history of hyperestrogenism, which may have many causes.

7. Reports indicate that there is a higher incidence of cancer of the endometrium occurring at an early age among patients with continuous unopposed estrogen stimulation of the endometrium, i.e., patients with the Stein-Leventhal syndrome or a long history of anovulation and/or amenorrhea.

8. It appears that the postmenopausal prehormone is androstenedione and that the notable postmenopausal estrogen is estrone.

a. Conversion of androstenedione to estrone is increased with age, massive obesity, and liver disease.

b. Increased production of the precursor androstenedione for conversion to estrone is noted in chronic anovulators, in polycystic ovarian disease, in certain functioning ovarian tumors, and in ovarian cortical stromal hyperplasia.

c. The significance of exogenous estrogens in the etiology of endometrial carcinoma is generally suspected but not completely understood.

9. In the endometrium, negative cytology does not suggest as reliably as it does in the cervix that the development of cancer is highly unlikely, because on cytologic evaluation the preinvasive lesions are not diagnosed with the same accuracy as they are in cancer of the cervix. Adenomatous hyperplasia should be considered a precursor lesion.

10. The first and most significant symptom is abnormal vaginal bleeding. In any age group it should be considered a sign of a potentially serious problem, and a fractional curettage should be carried out.

11. Pelvic examination may reveal a normal- or nearly normal-sized uterus for the stated age and parity. In most instances, there is some enlargement of the uterus, which may be of softer than normal consistency. The coexistence of fibroids may distort the estimation of uterine size. In more advanced cases, the uterus is definitely enlarged and softer than normal. Tumor may fungate out of the cervix and fragments may become detached during bimanual examination.

12. The diagnosis of endometrial carcinoma should not be difficult. Although the diagnosis may be made in the office by endometrial biopsy, a careful pelvic examination under anesthesia and a careful fractional curettage are mandatory for accurate clinical staging.

13. Pyometra may be the first manifestation of endometrial cancer because of blockage low in the endometrial cavity. In patients in the peri- and postmenopausal age groups who present with such a condition, an underlying carcinoma must be ruled out.

14. Adenocarcinoma of the endometrium is either localized or diffuse over the surface of the endometrium. Cancer arising in the endometrium tends to remain within the uterus for a long period of time.

a. As it grows it invades the myometrium and spreads toward the isthmus and the endocervix.

b. From the myometrium it spreads through the serosa to the peritoneal cavity, and from the endocervix it spreads to the pelvic nodes.

c. The lymphatics increase in amount as the serosa of the uterus is approached; deep penetration of the myometrium is associated with an increased incidence of positive node involvement.

d. Since the myometrium in the postmenopausal woman is much thinner than in the premenopausal patient, a little penetration of the myometrium may bring the cancer into contact with the lymphatics and account for the greater potency of endometrial cancer among postmenopausal women.

e. The high-risk group for extrauterine spread are those with involvement of the lower uterus or cervix, histologic Grade III lesions, deep myometrial invasion, or all three.

Endometrial Metaplasias

1. The differential diagnosis of endometrial carcinoma includes not only hyperplasia, but also a group of epithelial metaplasias. These have been classified as follows: morules, squamous metaplasia, papillary metaplasia, ciliated-cell or tubal metaplasia, eosinophilic metaplasia, mucinous metaplasia, hobnail metaplasia, and clear-cell metaplasia.

2. The significance of these metaplasias is that they may be mistaken for carcinomas. They are a benign finding.

3. Stromal invasion is the main criterion for distinguishing a typical hyperplasia from well-differentiated carcinoma.

Assessment of Myometrial Invasion

1. The most difficult determination to be made is the distinction between *penetration* (noninvasion) by cancer into pre-existing tongues of endometrium and the superficial myometrium or into islands of adenomyosis (which represents a deeper manifestation of the same phenomenon) and *true infiltration* of the myometrial stroma.

2. In penetration there are nests of tumors within the myometrium, and they are rounded, of fairly uniform size, and show residual benign endometrial stroma and/or glands at their periphery.

Papillary Serous Carcinoma

1. Although the existence of a papillary form of adenocarcinoma of the endometrium, often containing concentric microcalcification or some psammoma bodies, has been recognized for years, the clinical and pathological features of these tumors have only recently been fully characterized.

2. Histologically, these tumors are characterized by the presence of papillary structures with broad fibrovascular connective tissue cores. Foci of necrosis are frequently seen.

3. Since the tumors tend to be moderately to poorly differentiated, solid sheets of large, undifferentiated cells are almost invariably present.

4. Psammoma bodies are detectable in approximately 30 per cent of these tumors.

5. A very characteristic feature of this lesion is its tendency to infiltrate the myometrium within lymphatic or blood vascular channels.

a. This is often an unexpected microscopic finding, occurring in small, atrophic-appearing uteri.

6. Grossly normal-appearing uterine adnexa also frequently show extensive tumor emboli.

7. The prognosis is extremely poor for patients with a papillary serous carcinoma of the endometrium.

Clinical Staging of Carcinoma of the Corpus Uteri

Stage O	Carcinoma is situ. Histologic findings are suspect for malignancy; cases of Stage O should not be included in any therapeutic statistics.
Stage I	The carcinoma is confined to the corpus.
Stage IA	The length of the uterine cavity is 8 cm. or less.
Stage IB	The length of the uterine cavity is more than 8 cm.

Stage I Subgroups. It is desirable that the Stage I cases be subgrouped with regard to the histologic type of the adenocarcinoma, as follows:

G1	Highly differentiated adenomatous carcinoma
G2	Differentiated adenomatous carcinoma with partly solid areas
G3	Predominantly solid or entirely undifferentiated carcinoma
Stage II	The carcinoma has involved the corpus and the cervix but has not extended outside the uterus.
Stage III	The carcinoma has extended outside the uterus but not outside the true pelvis.
Stage IV	The carcinoma has extended outside the true pelvis or has obviously involved the mucosa of the bladder or rectum. A bullous edema as such does not permit a case to be assigned to Stage IV.
Stage IVA	Spread of the growth to adjacent organs
Stage IVB	Spread to distant organs

Management

1. *Stage O*

a. Carcinoma in situ. The management should be tailored to fit the needs of the patient, her age, and desire for future childbearing. In selected young patients with minimal disease, an alternative to hysterectomy may repeat curettage after 3 to 4 months or a course of progestational agents followed by repeat curettage.

2. *Stage IA, G1*

a. Total hysterectomy and bilateral salpingo-oophorectomy followed by postoperative vaginal radiation.

b. In patients in whom the histologic grade is G2 or G3, external pelvic radiation should be given preoperatively, followed by total hysterectomy, bilateral salpingo-oophorectomy, and vaginal radiation postoperatively.

c. If preoperative external radiation has not been given and the surgical specimen reveals a histologic grade of G2 or G3 (instead of G1) or moderate or extensive myometrial invasion (one-third or more myometrial penetration), postoperative external radiation should be given.

3. *Stage IB*

a. The same management as for Stage IA.

4. *Stage II*

a. Preoperative external pelvic radiation is followed in 6 weeks by a modified radical hysterectomy and pelvic node dissection, if possible. Otherwise, a total hysterectomy is chosen.

5. *Stage III*

a. If the lesion involves only the adnexal structures, preoperative x-ray therapy is followed by total hysterectomy and bilateral salpingo-oophorectomy. Postoperatively, vaginal radiation is given. An alternate plan is modified radical hysterectomy.

6. *Stage IV*

a. Primary therapy is external and intracavitary radiation therapy. The patient is evaluated to ascertain whether supplementary progestational agents should be used. If the cancer is limited to the pelvis but involves bladder, rectum, or both, the patient is evaluated for pelvic exenteration. External therapy may be employed before pelvic exenteration is selected. In certain instances, despite the presence of widespread disease, it is necessary to remove the uterus to control hemorrhage.

Alternate Plan of Therapy

1. Recently the protocol has been changed to include hysterectomy as the first step in the management of all stages of cancer of the endometrium.

2. All patients will receive vaginal radiation postoperatively, and the external therapy will be tailored to fit the needs of the patient.

3. This plan will allow a comparison between the value of preoperative and postoperative x-ray treatment.

Procedures for Different Types of Cancer

1. Distant Metastases

a. Primary progestational therapy is indicated. Depo-Provera 400 mg. intramuscularly a day for 7 days and then every 7 to 10 days, or Delalutin 250 mg. following the same schedule. In addition, Megace is given in doses up to 200 mg. by mouth a day.

b. Localized disease without response to progestational therapy is treated with x-ray therapy.

c. In the presence of widespread disease and no response to the treatment suggested above, chemotherapy is indicated.

d. Chemotherapy has not been particularly effective to date. However, combination therapy employing Cytoxan, Adriamycin, and platinum has shown some promise.

e. Progesterone therapy has been used for two decades. The conclusions about its efficacy are as follows:

(1) Response rate of patients with advanced and recurrent disease is 32 per cent.

(2) Response rate in well-differentiated tumors is 30 to 50 per cent as opposed to that in poorly differentiated tumors (0 to 15 per cent).

(3) Longest remission and best response are seen in patients in whom treatment is continued for at least 6 months.

(4) Optimum dose is not yet defined.

(5) Progesterone receptors are present in greatest numbers in well-differentiated tumors. This may be the explanation for diminished response in poorly differentiated cancer to progesterone therapy.

(6) The value of anti-estrogen, tamoxifen, is as yet unproven. Side effects are minimal, and tumor responses are seen in about 30 per cent of unselected cases.

2. Adenosquamous Cancer

a. The increasing frequency with which mixed adenosquamous cancer is detected in the endometrium adds a new dimension to treatment.

b. This cancer has both malignant-appearing glandular and squamous components.

c. Venous involvement is observed in one-half of the cases, and blood vascular and transtubal routes may be involved in the dissemination of the neoplasm.

d. The mean age at detection is 65.5 years.

e. The duration of symptoms tends to be short, and abdominal or distal spread is frequently observed.

f. These tumors respond poorly to ionizing radiation. The 5-year survival rate is 19 to 20 per cent.

g. The treatment is total hysterectomy and bilateral salpingo-oophorectomy.

3. Sarcoma of the Uterus

a. This is a very rare disease.

b. The main varieties are: leiomyosarcomas—true malignant neoplasms of smooth muscle cells (the most common form); endometrial stromal sarcomas, which are composed of rounded and fusiform cells arising from mesoblastic elements of the endometrium itself; mixed mesodermal tumors of the uterus, the counterpart in the adult of sarcoma botryoides of infants and children; and very rare forms such as fibrosarcomas and carcinocarcinomas (mixtures of leiomyosarcoma and endometrial carcinoma).

(1) One form of leiomyosarcoma arises within the myometrium and has a poor prognosis.

(2) The other form arises within a fibroid and has a better prognosis.

c. The diagnosis of malignancy is established by counting the number of mitoses per 10 high power fields (HPF). Tumors with fewer than 5 mitoses per 10 HPF are benign, those with higher mitotic counts are malignant. The prognosis for leiomyosarcomas with more than 10 mitoses per 10 HPF is poor, and metastases are frequent.

d. There are no characteristic symptoms of sarcoma of the uterus. Early bleeding does not occur unless polypoid lesions project into the endometrial cavity.

e. On physical examination the uterus is enlarged, suggestive of fibroids.

f. Rapidly enlarging masses in the uterus, especially of soft consistency, suggest sarcoma, but histologic study must be carried out to confirm this.

g. Treatment

(1) Total hysterectomy and bilateral salpingo-oophorectomy is the keystone of therapy.

(2) Combination chemotherapy (Cytoxan, actinomycin D, vincristine, and Adriamycin) has shown promise in controlling sarcoma. Platinum is now given in combination with other anticancer drugs and is proving effective in the treatment of sarcoma of the uterus. Among those patients with a cellular stroma, the addition of a progestational agent has proved of some benefit.

(3) Since it has been shown that sarcomas of the uterus have an increase in the estrogen receptors, tamoxifen has been recommended as a modality of therapy.

(4) There is controversy over whether progestational agents and tamoxifen should be given together, and it is probably better to use them in sequence rather than in combination.

CANCER OF THE FALLOPIAN TUBE

Basic Principles

1. This is the rarest carcinoma of the female genital tract.

2. The average age at diagnosis is 49 years.

3. The commonest form arises from the mucosa and forms papillary or medullary anaplastic lesions.

4. The metastatic pattern is similar to that for ovarian cancer.

5. The fallopian tube is commonly involved secondarily in advanced cases of endometrial and ovarian cancer.

6. There are usually no or only slight symptoms until the disease is advanced.

7. Only half the cases show the classic triad of bleeding, abdominal pain, and a pelvic or abdominal mass. Some cases present with a profuse, intermittent, watery discharge, the so-called hydrops tubal profluens.

8. A positive Pap smear in the presence of a negative curettage should alert the clinician to the diagnosis.

9. On pelvic examination an adnexal mass is present, with the corpus and cervix seemingly normal, but the exact diagnosis is rarely made preoperatively.

10. Staging for cancer of the fallopian tube is similar to that for ovarian cancer.

Treatment

1. On opening the abdomen, fluid or peritoneal washings should be sent for cytologic examination.

2. The treatment is similar to that for ovarian cancer.

OVARIAN CANCER

Basic Principles

1. Deaths from ovarian cancer have slowly increased over the last 40 years, and the rate is now 2.5 times that of 1930.

2. 1.4 per cent of newborn girls, or 1 of every 70, will develop cancer of the ovary at some time during their lives.

3. In 1989 the estimated number of new cases is 20,000. The age-specific incidence rates for ovarian cancer show a steady rise up to age 80, at which point they drop off slightly.

4. Cancer of the ovary is the leading cause of death from gynecological cancer. There are about 12,000 deaths a year from ovarian cancer.

a. It accounts for 25 per cent of gynecological cancers but for 50 per cent of all deaths from cancers of the female genital tract.

b. Ten out of every 1,000 women in the United States over age 40 years will develop ovarian cancer, and only one or two will be cured.

5. Early diagnosis is a matter of chance at present rather than of scientific method.

6. Common epithelial ovarian cancers spread along the surface of the peritoneum and organs and can involve structures in the upper abdomen.

7. Although it is stated that there are no early symptoms of ovarian cancer, a careful history will reveal vague abdominal symptoms and mild digestive disturbances which may be present for months before the diagnosis is made. In women over age 40 with a history of ovarian dysfunction and bouts of dyspepsia, indigestion, and abdominal pain, in whom no definite diagnosis can be made, it is important to rule out ovarian cancer.

8. What is interpreted as a normal-sized ovary in the premenopausal woman represents an ovarian tumor in the postmenopausal woman.

9. It is advisable to do a laparotomy when any pelvic mass has appeared after the menopause; when an adnexal mass in a woman of any age progressively enlarges beyond 5 cm. while under observation; for an adnexal mass 10 cm. or more in size; for a normal-sized ovary in the postmenopausal woman; and for masses which cannot be definitely diagnosed as either a fibroid or carcinoma.

10. Common epithelial ovarian cancers make up about 80 per cent of all ovarian cancers. Only 8 per cent occur in women under age 35, and most occur in women over age 40 years.

Classification (Histopathology)

1. Common primary epithelial tumors of the ovary (benign, borderline, or malignant)
Serous
Mucinous
Endometrioid

Clear cell tumor (mesonephroid)
Undifferentiated carcinoma
Mixed epithelial tumor
Brenner Tumor
No histology (unclassifiable)

2. Germ cell tumors
   Dysgerminoma
   Extraembryonal teratomas
   Adult teratomas
   Carcinoids
   Struma ovarii
3. Gonadoblastoma
4. Gonadal stromal (sex cord-mesenchymal) tumors
   Female type
     Granulosa cell tumor
   Male type
     Sertoli-Leydig
5. Tumors not specific for the ovary
     Lymphoma
6. Metastatic tumors
   Krukenberg
   Adenocarcinoma of large-intestinal origin
   Miscellaneous

Definitions of the Stages in Primary Carcinoma of the Ovary (Correlations of the FIGO, UICC, and AJCC nomenclatures)

These categories are based on findings at clinical examination and/or surgical exploration. The histologic characteristics are to be considered in the staging, as are results of cytologic testing as far as effusions are concerned. It is desirable that a biopsy be performed on suspicious areas outside the pelvis.

Stage I	Growth limited to the ovaries
Stage IA	Growth limited to one ovary; no ascites. No tumor on the external surface; capsule intact
Stage IB	Growth limited to both ovaries; no ascites. No tumor on the external surfaces; capsules intact
*Stage IC**	Tumor either Stage IA or IB but with tumor on the surface of one or both ovaries; or with capsule ruptured; or with ascites present containing malignant cells; or with positive peritoneal washings
Stage II	Growth involving one or both ovaries with pelvic extension
Stage IIA	Extension and/or metastases to the uterus and/or tubes
Stage IIB	Extension to other pelvic tissues
*Stage IIC**	Tumor either Stage IIA or IIB but with tumor on the surface of one or both ovaries; or with capsule(s) ruptured; or with ascites present containing malignant cells; or with positive peritoneal washings
Stage III	Tumor involving one or both ovaries with peritoneal implants outside the pelvis and/or positive retroperitoneal or inguinal nodes. Superficial liver metastasis equals Stage III. Tumor is limited to the true pelvis but with histologically verified malignant extension to small bowel or omentum.
Stage IIIA	Tumor grossly limited to the true pelvis with negative nodes but with histologically confirmed microscopic seeding of abdominal peritoneal surfaces

*In order to evaluate the impact of the different criteria for allotting cases to Stage IC or IIC on prognosis, it would be of value to know if rupture of the capsule was (1) spontaneous or (2) caused by the surgeon, and if the source of malignant cells detected was (1) peritoneal washings or (2) ascites.

Stage IIIB	Tumor of one or both ovaries with histologically confirmed implants of abdominal peritoneal surfaces, none exceeding 2 cm. in diameter. Nodes negative
Stage IIIC	Abdominal implants >2 cm. in diameter and/or positive retroperitoneal or inguinal nodes
Stage IV	Growth involving one or both ovaries with distant metastasis. If pleural effusion is present there must be positive cytologic test results to allot a case to Stage IV. Parenchymal liver metastasis equals Stage IV.

Treatment of the Common Epithelial Ovarian Cancer

1. Stage I

a. Aspiration of fluid for cytology

b. Total hysterectomy and bilateral salpingo-oophorectomy

c. Omentectomy

d. Appendectomy } optional
e. Instillation of P^{32} } optional
f. Chemotherapy } optional

2. Stages II, III, and IV

a. The same as for Stage I, if possible

b. Chemotherapy in Stages III and IV

Conservative Surgery (Unilateral Oophorectomy)

1. Conservative surgery may be considered if the following criteria are met in women under age 30:

a. Desire for childbearing

b. Stage IA negative pelvic and abdominal cytology

c. Low histologic grade

d. Full staging procedures have been carried out

e. Opposite ovary is clear histologically (wedge biopsy one-half of the surface epithelium)

2. In most instances the patient is best treated with total hysterectomy and bilateral salpingo-oophorectomy, omentectomy, and appendectomy.

Treatment of Nonepithelial Tumors

1. Germ Cell Tumors

a. *Dysgerminoma*

(1) In the presence of spread beyond the ovary, total hysterectomy, bilateral salpingo-oophorectomy, omentectomy, and biopsy of the para-aortic nodes. Postoperative x-ray therapy and combination chemotherapy should be given as indicated.

(2) In a young woman with a unilateral, encapsulated dysgerminoma, acceptable treatment includes a unilateral salpingo-oophorectomy, biopsy of the other ovary and of the para-aortic nodes, as well as cytologic examination of peritoneal fluid.

b. *Endodermal Sinus, Embryonal Teratoma, and Choriocarcinoma*

(1) Management is generally total hysterectomy and bilateral salpingo-oophorectomy.

(2) No strong argument can be made for the more radical procedure over a conservative management.

(3) The tumors are not radiosensitive.

(4) Combination chemotherapy has shown some encouraging results.

2. Gonadal Stromal Tumors—Granulosa Cell Tumors

a. In women over 35 years, treatment includes total hysterectomy and bilateral salpingo-oophorectomy.

b. In children and adolescents, the tumor is usually unilateral and encapsulated, and therefore unilateral salpingo-oophorectomy is sufficient treatment.

3. Gonadoblastoma

a. This is a rare tumor composed of germ-cell and gonadal stromal elements.

b. Most occur in patients who are intersexual with phenotype female habitus, who are amenorrheic and possibly virilized.

c. The malignancy rate is near zero, but the gonads are useless and both ovaries should be removed. The gonads should be removed in the presence of an XY chromosome pattern, even though the gonads are not enlarged.

Advanced Cancer of the Ovaries with Ascites

1. Ascites from carcinoma of the ovaries indicates the most advanced stage. Only palliative treatment is possible. Occasionally a patient may live for years.

2. Ascites of any appreciable degree produces mechanical symptoms, which are promptly relieved by paracentesis; this is indicated whenever symptoms of fullness, dyspepsia, and respiratory impairment are present. If surgical intervention is contemplated, this should be done expeditiously and is preferable to paracentesis.

3. If roentgenograms indicate accumulation of fluid in either or both chest cavities, thoracentesis is indicated.

4. All aspirations of abdominal or chest fluids should be sent to the laboratory for cytologic diagnosis.

5. After maximal drainage of ascites, abdominal and pelvic examinations are performed for evaluation of masses. Often a large ballotable abdominal mass is identified as a possible "omental cake." Under propitious circumstances, laparotomy is then indicated.

6. If large, fixed masses are palpated and surgery is not selected, P^{32} and/or radiation therapy have little to offer these patients.

7. A single alkylating agent is the treatment of choice. If the patient responds and then relapses, she should be evaluated for combination chemotherapy.

8. When mechanical interference with intestinal tract function occurs owing to neoplastic blockage of the bowel or infiltration of the bowel wall causing carcinomatous ileus, a long tube should be given a trial.

9. If the tube fails to relieve the obstructed bowel, the question of surgical intervention to relieve obstruction arises. Such procedures may entail bowel resection or by-pass procedures. Unfortunately, it is generally found that little can be done.

10. In unusual circumstances, when all factors indicate ovarian carcinomatosis and laparotomy is performed for palliation, it may be discovered that the cancer is indeed localized and totally excisable with bowel resection. A few patients operated on under such circumstances have survived for years free from evidence of active cancer.

CA-125

1. The work reported by Bast and colleagues on the use of monoclonal antibodies to monitor the course of epithelial ovarian cancer may someday be perfected so that it can be used for early diagnosis of ovarian cancer.

a. The murine monoclonal antibody OC-125 reacts with an antigen, CA-125, common in most nonmucinous epithelial ovarian cancers.

b. An assay has been developed to detect CA-125 in the serum. Progression or regression of disease correlates well with a rise or fall in the level of CA-125.

Other Markers

1. Alpha-fetoprotein (AFP) correlates very well with endodermal sinus tumors and is useful in monitoring the progress of the disease.

2. Human chorionic gonadotropin is found in the extraembryonal tumor choriocarcinoma.

Immunotherapy

1. *Immunization* implies a means of protection from disease rather than an active form of treatment.

2. Up until the present, all forms of immunotherapy have been nonspecific and unpredictable in their action.

3. With new technology and the introduction of monoclonal antibodies, however, greater specificity has been introduced.

In Vitro Testing of Ovarian Cancer

1. Chemosensitivity testing is done to improve therapy by means of an individual "selective" cytotoxic chemotherapy: a bioassay technique which facilitates drug selection.

a. This may be described as a quantitation of differential sensitivity of human tumor stem cells to anti-cancer drugs. In using this technique, the evaluator should expect no more than is achievable with studies of sensitivity of bacteria and antibiotics.

b. The current definition of sensitivity is an operational one. It has been shown, however, that there is a fairly high correlation between in vivo and in vitro sensitivity response.

Flow Cytometry

1. Flow cytometry has the potential to make a significant contribution to monitoring the response to tumor chemotherapy. By plotting the frequency of fluorescence intensity, the relative DNA content of cells can be displayed.

2. The relative number of cells in each phase of the cell cycle can be determined. DNA analysis can help to determine the best time to administer chemotherapy.

3. By staining bone marrow cells with a DNA stain, the percentage of abnormal cells in the S phase can be monitored.

4. A schedule can be determined to administer an S-phase–specific drug, maximizing the destruction of only abnormal S-phase cells.

Radiation Therapy

1. External radiation therapy has been phased out as a modality of therapy for the management of common epithelial ovarian cancer.

2. A prospective, randomized trial is under way at the Princess Margaret Hospital in Toronto.

a. They are giving the moving strip technique to all poorly differentiated Stage I tumors, along with tumors of Stages II and III with no gross residual or only a small amount of residual pelvic tumor. More extensive disease receives chemotherapy as the initial treatment.

3. There is a place for radiation therapy in the management of germ cell and gonadal stromal tumors.

Chemotherapy

1. Currently, triple chemotherapy is being used to treat common epithelial ovarian cancers. The drugs most commonly chosen are Cyclophosphamide, Adriamycin, and cisplatin. Cisplatin is probably the keystone of management by chemotherapy for patients with common epithelial ovarian cancer.

2. Germ-cell and gonadal stromal tumors being treated by chemotherapy require a combination chemotherapeutic regime.

a. In the past, vinblastine, actinomycin D, and Cytoxan were given for the treatment of these tumors. Later, Adriamycin was added to the regime. Currently, cisplatin has been used in the management of these tumors along with a combination of other chemotherapeutic agents.

Second-Look Operation

1. *Second-look laparotomy* is defined as an operation that is carried out after a stated interval following the initial and/or adjunctive therapy in the patient without evidence, clinical or otherwise, of disease.

2. Two groups of patients fall into this category.

a. The first includes patients with known disease that could not be adequately removed at surgery but that regressed after additional therapy; there is no longer any evidence of disease, either clinically or by laboratory testing or technological examination.

b. The second includes patients in whom all disease was removed at the time of the original operation, who received prophylactic chemotherapy for a stated interval of time, and who had no identifiable disease on examination.

3. The procedure for patients who have progression of disease during chemotherapy or whose disease is identified by any method at the time of scheduled surgery is called a *second operation* or an *exploratory laparotomy* rather than a second-look operation.

4. There are no hard data that prove that the second-look operation adds to the long-term survival of these cancer patients.

5. It is evident that, in some instances, disease is identified that can be removed, and, with additional therapy, longevity is increased.

45 Breast Diseases

Hugh R. K. Barber

CANCER OF THE BREAST

BASIC PRINCIPLES

1. One out of every ten women develops cancer of the breast (an incidence of 10 per cent).

2. There were approximately 142,000 new cases projected in the United States for 1989, and 43,000 deaths.

3. Among women in the United States who are 25 to 74 years of age, breast cancer is the leading cause of cancer mortality.

4. It is the leading cause of death from all causes in women 39 to 44 years of age. Every 15 minutes one woman dies of this disease.

5. Carcinoma is more common on the left than right side, in the outer than inner quadrant, in women without children, and in women who have not suckled.

6. The disease attacks both breasts successively in 4 per cent or more of cases.

7. It is five times more likely to occur in women who have familial histories of breast cancer.

8. The typical presentation is that of a lump in the breast which in the early stages is isolated, movable, and painless.

9. As the cancer advances, fixation, retraction of skin or nipple, ulceration, pain, erythema, and nodal axillary masses may appear.

10. Early detection depends on self-examination by women at monthly intervals and semiannual examination by physicians. The breast self-examination (BSE) should be performed monthly, one week after the menses.

11. To make an early diagnosis the physician must have a high degree of suspicion regarding all breast lesions, as well as a basic knowledge of the following factors:

a. The common types of breast lesion and their relative frequency

b. The age-periods at which these lesions usually occur

c. The characteristic symptom complexes

d. The various risk factors that increase a patient's chance of developing breast cancer

12. The most common types of breast lesion, and their frequencies, are: fibrocystic disease, 34 per cent; cancer, 27 per cent; fibroadenoma, 19 per cent; intraductal papilloma, 6 per cent; duct ectasia, 4 per cent; other types of lesion account for 11 per cent of cases.

13. *Patients at high risk* include: those over 40 years of age, those with family histories of breast cancer, nulliparous women or those with first parity after 34, women with previous histories of cancer in one breast, those with precancerous mastopathy-type fibrocystic disease, those with adverse hormonal milieu, those with lowered immunological competence, those with excessive exposure of the breast to ionizing radiation, those exposed to carcinogens, those with endometrial or ovarian cancer, those with high dietary intake of fat, those with chronic psychological stress, those living in the western hemisphere, and Caucasian women in the upper socioeconomic group.

14. *Biopsy* is mandatory in patients with:

a. True three-dimensional dominant lumps, even if diagnostic aids are negative—excluding cysts that can be safely aspirated under controlled conditions

b. Suspicious lesions found by diagnostic aids, even if there are no clinical findings

c. Serous, serosanguineous, bloody, or watery nipple discharge, even if there are no palpable masses and cytology and breast x-ray studies are negative

d. Other adverse signs—e.g., eczema of the nipple, unexplained retraction or elevation, suspicious axillary adenopathy, redness of the skin of the breast, underlying induration without signs of infection, unexplained skin dimpling, or a persistent dominant area of unexplained thickening of the breast

15. *X-ray studies* of the breast on a yearly basis are advised for all patients over 50 years of age, for those with symptomatic breasts that are difficult to diagnose clinically, for those with abnormal thermogram, for those with evident risk factors, preoperatively when a breast lump is present (except when the patient is under 25 years of age), after cyst aspiration, for multinodular breasts, for large pendulous breasts, for areas of thickening without a true mass, and for breasts with dense scar formation due to previous biopsies or trauma. The observed median survival time for cancer of the breast is 6 years for all ages; over 10 years for patients under 45 years of age; 9.5 years between 45 and 54; 6.5 years between 55 and 64; 5.2 years between 65 and 74; and 3 years at 75 and over.

16. A population that achieved a 5-year reduction in average age at first delivery might achieve a 30-per-cent decrease in the incidence of breast cancer.

17. Approximately 15 per cent of patients who survive the treatment of initial breast cancer for 3 or more years develop a cancer in the opposite breast.

18. Contralateral occult cancers are seen in about 25 per cent of patients with breast cancer recently proved on one side.

19. Thirty-five per cent of women with untreated breast cancer are known to survive for 5 years. Sixty-eight per cent of those who present with previously untreated localized disease and remain untreated survive for at least that long.

20. Unfortunately, some cancers still elude detection.

21. Some 10 per cent of cancers become apparent within a year of a negative examination.

22. Reliance for detection of these cancers must be placed on self-examination of the breast.

EARLY OR SMALL CANCER OF THE BREAST

1. Although primary breast tumors take time to grow, relating regional and subsequent systemic spread to time is not only misleading but inaccurate.

2. Breast cancer represents a heterogenous group of neoplasms; recent evidence suggests biological heterogeneity of cells making up individual breast cancers.

3. Despite this lack of uniformity, there are certain principles that apply to the growth of cancers, including those of the breast, and that provoke skepticism about clinical designations of "early" and "late":

a. Most breast cancers cannot be palpated until they measure at least 1 cm. A tumor of that size contains about 1 billion cells.

b. Genetic studies indicate that such a size requires thirty population doublings. Since doubling time may encompass 30 to 200 days, or more, it is apparent that a

Table 45-1. Clinical-diagnostic staging system of the American Joint Committee for Cancer Staging and End-Results Reporting: TNM classification

Primary tumor (T)

TX	Tumor cannot be assessed
TO	No evidence of primary tumor
TIS	Paget disease of the nipple with no demonstrable tumor NOTE: Paget disease with a demonstrable tumor is classified according to the size of the tumor.
T1*	Tumor 2 cm or less in greatest dimension
T1a	No fixation to pectoral fascia or muscle
T1b	Fixation to pectoral fascia, muscle, or both
T2*	Tumor more than 2 cm but not more than 5 cm in greatest dimension
T2a	No fixation to pectoral fascia or muscle
T2b	Fixation to pectoral fascia, muscle, or both
T3*	Tumor more than 5 cm in greatest dimension
T3a	No fixation to pectoral fascia or muscle
T3b	Fixation to pectoral fascia, muscle, or both
T4	Tumor of any size with direct extension to chest wall or skin NOTE: Chest wall includes ribs, intercostal muscles, and serratus anterior muscle but not pectoral muscle.
T4a	Fixation to chest wall
T4b	Edema (including peau d'orange), ulceration of the skin of the breast, or satellite skin nodules confined to the same breast
T4c	Both of above
T4d	Inflammatory carcinoma

Nodal involvement (N)

NX	Regional lymph nodes cannot be assessed clinically
NO	No palpable homolateral axillary nodes
N1	Movable homolateral axillary nodes only
N1a	Nodes not considered to contain growth
N1b	Nodes considered to contain growth
N2	Homolateral axillary nodes considered to contain growth and fixed to one another or to other structures
N3	Homolateral supraclavicular or infraclavicular nodes considered to contain growth, or edema of arm NOTE: Edema of the arm may be caused by lymphatic obstruction and lymph nodes may not then be palpable.

Distant metastases (M)

MX	Not assessed
MO	No (known) distant metastasis
MI	Distant metastasis present

*Dimpling of the skin, nipple retraction, or any other skin changes except those in T4 may occur in T1, T2, or T3 without affecting the classification.

tumor regarded as clinically early is, in truth, biologically late; with only ten to twenty more doublings it will cause the death of the host.

c. A small 0.5-cm. breast cancer detected by mammography, although regarded as early clinically, has already been through 27 doublings. Biologically it is a late tumor.

4. The most important consideration is when, if a tumor contains metastasizing phenotypes, metastasis begins.

5. Evidence suggests that when metastases occur, they do so within the first ten to twenty doubling times—i.e., at a stage of disease that is undetectable by current methods.

6. It has been estimated that 50 per cent of women with breast cancer measuring 1 cm. already have systemic disease.

Schematic Anatomic Staging Outline (Clinical Observations)

1. Stage I. Breast mass localized, all nodes negative.

2. Stage II. Breast mass localized, axillas positive.

3. Stage III. Breast mass locally extensive; axillas, supraclavicular, and internal mammary nodes positive.

4. Stage IV. Distant metastases.

5. The UICC and the AJCC have provided a TNM classification for cancer of the breast (see Table 45-1).

Treatment

1. Radical mastectomy, or modified radical mastectomy, and axillary node dissection is the preferred treatment. However, the procedure can be tailored to the extent of the disease and the needs of the patient.

2. Recommendations for surgery, radiation, and chemotherapy depend on the type, size, location, and extent of the tumor; the patient's age; relation to the menopause; and other pertinent factors.

DIFFERENTIAL DIAGNOSIS AND CHARACTERISTIC SYMPTOM COMPLEXES

1. Fibrocystic Disease

a. This is commonly bilateral and multiple.

b. It is characterized by dull, heavy pain, sensation of fullness, and tenderness.

c. Changes with menses are common.

d. Tenderness is common.

e. Axillary nodes should be normal.

f. There is no venous engorgement.

g. This disease occurs in women between 20 and 50 years of age.

2. Fibroadenoma

a. This lesion is very mobile, solid, firm, and well delineated.

b. It is the classic rubbery, slippery mass.

c. Fibroadenomas are multiple and bilateral in about 14 to 25 per cent of patients.

d. A fibroadenoma grows slowly and does not change with menses.

e. It occurs in women between 15 and 40 years of age.

3. Cystosarcoma Phylloides

a. This is a rare variant of fibroadenoma.

b. It may cause massive enlargement of the breast.

c. The skin is seldom involved and the axillas are usually clear.

d. Venous engorgement and skin inflammation may be present.

4. Galactocele

a. This typically occurs after lactation.

b. It is usually found beneath the areola.

c. It is occasionally tender.

d. A milky discharge is sometimes found.

5. Cyst of the Montgomery's Glands

a. This is essentially a sebaceous cyst involving periareolar glands, and presents under the areola. It is usually very small.

b. It may be fixed to the skin, but not to the chest wall.

6. Fat Necrosis

a. This usually results from trauma.

b. Skin dimpling and a firm, indistinct mass are very characteristic.

c. Fat necrosis may be very difficult to differentiate from cancer.

d. Occasionally the lesion is tender.

7. Mondor's Disease

a. This is caused by superficial thrombosis of veins overlying the breast, and may produce skin dimpling.

b. Typically, tenderness is present in early phases.

c. The lesion is self-limited and disappears with time.

8. Intraductal Papilloma

a. This presents with a serous (yellow), serosanguineous (pink), sanguineous (bloody), or watery discharge.

b. Usually no lump can be palpated.

9. Mammary Duct Ectasia (Comedomastitis)

a. This is usually subareolar.

b. It commonly manifests with nipple discharge.

c. The discharge is usually multicolored and sticky, bilateral, and from multiple ducts.

d. The patient may experience a burning, itching, or dull "pulling" pain around the nipple and areola. There may be palpable, tortuous, tubular swelling under the areola.

e. Nipple retraction, skin retraction, and a diffuse mass may be present.

f. There may be edema and axillary adenopathy.

g. This condition is very difficult to differentiate from cancer.

Treatment

Unless the diagnosis is obvious or there is regression of the lesion within a short time, a biopsy should be done and appropriate therapy selected. If any malignancy is found, tissue should be sent for estrogen receptor assay.

ALTERNATIVE TYPES OF TREATMENT

A current controversy over the surgical treatment of breast cancer has tended to divert attention from the importance of early diagnosis through breast self-examination (BSE) and periodic physical examination of the breasts by physicians aided by new diagnostic advances.

There is a definite trend toward less-radical operations for breast cancer. However, even when the breast cancer is found early, in at least 20 per cent of cases the cancer has already spread to adjacent lymph nodes. At present there is no completely satisfactory way to discern which tumors have already undergone limited extension, and which have spread beyond the confines of customary treatment. While studies continue in many disciplines on these exceedingly important questions, we must understand the natures and descriptions of the various methods of treatment of breast cancer that apply to the tumor itself.

1. Extended Radical Mastectomy or Supraradical Mastectomy. Surgical removal of the internal mammary chain of lymph nodes, the entire involved breast, the underlying chest muscles, and the lymph nodes in the axilla (armpit).

2. Halsted Radical Mastectomy. Surgical en-bloc removal of the entire involved breast, the underlying chest muscles, and the lymph nodes in the axilla.

3. Modified Radical Mastectomy. Surgical removal of the entire involved breast and many lymph nodes in the axilla. The underlying chest muscles are removed in part or are left in place after removal of the nodes in the axilla.

4. Simple Mastectomy (Total Mastectomy). Surgical removal of the entire involved breast. The underlying chest muscles and lymph nodes in the axilla are not removed.

Note: All of the above procedures remove the involved breast completely.

5. Limited Procedures. These have received a variety of names, including lumpectomy, local excision, partial mastectomy, tylectomy (comparable to lumpectomy). In all of these procedures the tumor is surgically removed, with a varying amount of surrounding tissue.

6. Treatment of Choice. For many years surgeons have preferred the Halsted radical mastectomy as the operation of choice for most cancers of the breast. More recently, some surgeons have preferred the modified radical mastectomy for early cancers, or a simple mastectomy for in-situ (extremely early and noninvasive) breast cancer. Subcutaneous mastectomy with subsequent implant has also been recommended for lobular carcinoma in-situ, but *not* for invasive cancer.

ADJUVANT THERAPY

1. Adjuvant therapy of breast cancer involves the use of cytotoxic drugs or endocrine therapy after definitive primary therapy. The aim is to eradicate occult metastatic disease that otherwise would be fatal.

2. Adjuvant chemotherapy and hormonal therapy are effective treatments for breast cancer patients.

3. From reports in the literature the following statements can be made:

a. For pre-menopausal women with cancer in the lymph nodes, regardless of hormone receptor status, treatment with established combinations of chemotherapy should be part of standard care.

b. For pre-menopausal patients with negative lymph nodes, adjuvant therapy is not generally recommended; but for certain high-risk patients in this group adjuvant chemotherapy should be considered.

c. For post-menopausal women with positive nodes and positive hormone receptor levels, tamoxifen citrate is the treatment of choice.

d. For post-menopausal women with positive nodes and negative hormone receptor levels, chemotherapy may be considered; but it cannot be recommended as standard practice.

e. For post-menopausal women with negative nodes, regardless of hormone receptor levels, there is no indication for routine adjuvant treatment. For certain high-risk patients in this group, adjuvant therapy may be considered.

f. Recently chemotherapy and/or tamoxifen have been recommended for all patients post operatively.

PREGNANCY-ASSOCIATED (PA) BREAST CANCER

1. The relationship between breast cancer and pregnancy is problematic. This association appears to account for between 1 and 2 per cent of all breast cancers and for 10 to 30 cases of breast cancer per 100,000 deliveries.

2. A thorough breast examination is particularly important at the obstetrical visit, since the progression of pregnancy results in increasing firmness, nodularity, and hypertrophy of the breast, which tends to obscure more subtle masses.

3. This, coupled with increasing radiographic density, results in increased difficulty in discerning malignant tumors in the breast during pregnancy and lactation. There is widespread reluctance to perform mammography during pregnancy, although the risk to the fetus with modern, low-dose mammography and shielding of the abdomen is minimal.

4. Needle aspiration of masses readily distinguishes cysts or galactorrhea cysts from solid tumors.

5. Delayed diagnosis and advanced disease are often characteristic of pregnancy-associated breast cancer. The prognosis, stage for stage, is the same for the pregnant as for the nonpregnant patient.

6. The major risks to the fetus during the treatment of breast cancer relate to staging procedures, surgery-induced miscarriage, fetal effects of radiation therapy and chemotherapy, and the rare chest x-ray or bone scan. Risks associated with the latter can be estimated by physics calculation.

7. A pregnant patient with breast cancer should receive the same treatment as a non-pregnant patient.

8. The management of the pregnancy depends on the trimester and on the shared judgment of the patient and her physician.

9. In general, abortion does not seem to be therapeutic.

46 Radiation Therapy in Gynecology

Hugh R. K. Barber

A working knowledge of the relevant physics, basic radiation biology, permissible radiation exposure, and the application of radioactive isotopes is important in the evaluation and management of clinical problems in oncology. Because of the great advances made in radiophysics, radiation therapy has become too complex for the average gynecologist. Proficiency in radiotherapeutic techniques demands teamwork between the different specialists, and competent radiotherapists and physicists. It is not within the province of this short discussion to create radiotherapists; certain fundamentals are emphasized so that the gynecologist may be an efficient member of the therapeutic team.

BASIC PRINCIPLES

1. All matter is made up of chemical substances, which can be divided into two kinds: *elements* and *compounds*.

a. An element is a distinct kind of matter which cannot be decomposed into two or more simpler kinds of matter.

b. A compound is formed when two or more elements combine together chemically to produce a more complex type of matter.

2. Atoms are the smallest particles of an element that can exist without losing the chemical properties of that element.

3. Molecules are the smallest particles of a compound that can exist without losing the chemical properties of that compound.

4. The atom is an electrical structure having three basic units: the *proton,* the *neutron,* and the *electron.* The *nucleus* contains the protons and neutrons, while the *orbits*—circular or elliptical—contain the electrons.

5. The simplest atom is that of the element hydrogen. This consists of a central nucleus comprising one proton, around which moves one electron.

6. The proton is a heavy particle carrying a positive charge. The electron is a very much lighter particle with a mass only 1/1,840 that of the proton, and with a negative charge of exactly equal magnitude (but of opposite sign) to that of the proton.

7. Therefore, almost all of the mass of the atom is in the nucleus, and the positive charge of the nucleus is balanced by the negative charge of the electron to make the atom as a whole electrically neutral.

8. The next simplest atom is that of the element helium. Its nucleus comprises two protons and two neutrons. Two orbital electrons move around the nucleus.

9. A neutron is a particle with a mass approximately equal to that of a proton, but with no electrical charge.

10. A *positron* has the same mass as an electron, but a positive charge that exists only while the positron in motion.

11. The nucleus of the helium atom, therefore, has a positive charge of 2 units (due to two protons) and a mass of approximately 4 units. The two positive charges of the nucleus are balanced by the two negatively charged electrons around the nucleus.

12. Every element has a *mass number* and an *atomic number* (Z).

a. The atomic number of an element is the number of protons in the nucleus (which is equal to the number of electrons around the nucleus) of an atom of that element.

b. The mass number of an atom is the total number of protons and neutrons in the nucleus. It gives a measure of the mass of the nucleus, or its *atomic weight*.

13. Protons and neutrons are known collectively as *nucleons* because they are found in the nucleus.

14. The atomic number is written to the left and below (subscript) the symbol for the element. Thus, for sulfur: $_{16}S$. The atomic mass is written above (superscript) and to the right, i.e., S^{32}. The mass number may also be written above the atomic number—i.e., $\frac{32}{16}$.

15. An *isotope* is a chemical element having the same atomic number as another (i.e., same number of nuclear protons) but possessing a different atomic mass (i.e., different number of nuclear neutrons).

16. *Isobar* is a term applied to two or more substances that have the same atomic weight but different atomic numbers.

17. A *radionuclide* is an atomic nucleus that will decay spontaneously into some other nuclear species, accompanied by the liberation of energy—a nuclear species that is radioactive.

18. *Bremsstrahlung* (from German, "braking radiation"—also called "brems rays") is a name applied whenever high-speed electrons, regardless of their source, are abruptly slowed down, and their energy converted to electromagnetic radiation. If the energy is large enough the electromagnetic radiation is in the x-ray region.

19. High-energy beta particles (see below), passing close to atomic nuclei and undergoing deceleration, also give rise to brems radiation.

TYPES OF RADIATION EMITTED

1. These radiations, whether emanating from natural or from artificial radioisotopes, are of three kinds, named after the first three letters of the Greek alphabet: (1) *alpha* rays (or particles), (2) *beta* rays (or particles), and (3) *gamma* rays (energy).

a. Alpha (α) particles are streams of high-speed helium nuclei (two protons and two neutrons packed tightly together) that have been ejected from radioactive substances.

b. Beta (β) rays are streams of fast-moving electrons (particles) ejected from radioactive substances with velocities that may be as high as 0.98 times the velocity of light. In soft tissues, beta rays can travel distances ranging from small fractions of a millimeter up to about one centimeter, producing ionization in their path.

(1) The beta particle comes from a neutron in the nucleus. Neutrons change into a proton and an electron. The electron is then ejected from the nucleus.

(2) Emission of the beta particle from the nucleus (beta decay) does not change the mass number (the total number of particles in the nucleus) but does increase the atomic number by one; i.e., $_{15}P^{32} \rightarrow {_{16}S^{32}} + {^{-}\beta^{0}}$.

c. Gamma (γ) rays come from radioactive substances. When they are produced by electrical machines, we call them x-rays. They differ fundamentally from alpha and beta radiations as they are not particles but waves, of the same type as light and radio waves, but with different properties of their very much shorter wave length.

RADIATION QUANTITIES AND UNITS

1. Activity is measured in *curies*.

2. Exposure is measured in *roentgens*.

3. Absorbed doses are measured in *rads*.

DEFINITIONS

1. **Roentgen (r).** This is a measurement of radiation exposure. It is defined as "that amount of x- or gamma radiation such that the associated corpuscular emission per 0.001293 gram of air produces, in air, ions carrying one electrostatic unit of quantity of electricity of either sign." One *milliroentgen* (mr) is 1/1,000 r.

2. **Rem (roentgen-equivalent-*man*).** This is defined as that quantity of radiation which produces the same biological effect in man as 1 r.

3. **Rad (radiation absorbed *d*ose).** This unit is defined as an energy absorption of 100 ergs per gram of any material (roughly equivalent to the roentgen).

4. **Curie (Ci).** This is the quantity of any radioisotope in which there occur 3.7×10^{10} disintegrations per second. The subunits of the curie are: millicurie (mCi) = 1/1,000 Ci, microcurie (μCi) = 1/1,000 mCi.

5. **mg.Ra (milligram radium).** This is used for radium only (1 mg. radium = 1 mCi radium = 8.2 rhcm).

6. **mg.Raeq. (milligram radium equivalent).** This is used for gamma-emitting radioisotopes which are applied in radiation therapy as substitutes for radium or radon. Defined as the activity which produces the same ionization in air by gamma radiation as 1 mg. of radium (1 mg.Raeq. = 8.25 rhcm).

7. **Linear Energy Transfer (LET)** is the energy released (usually in Kev, kiloelectron volts) per micron of medium (tissue) along the track of any ionizing particle.

8. **Bragg peak.** The rate of dissipation of the energy of a charged particle increases gradually as the particle slows down, and increases dramatically (the Bragg peak) just as the particle is coming to rest.

9. **Brachytherapy** (from the Greek *brachys*, short, and *therapy*). This term is used to distinguish the therapeutic use of an isolated radionuclide close to the tumor from its use at a distance from the tumor. For the latter, the term *teletherapy* (from the Greek *tele*, far) is used.

CHARACTERISTICS OF RADIATION

Basic Principles

1. Radiation can be defined as the propagation of energy through space or matter. In radiology, radiations can be divided into two main forms: corpuscular and electromagnetic. Radiations produce their effect principally by the process of ionization—the ejection of outer orbital electrons from atoms.

2. Corpuscular radiation consists of moving particles of matter. Electromagnetic radiation consists of a transport of energy through space as a combination of an electric and a magnetic field, both of which change in magnitude as a function of time and space.

3. X-rays and gamma rays are examples of these types of energy. Cesium, radium, cobalt, and x-irradiation are examples of this type of energy.

4. X- and gamma rays lose their energy in matter by three primary processes:

a. *Photoelectric absorption* and

b. *Compton scattering,* each of which results in the ejection of an orbital electron, while

c. *Pair production* involves a change of the photon energy into mass (a positive and a negative electron are formed).

5. Radiobiological effects on cells may include inhibition of cell division, chromosome mutation, and gene mutation. The energy of x-rays or gamma rays may cut through a chromosome, allowing the severed ends to join together with little change of function. The use of potentiators, such as hydroxyurea or actinomycin D, inhibits the chromosome from reforming.

Physical Aspects of High-LET Particles

1. Protons, helium ions, and heavy ions are heavy charged particles.

Table 46-1. Data on Permissible Radiation Exposure

The exposure in the United States for a 30-year period (reproductive life of average person)	*Rads*
For diagnostic radiology	4.1
For radioisotopes around us	1.4
For radioisotopes in body	0.8
For cosmic radiation	0.4
From luminous-dial watches	0.4
From nuclear testing	0.1
Total	7.2

a. These particles pass through matter and travel in nearly a straight line. They come to stop after passing through a certain depth of absorber, depending upon their initial energy.

b. The rate of energy loss of a decelerating high-LET particle increases sharply near the end of the range. There the dose reaches a peak, known as the "Bragg peak."

c. The dose falls off very rapidly beyond the Bragg peak.

2. Pi Meson (P ions), unlike other heavy charged particles, are unstable and have a very short half-life. They have not been used to treat gynecological malignancy on a limited trial.

3. Neutrons interact with tissue and release highly ionizing, heavy charged particles; most of the dose is contributed by recoiling protons from hydrogen in tissue. Current research with neutron therapy has promise, but has not had any significant effect on survival in the treatment of gynecological cancer.

Gross Effects of Intracavitary Radiation

1. Erythema—1 week
2. Exudation—2 weeks
3. Slough—6 to 8 weeks
4. Scarring—6 months
5. Contraction—1 year

Radiobiological Effects on Skin

For 6,000 r in 6 weeks, 250 Kv, HVL 2 mm. Cr, 10 × 10 cm^2 field. With supervoltage, approximately twice the doses are required to produce the same early effects.

1. Early Effects

First week	Faint (first erythema after 6 to 12 hours, fading in 2 to 3 days)
Second week	Sharply defined (second) erythema
Third week	Deepening erythema
Fourth week	Dry desquamation
Fifth week	Beginning moist desquamation
Eighth week	Complete moist desquamation
Twelfth week	Complete healing

2. Late Effects

3 months to years	Atrophy, telangiectasis, depigmentation, subcutaneous fibrosis

ADMINISTRATION OF RADIATION

Points of Reference Used in Calculating Dosages

1. Cervical cancers are not very sensitive tumors; high dosage must be used.

2. The adjacent normal tissue must be protected.

a. The function of the uterus and ovaries must be sacrificed, but it is often desirable to retain the sexual function of the vagina.

b. This is destroyed by shrinkage and fibrosis if too high a dosage is given.

Table 46-2. Radiation Contributions of Roentgenographic Diagnostic Procedures

Procedure	Skin Doses	Female
Chest film 14″ × 7″	100 mr	0.07 mr
Chest photofluoroscopic film	1,000 mr	0.70 mr
Pyelogram	1,200 mr	1,300 mr
Pelvimetry	12,000 mr	1,300 mr

Table 46-3. Point at Which Radiation Exposure Damages Fetus

Fetal Damage (Month of Gestation)	Rads
First	40
Second	90
Third	140
Fourth	200
Fifth	250
Sixth	350
Eighth	500
Tenth	600

No threshold for gene mutation. Estimates for doubling of the spontaneous mutation rate in man run from 10 R to 140 R.

Table 46-4. Historical Development of Regulations for Maximum Permissible Dose to the Whole Body

1931	1,000 mr per week	50 r per year
1935	500 mr per week	25 r per year
1946	300 mr per week	15 r per year
1958	100 mr per week	5 r per year

Currently 100 mr per week; 15 times as much for hands and feet; 1/10 as much for nonradiation workers

Table 46-5. Radioisotopes

Isotope	Symbol	Half-Life	Alpha	Beta	Gamma
Radium 226	^{226}Ra	1,620 years	+	+	+
Cesium 137	^{137}Cs	26.6 years	−	+	+
Cobalt 60	^{60}Co	5.4 years	−	+	+
Iridium 192	^{192}Ir	74.4 days	−	+	+
Phosphorus 32	^{32}P	14.3 days	−	+	−
Iodine 125	^{125}I	60.0 days	−	−	+
Radon 222	^{222}Rn	3.8 days	+	+	+
Gold 198	^{198}Au	2.7 days	−	+	+
Yttrium 90	^{90}Y	2.7 days	−	+	−

c. The bladder and rectum must be completely protected.

3. One method of avoiding damage to adjacent structures is to plan the radium dosage with reference to an imaginary point in the pelvis called *point A*. This method of delivering radiation therapy to the cervix was started in Manchester England at the Holt Radium Institute. (This is the basis for the Manchester method.)

4. Point A is 2 cm. from the central canal of the uterus and 2 cm. above the lateral fornix, and is in the middle of an area arbitrarily called the *paracervical triangle.*

5. Too large a dosage in this vascular area will cause ischemia and fibrosis with a risk of subsequent stricture of the ureter. This is, however, a very rare complication. The real limiting factor in intracavitary radiation is the sensitive loops of bowel lying in the pelvis.

6. The size of the tumor and the space available in the uterus and vagina vary from patient to patient.

a. Sometimes the uterine canal cannot be found because of the invasiveness of the tumor. The degree of lateral distension of the vaginal vault affects the dosage delivered to the pelvic wall.

b. The treatment of each patient must therefore be adapted to the conditions found on examination under anesthesia.

7. Afterloading technique is now commonly used. This means using a special tandem and colpostat which are first placed in position in the uterus and vagina and then loaded with radium, cobalt, or cesium.

a. The technique has been developed to allow the radiotherapist to take more time and care in inserting and adjusting the applicators without exposing himself to radiation while doing so.

b. It also allows more flexibility in dosage: one applicator can be unloaded, or the amount of radium in it altered, without interrupting treatment.

Preparation for Radiotherapy

1. Anemia must be corrected. It increases the anoxia of cancer and renders it less radiosensitive.

2. Local infection must be corrected. It is impossible to sterilize a septic fungating growth; some whole-pelvis radiation may be given as a preliminary to bring about some regression. Antiseptics and antibiotics may be needed.

3. If a pyosalpinx exists it should be removed surgically, and radiation delayed for a week. The presence of sepsis both increases tissue anoxia and endangers the patient's life. The very small mortality associated with radiotherapy is due to sepsis.

4. Intravenous pyelography is most important.

5. Bone scanning should be done as indicated.

6. Psychologically the patient should be prepared by a frank discussion of the treatment.

Postoperative Care

1. If there is a temperature elevation to 101°F or more for 12 hours, remove the radium.

2. The patient should remain flat and should use only one pillow. She may turn from side to side.

3. Place indwelling catheter in the bladder, with continuous drainage.

4. Ensure adequate fluid intake.

5. Give percodan or codeine and aspirin for discomfort.

6. Give Seconal to aid sleep.

7. Check any bleeding.

8. Give a low residue diet.

9. The exact time for removal of radioactive material should be placed on the order sheet.

Complications from Radiotherapy

1. Early

a. Variation in size and shape of the fornices and in extent of tumor

b. Dilatation of the cervical canal may sometimes cause a tear into the broad ligament.

c. Pyrexia

d. Frequency and dysuria

e. Proctitis, diarrhea, and bleeding
f. A whitish membrane may cover the vagina.
2. Late
a. Vaginal atrophy
b. Fibrosis of the ureter
c. Rectovaginal fistula and/or rectal drainage

Disadvantages of Megavoltage

1. Much higher cost for machine and installation

2. Beam shaping is more difficult. Despite these drawbacks, megavoltage is essential for up-to-date curative and palliative radiation therapy.

Colbalt 60 vs. Cesium 137

Isotope	*Half-Life*	*Gamma Lines*	*Corresponding Voltage of Electrical Generators*
Cobalt 60	5.24 years	1.7 and 1.33 Mev	2–3 M
Cesium 137	26.6 years	0.67 Mev	1–1.5 Mv

d. Avascular necrosis and spontaneous fracture of the femur have been observed.
e. Surface erythema, ulceration, and subcutaneous fibrosis

EVALUATION OF MACHINES FOR EXTERNAL RADIATION THERAPY

Units of Measure

1. 1 electron volt = 1 ev (the work done when an electron is accelerated by a potential of 1 volt)
2. 1 thousand electron volts = 1 kiloelectron volt = 1 Kev
3. 1 million electron volts = 1 Mev
4. 1 billion electron volts = 1 Bev

Advantages of Megavoltage

1. Less skin reaction, due to the lower surface dose. This is the most important advantage of megavoltage: it permits radiation therapy without bothersome skin reactions.

2. Greater depth doses, especially for small and medium-sized fields. This permits simple set-up—usually, opposing megavoltage fields are as satisfactory as multiple fields or rotational therapy with kilovoltage.

3. Lower doses to bones and less bone "shadowing." Less side scatter.

1. Advantages of Cobalt
a. Better skin sparing (surface dose about one-half that of Cesium 137)
b. Better field shaping (source diameter about one-half that of Cesium 137)
c. Higher output
2. Disadvantages of Cobalt
a. The source must be replaced every 2 to 5 years.
b. Room shielding is more difficult. Cobalt 60 is preferable.

X-rays and Gamma Rays vs. Electrons

1. Advantages of X-rays and Gamma Rays
a. Better skin sparing
b. Larger beams
2. Disadvantages of X-rays and Gamma Rays
a. Depth sparing is more difficult.
b. Lower output
c. Megavoltage electron-beam therapy is worthwhile only for very large institutions.

Linear Accelerator

1. In this machine, electrons from the filament of a vacuum tube are accelerated by the injection into the vacuum tube of electromagnetic waves all traveling in the same direction. Any electron is accelerated by an electromagnetic wave, and each wave imparts more energy.

Table 46-6. Irradiation Schedule for Specific Stages of Pelvic Cancer

Stage	*External RT, Whole Pelvis (Rads)*	*Intracavitary Parametrium Rads (Point A)*	*Max. Mg.–Hrs.*	*Ext. RT Booster (Rads)*	*Minimum Dose to Pelvic Wall (Rads)*
IA	None	3,500–3 wks,–3,500	9,000	None	None
IB, IIA	4,000 in 4 wks.	3,000–3 wks,–3,000	7,600	None	5,500
IIB	4,00 in 4 wks.	3,000–3 wks,–3,000	7,600	1,000 involved side wall	6,500
IIIA	4,000 in 4 wks.	3,000–3 wks,–3,000	7,600	None	5,500
IIIB, IV	4,000 in 4 wks.	3,000–3 wks,–3,000	7,600	1,000 involved side wall	6,500

Starting 2 to 3 weeks after completion of external radiation: if the cervical os is not identifiable, this step is replaced by additional 2,000 rads by multiple fields, followed by intravaginal radiation.

RT = radiation therapy

2. This gives an acceleration equal to the potential difference of several million volts. The linear accelerator is of practical use in radiotherapy—it can produce energies of up to 20 Mev.

3. Most linear accelerators used in gynecological work are in the range of 4 to 6 Mev. Although longer accelerators are needed to produce higher energies, the apparatus has become more compact than it used to be.

4. When energies above 20 Mev are required in radiotherapy, a *betatron* is used (see below).

Betatron

1. The betatron accelerates electrons in a spiral path instead of along a straight line; it can be made more compact than a linear accelerator.

2. In principle, it is a hollow evacuated ring (the "doughnut") lying in an electromagnetic field between the poles of a large electromagnet.

3. Electrons are injected into the doughnut and are then accelerated by programmed increases in the strength of the electromagnetic field.

4. This field both guides and accelerates the electrons, which may make hundreds of thousands of circuits around the doughnut before they reach maximum energy.

5. The electrons are finally directed to a target electrode, in colliding with which they produce X-radiation.

RADIATION THERAPY FOR GYNECOLOGICAL CANCERS

Cancer of the Cervix

Radiation therapy is the treatment chosen for Stages IIB, III, and IV. It is chosen for those patients in Stage IB who are poor operative risks.

Outline of Standard Pelvic Field for External Radiation

1. Superior Border: A transverse line at the upper end of L5. It is centered on the midline of the vertebral body.

2. Inferior Border: A transverse line at the lower edge of the obturator foramen (or pubic symphysis). It is centered on the midline of the pubic symphysis. In Stage IIIA (disease extending to the lower vagina), the lower edge of the pelvic field should be extended to include all disease, with at least a 1-cm. margin.

3. Lateral Border: Perpendicular lines on each side, through the center of the acetabulum (not the head of the femur).

WHOLE PELVIS IRRADIATION AND INTRACAVITARY CESIUM THERAPY

Cancer of the Endometrium

Fields are as outlined for cancer of the cervix.

Preoperative Radiation

1. Stage IA G1 (uterine cavity less than or equal to 8 cm., and/or well-differentiated malignancy: No preoperative radiation

2. Stage IA G2 or G3, IB G1, G2 or G3 (uterine cavity greater than 8 cm., and/or poorly differentiated malignancy): External radiation to pelvis including the upper vagina—4,000 rads

3. Stages II, III, IV: External radiation to pelvis including the upper vagina—4,000 rads

All patients receive vaginal radiation by insertion of radium, cesium, or cobalt, up to 2,000 rads, 0.5 cm. below the mucous membrane.

Postoperative Radiation

1. Stage IA G1 (speculum shows penetration of myometrium for more than one-third of its thickness):

a. External pelvic radiation 4,000 rads in 4 weeks, plus vaginal radiation by an applicator up to 2,000 rads 0.5 cm. below the mucous membrane.

b. If there is no penetration of the myometrium and the cancer is well differentiated, only intravaginal radiation is given.

2. Stages IA G2, IA G3, and IB G1 (or G2 or G3) (uterine cavity greater than 8 cm., and/or poorly differentiated malignancy): 4,000 rads in 4 weeks, plus intravaginal radiation

3. Stages II, III, and IV: External therapy of 4,000 rads in 4 weeks plus intravaginal radiation

A number of institutions have been carrying out primary surgery and tailoring the radiation to the pathology found at surgery.

Care of Patient Receiving External X-ray Therapy

1. These patients need close supervision.

2. Ambulatory patients appear to tolerate therapy better than those confined to bed.

3. The diet should contain adequate protein, vitamin B complex, and vitamin C.

4. Heat, sunlight, and irritating chemicals applied to the skin over the area of treatment are hazardous and may produce an accelerated or exaggerated skin reaction.

5. CBC should be checked each week.

6. The care of the patient should be shared by the radiation therapist and the referring physician.

Radiosensitization

Poorly oxygenated cells are particularly resistant to therapeutic irradiation. Several methods have been attempted to overcome this resistance. They include fractionation of radiation dosage, administration of hyperbaric oxygen, fast neutron therapy, and administration of chemical sensitizers.

1. *Fractionation* is used because it has been shown that after the first dose of a course of radiation the tumor begins to shrink, demand for oxygen is reduced, and the flow and distribution of the blood improves; some of the previously hypoxic cells are rendered more sensitive to the next dose of radiation.

2. *Hyperbaric oxygen* has been tried for over 20 years and has shown a slight, but definite, advantage. Oxygen tents or pressure chambers add to the work of the radiotherapist, and patients must spend longer periods under treatment. There are also side effects such as earache and sinus pain, oxygen convulsions, and claustrophobia.

3. *Neutrons* can now be accelerated with sufficient intensity for clinical use. They interact with tissues in a manner entirely different from that of gamma rays, such that the protective effect of hypoxia is largely overcome. Gamma rays interact only with electrons; electron recoil produces a sparse ionization and, therefore, low linear energy transfer (LET). Neutrons interact with nuclei; nuclear recoil produces a dense ionization from protons, alpha particles, and nuclei of carbon and oxygen—and thus a high LET. Fast neutron therapy is causing the disappearance of some tumors heretofore regarded as resistant.

4. *Chemical sensitizers* mimic the sensitizing effect of oxygen on hypoxic cells. They work by preventing the reuniting of a chromosome after it is cut in half by the radiation therapy. Many compounds have been found successful in vitro, including nitrofurantoin, metronidazole, and the more active misonidazole, which is neurotoxic. Some of the chemotherapeutic agents, such as actinomycin D and hydroxyurea, act as chemical sensitizers.

Safety Precautions

1. Physicians treating patients in whom radioactive sources have been inserted must be fully acquainted with the proper safety precautions. They must see that nurses and other staff take appropriate measures to protect themselves and any other visitors or patients who may come into contact with patients under treatment.

2. Special care must be taken to ensure that no pregnant staff or patients are exposed to radiation.

3. Warning signs must be displayed, and mobile lead screens put in place, around the patient's bed.

4. All excreta and bedding must be checked to ensure that no radioactive material is accidentally included with them during disposal. (Since radium has been phased out as a method of treatment, this type of accident is practically impossible.)

5. All staff involved in the treatment of these patients must wear film badges.

6. Patients should be isolated in treatment rooms with walls reinforced by lead or extra brick. In cases where patients are receiving cesium, however, distance (e.g., 6 feet) is adequate protection.

47 Chemotherapy

Hugh R. K. Barber

BASIC PRINCIPLES

1. In contrast to surgery and radiation therapy, chemotherapy (the treatment of cancer with drugs and hormones) can be used effectively for disseminated as well as for localized cancer.

2. Within the past two decades it has become clear that although chemotherapy was long considered largely a palliative procedure, capable of extending but not saving lives, certain kinds of cancer can now be cured by chemical treatment.

3. A major goal of current cancer chemotherapy is to achieve cures by prompt and vigorous treatment of these cancers. By "cure" is meant that the life expectancy of the treated patient is the same as "normal" life expectancy; specifically, the same as that of a matched cohort in the general population.

4. It has long been known experimentally that chemotherapy is more effective when tumor masses are small than when the tumor-cell burden is high.

5. The concept of the *first-order kinetic cell kill* by drugs (fixed-percentage kill rather than fixed-number kill per effective dose) means that, with a small tumor burden, total cell kill can be achieved with a reasonable number of repetitive doses which, with a large tumor cell burden, would still leave residual cells that would eventually develop "resistance" and start to grow again.

6. Immunotherapy is postulated to kill tumor cells by zero-order kinetics (fixed number of tumor cells).

7. In humans, the effect of chemotherapy on the host is based on the *cell-kill hypothesis.* In an attempt to represent cell kill, volume reduction is approximated because most clinical lesions can be measured only in two dimensions. As an example, oncologists refer to the *greater-than-50-per-cent objective response.* This criterion implies at least a halving of the product of perpendicular diameters of a tumor. In both human leukemias and solid tumors, duration of response and/or host survival represents the best clinical correlate of cell kill.

8. Combinations of chemotherapeutic drugs have been used with substantial success, particularly when each of the drugs used acted on the cancer cells in a different way. Major improvements in the treatment of certain types of cancer have been achieved both by the use of several of the active drugs simultaneously and by the use of different drugs in sequence.

9. The cumulative results of cancer treatment research have brought the tally of types of cancer that are so controllable as to be considered curable to 11 out of the 100 or more different forms.

a. These are: acute leukemia in children, Hodgkin's disease, histiocytic lymphoma, skin cancer, testicular carcinoma, Wilms' tumor, Burkitt's lymphoma, retinoblastoma, and choriocarcinoma.

b. Eleven additional types of cancer have shown significant improvement in survival. These are ovarian carcinoma, breast carcinoma, adult acute leukemias, multiple myeloma, endometrial carcinoma, prostatic cancer, lymphocytic lymphomas, neuroblastoma, adrenal cortical carcinoma, malignant insulinoma, and osteogenic sarcoma.

CELL KINETICS

1. Cellular reproduction (cell division cycle, or cell kinetics) is divided into five phases:

Growth 1 (G1)—postmitotic; takes at least one-half the life cycle of the cell

Synthesis (S)—DNA content is doubled; takes up about 30 per cent of the cycle

Growth 2 (G2)—occurs just before mitosis; takes up about 20 per cent of the cycle

Mitosis (M)—takes up about 1 per cent of the cycle

Growth 0 (G0)—the resting, or nondividing, phase of the cell. The length of the G0 phase is variable and depends upon the type of cancer. The cell is relatively resistant to attack by the anticancer drugs during this phase.

2. Studies on cell kinetics reveal that certain anticancer drugs have more predictable effects than others on different phases of the cell.

3. Approximately 40 to 80 per cent of the marrow stem cells are in G0 at any given time. When chemotherapeutic agents cause a decrease of white blood cells, the resting marrow cells temporarily enter the cell cycle and proliferate rapidly.

4. Studies have shown that a given dose of drug kills the same percentage of cells that are in cycle, no matter how many are present.

a. For example, the same dose will kill 90 per cent of 100,000 leukemic cells or 90 per cent of 100 cells, whichever number of leukemic cells is present in the animal.

b. Therefore, 1,000,000 cells can be reduced to 10,000 and 10,000 reduced to 100, and 100 to 10 or less, and then 10 cells to 0.

c. By the institution of an intermittent schedule to allow for recovery of normal cells, cures can be produced if the dose is large enough so that the percentage of cell population killed outpaces the multiplication of surviving cancer cells.

d. If each dose of the anticancer chemotherapy does not reduce the cell population by at least 75 per cent, the continuing multiplication of surviving cancer cells will outpace the inhibiting effect of the drug and will soon kill the animal.

5. Cancer-cell population studies have concluded that each tumor cell divides into two cells once each generation time, i.e., the time for one entire division cycle.

a. The time required for this cycle is about the same for all cells in a given population of cells.

b. Since each tumor cell divides into two cells at each generation time it is evident that by ten generations, a single cell proliferates into 1,000 (10^3) cells. Therefore, the growth of many cells following this pattern of growth will result in a thousandfold increase every ten generations.

c. The growth pattern is referred to as *exponential,* or *logarithmic.*

d. By charting the log cells against time the pattern is charted as a smooth curve.

6. In order to be detected, a tumor must have a volume of at least 1 cubic centimeter—consisting of about 10^9 cells (one billion, or 1,000,000,000).

7. The volume of cells necessary to kill a patient (critical volume) is $10 \times 10 \times 10$ cm., or about 10^{12} cells (one trillion).

8. Since these values are a thousandfold (10^3) apart, their separation in time represents ten generations of growth.

9. If treatment reduces the cell population from 10^{12} to 10^6 in acute lymphatic leukemia, the patient is in remission but is not cured.

10. The goal of anticancer chemotherapy is to reduce the last million cells

(10^6) to zero. It is accepted that 100-percent cell kill is necessary to cure leukemia.

CHEMISTRY, MECHANISMS OF ACTION, TOXICITY, METHODS OF ADMINISTRATION, AND USES

The central dogma of molecular biology deals with the genetic material deoxyribonucleic acid (DNA), the replication of DNA to produce more DNA, the transcription of DNA into ribonucleic acid (messenger RNA), and the translation of RNA into protein. (Amino acids in the cytoplasm are activated by enzymes and transferred by transfer RNA to a ribosome, at which point the message is read off and the completed protein released.)

CALCULATION OF DOSES ON BODY SURFACE AREA

There is increasing evidence that calculation of doses based on body surface is important in relating tolerated and effective doses in animals to those in man. Calculating by the body surface area helps to minimize the apparent dose differences between children and adults. Nomograms, from which body surface areas can be calculated when height and body weight are known, are available (*CA—A Cancer Journal for Clinicians,* May/June 1977, vol. 27). When doses are expressed in mg./Kg., the following formula can be used to convert roughly to mg./m.^{2}: mg./Kg. $\times$ 40 = mg./m.^{2} Depending on the drug, there may be an upper limit to the single dose given to patients weighing more than 70 Kg.

A brief outline is given of the principal groups of anticancer drugs used in practice.

DIFFERENCES BETWEEN CANCER GROWTH AND NORMAL TISSUE GROWTH

1. All living things have an inherent capacity to multiply. They seek multiplication for a variety of reasons. In humans, a cellular brake is required to prevent overgrowth for the benefit of the community of cells. In vitro, this appears to be controlled by an unknown feedback mechanism, probably resulting from contact phenomenon when cells are crowded.

2. In cancerous growth, cells no longer cease multiplying when they reach a critical mass; the uncontrolled growth leads to death of the host.

3. In the early phases of growth, tumor cells grow exponentially. But as tumor mass increases, the time needed for a tumor to double its volume increases—i.e., the growth follows a Gompertzian curve. It is likely that the increase of doubling time is related to crowding and the loss of nutrient supply.

Skipper Model (Skipper Hypothesis)

1. The survival of an animal with cancer who is receiving chemotherapy is related inversely to either the number of cancer cells inoculated (for lab study) or the number remaining after therapy.

2. A single leukemia (or cancer) cell is capable of multiplying and killing the host.

3. A given drug kills a constant fraction (percentage) of cells, not a constant number, regardless of the number of cells present at the onset of therapy.

4. The dosage of a drug and its ability to eradicate cells are related.

5. Conclusion: Good results are most likely if therapy is started before the tumor reaches an overwhelming volume.

Commonly Used Criteria for Objective Response and Disease

1. Complete response: Complete disappearance of all demonstrable disease

2. Partial response: Reduction by more than 50 per cent of the sum of the products of the longest perpendicular diameters of discrete measurable disease, with no demonstrable disease progression elsewhere.

3. No response: No change in the size of any measurable lesion, or less than 50-per-cent reduction of measurable disease as defined above.

4. Progression. More than 50-per-cent increase in the sum of the products of the largest perpendicular diameter of any measurable lesion.

PRINCIPAL GROUPS OF ANTICANCER DRUGS USED IN PRACTICE

ANTIMETABOLITES

Folic Acid Antagonists

Chemistry

1. These are derivatives of folic acid.
2. The component parts of the folic acid molecule are:
   a. Plexidine nucleus
   b. *p*-Aminobenzoic acid
   c. Glutamic acid
3. Folinic acid is the formyl-containing analogue of reduced folic acid. It is called *synthetic citrovorum factor of leucovorin.*

Mechanism of Action

1. A drug of this type blocks folic acid and reductase to prevent availability of a single carbon fragment. This blocks purine ring biosynthesis.
2. By a lesser action it inhibits methylation of deoxyuridylic acid to thymidylic acid, blocking pyrimidine synthesis.

Toxicity

1. Mouth lesions
2. Ulceration of the gastrointestinal tract
3. Bone marrow depression
4. Susceptibility to infection
5. Alopecia
6. Hyperpigmentation
7. Teratogenic properties
8. Toxicity enhanced by impaired kidney function

Method of Administration and Dosage

1. 4 Amino-N^{10}-methylpteroylglutamic acid: oral 2.5–5.0 mg./day
2. Amethopterin (methotrexate): I.V. or I.M. 5–25 mg./day for 5 days

Uses

1. Choriocarcinoma
2. Cancer of the ovary
3. Cancer of the breast
4. In combination with other anticancer drugs for treating cancer of the cervix

PURINE ANTIMETABOLITES

Chemistry

1. 6-Mercaptopurine (6 MP) (Purinethol)

Mechanism of Action

1. Blocks purine ring biosynthesis
2. Inhibits interconversion of purines

Toxicity

1. Leukopenia
2. Thombocytopenia
3. Stomatitis
4. Nausea and vomiting (about 25 per cent of adults)

Method of Administration

Usual dose: 2.0–2.5 mg./Kg./day orally or 500 mg./m.^{2}/day intravenously for 5 days every 10 to 14 days

Uses

1. Acute lymphatic leukemia
2. Acute granulocytic leukemia
3. Chronic granulocytic leukemia
4. Occasionally in choriocarcinomas

PYRIMIDINE ANTIMETABOLITE

Fluorouracil (5-FU)

Mechanism of Action

1. Blocks thymidylate synthetase

2. Inhibits methylation of deoxyuridylic to thymidylic acid, blocking pyrimidine synthesis

Toxicity

1. Myelosuppression
2. Stomatitis
3. Gastrointestinal ulceration
4. Nausea and vomiting
5. Alopecia
6. Cerebellar ataxia (uncommon)
7. Diarrhea
8. Dermatitis
9. Skin hyperpigmentation

Method of Administration

1. 12 mg./Kg./day × 3 days
2. Smaller dose, 1–2 times weekly for maintenance

Uses

1. Bladder carcinoma
2. Breast carcinoma
3. Colorectal carcinoma
4. Gastric carcinoma
5. Hepatoma adenocarcinoma
6. Ovarian carcinoma
7. Pancreatic adenocarcinoma

GLUTAMINE ANTAGONISTS

Azaserine (O-diazoacetyl-1-serine)
DON (6-diazo-5-oxo-1-norleucine)

Chemistry

1. These are diazo compounds, closely related in structure to glutamine.
2. They are derived from both filtrates of a *Streptomyces.*

Mechanism of Action

1. Interference in the donation of an amino group by glutamine to various biochemical needs in the body; blocks the conversion of formyl glycineamide ribonucleotide (FGAR) to formyl glycineamidine ribonucleotide (FGAM)

2. A step in purine biosynthesis in which glutamine acts as an amine donor under the influence of an amidotransferase

Toxicity

1. Mouth lesions
2. Gastrointestinal tract disturbances
3. Leukopenia
4. Thrombocytopenia
5. Liver damage

Methods of Administration and Dosage

1. Azaserine: I.V. 5–10 mg./Kg./day; oral × 10 or more
2. DON: I.V. 0.2 mg./Kg./day

Uses

1. Choriocarcinoma (rarely now)
2. Childhood acute leukemia

POLYFUNCTIONAL ALKYLATING AGENTS

Chemistry

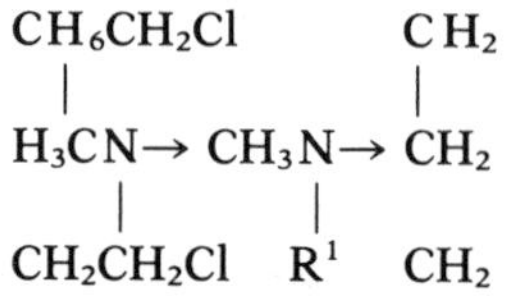

$$\begin{array}{ccc} CH_6CH_2Cl & & CH_2 \\ | & & | \\ H_3CN\rightarrow & CH_3N\rightarrow & CH_2 \\ | & | & \\ CH_2CH_2Cl & R^1 & CH_2 \end{array}$$

Mechanism of Action

1. Important sites of action appear to be on the nucleic acids, probably within the nucleus; this is suggested by the following observations:

a. These agents are mutagenic.
b. They are carcinogenic.
c. They preferentially deactivate DNA-containing viruses.
d. They inactivate the pneumococcal and *H. influenzae* transforming principles.

2. Alkylation (insertion of an alkyl group) may interfere with synthesis of cross-linking in a number of places; it prevents H bonding between chains of DNA.

3. A monofunctional compound produces nuclear energy by a sheet mass effect.

Such a compound has only one active alkyl group.

4. Polyfunctional agents are 50 to 100 times more active than the monofunctional group.

a. They are cross-linking agents.

b. Reactive atoms bridge across two chromosomal strands or react at two points on a chromosome.

Toxicity

1. Delayed deaths may occur 3 to 7 days after exposure to LD50.
2. Decrease in antibody production
3. Increased susceptibility to infection
4. Diarrhea
5. Ulceration of the gastrointestinal tract
6. Hemorrhagic cystitis
7. Involution in size of lymph nodes, thymus, and spleen
8. Progressive decrease of leukocytes and platelets in the peripheral blood
9. Decrease in spermatogenesis
10. Teratogenic effect

Methods of Administration and Dosage

1. Mechlorethamine HCl (HN_2CHl, Mustargen): I.V. 0.4 mg./Kg., single or divided doses

2. Chlorambucil (Leukeran): Oral 0.1–0.2 mg./Kg./day (6–12 mg./day)

3. Melphalan (Alkeran) (L-phenylalanine mustard, L-PAM) (L-Sarcolysin): Oral 0.2 mg./Kg./day × 5, 2–4 mg./day maintenance

4. Cyclophosphamide (Endoxan, Cytoxan): I.V. or Oral—200 mg./day I.V. for 5 days, or 50 mg./BID orally

5. Triethylenethiophosphoramide (TSPA, thiotepa): I.V. 0.2 mg./Kg. × 5 days

6. 1,4 Dimethanesulfonyloxybutane (busulfan, myleran): Oral 2–6 mg./day 150–250 mg./course

7. Nitrosourea alkylating agents:

a. 1,3-bis (2 chloroethyl)-1-nitrosourea (BCNU): I.V. 100 mg./m.^{2} every 6 weeks

b. Next course, in 4 to 6 weeks: Chloroethyl-cyclohexyl-nitrosourea (CCNU): Oral 120–150 mg.m.^{2} every 6 weeks

Uses

1. Carcinoma of the ovary
2. Hodgkin's disease
3. Lymphomas
4. Burkitt's tumor
5. Multiple myeloma
6. Cancer of the breast
7. Neuroblastoma
8. Carcinoid
9. Leukemias

ANTIBIOTICS

Mechanism of Action

Each antibiotic agent forms a complex with DNA involving selective binding at the guaninecystosine segments, with a specific block in the DNA-dependent RNA synthesis (inhibits formation of messenger RNA [mRNA]).

Toxicity

1. Damage to bone marrow and intestinal epithelium
2. Nausea and vomiting
3. Diarrhea
4. Skin eruption

Methods of Administration and Dosage

1. Actinomycin D or dactinomycin (Cosmegen): I.V. 0.01 mg./Kg./day × 5 days or 0.04 mg./Kg. weekly

2. Daunomycin: I.V. 0.8–1.0 mg./Kg./day × 3 to 6 days; total dose never to exceed 25 mg./Kg.

3. Mitomycin C (Mutamycin): I.V. 0.06 mg./Kg. × 2 weekly if blood counts permit

4. Adriamycin: I.V. 50–75 mg./m.^{2} in single or divided doses every 2 weeks

5. Mithramycin: I.V. 25 μg/Kg. every other day × 3 doses.

Uses

1. Lymphomas
2. Leukemias
3. Solid tumors
4. Embryonal tumors
5. Trophoblastic disease
6. Carcinoid
7. Lower calcium level (mithramycin)

ADRIAMYCIN (ADRIA)

Adriablastina, Doxorubicin

Toxicity

1. Gastrointestinal
2. Hematologic
3. Cardiac

 a. Electrocardiogram changes may occur, such as sinus tachycardia, T-wave flattening, ST-segment depression, voltage reduction, and arrhythmias. These are indications to stop or defer treatment.

 b. Congestive heart failure secondary to cardiomyopathy

4. Alopecia
5. Dermatitis
6. Red urine (not hematuria)

Administration

1. 60 to 75 mg./m.^{2} I.V., single dose q.3 weeks

2. 30 mg./m.^{2} I.V., single dose for 3 days every 4 weeks. Administer through running I.V. infusion.

3. Do not give to patients with significant heart disease; reduce dosage in patients with impaired hepatic function.

4. The total cumulative dose of adriamycin should not exceed 550 to 600 mg./m.^{2}, since the risk of congestive heart failure increases markedly above this level. A small cumulative dose (500 mg./m.^{2}) should be used when multiple drugs are included in the therapy. It is important to follow for EKG abnormalities and signs of heart failure.

Uses

1. Ovarian cancer
2. Embryonal tumors
3. Sarcomas
4. Breast carcinoma

MITOTIC INHIBITORS

Vinka Alkaloids

Chemistry

1. Dimeric indole-dihydroindole alkaloids
2. Periwinkle plant

Mechanism of Action

These agents arrest mitosis in the metaphase by destroying the spindles in cell nuclei.

Toxicity

1. Nausea and vomiting
2. Diarrhea
3. Leukopenia
4. Neurotoxic paresthesias
5. Palsies
6. Peripheral neuritis
7. Alopecia
8. Ileus

Methods of Administration and Dosage

1. Vinblastine (Velban): I.V. 0.1–0.15 mg./Kg. weekly

2. Vincristine (Oncovin): I.V. 0.03–0.075 mg./Kg. weekly

Uses

1. Choriocarcinoma
2. Lymphoma
3. Leukemia
4. Hodgkin's disease

ENZYMES

L-asparaginase

Normal cells can synthesize their own supplies of asparagine. It appears that asparagine-dependent cells lack an enzyme, asparagine synthetase, which in normal cells converts aspartic acid to asparagine. Certain types of leukemia (such as acute lymphoblastic) have an asparagine dependence. This provides an explanation for the effect of L-asparaginase. The tumor activity of L-asparaginase is also found with transplanted rat tumors and with primary dog lymphosarcoma. The final indications for the use of the enzyme in the treatment of malignancy remain to be determined.

Method of Administration and Dosage

1. L-asparaginase: I.V. 50–200 I.U./Kg./day or 200–1,000 I.U./Kg. 3–7 days each week for 28 days

Uses

Acute lymphoblastic leukemia

NONALKYLATING AGENT THERAPY

Hexamethylmelamine (HMM, HXM)

Mechanism of Action

Although hexamethylmelamine structurally resembles triethylenemelamine (TEM), a known alkylating agent, it is thought not to act as an alkylating agent at first, but more like an antimetabolite.

Toxicity

1. Gastrointestinal tract disturbances
2. Myelosuppression
3. Neurologic disturbances
4. Alopecia
5. Dermatitis

Dose

8 mg./Kg./day, P.O.

Cisplatin Dianmine Dichloride (CPDD)

Mechanism of Action

Upon loss of a chlorine atom, this drug binds to DNA, high-molecular-weight RNA, and transfer RNA. The resulting inhibition of DNA synthesis persists for several days after administration of the drug. It is a cell-cycle-nonspecific agent (i.e., it works at all points in the cell cycle).

Cisplatin appears to be an alkylating agent. It is a DNA-binding agent and appears to act at all points in a cell cycle. It may also unmask tumor-associated antigens on the tumor cell and set up an antigen-antibody immune response.

Toxicity

1. Nephrotoxicity
2. Tinnitus and hearing loss
3. Nausea and vomiting
4. Myelosuppression

Dose

50 mg./m.^{2}, I.V., × 3 every 28 days, with mannitol diuresis

Carboplatinum (Paraplatinum) Cis-drammine 1,1-cyclobutane Dicarboxylate Platinum II

Mechanism of Action

Reacts with nucleophilic sites on DNA, causing predominantly intrastrand and interstrand cross-links rather than DNA-protein cross links. These cross-links are similar to those formed with cisplatin but are formed later.

Toxicity

Reduces the dose-limiting adverse effects of cisplatin (nephrotoxicity, neurotoxicity, nausea, and vomiting).

1. Myelosuppression
2. Anemia
3. Rarely, hypersensitivity

Indications

Is indicated for the palliative treatment of patients with ovarian carcinoma that is recurrent after prior chemotherapy, and including patients who have been previously treated with cisplatin. Is also used as a first line drug.

Dose

360 mg./m.^{2} as a single agent. Prehydration and posthydration are not required. Can be infused over 15 minutes or longer.

BLEOMYCIN SULFATE

Mechanism of Action

Although the exact mechanism of action of bleomycin sulfate is unknown, current evidence suggests that the main mode of action is the inhibition of DNA synthesis. There is some evidence of lesser inhibition of RNA and protein synthesis.

Toxicity

The most frequent presentation is pneumonitis, occasionally progressing to pulmonary fibrosis. Approximately 1 per cent of patients treated have died of pulmonary fibrosis.

Idiosyncratic Reactions

Reaction may be immediate or may be delayed for several hours, and usually occurs after the first or second dose. It consists of hypotension, mental confusion, fever, chills, and wheezing.

Side Effects

The integument and mucous membranes are the sites of the most frequent side effects, which are reported to occur in approximately 50 per cent of treated patients. These consist of erythema, rash, striae, desquamation, hyperpigmentation, and tenderness of the skin. Hyperkeratosis, nail changes, alopecia, pruritis, and stomatitis have also been reported.

Dose

1. For patients with squamous cell carcinomas, lymphosarcoma, reticulum cell sarcoma, or testicular carcinoma: 0.25–0.50 I.U./Kg. (10–20 I.U./m.^{2}) I.V., I.M., or subcutaneously, weekly or twice weekly.

2. Pulmonary toxicity appears to be dose-related, with a striking increase when the total dose is over 400 I.U. When bleomycin is used in combination with other antineoplastic agents, pulmonary toxicities may occur at lower doses.

ETOPOSIDE (VP-16-213, VePesid)

Etoposide (VP-16-213) is a semi-synthetic derivative of podophyllotoxin used in the treatment of certain neoplastic diseases. (*synonyms:* Epipodophyllotoxin VP-16-213, Exoposide, VePesid)

Mechanism of Action

1. Etoposide has been shown to cause metaplasia arrest in thick fibroblasts. Its main effect in mammalian cells, however, appears to be at the G2 portion of the cell cycle.

2. Two different dose-dependent responses are seen:

a. At high concentrations, lysis of cells entering mitosis is observed.

b. At low concentrations, cells are inhibited from entering the prophase. The drug does not interfere with microtubular assembly.

3. The predominant macromolecular effect of etoposide appears to be DNA synthesis and inhibition.

4. See *Physician's Desk Reference* (PDR) for dosage schedule.

Toxicity

1. Myelotoxicity is most often dose-limiting, with granular site nadirs occurring 7 to 14 days, and platelet nadirs occurring 9 to 16 days, after drug administration. Bone marrow recovery is usually complete by day 20. No cumulative toxicity has been reported.

2. Gastrointestinal disturbances (nausea, vomiting)

3. Alopecia (reversible—sometimes progresses to total baldness)

4. Hypotension (usually temporary)

5. Allergic reactions (anaphylactic—chills, fever, tachycardia, bronchospasm, dyspnea, hypotension)

6. Peripheral neuropathy (reported in a small number of cases)

7. Central nervous system toxicity (somnolence and fatigue—about 3 per cent of the patients)

8. Other toxicities include aftertaste, hypertension, and rash. There has been one report of radiation recall dermatitis.

Dose

I.V. 50–100 mg./m.^{2}/day, days 1 to 5, or 100 mg./m.^{2}/day, days 1, 3, and 5, every 3–4 weeks in combination with other drugs approved for use in the disease to be treated.

Dosage should be modified to take into account myelosuppressive effects of other drugs in combination or the effects of prior x-ray therapy or chemotherapy which may have compromised bone marrow reserve.

METHODS OF TREATMENT

Two methods are selected more often than any others for the administration of chemotherapeutic drugs: the continuous, or maintenance, method, and the intermittent plan.

The intermittent plan is being used more and more. It is based upon Bruce's observation that chemotherapeutic agents lower the white blood count, causing the resting marrow stem cells to temporarily enter the cell cycle and proliferate rapidly in the presence of the intermittent chemotherapeutic regime.

48 Pediatric and Adolescent Gynecology

Hugh R. K. Barber

1. The adolescent patient poses special problems in the delivery of health services to women. The adolescent gynecologic patient provides the physician with an unusual opportunity to introduce young women to a medical program that can be both preventative and educational.

2. The problems encountered are attitudinal on the part of the practicing physician, emotional on the part of the adolescent patient herself, and related to the environment in which the program of health care is delivered.

3. The background for understanding the management of adolescent gynecologic problems should be rooted in an understanding of the mechanisms of growth and development and puberty.

4. Unfortunately, adolescent female medicine has not been identified as a separate speciality. It is recognized that it should be, but, at present, very few private practices or hospitals have structured special units for these patients. Therefore, it is important to reserve special time for interviewing and managing the adolescent female.

5. It is best to have patients of similar age visit the office at the same time. Depending on the situation, it may be helpful if the patient is accompanied by a parent, preferably the mother or a close female relative.

HISTORY AND PHYSICAL

General Considerations

1. Puberty represents a period of transition from childhood to sexual and reproductive maturity. The accompanying physical and psychological changes often have major social implications.

2. The major determinant of the timing of onset of puberty is probably genetic, but nutrition, physical health, environment, and social and psychological factors influence the age of onset and the rate of progression of pubertal changes.

3. Puberty progresses sequentially until adult sexual characteristics are obtained.

4. Ethnic and geographic considerations affect the time of appearance of sexual characteristics, but in the United States the following landmarks are recognized: the initiation of breast development at age 10.8 years; the appearance of pubic hair at 11 years; the onset of menstruation between 12.6 and 12.9 years; and peak height velocity is achieved at about 12 years.

Progression of Puberty

1. Puberty is usually an orderly process of events beginning at about age 8 or 9. A spurt in growth is usually the first step noted in this orderly progression.

2. Menarche, or the onset of menses, occurs two years after the onset of puberty, which normally lasts for between 4 and 8 years. Puberty begins about 2 years earlier in girls than in boys. The age of menarche

appears to have fallen gradually during the last few decades.

History and Physical

1. The average adolescent is anxious and concerned about any examination, particularly the gynecologic one. The patient fears only not the discomfort that may accompany it but also the possibility of the discovery of an abnormality or a serious illness.

2. Almost universally, the female adolescent expresses concern over the interview and the vaginal examination, considering the latter an invasion of privacy. It is very important that the physician approach this examination with empathy, but it is of the utmost importance that the physician not be condescending to the adolescent patient.

3. The initial interview should be done in a private room with only the patient present. The physician must impress upon the patient that she is his or her patient and that there is a confidentiality that will be respected. It is essential for the physician to establish rapport with the young patient.

4. Having done this, a cooperative and intelligent interaction develops which evolves into mutual respect. This establishes the ideal patient-physician relationship.

5. The history should be taken in a professional but relaxed atmosphere. The patient should obviously be asked about her past history, her menstrual history, and whether she has had any type of treatment. Operations should be discussed with the patient. Questions concerning sexual activity should be kept to the end of the interview when a physician-patient relationship has been developed.

6. The patient must be assured of the confidentiality of the interview.

Physical

1. All procedures and examinations to be performed should be carefully explained to the patient. Since the adolescent is particularly sensitive to body image, sexuality, and sex structures, she requires a careful explanation and a measure of reassurance regarding gynecologic matters to avoid embarrassment and the development of a distorted self-image.

2. The physician should take the opportunity at the initial visit to inform the patient of the importance of regular checkups. It is a time to stress the idea of lifestyle based on moderation in all respects.

3. At the initial examination, the physician can counsel the adolescent and introduce her to meaningful information concerning sexuality, contraception, pregnancy, venereal disease, and the importance of the health maintenance examination throughout her life.

4. As far as the physician is concerned, the management of adolescent gynecologic problems should be based on the sound understanding of normal sexual maturation, growth, and development, and the influence of medical and behavioral disease on these problems.

5. When the adolescent patient is examined, a small speculum should be used, cotton tip applicators should be available to obtain material from the vaginal wall for study under the microscope, and the adolescent should be properly draped and comfortable, with a female nurse or relative nearby and visual aids handy for the patient to follow the examination.

6. The physician should explain to the patient why the examination is being performed and what information is being obtained. It is important to describe the anatomy so that the adolescent may learn more about her body.

7. A bi-manual rectal examination often suffices. The ovaries do not come down into the pelvis in the adolescent until the time of puberty.

8. Need for a Papanicolaou smear should be based on whether the patient is sexually active, has been pregnant, is using oral contraception, or, on examination, whether there is a cervical erosion or eversion. The patient who has been exposed to diethylstilbestrol should also have a Papanicolaou smear carried out.

HYPOTHALAMIC-PITUITARY-GONADAL-HORMONAL RELATIONSHIPS

1. Control of reproductive function arises from a complex interplay involving the central nervous system, the hormones, and all of the organs concerned.

2. Maturational changes appear to affect primarily the hypothalamus. During infancy and pregnancy, the secretion of gonadotropin-releasing hormones (GnRH) is minimal.

3. It has been shown that small amounts of ovarian steroids have an inhibitory influence, presumably on the hypothalamus.

4. The pituitary secretion of an adrenal-androgen–releasing hormone is associated with a significant rise in such adrenal-androgens as dehydroepiandrosterone-sulfate (DHEA-S).

5. During the pre-pubertal period the pituitary response to exogenous GnRH is to release follicle-stimulating hormone (FSH), but little or no luteinizing hormone (LH).

6. When maturity is achieved, there is a pulsatile release of GnRH on the arcuate nucleus. Gonadotropin-stimulating steroid secretion also rises. Somatic growth and secondary sex characteristics are stimulated.

ABNORMAL ENDOCRINE FUNCTION

Abnormal function of the reproductive endocrine system may manifest itself in a number of ways, including genital ambiguity, precocious puberty, delayed or absent pubarche, primary or secondary amenorrhea and hirsutism in the female, galactorrhea, and infertility.

PRECOCIOUS PUBERTY

1. *Precocious puberty* is defined as puberty before the age of 8 years in girls.

2. Precocious puberty may be isosexual or heterosexual in nature. The events in heterosexual precocity usually involve phenotypic changes in the female that are predominantly androgenic in nature.

a. Isosexual precocity may be of two types, that is, true constitutional precocity or pseudoprecocity.

(1) The culmination of the progression of these events, in the female, is menarche. *True constitutional precocity* is defined as a progression of events that culminates in menarche prior to the age of 8 years.

(2) Precocious pseudopuberty implies the premature appearance of one or more secondary sexual characteristics without the development of normal reproductive capacity.

(3) It has been observed to occur in association with significant disease. Central nervous system disorders are the most common associated cause and usually involve lesions in close proximity to the hypothalamus.

(a) These lesions include a variety of neoplastic and non-neoplastic conditions as well as encephalitis, meningitis, hydrocephalus, and hypothalamic hematoma.

(b) Only about 4 per cent of precocious pseudopuberty in girls results from intracranial tumor.

3. In all forms of sexual precocity the patients initially will be tall for their age, but, because their epiphyses close prematurely, they will ultimately be shorter than average for their age.

4. A careful history is very important in the evaluation of these patients. A history should include statements regarding birth trauma, neonatal anoxia, familial history, and inflammatory disease to the brain. In addition, a good review of the growth and development of the child should be obtained. At physical exam, rectal examination should be carried out. The palpation of ovaries in the prepubertal age group may be difficult since the ovaries are intra-abdominal.

5. Gonadotropins and gonadal steroidal hormones should be measured to distinguish true precocity from pseudoprecocity. In true precocity, all hormone levels are within normal adult limits. In pseudoprecocity the levels of serum estrogen and androgen are elevated.

6. A vaginal smear for the presence of estrogen is a valuable study.

7. Diagnostic x-ray studies should include a skull film and a survey of the bones for the evaluation of bone age.

8. A CT scan gives very valuable information.

9. Having made a decision about whether pseudoprecocity or true constitutional precocity is the condition presented, a treatment plan can be structured.

a. In pseudoprecocious puberty, the pathology should be identified and treated.

b. The treatment of true constitutional precocious puberty should be based on supportive principles and specific pharmacologic principles.

(1) Pregnancy must be prevented if the patient is ovulating and counseling is helpful to aid the patient in her psychosexual adjustment. The agent of choice for treating true constitutional precocious puberty is medroxyprogesterone acetate, given intramuscularly every three to four months.

DELAYED ADOLESCENCE

1. Patients with delayed sexual maturation are either *eugonadal* (with signs of ovarian function) or *hypogonadal* (with evidence of ovarian failure).

a. Hypogonadal patients are either hypogonadotropic or hypergonadotropic, depending on their gonadotropin levels. Those who have an increased secretion of gonadotropins are further screened for normal chromosomal components.

2. Diagnosis is based on neurological, physical, and pelvic examinations, measurement of gonadotropin levels, karyotype, and endocrine profiles.

3. Therapy is simply gonadal steroid replacement with estrogen and progesterone.

AMENORRHEA

1. Amenorrhea is the complete absence of menstruation in patients within the reproductive span of life. It is not a diagnosis but a symptom. Amenorrhea is divided into primary and secondary amenorrhea.

a. *Primary amenorrhea* is usually defined as the absence of menses by the age of 17 years.

b. *Secondary amenorrhea* is the absence of menses for more than 150 days in a patient who has menstruated regularly in the past.

2. The absence of menstruation is to be regarded as physiologic prior to puberty, during pregnancy and lactation, and after the menopause. It is also expected during the administration of certain drugs.

3. By far the most common cause of amenorrhea in a woman in the reproductive years is pregnancy.

4. Chromosomal abnormalities account for approximately 30 to 40 per cent of all cases of primary amenorrhea.

5. Other etiologies for amenorrhea include malnutrition, delayed puberty, systemic illnesses, central nervous system lesions, tumors, and psychogenic, anatomic, hypothalamic, and metabolic disorders.

6. The patient with primary amenorrhea should have an accurate diagnosis made.

7. Estrogen-deficient individuals with a genetic abnormality and the absence of the Y chromosome should be treated with hormonal therapy in a cyclic manner to ensure sexual maturation. The adolescent female with a Y chromosome should have her abdomen explored and the gonads containing the Y chromosome, as seen in testicular tissue, removed. These patients should receive supplemental therapy.

8. The presence of demonstrable endocrinopathy requires specific therapy. Therapy for a congenital absence of the vagina or uterus requires no surgical treatment unless the patient is desirous of having reconstruction done.

9. Endocrine therapy, per se, should be employed when a diagnosis has been established.

Secondary Amenorrhea

1. Secondary amenorrhea is defined as the absence of menses for more than 5 months in a patient who has had regular menstrual periods.

2. It is to be differentiated from oligoamenorrhea, in which the patient has regular periods, most commonly occurring every 2 to 5 months.

3. The three most important diagnoses to be ruled out immediately in any patient with secondary amenorrhea are pregnancy, pituitary tumor, and premature menopause.

4. The patient with secondary amenorrhea should have a very careful work-up to document the site of the pathology.

5. Therapy depends on the etiologic diagnosis and should be appropriate for the patient's chief complaint.

DYSFUNCTIONAL UTERINE BLEEDING (DUB)

1. Most adolescent girls have anovulatory menstrual periods for the first 2 to 3 years after menarche; approximately 2 per cent of adolescents ovulate in the first 6 months and 18 per cent do so by the end of the first year after menarche.

2. This bleeding is not considered pathologic unless the menses lasts for more than 7 days, and anemia is present.

3. The usual etiology of DUB is an immature hypothalamic pituitary axis. Other causes include psychogenic factors, juvenile hypothyroidism, and coagulation disorders.

4. Therapy is cyclic hormone manipulation with estrogens and progestins.

DYSMENORRHEA

1. Dysmenorrhea, or painful menstruation, is a symptom and not a disease. Dysmenorrhea may be the most common of gynecologic symptoms.

2. *Primary dysmenorrhea* occurs in the absence of a significant pelvic lesion. It is essential, or functional, dysmenorrhea and is caused by factors intrinsic to the uterus.

a. Primary dysmenorrhea is generally associated with ovulatory cycles and appears to be caused by an excessive production of endometrial prostaglandins, which stimulate painful uterine contractions.

b. The principle treatment of primary dysmenorrhea is administration of prostaglandin inhibitors.

c. Progesterone may occasionally relieve dysmenorrhea without necessarily inhibiting ovulation.

d. In very severe cases, ovulation may be inhibited by oral contraceptive drugs.

3. In *secondary dysmenorrhea,* pelvic disease can be demonstrated. Adolescents may have endometriosis and chronic pelvic inflammatory disease. The treatment of secondary dysmenorrhea should be directed at the pathology behind it.

GYNECOLOGIC TUMORS IN CHILDHOOD AND ADOLESCENCE

The term *childhood,* or *adolescent, gynecologic tumor* is used to indicate any new growth (benign or malignant) occurring between birth and age 16 years. It implies the growth of newly formed cells derived from normal body cells or their preceding developmental cells of origin. A benign neoplasm is a tumor that does not destroy the host. A malignant neoplasm, if left untreated, destroys the host.

Vulvar Tumors

1. Any variation in the area of the vulva considered abnormal by parents or the adolescent should result in a visit to the doctor.

2. Both benign and malignant tumors of the vulva are rare in children.

3. An overall knowledge of their significant pathology as well as the variations that can exist in this area is most important. It serves as a basis for an informed, intelligent decision (both diagnostic and therapeutic) about pathologic conditions arising in the vulva.

a. White lesions are uncommon but may occur, and they usually represent a thinning of the integument in the area. Biopsy readily establishes the diagnosis. The most common of these is lichen sclerosus and it is usually self-limiting. Cortisone creams may be used to control itching.

b. Granulomatous lesions are of two varieties, pyogenic granulomas and the nonspecific, chronic granulomatous lesions. Biopsy will exclude the more serious problems.

c. Tumors of the vulva may originate in the labia, vulvar glands, vestibule, or clitoris. They may remain localized or they may extend locally or to distant lymph nodes and organs.

d. Benign tumors of the vulva in the child or adolescent run the whole gamut seen in the adult. The most common benign lesion of the vulva is the hemangioma. Hemangiomas may be single or multiple. The majority are manifested as a local swelling. Lymphangiomas have a basic histology that is not unlike a hemangioma except that the tumor sinuses are filled with lymph instead of blood.

(1) Conservative treatment for both is the best method of management, with surgical intervention only when necessary.

e. Hidradenomas are derived from apocrine sweat glands and are found in the labia. They are benign and respond to simple excision if their size becomes a problem.

f. Also present may be fibromas, lipomas, and granular cell myoblastomas.

g. Cysts of the canal of Nuck originate as cystic dilatation of the closed end of the hernia sac with atrophy of the proximal portion. This origin is indicated by the bleeding of fibrous tissue proximally into the inguinal canal. They are usually found in the inguinal region or in the labia majora. Unless their size dictates, there is no need for treatment.

h. Periurethral cysts usually occur when the periurethral glands become infected and there is a closure of the proximal end leading into the urethra. They are occasionally seen in adolescence.

i. Condylomata acuminata (venereal warts), once rarely seen, are quite common now and have become more aggressive in their growth patterns since the sexual revolution. They are best handled by podophyllin or cauterization. Laser ablation is being used with increasing frequency to treat them.

j. Carcinoma of the vulva in children is extremely rare, but in situ lesions are being reported with increasing frequency among teenagers who are and have been exposed to multiple partners. Currently these lesions are best handled by the use of laser ablation.

Vaginal and Hymenal Tumors

1. Congenital cysts of the hymen are occasionally seen which measure 2 to 8 mm. in diameter. One of the more common conditions arising in the adolescent gynecologic patient is the congenital obstruction of the lower vaginal tract by an imperfect hymen presenting as a bulging membrane.

2. Prior to 1970, adenosis vaginae was considered a benign disease. A new dimension has been introduced, however, by the work of Herbst and Scully. Although it is still considered a benign disease, it is important to rule out any evidence of clear-cell carcinoma. Epidemiologically, an association has been established between the treatment of mothers of girls with adenosis vaginae with diethylstilbestrol during pregnancy and the later development of adenocarcinoma in their daughters.

3. Carcinoma of the vagina is extremely rare in childhood, but a few cases have been reported. Since 1970, the number of cases reported has increased to about 400. They are associated with the use of in-utero stilbestrol for pregnancy problems in the mother.

4. Sarcoma of the vagina (sarcoma botryoides), which is really rhabdomyosarcoma, is one of the tumors seen classically in children. While occasionally seen a few days after birth, most cases develop before the age of 5 years.

a. The lesion originates in the subepithelial layers of the vagina and extends within the limits of the vagina. When seen in the vagina, it usually starts as a small, broad-based polypoid mass and, as it grows, it takes on the typical appearance of lobulated masses of vesicular hemorrhagic polyps, which soon fill the vagina and project through the vaginal introitus.

b. Prior to the advent of chemotherapy, they were very difficult to treat. In spite of radical surgery, distant metastases often occurred. Currently the management is by a combination of surgery and chemotherapy, and results have been greatly improved.

Tumors of the Cervix

1. The cervix gives rise to both benign and malignant lesions in children and adolescents. The commonly seen benign lesions are polyps, squamous papillomas, adenosis, hemangiomas, leiomyomas, hypertrophy and hyperplasia of the cervical glands, condylomas, leukoplakia, and endometriosis.

2. While undue concern usually occurs when these lesions are discovered, biopsy, and/or removal when indicated, promptly resolves the anxiety.

3. Dysplasia and carcinoma in situ of the cervix are being recorded with increasing frequency in the under-20 age group. With the spread of the sexual revolution, more teenage girls are taking the pill and starting intercourse at an earlier age, often with multiple partners.

a. The epidemic of human papilloma virus that is currently spreading across the United States seems to play a very significant role in the production of these lesions.

4. Cancer of the cervix in children is rarely diagnosed, and, when it is, it is usually clear adenocarcinoma related to the use of diethylstilbestrol in utero.

5. Sarcoma botryoides may also arise from the cervix. It has the same prognosis and requires the same treatment as that found in the vagina (see "Vaginal and Hymenal Tumors," above).

Tumors of the Uterine Fundus

1. Uterine tumors are extremely rare, but the majority reported are malignant. The main benign tumors are fibroids, endometriosis, and polyps.

2. Although the invasive type of endometrial cancer encountered in adults is practically unknown in the teenage patient, dysplasia and carcinoma in situ have been reported.

3. It usually occurs in, but is not necessarily caused by, a continuous, uninterrupted stimulation of the endometrium by estrogen.

4. The patient has some or all of the following findings: hirsutism, obesity and anovulation, amenorrhea followed by hypermenorrhea, and infertility. These patients are usually managed by a hormonal regime, but a firm diagnosis has to be made before starting treatment.

5. Primary sarcoma of the uterus in the adolescent is occasionally seen, fortunately only rarely. It is treated with the same aggressive management carried out in the adult.

Ovary

1. Common epithelial ovarian cancer is extremely rare before age 20. However, in the last few years, an increasing number of epithelial tumors have been seen in women in their twenties and, occasionally, among teenage girls.

2. The ovarian cancers that are found in childhood almost always arise from the germ cell or gonadal stromal cell. The malignant germ-cell tumors are generally encountered in childhood or among adults. Malignant changes arising in dermoid cysts are also extremely rare.

3. Having made the diagnosis, the question of management is raised and rightfully so in view of the young age of the patient.

a. The most common benign germ-cell tumor is the cystic teratoma (dermoid), and the most common malignant germ-cell tumor is the dysgerminoma.

b. Fortunately, it is usually possible to treat both conservatively.

c. The dermoid cyst can usually be shelled out with a complete preservation of the ovary.

d. For the dysgerminoma, if it is confined to the ovary and there is no positive cytology, no involvement of the opposite ovary, and no spread to the para-aortic nodes, a unilateral salpingo-oophorectomy can be carried out.

e. If the dysgerminoma has spread beyond the ovary, the patient should then be treated with total hysterectomy and bilateral salpingo-oophorectomy followed by either irradiation or chemotherapy.

4. The other germ-cell tumors are the endodermal sinus tumor, choriocarcinoma, and embryonal teratomas, which in the past were treated with very aggressive surgical means (hysterectomy and bilateral salpingo-oophorectomy).

a. However, due to developments in the last few years, if the tumor is confined to the ovary in which it arose and there is no evidence of positive cytology or spread, the patient can be treated by a unilateral salpingo-oophorectomy followed by triple or quadruple chemotherapy.

b. It is best not to use cyclophosphamide if preservation of the opposite ovary is desired, because this cytotoxic drug may destroy ova in the remaining ovary. Pregnancies have been reported among adolescent girls who have been treated with this conservative approach.

Gonadal Stromal Tumors (Sex Cord Mesenchymal Tumors)

1. The most common feminizing tumor in this group is the granulosa cell, and the most common masculinizing tumor is the Sertoli-Leydig cell tumor.

2. Only 25 per cent of each of these tumors functions with the production of hormone.

3. They are rarely bilateral (perhaps 5 per cent are) and only about 25 per cent are malignant.

4. It is possible to manage these patients conservatively if the tumor is confined to the ovary. Once it has spread from the ovary, the patient should have a total hysterectomy, bilateral salpingo-oophorectomy, and either radiation therapy or chemotherapy.

SUMMARY

1. Children and adolescents share the problems of adults. The term "little people" should be used when evaluating new growths in the pediatric and adolescent patient.

2. The small size of the child or adolescent markedly limits the available room for growth of a tumor. This results in grotesque deformity produced by only moderate-sized tumors.

3. The tumors parallel the rapid growth of children and usually possess a high degree of malignancy which results in rather fast clinical deterioration of the child or adolescent.

4. The margin of safety in giving treatment is smaller than in adults, since radical surgery and radiation therapy may have far-reaching effects on the patient's future development.

5. In dealing with problems in this age group, the same principles for judging operability, indications, and contraindications must be followed as in the treatment of the adult.

6. This approach offers the patient the maximal opportunity for treatment without an inordinately high morbidity and mortality.

7. However, if there is any chance for survival, comprehensive treatment must be carried out in a reasonable period of time.

8. The age-old tenet of medicine of not inflicting harm must be respected, and this broad principle, applicable to all disciplines in medicine, continues to serve as a guide for clinical judgment in the management of the pediatric and adolescent patient.

SEXUALITY

Sexuality is a pervasive force in society today. More precise biological and behavioral knowledge can only enhance the positive force that sexuality exerts on our civilization.

1. Sexual development begins with the determination of genetic (chromosomal) sex and has its fulfillment in sexual activity. In between these two periods of development is a series of stages of definition: gonadal sex, genital sex, nursery sex, legal sex, hormonal sex, and sexual orientation.

2. By the mid-teens, the female has achieved physical sexual maturity and is capable of sexual function and procreation.

3. Behaviorally, the adolescent has considered and acted on the emotional complexities of dependence and independence, passivity and aggression, the markedly different interpersonal relationships demanded by peers and the family, and other important aspects of individuality and self-interest.

4. Psychological growth has been divided into the stages of basic trust, autonomy, and initiative in childhood, and identity in the adolescent. Identity is that period when the individual differentiates from parental beliefs and value systems.

5. This should not be confused with the earlier stage of gender identity. By their late teens most girls have acted on erratic impulses which may take the form of masturbation or coitus.

6. The last two levels of sexual development are sexual orientation and sexual activity. By the late teens, the female has developed her sexual orientation.

7. The majority opt for an interpersonal sexual relationship and most choose heterosexuality. A minority choose homosexuality and some become bisexual.

8. A very small number choose not to relate overtly to sex and are termed *asexual.* The asexuality may be fashioned by religion or other interests.

CONTRACEPTION IN ADOLESCENCE

1. It is now a matter of record that teenagers are engaging in intercourse at younger and younger ages, most without using any form of contraception.

2. It is very unusual for a girl of 14 or 15 years of age to request a contraceptive from a doctor unless she is specifically questioned about menstrual periods and her sexual history. This may establish the rapport that leads into the discussion of contraception.

3. The college student of 18 or 19 is more likely to seek gynecologic care on her own. The physician is often faced with this dilemma when providing care to the adolescent patient. Prescribing a contraceptive without any discussion implies approval of a particular form of behavior, whereas denying contraception sets up the physician as a harsh "parent figure" who can later be blamed for an unwanted pregnancy.

4. Successful contraceptive use among adolescents depends on many factors. Medical, social, psychological, and economic issues all exert independent influences on young patients.

a. Medical concerns are important in the choice of any therapeutic regime, but they may be secondary or of minor importance in the selection of a contraceptive method that an adolescent will utilize successfully. Successful contraceptive use depends on resolution of both the medical and nonmedical concerns of the patient.

5. Contraceptives may be prescribed, demonstrated, and sold in most states of the United States without restriction.

a. Occasionally the law stipulates parental consent, minimum age, relevance to marriage, and parenthood. All states have family planning policies or laws. The physician should familiarize himself with the laws of his or her state.

6. Among 15- to 19-year-old women, two-thirds of all pregnancies are unintended. The most common reason given by adolescents for not using contraception is that they did not expect to have intercourse. Less than 10 per cent fail to use contraception because their partners object.

7. The reasons teenage girls give for delay in seeking professional help from family planning clinics are numerous and complex.

a. The two most common reasons given are that the patient "did not get around to it" or that she was afraid that her family would find out that she was using contraception.

Post-Coital Contraception

1. Since most teenagers do not use any form of birth control during their first sexual contact, it is important that they know that there is an option available to them.

2. Post-coital contraception is largely an emergency measure. Stilbestrol was formerly used at a dose of 25 mg. per day for 5 days. It made almost all patients intensely ill. Word got around that it was a devastating drug to take, and most women avoided it, even though they believed it would prevent pregnancy.

3. Ethinyl estradiol (2 mg. a day for 4 or 5 days) is now being used. Currently, a combined preparation (ethinyl estradiol, 100 μg. plus norgestrel, 500 μg.) is given in two doses, 12 hours apart. This hormonal interception interferes with endocrine balance and disturbs endometrial development. Treatment should be given within 48 hours of coitus.

The Condom

1. The sexual revolution has led to an epidemic of sexually transmitted diseases. Teenage girls who are having intercourse with more than one partner probably are best served by use of condoms.

2. A teenage girl can carry the condoms in her pocketbook and apply them to the penis of her partner during foreplay. This is a very good form of contraception and provides some protection against some sexually transmitted diseases.

Hormonal Contraception

This is the most effective form of birth control presently available. It has the same risks and side effects in the adolescent as it has in the adult. One major problem in the use of oral contraception in adolescents is the associated high rate of failure to take the pill and the high discontinuance rate. These occur in spite of intensive individual counseling and educational programs.

The Diaphragm

1. The diaphragm is a mechanical barrier between the vagina and the cervical canal. A contraceptive jelly or cream should be placed on the cervical side of the diaphragm before insertion. The diaphragm carries the disadvantages of requiring being fitted by a physician or a trained paramedical person and the necessity of anticipating the need for protection and privacy for its insertion.

2. Failure may result from improper fitting or placement and dislodgement of the diaphragm during intercourse. It has not been widely accepted by adolescent patients.

49 Rape

Hugh R. K. Barber

The word *rape* is derived from the Latin *rapere,* meaning to steal, seize, or carry away.

Rape is one of the most heinous crimes in the history of the world. Unfortunately, the courts have not properly addressed the problem and, for a variety of reasons, little progress has been made in controlling this monstrous crime.

Recently, FBI reports indicate that there are about 200,000 rapes and attempted rapes nationwide per year and that this figure may indeed represent only about 50 per cent of the problem.

The American Heritage Dictionary defines *rape* as the crime of forcing a female to submit to sexual intercourse. The FBI Uniform Crime Report states the legal definition: carnal knowledge through the use of force or threat of violence.

Sexual assault is a term used to describe manual, oral, or genital contact with the genitalia of the victim without the victim's consent. Rape and incest are coital forms of sexual assault. The primary motive of rape is aggression.

Common-law rape is defined as unlawful carnal knowledge of a woman not the wife of the perpetrator without her consent.

Statutory rape comprises those crimes of intercourse where the victim is judged incapable of consenting; that is, where the victim is underage or mentally subnormal. Included in this are patients whose consciousness has been altered by illness, sleep, drugs, or alcohol.

Force includes duress and intimidation; it need not involve physical violence. Yet the courts may require proof of actual resistance by the victim and not just the refusal to consent.

Sexual assault happens to people of all ages, races, and socioeconomic groups. But the very young, the very old, and those with physical and mental infirmities are particularly susceptible.

The typical rapist is a disturbed, compulsive, violent man who becomes sexually excited by the mortal fear of his victim. He rarely is a psychotic.

Rape is usually motivated by a wish to terrorize and humiliate the woman and is really the outcome of a frustrated seduction in the mind of the rapist. Often the rapist or potential rapist is concerned about his abnormal impulses and wants help.

As reflected in reports, rape is the fastest-growing violent crime in the United States. Reported sexual assaults increased 115 per cent between 1965 and 1974. It is estimated that up to ten times as many sexual assaults are committed as are reported. If this is true, then sexual assault is one of the least-reported crimes.

The average likelihood of serious personal attack on a female in this country, on a given day , is 1 in 12,000; the greatest risk is to females in the lower socioeconomic groups. One woman in ten is the victim of an attempted or actual rape during her lifetime. In 85 per cent of these assaults, the victim is beaten or intimidated with the display of life-threatening physical force. One in four victims is subjected to group rape, and is likely therefore to suffer even more direct physical violence and more extreme humiliation than other rape victims.

Approximately one-half of all rape victims are assaulted in their homes. Contrary to popular belief, rapists pay little attention to appearance. A woman's sexual allure has little to do with her being chosen as a victim.

A very disturbing fact is that the incidence of rape in women over 60 has increased by 800 percent during the last 15 years.

CHARACTERISTICS OF VICTIM AND RAPIST

The relationship of rapist to victim is: stranger 42.3%, recognized person 9.6%, acquaintance 14.4%, close neighbor 19.3%, close friend or boyfriend 6%, family friend 5.3%, relative 2.5%, no information 0.6%.

Violence used: no physical force 14.9% (but includes threat, display of weapon and intimidation), roughness 28.5%, beaten before rape 21.8%, beaten before, during and after 2.9%, beaten brutally before, during and after 9.8%, and choked 11.5%.

The previous criminal record of the rapist: 20.5% against property, 10% against the person, 11.3% for public disorder, 2.7% other, 4.5% forcible rape, 51% none.

Rapists' occupations when known include 53.9% unskilled laborers, 28.2% unemployed, 11.5% students, and 6.4% all other occupations.

Sexual aggressiveness in men is often excused by the myth of a spontaneous, uncontrollable sex drive. In fact, most rapes are premeditated.

THE RAPE TRAUMA SYNDROME

The *rape trauma syndrome* is outlined under seven categories:

1. **Acute Phase Disorganization**
   - **a.** Shock
   - **b.** Disbelief
2. **Expressed Affective Impact**
   - **a.** Anxiety
   - **b.** Fearfulness
   - **c.** Sobbing
   - **d.** Smiling
   - **e.** Shaking
   - **f.** Restlessness
3. **Controlled Affective Impact**
   - **a.** Calmness
   - **b.** Composure
   - **c.** Silence
4. **Mood Swing**
   - **a.** Humiliation
   - **b.** Degradation
   - **c.** Guilt
   - **d.** Shame
   - **e.** Embarrassment
   - **f.** Self-blame
   - **g.** Anger
   - **h.** Vengefulness
   - **i.** Fear of another assault
5. **Physical and Physiological Symptoms**
   - **a.** Exhaustion
   - **b.** Sleep disturbance
   - **c.** Soreness
   - **d.** Bruising
   - **e.** Skeletal muscle tension
   - **f.** Gastrointestinal irritability
   - **g.** Appetite disturbance
   - **h.** Genitourinary disturbances
6. **Thought Processes**
   - **a.** Denial
   - **b.** Undoing
   - **c.** Obsessing
7. **Long-Term Process of Reorganization**
   - **a.** Reorganization of lifestyle
   - **b.** Some affective reaction
   - **c.** Mood swings
   - **d.** Physiological reactions
   - **e.** Dreams and nightmares
   - **f.** Fears and phobias

MEDICAL EVALUATION

Initial Management

Any alleged or suspected victim of rape should be seen promptly. The nursing and physician personnel should treat the victim with nonjudgmental medical support.

The woman should be asked whether she would like to see a clergyman of her faith. If there is a local group organized to aid rape victims, they should be called so that one of their volunteers can come to help the victim.

It is important to give the victim a careful explanation of procedures to be performed and the reasons for them. This often helps to allay the victim's anxiety, fear, and mistrust. After this explanation it is important to secure a written consent from the patient, her guardian, or her next-of-kin for the gynecological examination, photographs, and the release of pertinent information to the authorities. The police should be notified.

Rape is a crime. The law may require that the physician report any injury inflicted in violation of the penal code. It may be impossible to know if an injury is a result of a penal code violation; reasonable belief warrants reporting. This would indicate reporting, therefore, when the victim claims sexual assault and the physician has reason to believe that there has been an assault.

In addition to state law, many cities have ordinances requiring physicians to report sexual assault to multidisciplinary groups that manage these complaints. In cases involving younger (adolescent) patients, reports must be made also to the relevant welfare agencies.

The history taking should be very thorough. It is good medical practice to have the victim describe the offense in her own words. This allows her to ventilate. By listening carefully to the patient's story, the physician can give her a sense that she is safe and is being helped.

The history should include a complete description of, and/or the identity of, the perpetrator; a description of the resistance offered; the type of sexual contact; the time and place of the assault; and whatever the victim knows about any witnesses who may have been present.

It is important to obtain the history of the last menstrual period and whether it was normal, and a description of the patient's contraceptive habits. The last voluntary sexual experience should be appropriately documented. It is important to have a female nurse present throughout the history taking and physical examination. At the end of the history taking the nurse should co-sign the history and the physical examination report, stating that they are accurate accounts of what the patient said and what was found.

Physical Examination

1. The physician should evaluate the patient's general appearance; whether she is calm, agitated, or confused; and should try to see whether she has been taking drugs or alcohol.

2. Bruises, lacerations, tears, and foreign bodies should be described accurately and treated appropriately.

3. An ultraviolet light may be used before the collecting of evidence. Wood's lamp causes semen to fluoresce, and thus indicates areas of the body or clothing from which evidence can be taken. All prostatic secretions are fluorescent, even when dry.

4. All specimens obtained should be labeled as to where they were found. The physician should initial all specimens; the chain of evidence goes from the patient to the physician, and then from the physician to the receiving person in the police department.

5. Sexual intercourse is defined as the slightest degree of penetration of the vulva by the penis. Entry of the hymen is not necessary.

6. A water-moistened, non-lubricated warm speculum or vaginoscope should be used to inspect the vagina and cervix. The samples taken include vaginal smear for acid phosphatase determination, vaginal smear to determine the presence of semen, blood antigen, cervical and rectal cultures for gonorrhea, blood samples for serological testing, fingernail scrapings, pubic-hair combings, remnants of clothing, and medical photographs of lesions or bruises. It is wise also to obtain corresponding samples from the mouth.

7. Salivary tests are used for secretor and antigen typing of the victim. Have the victim chew a dry 2-by-2-inch piece of gauze, and then place the gauze in a Petri dish for cooling and air drying.

8. It is vitally important that the physician personally turn over all specimens and clothing obtained to an appropriate technician or police officer and get signed receipts for all material submitted. This is vital for the medical-legal aspects of the case.

PROTECTING THE VICTIM

In any case of alleged or suspected rape there are three particular problems that the physician must address: the possibility of any venereal diseases' having been contracted, the possibility of pregnancy, and the immediate and delayed psychological sequelae.

The patient should be offered prophylaxis against venereal disease. This can be given in the form of probenecid, 1 g. orally, followed by 4.8 million I.U. of penicillin G benzathine. Penicillin-sensitive patients may be given tetracycline 500 mg. orally 4 times daily for 15 days.

The patient should be offered treatment to intercept a pregnancy. (Pregnancy occurs in fewer than 1 per cent of female rape victims.) This includes diethylstilbestrol (DES) 5 mg. orally daily for 25 days if the assault occurred in the follicular phase of the menstrual cycle, or 25 mg. orally daily for 5 days if it occurred in the luteal phase. Medroxyprogesterone acetate, 100 mg. I.M. as a single dose, and conjugated equine estrogens, 40 mg. I.V. as a single dose, have also proved to be effective.

The patient must be told that if this treatment does not intercept the pregnancy she will be offered an induced abortion. She must be told that if she chooses not to have an abortion and the offspring is a girl there are likely to be problems (i.e., a DES-exposed female in utero). It should be pointed out that there are well-documented cases of adenosis and clear adenocarcinoma of the vagina and cervix in females whose mothers used DES.

The emotional management of these patients is very important. There are two stages of reaction to rape: The first, a period of acute disorganization of personality, lasts from a few days to a few weeks. It usually overlaps the woman's transition into the second, or reorganization, phase.

It is important to supply psychological support over an extended time. About 10 per cent of rape victims develop overwhelming fears, particularly of being left alone or of being in enclosed places. There is a change in the libido in 5 to 15 per cent of these patients; this often has an adverse impact on a victim's marriage.

It is important to refer these patients to support groups, which can provide immediate post-evaluation counseling and a stable fabric of social support. This support may include group sessions with other victims; opportunities to reenact the traumatic episode in the company of understanding, objective individuals; and other assistance in converting feelings of rage and shame to healthy anger.

RAPE AND THE COURTS

A rape case boils down to one individual's testimony against another's. The plaintiff often receives harsher treatment in court than the defendant. The reasons for this are complex; they involve the rules of evidence and their interaction with society's attitudes toward women and sexuality.

Society takes confused attitudes toward rape. On one extreme are laws that dictate life imprisonment or death for convicted rapists in fourteen of the fifty states; at the other is the still widely-held belief that rape is the victim's fault.

The main issues in a rape case are to prove that the assault occurred, that it occurred without the victim's consent, that the victim resisted, and that the defendant was the rapist. The defendant is innocent until proved guilty; therefore the burden of proof falls on the prosecution, for whom the rape victim is a complaining witness.

Nothing can be said in court about any prior arrest of the defendant for similar offenses, or about his sex life. The victim, however, may find her credibility attacked in many ways. Since defense tactics are apt to rely largely on the idea that rape is a woman's fault, the victim may have her own character and personal life put on trial to such an extent that she begins to doubt or blame herself. To make matters worse, a married victim's husband may be embarrassed and angry over his wife's wish to pursue the case in court. Many trials end with rape victims, emotionally exhausted by their courtroom ordeals, devastated to see their attackers go free.

Rape is a shattering experience for many women. It is not merely a sexual assault but a violent crime maliciously directed against a woman. It may utterly disrupt her physical, emotional, social, and sexual life. Legal and health professionals, whether working separately or in interdisciplinary teams, must recognize the gravity of this crime and must treat its victims with all requisite understanding.

50 Climacteric, Menopause, and Aging

Hugh R. K. Barber

1. The climacteric, perimenopause, and menopause are often confused.

2. The *climacteric* is that phase in the life of a woman which marks the interval of transition from reproductive age to the age at which reproductive function is lost. This stage is characterized by progressive endocrine changes that lead to menopause, the final menstrual period that signals the end of cyclic ovarian function.

3. The *perimenopause* is defined arbitrarily to include the last few years of the climacteric and the first year after the menopause. The term *post-menopausal* is employed to describe the period following this interval.

4. *Menopause* is the cessation of menses due to failing ovarian function. It is the last menstruation which occurs during the climacteric. When the menopause is discussed, the discussion really concerns the climacteric.

5. The climacteric (meaning "critical period") is a time in the later years of reproductive life when changes occur in association with diminished gonadotropin function.

a. The term covers the perimenopausal years and the general syndrome which includes all the metabolic and psychological changes in these years. The climacteric has neither precise beginning nor end and may extend over many years. Therefore, the climacteric includes three periods of time. The *pre-menopause* includes the 4- or 5-year period before the menopause. During this time there are symptoms of decreased ovarian function, such as anovulation and irregular bleeding. The next interval is the menopause, which is the final menstruation occurring as part of the climacteric. The post-menopause describes the time of life that follows the menopause. There is a difference of opinion as to whether post-menopause should be defined to include the remainder of a woman's life or just the period in which the climacteric symptoms take place.

BASIC PRINCIPLES

1. In the United States there are approximately 30 million women who have experienced or who are now undergoing menopause. The average age at menopause is slightly over 51 years.

2. The average woman spends one-third of her life in an estrogen-deprived environment.

3. In almost all women over 50 years of age, estrogen levels fall, upsetting the hypothalamic-pituitary balance. The absence of neuroendocrine manifestations by no means guarantees that metabolic disturbances due to estrogen deprivation are not present.

4. The metabolic changes consist essentially of alpha/beta-lipoprotein reversal and elevation of estrogen and triglycerides—factors believed operative in producing atheriosclerosis and arteriosclerosis. These metabolic disturbances are also manifested by greater calcium and hydroxyproline excretion in the urine, evidenced by diminution of bone density and by osteoporosis.

5. There are two types of menopause, spontaneous and artificial.

a. In *spontaneous* or *physiologic menopause,* ovarian failure is heralded by decreased frequency of ovulatory cycles and resultant menstrual irregularities, abnormal bleeding, and infertility.

b. Removal of the ovaries prior to menopause may precipitate an *artificial* menopausal syndrome. At this time, the patient's ovaries may have been going through a period of deterioration and decreased function so that the withdrawal of estrogens may not produce such a dramatic estrogen withdrawal effect. Most hysterectomies with oophorectomies are carried out in the late perimenopausal or menopausal interval. The ovary will become too old to function but never becomes too old to form a tumor.

POST-MENOPAUSE

1. During the post-menopausal period the pituitary responds to ovarian failure with increased activity. This results in elevated levels of follicle-stimulating hormone (FSH) and increased production of growth hormone. The pituitary may also stimulate increased androgen production by way of the adrenal cortex. Despite the loss of ovarian function and the important follicular production of estradiol, estrogen—principally estrone—is produced from androstenedione in an extraglandular, extrahepatic conversion called *aromatization.* The androgenic substances excreted mainly by the adrenal glands are converted in the peripheral fat to estrone. The estrone is probably incorporated into the endometrial cells and converted to estradiol with a function similar to that seen in premenopausal women.

2. The endometrium responds to ovarian failure by remaining in the proliferative phase. Progesterone is not present, and, therefore, if there is a continuous, uninterrupted stimulation by estrogen, the endometrium may become hyperplastic.

3. In some women there is a fairly rapid atrophy of the vaginal mucosa, particularly at the introitus. However, in some there is little change for a long period after the menopause. Coital activity seems to prevent some of this atrophy, though not completely. A certain number of women develop an atrophic urethritis and trigonitis.

a. This is often diagnosed as cystitis but is not helped by antibiotics or sulfa drugs. It is helped by the use of estrogen, either in the form of a local cream or by mouth.

4. Small, asymptomatic cystourethroceles and rectoceles may enlarge and become symptomatic. Vaginal relaxation is also another problem in elderly women and may occur in the form of prolapse as well as the above-mentioned rectocele and cystocele.

a. The value of hormone therapy in relieving the symptoms is controversial but worth a trial.

EPIDEMIOLOGY

1. Women outnumber men in the age group 65 and above. With advancing age, the ratio becomes more extreme; beyond 85 there are only 45 men per 100 women.

2. The average age of women at menopause in the United States is approximately 51.4 years with a standard deviation of ±3.8 years.

3. Since the age of onset of puberty has steadily declined, there is an average reproductive span of approximately 37 years, followed by a post-menopausal interval of 28 to 30 years or longer. Therefore, American women now spend about one-third of their lives with reduced ovarian function. This number is even larger when women with premature ovarian failure and premenopausal castration are included.

4. The age of menopause in the United States appears to be unaffected by race, socioeconomic status, education, physical characteristics such as height and full-skin thickness, or age at last pregnancy.

5. Cigarette smoking does appear to be related to an earlier natural menopause. Nicotine may have a direct effect on the central nervous system or on the gonads, and the content of cigarette smoke produces certain hepatic enzymes that may affect the metabolism of steroid hormones.

6. Contrary to common belief, the age at menopause has been constant for several centuries and does not vary from one population to another. It may be true that the menopause in human beings is essentially an invariant biological trait. No single theory has been advanced to explain this observation.

CLINICAL SYMPTOMS OF THE MENOPAUSE

The symptoms frequently associated with the menopause and estrogen deficiency are: vasomotor instability ("hot flashes"), genital atrophy, osteoporosis, atherosclerotic heart disease, and psychological changes.

VASOMOTOR SYMPTOMS

1. The patient usually reports that she has flushes and/or flashes. Frequently they occur during sleep and wake the patient. The patient complains of night sweats, insomnia, and fatigue.

2. Other symptoms reported by the patient in the climacteric include nausea, dizziness, headaches, palpitations, diaphoresis, depression, anxiety, and irritability. Most of the symptoms occur in the early menopausal years. However, about one-quarter of the post-menopausal women will experience symptoms for five or more years.

3. Vasomotor symptoms have been explained as being due to instability in the autonomic nervous system. These women have a marked diminution of estrogen production, elevated levels of FSH, and surges of LH and beta-endorphins which correlate with the occurrence of flushes. On monitoring these patients, there is a surge of LH prior to the flash.

4. Effective and predictable control of vasomotor symptoms results from adequate estrogen replacement, which acts as a suppressant of the hypothalamic overactivity. There are contraindications to estrogen therapy. In such women, progesterones, clonidine, tranquilizers, and, occasionally, vitamin E have provided symptomatic relief.

ATHEROSCLEROTIC HEART DISEASE

1. *Arteriosclerosis* is a general term referring to the thickening and hardening of arterial walls. *Atherosclerosis* is a particular type of arteriosclerosis characterized by patchy deposition of fatty streaks and fibrous plaques on the walls of the larger arteries.

2. The pathogenesis of atherosclerosis includes endothelial injury, intimal and smooth muscle proliferation, and alteration in lysosomal function. In the subsequent healing process, deposition of lipids (mainly cholesterol) leads to the formation of streaks and plaques. These lesions progress with age.

3. The most common clinical problem of arteriosclerosis is ischemic coronary disease, the leading cause of death in both sexes after the age of 45. The factors that increase the chance of acquiring arteriosclerotic heart disease, apart from aging itself, are hypertension, diabetes mellitus, hyperlipidemia, smoking, and obesity.

4. Studies on the preventative effect of estrogen on heart attacks have provided variable results. Recently, some studies have suggested that estrogens in lower doses might be beneficial.

5. Cholesterol and triglyceride concentrations increase with age, and there is an augmented risk of coronary artery disease associated with cholesterol concentrations greater than 220 to 250 mg. per dl.

a. An increase in cholesterol values is associated with increased concentration of low density lipoproteins (LDL), whereas a rise in triglyceride values is associated with increased concentrations of very low density lipoproteins (VLDL).

b. High density lipoproteins (HDL), which carry about 20 per cent of cholesterol, seem to protect against the development of arterial sclerosis. A low HDL concentration appears to be a more potent risk factor for coronary artery disease than a high concentration of cholesterol or LDL. The addition of a progestin, medroxyprogesterone acetate (Provera), 10 mg. daily, helps augment the favorable effects of estrogen, whereas progestins that have an androgenic effect adversely affect HDL levels.

MENOPAUSAL OSTEOPOROSIS

1. Osteoporosis has been termed the "silent disease," and the reason for this is that the first identification of it may result from a broken bone.

2. Osteoporosis is not a disease per se but rather it is the end result of severe, prolonged bone loss. By bone loss is meant the gradual thinning and increased porosity of bone (hence the term *osteoporosis*) that occurs naturally with aging but that can be influenced by a variety of factors.

3. Osteoporosis is a painful, disfiguring, and debilitating process. It is a woman's issue. Osteoporosis cannot be cured but it can be prevented.

4. One out of every four women may develop osteoporosis. It is impossible to accurately predict exactly who will suffer from osteoporosis, but there are certain factors that seem to increase the risk of developing the condition.

5. Osteoporosis is more likely to develop in: thin women, small women with small bones, white women with fair complexions, Oriental women, women who have their ovaries removed by surgery, women who have x-ray treatment that causes their ovaries to stop making estrogen, women who have never been pregnant, women whose grandmothers, mothers, or sisters have osteoporosis, women who eat a diet that contains only a small amount of calcium, women who smoke, women who are not physically active, and women who drink excessive amounts of alcohol.

Bone Formation

1. Bone is living tissue and is constantly being broken down and reformed, like all tissues in the body. Bone formation is needed for growth, for repair of microscopic fractures that result from everyday stress, and for the replacement of worn-out bone.

2. Bone formation begins with bone breakdown. Bone-absorbing cells called *osteoclasts* dig microscopic cavities in the inner surface of the bone. Next, bone-building cells called *osteoblasts* begin filling in these cavities with new bone cells. These cells begin the bone rebuilding process by first producing the collagen matrix. This is followed by the laying down of calcium and phosphorus crystals within the matrix, a process called *bone mineralization.* Each year, between 10 and 30 per cent of the entire skeleton is remodeled in this way.

Bone Types

1. Structurally, there are basically two different types of bone, that is, *cortical* and *trabecular.* Cortical bone is very dense and solid. The long, hard bones of the arms and legs are mostly of this type.

2. Trabecular bone, on the other hand, is much more porous, honeycombed with many minute spaces. The vertebral bones are mainly made up of trabecular bone.

3. Every bone consists of both types, with the porous trabecular on the inside and solid cortical bone on the outside. The proportion of this mixture differs from bone to bone.

4. Spinal vertebrae are mostly porous, trabecular bone, with a thin cortical shell. Since osteoporosis affects trabecular bone more than cortical bone, the spine is one of the first areas to be affected.

5. A woman may, on sudden motion or in lifting a child or heavy object, have a sudden pain in her back which over the next few days improves. This pain may represent a fracture in an osteoporotic bone.

6. Osteoporosis of the vertebrae may account for some of the chronic back pain that women have that is often diagnosed as a gynecologic disorder. It may also account for the decrease in height in women with age and also contributes to the so-called dowager hump.

7. Osteoporosis accounts for about 125,000 fractures of the hip each year, and this is associated with approximately 20,000 deaths.

Bone Robbers

There are certain foods and substances that can increase bone loss. These are: excess protein, salt-loaded and salt-restricted diets, coffee, oxalates and phytates, fiber, diets, fasting, stress, and excess vitamin A.

Prevention

1. Simple changes in lifestyle may help avoid osteoporosis: the patient must get enough calcium and vitamin D, be active but not to excess, avoid alcohol, eat a well-balanced diet, and stop smoking.

2. Simple physical activity cuts down on bone loss after the menopause. Jogging, bicycle riding, and tennis are good exercises. Walking is also a good activity. Swimming is not particularly good for preventing osteoporosis, but it is a safe exercise for women who already have the condition. Antigravity exercises are the best at preventing osteoporosis.

Diagnosis

1. Conventional x-rays cannot diagnose bone loss until about 35 per cent of the mass has been lost.

2. Photon densitometry is one of the most accurate ways of making a diagnosis. Bone loss can also be diagnosed by CT scan using special equipment.

PSYCHOLOGY

1. The effect of estrogen on the psychological state of the post-menopausal woman is a controversial subject. Although it is generally stated that depression, irritability, and fatigue may occur at the time of the menopause, epidemiological studies do not correlate them significantly with actual age of the menopause.

2. Studies indicate that the hot flashes which contribute to insomnia may result in depression, irritability, and fatigue.

3. Atrophic vulvitis and vaginitis often result in a decreased libido.

4. Many of these symptoms are self-limiting, but, if there is no contraindication to estrogen therapy, it often corrects these problems.

ESTROGEN THERAPY AND ENDOMETRIAL CANCER

1. Originally the idea of a relationship between estrogenic hormones and endometrial cancer was generated by a great deal of circumstantial evidence. Repeated studies revealed that women with endometrial cancer appeared to show a greater prevalence of obesity, nulliparity, infertility, and dysfunctional bleeding.

2. It is been shown that, with careful screening of patients prior to the onset of estrogen therapy (particularly by use of an endometrial biopsy) the incidence of carcinoma of the endometrium is not significant. The addition of progesterone for approximately 10 to 13 days has decreased the incidence of carcinoma of the endometrium below that in a control group.

3. Gambrell has advocated the progestin challenge test. A progestational agent is given to the patient for a stated period of time. If there is withdrawal bleeding, it is felt that the patient has sufficient estrogen and is at risk of developing carcinoma of the endometrium unless treated with a progestational agent.

4. It is the height of professional integrity to provide estrogen therapy when indicated and to withhold estrogen therapy if there is a contraindication or if it is not needed.

ERRORS IN TREATING THE MENOPAUSAL WOMAN

Four errors are commonly made in treating the post-menopausal woman.

1. Abnormal bleeding in women in their 40's is often labeled menopausal. These women should undergo thorough investigation, and any abnormal bleeding should have an aspiration, biopsy, or curettage to rule out carcinoma. A thorough pelvic examination is indicated.

2. Hot flushes and hot flashes can be due to other reasons than estrogen deficiency. They can be due to stress or tension as well as to metabolic disorders.

3. Amenorrhea may be considered to be due to the menopause when, in reality, it may result from pregnancy or another cause.

4. Women with estrogen deficiency are often treated for vaginitis without any attempt to restore the vaginal epithelium by exogenous estrogen. Vaginitis occurring in the menopausal or post-menopausal woman must be investigated and an attempt made to identify whether it is due to atrophic vaginitis.

SUMMARY

1. The climacteric is that phase in the life of a woman which marks the interval of transition from the reproductive age to the age at which reproductive function is lost.

2. Menopause is a cessation of menses due to failing ovarian function. It is the last menstruation which occurs during the climacteric.

3. The basic change in the climacteric is the loss of ovarian function and the resultant diminution in estradiol production. Estradiol is the principal estrogen present in women in the pre-menopausal period, whereas estrone, a much less potent estrogen, accounts for most of the circulating estrogen in the post-menopausal woman.

4. There are many atrophic changes in the genital and urinary systems that are directly related to estrogen deficiencies. These symptoms and signs can be reversed with estrogen therapy.

5. Estrogen therapy should be given if there is any indication for it and no contraindication against it. It improves the quality of health and may help control loss of bone and cardiovascular changes.

6. The danger of carcinoma of the endometrium has been overstated, and by combining estrogen with progesterone therapy the possibility of having endometrial carcinoma develop becomes small.

7. *Aging* is a biological term used to identify changes taking place over time which end in death. These changes are determined by heredity and modified by lifestyle and environment.

8. The theories of aging include biological theories, genetic factors, lipofuscin deposition, autoimmune reactions, and immunological changes.

9. There are changes within the body and to the physical appearance in aging. There is a loss of nerve cells, hardening and narrowing of the arteries with arteriosclerosis, and a progressive decrease in endocrine function.

10. Changes in temperament and behavior in old age are accepted as inevitable. Stereotyping of the aged results from prejudice and ignorance. As applied to the elderly, the prejudice is known as *ageism.*

11. It is an interesting observation that women can function sexually much better than men in old age, whereas men retain the power of reproduction despite a decrease in their sexual performance.

12. Disease and disability become more and more common as humans age. In the older age groups, close to 100 per cent have conditions which, to some extent, limit their activity. Most elderly patients have more than one symptom or disease process. Many diseases manifest themselves after 65 because they are consequences of changes in the body brought on by slow, progressive conditions. It is not because people are old that they become sick; it is because the disease process has time to develop for so long a period.

13. The use of biofeedback in managing the elderly is increasingly common. Biofeedback is the use of behavior therapy in the treatment of medical problems.

a. It has been a therapeutic method for a long time, especially in the treatment of obesity and excessive smoking.

b. Biofeedback is a kind of behavior therapy in which one specific bodily function is treated. It has been used to control heart rate and to lower blood pressure.

c. Biofeedback techniques have been successfully used with elderly patients suffering from stroke and from incontinence.

Index

A "t" after a numeral indicates a table.